Cancer of
the Cervix

Cancer of the Cervix

Hugh M. Shingleton, MD
J. Marion Sims Professor of Gynecology Emeritus
University of Alabama at Birmingham
Birmingham, Alabama
National Vice President for Detection and Treatment
American Cancer Society
Clinical Professor of Gynecology
Emory University
Atlanta, Georgia

James W. Orr, Jr., MD
Clinical Professor of Obstetrics and Gynecology
University of South Florida
Tampa, Florida
Director
Division of Gynecologic Oncology
The Watson Clinic
Lakeland, Florida

With a Foreword by Felix N. Rutledge

J. B. LIPPINCOTT COMPANY
Philadelphia

Acquisitions Editor: Lisa McAllister
Sponsoring Editor: Emilie Moyer Linkins
Project Editor: Ellen M. Campbell
Indexer: Lynne E. Mahan
Interior Designer: Doug Smock
Cover Designer: Paul Moran
Production Manager: Caren Erlichman
Production Coordinator: Mary Clare Malady
Compositor: Pine Tree Composition, Inc.
Printer/Binder: Quebecor/Kingsport
Color Insert Printer: Walsworth Publishing Company

6   5   4   3   2   1

Library of Congress Cataloging-in-Publications Data
Shingleton, Hugh M.
    Cancer of the Cervix / Hugh M. Shingleton, James W. Orr, Jr.;
with a foreword by Felix N. Rutledge.
        p.   cm.
    Includes bibliographical references and index.
    ISBN 0–397–51355–0 (alk. paper)
    1. Cervix Uteri—Cancer.   I. Orr, James W.   II. Title.
    [DNLM: 1. Cervix Neoplasms—therapy.   2. Cervix Neoplasms––diagnosis.   WP 480 S556c 1995]
    RC280.U8S47   1995
    616.99′466—dc20
    DNLM/DLC
    for Library of Congress   95–2244
                                                          CIP

∞ This Paper Meets the Requirements of ANSI/NISO Z39.48-1992
(Permanence of Paper).

The authors and publishers have exerted every effort to ensure that drug selection and dosage set forth in this text are in accord with current recommendations and practice at the time of publication. However, in view of ongoing research, changes in government regulations, and the constant flow of information relating to drug therapy and drug reactions, the reader is urged to check the package insert for each drug for any change in indications and dosage and for added warnings and precautions. This is particularly important when the recommended agent is a new or infrequently employed drug.

DEDICATION

Few academic physicians excel both in teaching and in the practice of their particular discipline. Hazel Gore, M.B., B.S., an exceptionally gifted gynecologic pathologist, has left a mark first at Harvard University and more recently at the University of Alabama at Birmingham. Her energy, her infectious enthusiasm, and her uncompromising pursuit of excellence have benefited patients, students, and colleagues. We recognize her for her contributions to this book and for the very high standards she has set.

FOREWORD

These two leading authorities collaborate again on a book which should prove useful for students and practitioners. This volume presents the latest knowledge about the etiology and genesis of carcinoma of the cervix.

Cancer of the Cervix is recommended for practicing obstetricians and gynecologists as well as specialists in gynecologic oncology. It is clear and well written, and serves as a reference for a variety of health care providers. The range of information is useful for all physicians whom women consult, even for nonspecific complaints, since most types of physical examination provide opportunities to detect gynecologic cancers. This book is more than ample to sharpen our recognition skills and bring us up-to-date with this disease. Management of patients with unsubstantiated evidence of cancer or those with well-established diagnoses is presented clearly and in sufficient depth to be appreciated by the student or the clinically experienced practicing physician. The use of color photographs adds to its overall quality.

While this is a relatively compact volume, its contents are comprehensive. The continuity is excellent. Presentations are succinct, material no longer pertinent is excluded, and the format is easy to follow. Still, it provides comprehensive coverage of one of the most important gynecologic cancers. The authors have been judicious in the selection of their material and have dealt with controversial topics by stating their opinions, not by laboriously debating issues. Each chapter has a well-annotated bibliography. The solid opinions and judgment of Dr. Shingleton and Dr. Orr are supported by extensive clinical experiences.

Especially valuable is Chapter 14, which deals with the psychological and sexual effects of cervical cancer and its treatment. Sexual function is altered; for younger patients, loss of reproduction must be discussed. The effects of standard and radical operations are deliberated. This is appropriate. Resection in cancer of the cervix re-sults in some shortening of the vagina. Less frequently, total removal with exenteration is required. Although vaginal reconstruction is offered, the patient must still adjust to less than normal connubial relations. Irradiation in cancerocidal doses induces vaginal dryness and reduces mucosal pliability. These changes must be explained to the patient. Sometimes the primary care physician inherits this assignment. This valuable chapter is often omitted from textbooks of this type.

Chapter 6, "Diagnosis, Staging, and Selection of Therapy for Invasive Tumors," is also important. The new methods of radiologic imaging for detecting metastasis and discovery of organ damage due to the cancer are thoroughly discussed. Surgery or irradiation are equally successful for treating early stage cancer of the cervix, but not when metastases have developed. It is important to investigate the boundaries of the cancer to be able to make this selection properly. The chapter explains why certain patients are chosen for surgical techniques rather than more frequent treatment with radiation.

In the opening paragraph of Chapter 8, "Radiation Therapy," it is stated that gynecologists need to develop a basic understanding of irradiation treatment to allow better communication with the consulting radiotherapist. The authors provide an easily understandable review of the principles of radiation therapy, including an explanation of terminology. With this understanding, the gynecologist can now choose to participate in the deliberations of treatment planning.

For the generalist and the obstetrician/gynecologist, this book will stand alone as a ready reference for the desk. The medical student should certainly read it. For those with special interest in gynecologic oncology, I would consider this work a must.

Felix N. Rutledge, M.D.
Houston, Texas

PREFACE

Worldwide, cervical cancer continues to be an important cause of morbidity and mortality. While the refinement of cytologic screening techniques and programs for early detection have been associated with a decreasing risk of invasive disease in the United States, diagnostic and management problems associated with precursor lesions have become more important. Innovations in radiotherapeutic planning and treatment including 3-D dosimetry, high-dose afterloading, and neutron therapy also represent potentially important advances for treatment of women with invasive cervical cancer. The results from surgical staging have engendered a better understanding of cervical tumor biology as well as altering specific treatment techniques.

The classic radical hysterectomy and pelvic lymphadenectomy developed by pioneers Clark, Wertheim, Bonny, and Meigs remains an important part of surgical treatment, and recent reports have addressed important methods to decrease morbidity. Refinements in ultraradical surgery for persistent or recurrent carcinoma include neovaginal reconstruction, the use of continent conduits, and low rectal reanastomosis.

This text has evolved from a combined experience of more than five decades of management of patients with cervical cancer. We believe our opinions reflect an extensive clinical experience as well as a thorough review of recent literature. The 1983 edition of this monograph has been dramatically revised to incorporate the newer techniques of diagnosis, staging and management evolving in the 80's and 90's. It is intended to provide precise guidelines for the diagnosis and treatment of patients with premalignant or malignant disease of the cervix to residents, fellows, and practitioners.

As with any publication, a number of people have invaluably assisted in the preparation of this text. Josephine Taylor prepared tables, figures, photographs, and drawings, and assisted with historic material. Sylvia Foltz has devoted extensive energy to manuscript preparation. Dr. Cheryl Dee and the library staff at The Watson Clinic provided invaluable assistance in referencing this text. Obviously, our wives, Lucy Shingleton and Pamela Orr, have allowed us time to develop this text and devoted specific attention to the details of the manuscript.

We are certainly grateful to the many clinicians and researchers in the field of gynecologic oncology, radiation therapy, and medical oncology for their dedication and quality care of the gynecologic cancer patients at our institutions. We also are indebted to the resident physicians and oncology fellows who have contributed so much of their time and energy to the treatment of these patients.

Hugh M. Shingleton
James W. Orr, Jr.

CONTENTS

13
Recurrent Cancer: Radiation Therapy, Chemotherapy, and Other Treatment . . .

14
Social, Psychological, and Sexual Aspects of Cervical Cancer
and Its Treatment . . . .

Cancer of the Cervix

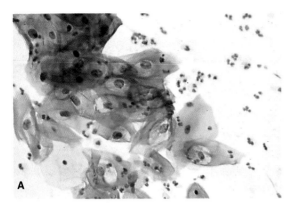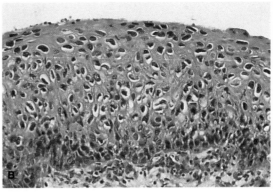

COLOR FIGURE 3-1. Low-grade squamous intraepithelial lesion. (**A**) Pap smear including intermediate and superficial squamous epithelial cells with enlarged atypical nuclei, hyperchromatic, with coarse chromatin. There is perinuclear clearing surrounded by a dense zone of cytoplasm. Nucleus is usually towards the periphery. This is the cytologic pattern of human papillomavirus (HPV) effect. (**B**) In this section of cervix, there are large squamous cells with enlarged atypical nuclei surrounded by a clear perinuclear zone, koilocytosis (or koilocytotic atypia), HPV effect. Only rare cells are binucleate. The appearance of the exfoliated cells may be correlated with the histologic pattern.

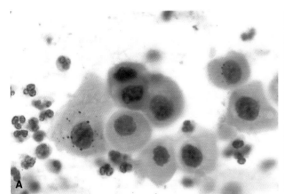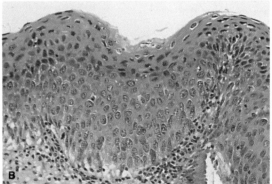

COLOR FIGURE 3-2. High-grade squamous intraepithelial lesion (moderate dysplasia). (**A**) Cells in the Pap smear have nuclei of varying size, well demarcated and hyperchromatic. There is increased nuclear-cytoplasmic ratio, with the nucleus occupying half of the cell area to about three quarters. The cytologic pattern is that of moderate dysplasia. (**B**) In this section of cervix, proliferative activity with atypical cells, increased nuclear-cytoplasmic ratio, and loss of polarity involves the lower two thirds of the epithelium. There is some surface differentiation. This pattern of moderate dysplasia correlates with the Pap smear.

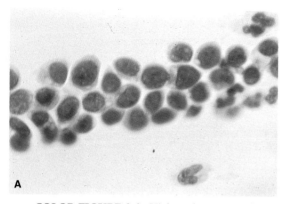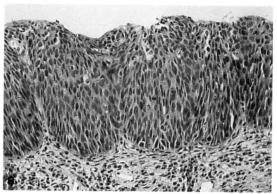

COLOR FIGURE 3-3. High-grade squamous intraepithelial lesion (squamous carcinoma in situ). (**A**) Strands of malignant squamous cells, with well-demarcated hyperchromatic nucleus surrounded by a thin rim of cytoplasm in a Pap smear with "clean" background consistent with origin from squamous cell carcinoma in situ. (**B**) Cells in the surface squamous epithelium in this biopsy are all atypical, with loss of polarity. Nuclei are at right angles to the basal layer, and only rarely is there a suggestion of surface differentiation. This pattern of squamous cell carcinoma in situ correlates with cells in the Pap smear.

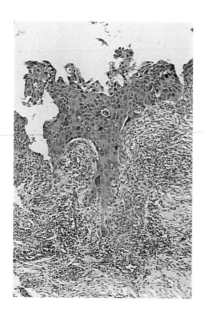

COLOR FIGURE 3-4. Microinvasive squamous cell carcinoma. A prong of malignant cells with large irregular nuclei and minimal differentiation is extending from the surface malignant epithelium into the underlying cytoplasm and is surrounded by inflammatory cells. This is the classic pattern of early microinvasive squamous cell carcinoma.

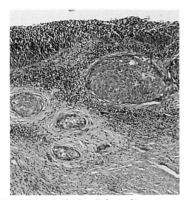

COLOR FIGURE 3-5. Small foci of invasive squamous cell carcinoma invading stroma, deep to surface squamous cell carcinoma of the cervix, compressing adjacent stroma. The focus just beneath the surface epithelium has split away from the adjacent stroma. A few flattened cells remain attached to the stroma. These may be split-off cancer cells, but this is the type of focus wherein the possibility of lymphvascular space extension might be considered and further investigated. The small space at the edge of the next focus appears to be shrinkage artifact, and the other focus is just stromal invasion. Although this is consistent with microinvasive carcinoma, such a diagnosis could not be made without knowledge of what is elsewhere in the cervix.

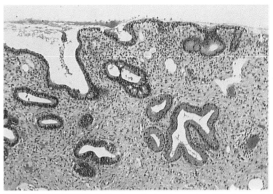

COLOR FIGURE 3-6. A typical columnar epithelium with minimal nuclear pseudostratification is on the surface to the left; there are some glands lined by similar epithelium, including two clusters. Immediately beneath one atypical group and to the right of some single atypical glands is a group of physiologic endocervical glands (clefts). The hyperchromatic glands are adenocarcinoma in situ.

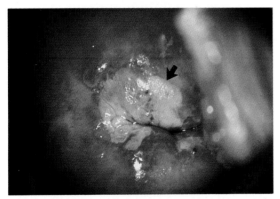

COLOR FIGURE 3-7. Low-grade squamous intraepithelial lesion. Acetowhite epithelium with well-demarcated borders extends from the 7 o'clock position around (and covering) much of the anterior lip. The surface changes (*arrow*) in one area suggest a flat condyloma. (Courtesy of Kenneth D. Hatch, MD, University of Arizona, Tucson, AZ.)

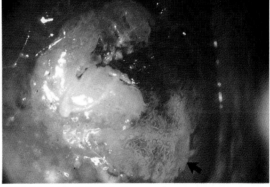

COLOR FIGURE 3-8. Low-grade squamous intraepithelial lesion. Acetowhite lesion occupies most of the transformation zone. On the posterior lip (*arrow*) a fine mosaic is present. (Courtesy of Kenneth D. Hatch, MD, University of Arizona, Tucson, AZ.)

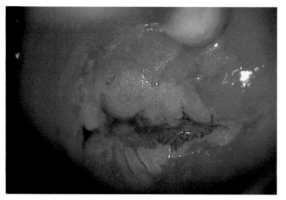

COLOR FIGURE 3-9. High-grade squamous intraepithelial lesion. The acetowhite lesion on the anterior lip contains extensive punctation and mosaic patterns. (Courtesy of Kenneth D. Hatch, MD, University of Arizona, Tucson, AZ.)

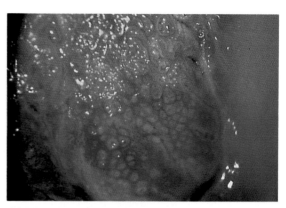

COLOR FIGURE 3-10. High-grade squamous intraepithelial lesion. A coarse mosaic pattern is present, with some punctation. (Courtesy of Kenneth D. Hatch, MD, University of Arizona, Tucson, AZ.)

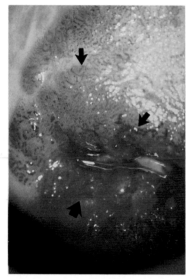

COLOR FIGURE 3-11. Probable microinvasion. Atypical vessels (*arrows*) of various shapes run parallel to the surface in a transformation zone that also contains coarse punctation. Such vessels suggest superficial invasive disease. (Courtesy of Kenneth D. Hatch, MD, University of Arizona, Tucson, AZ.)

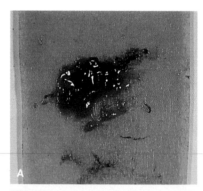

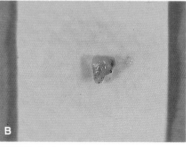

COLOR FIGURE 3-16. (**A**) Endocervical curetting sample on Histowrap. (This may also be placed on a square of paper towel or Telfa). After it adheres (a few seconds), it is placed gently in fixative; after fixation, it is removed as a globule for processing. (**B**) Colposcopically directed cervical biopsy on Telfa (this may also be placed on a square of paper towel or histowrap). After it adheres, it is placed gently in fixative; after fixation, it is removed for processing.

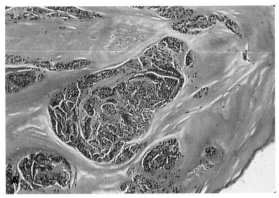 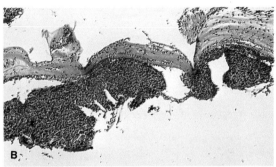

COLOR FIGURE 3-17. (A) A good example of a "negative" endocervical curettage. The specimen is adequate and there are numerous strips of unremarkable endocervical columnar epithelium amid mucus. (B) A good example of a "positive" endocervical curettage. Partly attached to a strand of mucus with inflammatory cells is an irregular strip of atypical epithelium, dysplastic/?neoplastic. This is at least high-grade squamous intraepithelial lesion, but from this singular focus, the possibility of invasive carcinoma cannot be ruled out.

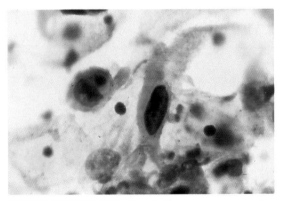 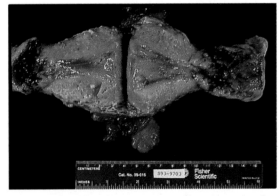

COLOR FIGURE 5-2. Papanicolaou smear from patient with invasive squamous cell carcinoma. Malignant squamous cells have a large irregular nucleus, increased nuclear cytoplasmic ratio, and either basophilic or eosinophilic cytoplasm. A normal superficial squamous epithelial cell is at the left.

COLOR FIGURE 5-3. Squamous cell carcinoma involves both anterior and posterior endocervix and extends from lower segment/endocervical junction outward to the portio. There is some exophytic tumor in the proximal part but most is superficially ulcerated and appears to be largely endophytic.

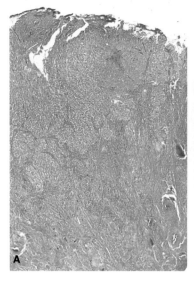

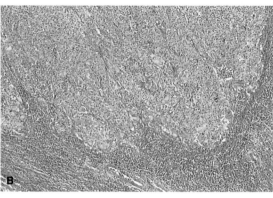

COLOR FIGURE 5-4. (**A**) In this invasive squamous cell carcinoma, groups of malignant squamous cells are extending into the cervical stroma. (**B**) An inflammatory response is evident at the infiltrating margin.

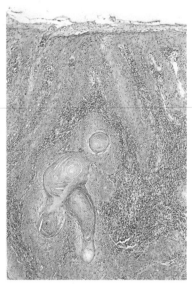

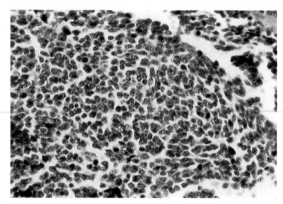

COLOR FIGURE 5-6. Classic small cell carcinoma, formed by fairly uniform small cells with high nucleus-cytoplasm ratio, histologically similar to small cell carcinoma of the lung.

COLOR FIGURE 5-5. Within the invasive squamous cell carcinoma is a large lobulated mass of keratinizing squamous cells with central keratinization, a so-called epithelial pearl.

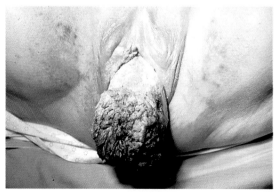

COLOR FIGURE 5-7. Verrucous carcinoma (occurring with uterine procidentia) with a fungating warty appearance.

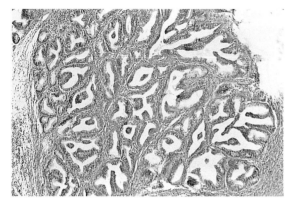

COLOR FIGURE 5-8. Well-differentiated adenocarcinoma of mucinous (endocervical) type.

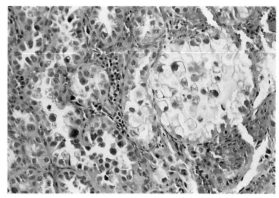

COLOR FIGURE 5-9. Clear cell adenocarcinoma, in which cells have clear or finely granular cytoplasm; some cells are of hobnail type, in which hyperchromatic nuclei surrounded by very scanty cytoplasm push into the gland lumen.

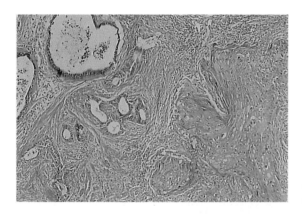

COLOR FIGURE 5-10. Adenocarcinoma and invasive squamous cell carcinoma, growing as two separate tumors.

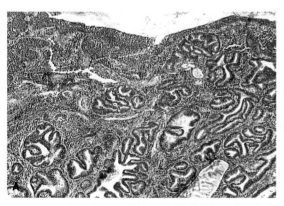
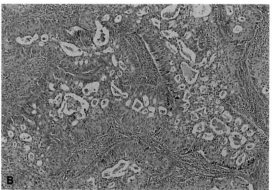

COLOR FIGURE 5-11. (**A**) Well-differentiated adenocarcinoma of endometrioid type is invading the endocervical stroma, whereas on the surface there is carcinoma in situ, which also involves some relatively superficial clefts. These are two separate tumors. (**B**) Adenosquamous carcinoma with small glandular spaces and malignant squamous epithelial component.

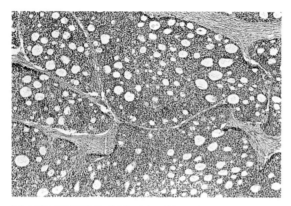

COLOR FIGURE 5-12. Adenoid cystic carcinoma with large groups of fairly uniform cells, in which are small round lumens.

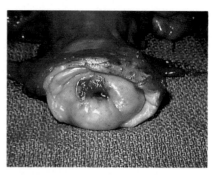

COLOR FIGURE 6–1. A one-quadrant superficial ulcerative carcinoma. Maximum depth of invasion in this tumor was 8 mm. (Shingleton HM, Orr JW Jr. Cancer of the cervix: diagnosis and treatment. New York: Churchill Livingstone, 1987:99.)

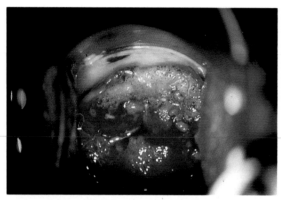

COLOR FIGURE 6–2. An exophytic squamous cell carcinoma involving the entire cervical circumference. (Shingleton HM, Orr JW Jr. Cancer of the cervix: diagnosis and treatment. New York: Churchill Livingstone, 1987.)

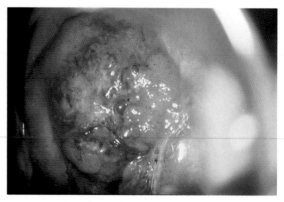

COLOR FIGURE 6-3. Adenocarcinoma of the cervix. The Stage IB lesion demonstrates disturbed surface contour and atypical surface blood vessels.

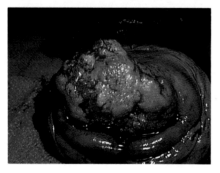

COLOR FIGURE 6–4. A radical hysterectomy specimen, in which a large polypoid adenosquamous carcinoma extends from the endocervical canal. (Courtesy of Dr. J. Max Austin Jr, Birmingham, Alabama.)

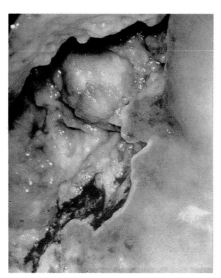

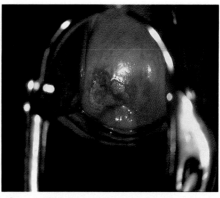

COLOR FIGURE 6–6. An ulcerating squamous cell carcinoma of the cervix in a 32-year-old pregnant woman. (Shingleton HM, Orr JW Jr. Cancer of the cervix: diagnosis and treatment. New York, Churchill Livingstone, 1987.)

COLOR FIGURE 6–5. An advanced-stage ulcerative squamous cell carcinoma. Note the necrotic exudate replacing the cervix. (Giuntoli RL, Atkinson BF, Ernst CS, Rubin MM, Egan VS [eds]. Atkinson's correlative atlas of colposcopy, cytology, and histopathology. Philadelphia, JB Lippincott, 1987:175, with permission).

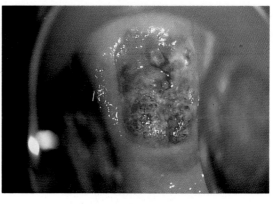

COLOR FIGURE 6–7. Atypical vessels in a squamous cell carcinoma of the posterior lip of the cervix. The surface contour is also altered. (Shingleton HM, Orr JW Jr. Cancer of the cervix: diagnosis and treatment. New York, Churchill Livingstone, 1987.)

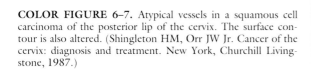

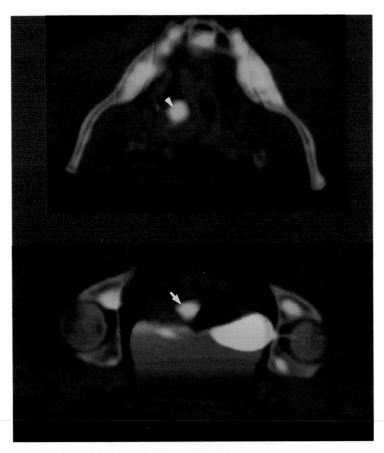

COLOR FIGURE 6–16. Patient referred for assessment of primary cervical carcinoma. Clinical evaluation included examination under anesthesia. Stage 1B CT scan demonstrated disease at the primary site but no pelvic node disease was identified. Registered CT-PET-FDG image showed clearly the primary disease and the isolated external iliac nodal spread. Histologic examinations after radical hysterectomy and lymphadenectomy confirmed the registered CT-PET-FDG findings (PET-FDG shown in *green.*) *CT,* computed tomography; *PET,* positron emission tomography; *FDG,* 2-[18F]fluoro-2-deoxy-D-glucose. (Courtesy of Dr. K.S. Raju and Dr. W.L. Wong, Department of Gynaecology and Radiology, United Medical and Dental Schools of Guy's and St. Thomas's Hospitals, University of London.)

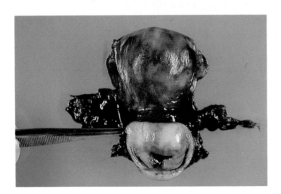

COLOR FIGURE 7–7. Excised uterus with wide vaginal cuff and parauterine tissues. The ovaries were not removed in this patient.

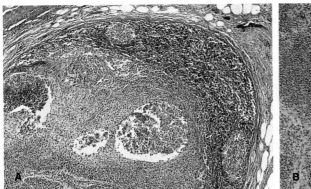
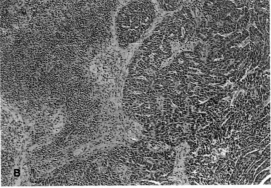

COLOR FIGURE 7–11. **(A)** Squamous cell carcinoma with focal necrosis metastatic to lymph node. **(B)** Adenocarcinoma, moderately well- to well-differentiated, metastatic to lymph node.

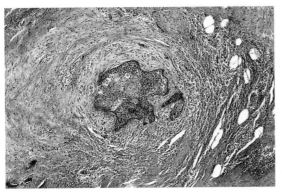
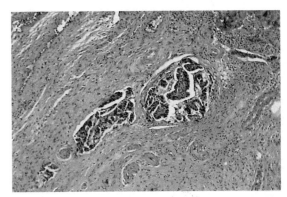

COLOR FIGURE 7–12. Venous extension of squamous cell carcinoma, now enveloped by organized thrombus within parametrial tissue. At the right is a small focus of tumor within a lymphvascular space.

COLOR FIGURE 7–15. Adenocarcinoma of cervix, extending within a lymphvascular space.

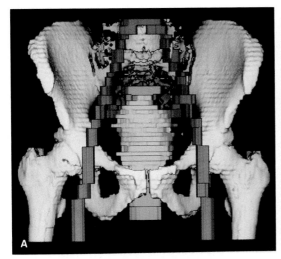
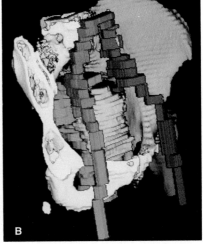

COLOR FIGURE 8–9. Computed tomograph dosimetry reconstruction of the vaginal (*blue*), cervix-uterus (*yellow*), rectum (*green*), and nodal tissue (*orange*) in an anterior (**A**), oblique (**B**), and lateral

(*continued*)

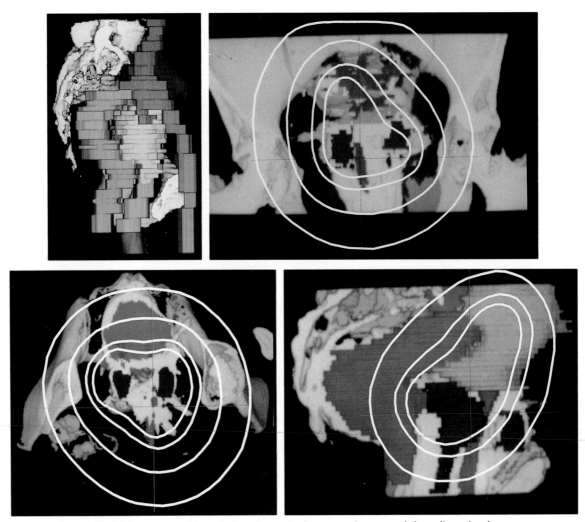

COLOR FIGURE 8–9. *(Continued)* **(C)** view. **(D)** Isodose curves in a coronal three-dimensional reconstruction of the pelvix with a Fletcher applicator (*dark blue*) in place. Cross-hairs intersect at the cervix with the uterus (*yellow*) above, the rectum (*green*) behind, and the bladder (*red*) anterior. The 3000-, 2000-, and 1000-cGy isodose curves are depicted after ^{137}Cs loading. **(E)** An axial plane with the cervix at the cross-hairs and the 3000-, 2000-, 1000-, and 500-cGy isodose curves. **(F)** The sagittal plane as visualized through the three-dimensional virtual simulator. (Images generated with a Picker-Varian virtual simulator; courtesy of Dr. A. Wiley an Dr. J. Stephenson, Watson Clinic, Lakeland FL.)

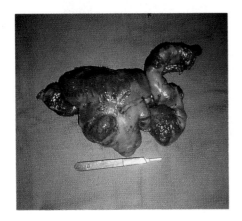

COLOR FIGURE 11–6. Marked radiation damage to small bowel in a young woman given postoperative whole-pelvis radiotherapy (50 Gy) after radical hysterectomy. Surgical resection of the matted bowel was required. Long-term hyperalimentation was necessary in this patient and a "short bowel" syndrome occurred, with permanent partial disability. (Courtesy of Dr. E.E. Partridge, The University of Alabama at Birmingham.)

Cancer of the Cervix by Hugh M. Shingleton and James W. Orr, Jr.
J. B. Lippincott Company, Philadelphia, © 1995.

1

Historical Aspects, Pathogenesis, and Epidemiology

HISTORY

The Disease

The first reference largely devoted to gynecology as a recognized and practiced field of medicine (Table 1-1) is found in the Kahun papyrus (2000 B.C.). Specific aspects of gynecologic medicine were not detailed nor were there descriptions of surgical techniques or specific reference to cancer. The first reference to cancer of the uterus appears in a description of diseases of women in the writing of Hippocrates (about 450 B.C.), which describes a poor prognosis. The Hindus, in the fifth century B.C., were among the first to develop surgical technique. Existing texts suggest that they developed procedures to remove tumors; one such text describes tumors of the vagina and cervix in a chapter devoted to the diseases of the generative organs. The Romans practiced gynecology, and it is thought that their knowledge was largely gained from the medical practices of Greece and Alexandria. The works of Galen and Celsus suggest that vaginal specula were used as early as the first century A.D. (Mann 1887). Two specula were found in Pompeii and Herculaneum, cities that had been destroyed by an eruption of Mount Vesuvius in A.D. 79. Cancer of the uterus was described by Galen in his work, *De Morbis Mulierum*, and in concurrence with his predecessors, he predicted a poor outcome (Mettler 1947).

Aetius of Amida practiced in Alexandria in the sixth century A.D. and may have had dissecting rooms. He published four books that are collectively known as *Medici Graeci Tetrabiblos* (Jameson 1936). In the fourth discourse of the fourth book, "On the rationale of conception and parturition and diseases of women,

especially those of the uterus and mamma," he accurately describes the structure and function of the uterus and ovaries, indicating an in-depth knowledge of anatomy and physiology. One chapter, "De cancris uteri," written by Archigenes, includes descriptions of the appearance of the cervix, the symptoms of pain, discharge, and bleeding, and categorizes uterine cancer into ulcerative and nonulcerative types (Jameson 1936).

Little was written about cervical cancer until the time of the Renaissance. The *Medieval Woman's Guide to Health* in the early fifteenth century includes this information: "cancers and festerings of the womb come from old injuries of the womb that have not healed well, but that kind of sickness we will hardly mention because doctors say that, regarding hidden cancers, it is better that they should be uncured rather than cured or treated." A recipe for ointment follows, with which the patient was to be anointed "inside" (Rowland 1981). Ambroise Paré (1510–1590), eminent in the history of both gynecology and surgery, recommended use of the vaginal speculum to expose and evaluate the malignant cervix (Mann 1887). Astruc (1762), in *A Treatise on the Diseases of Women*, described uterine cancer and recommended methods of treatment. In 1793, Matthew Baillie included descriptions of diseases of the uterus and cervix in his textbook of morbid anatomy, and gave a detailed account of cancer of the cervix. An excerpt from his text included this description: "There is no enlargement of the uterus; ulceration continues until a great part of the uterus is destroyed. The disease begins in the cervix, and when it has made a great progress, the contiguous parts, as the rectum and the urinary bladder, are often involved in it" (Ricci 1950).

TABLE 1-1
Milestones in History Regarding Cervical Cancer

YEAR	EVENT	YEAR	EVENT
2000 B.C.	Gynecologic medicine described in Egyptian Papyrus	1903	**Cleaves** used intrauterine application of radium for treatment
450 B.C.	**Hippocrates** referred to cancer of the uterus	1905	**Abbé** first to report long-term survival after radium treatment
A.D. 600	**Aetius of Amida** described cancer of the uterus	1906	Laboratoire Biologique du Radium established in Paris as a center for research
1575	**Paré** recommended amputation as treatment of cancerous cervix	1910	Beginning of development of special hospitals or clinics for the treatment of cancer, including:
1652	**Tulpius** performed cervical amputation as treatment		Radiumhemmet in Stockholm (1910)
1793	**Baillie** described invasion of bladder and rectum by cervical cancer		Radium Institute of London (1911)
1801	**Osiander** used mass ligature amputation of the cervix		Institute of Radium of Paris (1913)
1822	**Sauter** performed first successful total vaginal hysterectomy as treatment (patient survived four months)		Memorial Hospital in New York (1915)
		1915	American Radium Society founded
1829	**Récamier** described the process of metastasis	1917	Radiation treatment regimen introduced by **Forssell** (Stockholm Method)
1846	**Sims** and **Huguer** used galvanocaustic loops for cervical amputation	1922	Radiation treatment regimen introduced by **Regaud** (Paris Technique)
1847	**Virchow** described stromal invasion by nests of tumor cells	1925	**Von Hinselmann** introduced colposcopy for diagnosis
1872	Strong caustic chemicals, applied to the cervix to destroy local growth, came into vogue, replacing hot cauteries	1934	Radiation treatment regimen introduced by **Paterson** and **Parker** (Manchester Technique)
1878	**Schröder** introduced high surgical amputation of the cervix	1935	**Bonney** reported improved results with radical surgical treatment
1895	**Clark** and **Rumpf** performed extended abdominal hysterectomy with removal of the pelvic nodes as treatment	1943	**Papanicolaou** and **Traut** developed exfoliative cytology for diagnosis and screening
1895	**Roentgen** discovered x-rays	1948	**Brunschwig** reported ultraradical surgical approach for advanced and recurrent cancer
1896	**Becquerel** described the radioactivity of minerals containing uranium and thorium	1950	First commercial linear accelerator (by Varian Brothers—Magnatron)
1898	The **Curies** isolated radium from pitchblende; shared Nobel Prize for Physics (1903) with **Becquerel**	1951	**Meigs** proved that a radical surgical approach for early stage cancer could equal radiation results, with acceptable complications
1898	**Wertheim** devised extended abdominal hysterectomy and node sampling as treatment	1951	^{60}Co teletherapy introduced (M.D. Anderson Hospital)
1902	**Schauta** performed radical vaginal hysterectomy for treatment	1963	Introduction of Fletcher-Suit afterloading intracavitary applicator

Modified from Shingleton HM, Orr JW Jr. Cancer of the cervix: diagnosis and treatment. New York, Churchill Livingstone, 1987:2.

John Clarke in 1812 reported a peculiar degeneration of the cervix, which he labeled "cauliflower excrescence" (Ricci 1945). Although this condition had been described by other physicians, doubt remained about the nature of the tumor and its correct classification. Observations were based on macroscopic appearance, and nomenclature such as "schirrous enlargement" and "cervical ulceration" was used. Although Virchow was said to have been the first to make the association between these conditions and cervical cancer,

Hooper first published it in 1832. Bennet further described the differentiation between benign and malignant cervical changes in 1845. Sarcomatous lesions were distinguished from epithelial lesions, and a classification of cervical diseases evolved. The advent of the technique for light-microscopic examination of tissues led to the publication in 1872 of a more precise classification of cervical cancer by Thomas (Ricci 1945).

In addition to clinical recognition and classification of cervical cancer at this time, some observations were also made regarding its incidence. In 1844, Samuel Ashwell (Guy's Hospital, London) observed that most of the patients with cervical cancer were "dark complexioned" (Ricci 1945). In 1872, the deaths from cervical cancer in black and white women in South Carolina were reported; it was apparent that the mortality rates were higher in black women.

Theories of the possible causes of cervical cancer were also recorded. Many physicians in the early nineteenth century shared the opinion that the disease was stress-related; however, others suggested that injuries, particularly those related to parturition, preceded cancer. In 1861, von Scanzoni was the first to observe that the disease was more frequent in city dwellers and thus possibly related to the manner of living (Ricci 1945). The "excessive sexual excitation," which he considered a feature of women with the disease, may have reflected Victorian ideas of morality. Other etiologic factors proposed included cervical inflammation, the abuse of purgative medicines, and the presence of hemorrhoids. Many believed in a constitutional factor but others regarded the disease as being dependent on local factors (Ricci 1945).

By the beginning of the twentieth century, medical opinions suggested that untreated cervical lacerations were an important etiologic factor in the later development of cervical cancer. This theory was supported by the observations of many gynecologists who noted cervical cancer to be rare in nulliparous women. It was thought that heredity, injury, irritation, occupation, stress, and race were predisposing factors, and that cervicitis, erosions, and unhealed lacerations were precancerous conditions. Many physicians advocated prompt treatment of these conditions to prevent the development of cancer. The importance of early diagnosis was recognized and the investigation of early symptoms such as abnormal bleeding and discharge was advocated. Carstens, at the turn of the century, advocated the education of women to recognize symptoms and to seek medical advice promptly (Schmitz 1955). Although some physicians recognized the importance of light microscopy as an aid to diagnosis, others thought that this technique was unreliable. During the first half of the twentieth century, there developed an increasing awareness of the various forms of pelvic cancer and their histologic diagnosis and classification. Novak (1940) made a major contribution to the subject of tumor pathology with publications on the diagnosis of early cervical cancer and its differentiation from inflammatory lesions.

The regular examination of those women considered to be in a high-risk category was advocated at this time. Schiller's test and microscopic examination of biopsy specimens from suspicious areas of epithelium were employed. The colposcope, first introduced by Von Hinselmann in 1925, subsequently became a widely used tool for the diagnosis of cervical cancer in Europe. Exfoliative cytology of vaginal secretions, first described in 1943 by Papanicolaou and Traut, provided an economical method to screen large numbers of women for cervical cancer and premalignant lesions. These two methods of detection developed on opposite sides of the Atlantic, and the benefits of combined use were not appreciated for a quarter of a century.

Treatment

The earliest specific reference to treatment of uterine cancer is recorded in the works of Hippocrates. Advanced disease was recognized as incurable, and the only treatment was one of local fumigation for symptomatic relief. Aetius (Jameson 1936) indicated that the disease could be "mitigated and alleviated" by baths, poultices, and irrigations consisting of various herbs and other concoctions. Astruc's treatise of 1762 describes nonsurgical methods of treatment; bloodletting, purging, control of the diet, and direct injection into the tumor with such things as an extract of nightshade were recommended. Narcotics, such as opium, were given internally or injected directly into the uterus for relief of pain. Some of these techniques, although ineffective and potentially harmful, persisted into the nineteenth century. After 1830, Duparcque and others advocated the application of leeches to the cervix. At the same time, some physicians favored the application of red-hot irons or other powerful caustics. In the latter part of the nineteenth century, local applications of caustics such as gold, zinc chloride, creosote, nitric acid were advocated as therapy. Injections of silver nitrate, mercuric chloride, and pure alcohol into the parametrial tissues were also used. Advocacy of surgical treatment began in the sixteenth century, when Paré recommended amputation of the cancerous cervix as treatment. This procedure was first successfully performed by Tulpius of Amsterdam in 1652 (Ricci 1990).

Between 1801 and 1802, Osiander performed excision of the cervix in eight patients. Struve, a pupil of Osiander, presented a dissertation in 1802, outlining the procedure and advocating its use as a treatment for cervical malignancy. Between 1810 and 1840, many reports of cervical amputation using specially designed instruments appeared, some claiming cures (Ricci 1990). The survival rate was so poor, however, that in 1854 C. D. Meigs commented, "If the cervix was cut off and the woman recovered, it affords the most uncontestable proof that the operation was unnecessary."

In 1822, Sauter performed the first successful vaginal hysterectomy for malignancy. In 1856, West reviewed the literature and reported 25 authentic cases of vaginal hysterectomy as treatment; 22 of these women died postoperatively from shock, hemorrhage, and peritonitis (Ricci 1990). The high mortality led one surgeon, de L'Isere, to comment, "This statistical and funereal record of extirpations of the uterus is fitter than any course of reasoning to deter the practitioner from so redoubtable an attempt" (Ricci 1945). Because of the high mortality, surgical treatment temporarily fell into disfavor.

The 1870s heralded a new interest in surgical treatment for cervical carcinoma. In 1878, Freund performed a total abdominal hysterectomy, using anesthesia and antiseptic measures while paying careful attention to hemostasis. By 1882, 95 patients treated by this surgical procedure had been reported. Of the 95 cases, 65 died from surgical complications, whereas 30 survived the procedure but later died with recurrent disease. These results and those of McGraw in 1879, who reported the effects of limited surgery, strongly suggested the need for more extensive surgical procedures to improve cure rates.

The development of radical vaginal hysterectomy preceded that of the radical abdominal operation as treatment for cervix cancer. Karel Pawlik, chief of the Gynecologic Clinic at the University of Prague, performed a radical vaginal hysterectomy as early as 1888. Friedrich Schauta, who was teaching and practicing in Prague at that time, was aware of Pawlik's work. One of Schauta's assistants, Ernst Wertheim, followed Schauta to the first obstetric and gynecologic clinic in Vienna and remained with him until 1897. Schauta, influenced by the work of Schuchardt and using his paravaginal incision, performed his first radical vaginal hysterectomy in l901.

Experimental studies by Ries (1895), based on the ideas proposed by Halsted in the treatment of breast cancer, suggested the feasibility of total abdominal hysterectomy combined with the removal of the iliac lymph nodes and part of the broad ligament as a primary surgical procedure. He performed this operation only on cadavers and animals, however. In the same year, radical abdominal procedures were first performed on living patients in Germany by Rumpf and in America by J. G. Clark, a young physician at Johns Hopkins Hospital. During a 12-month period, Clark performed 12 such operations, each with some technical variation. Lymph nodes were removed in some cases, whereas in others he widely excised the vaginal cuff, removing as much parametrium as possible (Clark 1913).

In 1912, Wertheim published the results of 500 radical hysterectomies performed between 1899 and 1912. Wertheim's technique emphasized removal of the uterus and the medial portion of the parametrium and paracolpos. The pelvic lymph nodes were removed only if enlarged and suspicious for metastasis. In 1913, Wertheim was to have presented his operative experience at a meeting in Halle an der Saale but after the

radium therapy results were presented, the less morbid technique appeared so superior that Wertheim withdrew his paper.

In the early years of surgery for cancer of the cervix, proponents of the vaginal method, principally Dr. Schauta, believed that there was less mortality associated with that approach. Wertheim and his followers, however, believed that the percentages of cures were greater with the abdominal method. The fact is that prior to 1913, the operative mortality was very high from both procedures (23% Wertheim, 19% Schauta), while the percentages of cures were quite poor (25% Wertheim, 17% Schauta), albeit for advanced cases in an era before effective antibiotics and blood banking (Clark 1913).

Once techniques were developed to radically excise the primary lesions, attention turned to the regional lymphatics, which were known to be sites of metastasis. Emphasis shifted toward sampling and, later, toward methodical lymphadenectomy as a part of the operative procedure. This made the abdominal route the preferred one since the lymphadenectomy could not be performed in conjunction with the vaginal operation. In the last half of the twentieth century, sporadic reports advocating the vaginal route have continued, mostly in Europe. Ernst Navratil, writing in 1963 in Meigs's classic textbook on surgical treatment of cervical cancer, compared his own use of the Schauta-Amreich operation to Meigs' abdominal operations (Table 1-2), reporting that the survival was the same for the two methods. In the United States, Milton McCall (1962) was a great advocate of the use of vaginal radical hysterectomy; however, radical abdominal hysterectomy with the pelvic lymphadenectomy gained ascendancy and still enjoys that status. Massi (1993) has recently published a series comparing the two approaches.

RADIATION THERAPY

In 1895, W.C. Röentgen, working with a Hittorf-Crookes tube in his laboratory at the University of Wurtzburg, observed fluorescence in crystals of barium platinocyanide that were located too far from the tube for the fluorescence to be due to the known properties of cathode ray tubes. At the January 1886 meeting of the French Academy of Sciences, the details of Röentgen's discoveries were described and demonstrated by Poincaré. Becquerel deduced that there was a spontaneous emission of radiation from uranium sulfate crystals, later named "Becquerel rays." Marie Curie assayed many materials and carried out extensive chemical separations for her doctoral thesis, eventually discovering and reporting the radioactivity (her term) of polonium in July 1888 and of radium in

TABLE 1-2
Comparison of Schauta-Amreich with Radical Abdominal Operation
for Stage IB Cervical Cancer

STUDY	PATIENTS (N)	5-YR SURVIVAL (%)	PROCEDURE
Meigs (1940–1949)	84	81.0	Radical abdominal operation with lymphadenectomy w/o radiation
Navratil (1947–1956)	294	83.3	Schauta-Amreich post-op irradiation

Navratil E. VI. Radical vaginal hysterectomy. 1. The Schauta–Amreich operation. In: Meigs JV, Sturgis SH (eds). Progress in gynecology. New York, Grune & Stratton, 1963:564; with permission.

1889. In 1899, Sjoegren and Stenbeck first used radiation therapy for cancer treatment.

Brachytherapy was given its name by Forssell because of the short distance implied in the use of radioactive sources placed in close proximity to the region to be treated. Radium was first used for treatment of cervical cancer in New York City in 1903 (Cleaves) and the first radium hospital opened in Stockholm in 1910. The Stockholm method was introduced in 1917 (Forssell), the Paris method in 1923 (Regaud), and the Manchester method in 1934 (Paterson).

In 1963, Suit introduced afterloading intracavitary applicators. The concept of remote afterloading was developed at the Radiumhemmet by Sievert (1937). The use of high intensity sources in remote afterloading was introduced by Henschke in the 1960s (Stitt 1992). High dose rate therapy was first reported by O'Connell (1965).

The earliest supervoltage unit (1 mV) was placed in use for patients in 1937 at St. Bartholomew's Hospital, London. When fabricated and installed, this unit included a 30-foot evacuation x-ray tube containing the cathode and anode for x-ray production. St. Bartholomew's acquired a 15 meV linear accelerator in 1960. The first medical linear accelerator was operated at 8 mV and was installed at the Hammersmith Hospital in England in 1953. In the United States, Fletcher installed a design by Grimmet using cobalt 60 at the M.D. Anderson Hospital, Houston, in 1951. A 5 mV linear accelerator was installed at Stanford University; Kaplan treated the first patient in 1956.

The term *conformational radiation therapy* was first used by Takahashi (1961) to denote techniques designed to cause the high dose ratio to be matched closely to the irregular shape of the treatment volume. In 1979, McShan and colleagues described computerized three-dimensional treatment with interactive color graphics.

Futh was the first to report radiation-induced rectal strictures and fistulas.

RE-EMERGENCE OF SURGICAL THERAPY

When compared with the results of radiation therapy, radical surgery did not appear to be a safe and effective form of treatment until the reports of Bonney (1935), Taussig (1943), and J. V. Meigs (1944). Between 1907 and 1935, Bonney performed 483 radical operations. His operative morality rate was 20% for his first 100 operations but fell to 9.5% for his last 200 cases. His 5-year cure rate was only 20%; however, cure rates were higher when patients who were lost to follow-up or dead from other causes were excluded. Taussig (1943) reported the results of combined radiation therapy and iliac lymphadenectomy for cases of cervical cancer with involvement of the medial parametrium and upper third of the vagina; his operative mortality rate was 1.7% for 175 cases treated between 1930 and 1942. The 5-year survival rate was 38.6%, compared with 22.9% for 118 cases treated with radiation therapy alone. The low primary surgical mortality and the improved 5-year survival convinced Taussig of the value of this procedure. In patients with early invasive carcinoma treated surgically, Meigs (1944) reported excellent long-term survival and a reduced rate of complications that compared favorably with those of radiation therapy. He was a proponent of pelvic lymph node dissection, using the technique described by Taussig. In 1951, Meigs reported the results of 100 operations combining radical parametrial resection, hysterectomy, and pelvic lymphadenectomy. Despite a quarter of the women having stage II disease, the reported 5-year survival was 75%. He had no operative deaths in his last 100 patients. Metastases in lymph nodes were encountered in 22.4% of patients and were associated with a decreased survival (26.3%). Meigs' operative technique is that used by American gynecologic oncologists and differs from Wertheim's in the wider resection of the parametrial tissues and the routine performance of a more thorough pelvic lymphadenectomy.

SURGERY FOR RECURRENT CANCER

Brunschwig (1948) reported an ultraradical operation for the treatment of advanced and recurrent cancer, which he first performed in 1946. It consisted of an en bloc resection of the uterus, cervix, vagina, and the adjacent pelvic organs with urinary and fecal diversion. Initially, there was high mortality and morbidity and few survivors. In ensuing years, improvements in perioperative intensive care, diversionary procedures, and methods of pelvic reconstruction have reduced operative mortality rates to 8% to 12% and attained 5-year survival rates of 30% to 50% in selected patients (Hatch 1990). Pelvic exenteration became an option in the management of the patients who developed central pelvic recurrence. Improved radiotherapeutic techniques and equipment have reduced the need for this operation; high-energy teletherapy equipment, introduced in the 1950s, and high-dose brachytherapy have led to improved pelvic control of tumors with fewer complications.

Controversy between those who advocate radiation therapy and those who recommend radical pelvic surgery for primary treatment of early invasive carcinoma of the cervix has persisted through the years. However, a continuing process of advancement in new and existing surgical and radiotherapeutic techniques, coupled with a greater understanding of tumor biology, has led to a more individualized approach, with the recognition that both modalities have a place in the treatment of this disease.

The shift toward early stage lesions in recent years has resulted in radical surgery eclipsing radiation as the most common modality for therapy, as demonstrated in an American College of Surgery Patterns of Care study, representing 45% of the cases of invasive cervix cancer treated in the United States in the years 1984 and 1990 (Shingleton 1994).

TREATMENT OF PREMALIGNANT LESIONS

From line drawings in the German literature of the nineteenth century, P. A. Younge concluded that preinvasive lesions had been recognized at that time although their significance was not determined (personal communication, 1952). Cancerous squamous epithelium was noted by Williams in 1886, and incipient carcinoma (later termed carcinoma in situ) by Rubin 1910 and 1918 (Graham 1962). Pemberton and Smith (1929) recognized a precancerous lesion and were taking biopsies about that time. The beginning use of vaginal smears increased the numbers of cervical biopsies, as did the increasing knowledge of the significance of colposcopic observations following correlation with histologic examination of the whole cervices (Hinselmann 1933).

The relationship of carcinoma in situ and its precursors was discussed at length in the 1950s, and slowly a relationship was accepted, laying the basis for subsequent management of these earlier lesions. Few contemporary authors disagree regarding the need for treatment in patients with high-grade premalignant lesions; however, individual bias determines the type of treatment in most cases. Surgical methods (cold knife, electrosurgical, or loop diathermy conization, hysterectomy) and local ablative methods (diathermy, cryo-surgery, and laser therapy) are favored, depending on the physician's expertise and the treatment modality available. Many questions regarding the efficacy or need for treatment of patients with "low-grade" premalignant lesions still exist.

PATHOGENESIS

Squamous Cell Cervical Cancer

The literature concerning the etiology of cervical squamous cell carcinoma is voluminous and summaries are available (Gissmann 1989, Kessler 1990, Blomfield 1991, Meanwell 1991). Studies of 10 to 20 years ago linked herpes simplex type II viruses to cervical cancer and its precursors, primarily on a serologic or immunohistochemical basis; evidence of their linkage was mostly indirect. A report by Macnab (1987) states that herpes simplex viruses have no strong or proved role in cervical carcinogenesis other than as possible mutagens. Kessler (1990) disagrees, stating that herpes viruses satisfy the criteria for a viral etiology of cervical cancer better than papillomaviruses, for example.

During the past decade, evidence has accumulated implicating the human papillomavirus (HPV) as a possible viral etiologic agent. As a member of the family of DNA tumor viruses, the papillomaviruses colonize mucosal or cutaneous epithelium and induce hyperproliferation, resulting in warts. The genetic structure of the virus is a small circular double-stranded DNA sequence (de Villiers 1989, zur Hausen 1991). More than 70 HPV types have been defined, based on significant differences in their DNA sequences. Controversy still exists regarding the nature and importance of HPV infection in the development of invasive carcinoma of the cervix. It is fairly well accepted that HPV is a major contributor to the development of the precursor squamous intraepithelial lesions (SIL), and HPV cytologic changes are included in the terminology of the Bethesda classification system for cervical cytology (Tabbara 1992). Koilocytosis, however, and the other pathognomonic changes attributed to HPV do not alone define those patients who are destined to develop cervical cancer. Most individuals with these HPV changes never develop either in situ or invasive carcinoma but undergo spontaneous regression within 1 year in 63.6% of low-grade SIL and 38.2% of high-grade SIL (Syrjanen 1992). Most prevalence studies find that 6% to 40% of cytologically normal controls have demonstrable HPV-16 or HPV-18 DNA in cervical smear samples (de Villiers 1989, van den Brule et al 1989, Butterworth et al 1992). This epidemiologic reality has tempered enthusiasm for widespread cervical screening to identify the presence of HPV DNA.

Evidence supporting the association of human papillomaviruses with cervical neoplasia, especially types 16 and 18, includes serologic studies (Baird 1983, zur Hausen 1991), cytologic studies (Wagner et al 1984), and histologic studies of genital condylomas and precursor lesions of cancer (Crum and Levine 1983, Okagaki 1984, Mazur et al 1984), and invasive tumors (Gissman et al 1984), in addition to colposcopic–histologic correlation studies (Grunebaum et al 1983).

One of the early events in the initiation of cervical dysplasia and carcinoma may involve interactions of the HPV with specific genes that control cell growth (Howley 1991). The E6 and E7 proteins synthesized by HPV 16 and HPV 18 can bind to the gene products of the retinoblastoma (Rb) and p53 tumor suppressor genes (Jones et al 1990, Scheffner et al 1990). These interactions result in the loss of normal Rb and p53 gene-product function, removing two inhibitory influences on cellular proliferation and concomitantly providing HPV-infected cells with a growth advantage (personal communication, VV Baker, MD, University of Texas–Houston, Health Science Center 1992).

In studies of other infectious organisms, Hare and coworkers (1982) and Schachter and associates (1982) reported the common relation of *Chlamydia trachomatis* infections and carcinoma in situ (CIN); however, no additional studies have been reported substantiating this finding. Macnab (1987) believes that human cytomegaloviruses may have a role in human tumorigenesis, whereas Meanwell (1991) suggests that the accumulated literature incriminates Epstein-Barr viruses in cervical carcinogenesis just as other data incriminates HPV.

THE MALE FACTOR IN CARCINOGENESIS

Skegg and colleagues (1982), addressing the male factor in etiology of cancer of the cervix, note that the sexual background of the male partners of the woman may be important. They comment that in some societies a woman's risk of developing cancer of the cervix depends less on her own behavior than that of her partner; male sexual behavior, particularly in relation to prostitution, may have clear relevance to the high

incidence of this disease in Latin America. If it is true that men carry the etiologic agent, then it would be important to know whether they do so for short or long periods. Some believe that husbands of women with cervical cancer may carry some increased risk to their subsequent wives or sexual partners (Kessler 1976, 1990). The difficulty of proving such a hypothesis is apparent, however.

CIGARETTE SMOKING AND CERVICAL CANCER

Harris and coworkers (1980) found a graded association between smoking and increased severity of cervical atypias, which persisted (although weakened) when the analysis was controlled for number of sexual partners, pregnancy outside marriage, and years of contraceptive use. Studies of smokers versus nonsmokers (Lyon et al 1983) noted a relative risk of 3.0, comparing the former to the latter. In Hellberg and associates' (1988) interesting study, blood samples and cervical mucus samples of 35 women with CIN were analyzed for levels of nicotine and cotinine. Both agents, especially nicotine, were strongly concentrated in cervical mucus when compared with serum levels and may represent a mechanism for the association of cervical neoplasia and smoking. This subject is well reviewed in Meanwell's work (1991) and is substantiated by the reports of the investigative groups of Hellberg (1988), Winkelstein (1984), Gram (1992), and others.

ORAL CONTRACEPTIVES AND CERVICAL CANCER

Meanwell (1991), summarizing the literature to date, estimated that at least 60 million women in the United States regularly take oral contraceptive pills. The number of anytime users is probably far greater. Although many women believe that birth control pills may cause cancer, Meanwell concludes that one cannot make a firm statement relative to the role of these substances in the cause of cervical cancer. He suggests that birth control pill users should be subjected to regular cervical cancer screening. Beral and coworkers' (1988) study of 47,000 women followed since 1968 revealed that women using oral contraceptives for more than 10 years had a four times greater incidence of cervical cancer when compared with those who never used oral contraceptives. In contrast, Brinton and associates' (1986) study of 479 invasive cervical cancer patients and controls in five American and British geographic areas suggested a lower relative risk (1.5 times overall), whereas those using birth control pills for 5 years or more had a twofold risk over nonusers. These and other studies that require controlling for important variables (e.g., time intervals since the last cervical smear, sexual behavior of the individuals, and the role of the male partner) are difficult to interpret.

ROLE OF IMMUNOSUPPRESSION

Schneider and colleagues' (1983) report concerned renal transplant recipients in whom a few developed CIN and cervical condylomata (4.5% and 4%, respectively). They noted a lag time from transplantation to the diagnosis of condylomata of 22.4 months and a lag time from transplantation to the diagnosis of CIN of 38 months. They thought this suggested that condylomata were precursors of cervical cancer. Sillman and associates (1984) reported 20 immunosuppressed women, all with histologic evidence of koilocytes in the upper strata of areas of mild to moderate dysplasia. Twelve of the 20 patients had unusually persistent and recurrent intraepithelial neoplasia and represent an accelerated version of the long-term course of such lesions in immunocompetent people. Castello and coworkers (1986) studied the cellular immune response of 58 patients with cervical cancer, evaluated by studying T-cell populations. A significant T-cell depression was observed in all patients, some of whom had severe dysplasia or carcinoma in situ, some had microinvasive carcinoma, and some had invasive carcinoma. These results support the idea that cell-mediated immunity is a factor in the development of cervical cancer.

Maiman (1990) and Schäfer (1991) and their coworkers addressed the subject of cervical neoplasia as associated with human immunodeficiency virus (HIV) infections. Neuman found that 19% of women with invasive carcinoma younger than age 50 were HIV positive, including a 16-year-old with stage IIIB disease. It was noted that HIV-positive patients seemed to have more advanced invasive disease than the HIV-negative patients and that the disease responded poorly to therapy. Schäfer and colleagues concluded that the increased frequency of cervical neoplasia in women with HIV infections is related to the degree of immunosuppression. One hundred eleven HIV-positive women were compared with 76 HIV-negative female intravenous drug users and 526 female controls in outpatient clinics. Twenty-one percent of the HIV-positive patients had dysplasia or neoplasia (five invasive cases), whereas the HIV-negative drug users had a 9% incidence of precancer and the outpatients had 4% (two invasive cases).

Adenocarcinoma

The etiology of cervical adenocarcinoma is less clear. Dallenbach-Hellweg (1984) suggested an association between continuous use of oral contraceptive pills and the increased incidence of adenocarcinoma of the cervix, stating that 82% of a study group with adenocarcinoma or adenocarcinoma in situ had taken oral contraceptive pills, whereas only 40% of women with squamous cell carcinoma younger than age 50 had used them. In the women with cervical adenocarcinoma taking oral contraceptives, microglandular hyperplasia was diagnosed either before or coincident with the adenocarcinoma. Dallenbach-Hellweg was able to produce adenocarcinoma of the cervix in two of 12 rhesus monkeys treated for 10 years with medroxyprogesterone acetate in doses 50 times that prescribed for women and concluded that long-term use of synthetic gestagen may be causally related to development of cervical adenocarcinoma in humans. These studies have not been corroborated by other investigators, especially in reference to the induction of adenocarcinoma by synthetic hormones.

Valente and Hanjani (1986) addressed the subject

TABLE 1-3
Adenocarcinoma of the Cervix Associated With Human Papillomavirus, Using Southern Blot Method

STUDY	YEAR	CASES (N)	HPV-16	HPV-18	HPV(%)
Fukushima, et al	1985	4	1	0	25 (1/4)
Yoshikawa, et al	1985	3	0	1	33 (1/3)
Smotkin, et al	1986	2	1	0	50 (1/2)
Tsunokawa, et al	1986	3	1	1	66 (2/3)
de Villiers, et al	1986	6	2	0	33 (2/6)
Lorincz, et al	1987	9	4	2	89 (8/9)*
Wilczynski	1988	11	2	5	63 (7/11)
		38	11 (29%)	9 (24%)	58 (22/38)

*Other HPV.
HPV, human papillomavirus.

TABLE 1-4
Adenocarcinoma in Situ Associated With Human Papillomavirus
Using in Situ Hybridization

					HPV	
STUDY	YEAR	CASES (N)	HPV-16	HPV-18	(%)	(n)
Farnsworth, et al	1989	17	5	10	88	(15/17)
Tase, et al	1989	10	2	5	70	(7/10)

*One case contained both HPV-16 and 18
ACIS, adenocarcinoma in situ; *HPV,* human papillomavirus

of endocervical neoplasia in long-term users of oral contraceptives. Comparison was made of the clinical pathologic features of 7 women with endocervical neoplasia, all of whom were long-term pill users and all 33 years of age or younger. Pathology on these women was compared with seven similar cases of neoplasia in non–pill users. The entity known as microglandular hyperplasia is common in pill users and also occasionally seen in pregnant women. There is no evidence, however, that this is a premalignant lesion (Kyriakos et al 1968). Based on his own study and a review of the pertinent literature, Valente concluded that there is no convincing evidence for a direct link of oral contraceptive use with cervical neoplasia. The increased risk suggested by several epidemiologic studies of pill users does not stand the test of statistical significance and is confounded by sexual factors that cannot be sorted out in a study of large populations (Stubblefield 1984).

Parazzini and LaVecchia (1990), addressing the rising frequency of adenocarcinoma as compared with squamous cell carcinoma in both the United States and northern Europe, observed that this trend is generally restricted to women younger than age 35. They believe that this suggests a potential role for sexually transmitted and possibly viral factors (Tables 1-3 and 1-4).

EPIDEMIOLOGY

Studies of Squamous Cell Carcinoma

The first observations related to the incidence of cancer of the cervix are traditionally attributed to Rigoni-Stern (1842), an Italian physician who examined the records of deaths in Verona, Italy, from 1760 to 1839. He is said by some to have noted that the prevalence of uterine cancer was higher in married than in unmarried women and that the rates increased steadily between the ages of 30 and 60 years. He also is quoted

to have said that uterine cancer was less common in unmarried women and was extremely rare in nuns, a finding confirmed by a report published by Gagnon (1950). Skrabanek (1988), addressing the subject of the epidemiology of the disease, concluded that the evidence on prevalence of cervical cancer in nuns and prostitutes is of poor quality and neither supports nor refutes the belief that this is a venereal disease. Meanwell (1991) states that Rigoni-Stern's remarks related to breast cancer; he attributes the observation of a sexual link in the etiology of cervical cancer to Logan (1953), who stated that the lowest rates of cervical cancer were among single women and the highest rates among parous and widowed women.

In 1906, Vineberg indicated that Jewish women had a decreased incidence of cervical cancer despite being a part of the lower socioeconomic classes residing in New York City. From his case records between 1893 and 1906, Vineberg observed a 20-fold difference in the number of cases of cervical cancer in non-Jewish as compared with Jewish women. Later studies on Jewish and non-Jewish populations conducted in the United States, Europe, and Israel confirmed his findings. The inference that circumcision of the Jewish males may be a contributing factor prompted the examination of other ethnic groups such as Moslems, who also practice circumcision. The results of these investigations suggest that the variation in incidence between the compared ethnic groups cannot be attributed solely to circumcision but may be due to associated cultural differences or other factors.

INCIDENCE, MORTALITY, AND END RESULTS WORLDWIDE

Cancer of the cervix is an important cause of death in women worldwide; in many countries, it is the major cause of death in women due to cancer (Meanwell 1991). Despite the considerable effort and costly healthcare resources expended on women who have abnormal Papanicolaou smears, the total contribution of cervical neoplasia to cancer-related morbidity may be the largest of any neoplastic process.

The highest incidence of the disease is in Central and South America, Southeast Asia, Eastern Europe, and India (Fig. 1-1). Countries with low rates of this disease are Israel, Kuwait, Spain, and Ireland. Mortality (Figs. 1-2 and 1-3) reasonably parallels incidence; it is highest in Central and South America and lowest in Italy, Spain, Israel, Greece, and Malta.

Reeves and coworkers (1984) indicated that cervical cancer affects one in every 1000 Latin Americans. In their case control studies in Panama, the same variations existed as in other countries. Although the incidence rate for the country was 28.4 per 100,000, the Herrera Province had a rate of 79 per 100,000. The increased risk for women in this province was maintained despite changes in regional location, and these women apparently contracted or exhibited the disease at an early age. The reasons for the varying rates in different world locations are unclear.

Incidence rates for different populations within the United States and survival rates by race and year comparing black and white populations in the United States are depicted in Figures 1-4 and 1-5. Presumably, most of these differences are attributable to socioeconomic factors such as low income, early onset of sexual intercourse, and multiple sexual partners, yet other factors should also be considered. Regarding 5-year survival (see Fig. 1-5), there has been a slight gain among blacks, whereas the rates have not changed for whites; however, survival for blacks with this disease continues to be worse.

Sasieni (1991) reported age-specific death rates for cervical cancer in England and Wales, 1950 to 1990. Mortality rates have considerably improved; not only have rates for women younger than age 40 stabilized, but mortality in women aged 40 to 49 has decreased considerably. He attributes this encouraging trend to increased screening in the past decade.

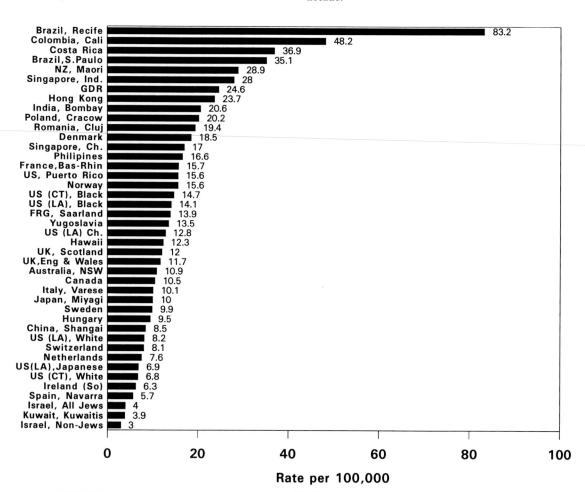

FIGURE 1-1. Age-standardized incidence rates per 100,000 for cancer of the cervix (42 countries on five continents). (Data from Whelan SL, Parkin DM, Masuyer E. Patterns of cancer on five continents. Lyon: International Agency for Research on Cancer, 1990)

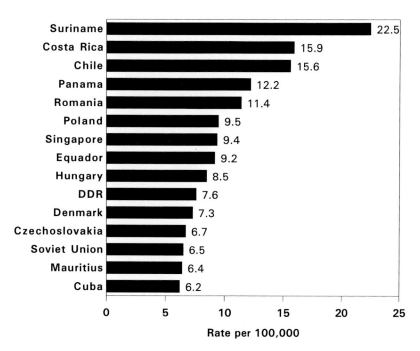

FIGURE 1-2. Fifteen countries with the highest mortality rates for cancer of the cervix, 1984–1986. (Data from Boring CC, Squires TS, Tong T. Cancer statistics, 1991. CA Cancer J Clin 1991; 41:19)

Studies of Adenocarcinoma of the Cervix

Although a great deal is known of the epidemiology of squamous cell carcinoma, less is known about that of adenocarcinoma of the cervix. Horowitz and associates' (1988) study noted a statistical significance in risks between the two types of lesions regarding the likelihood of squamous cell carcinoma in patients who (1) are unemployed, (2) come from a family with an income of less than $6000 per year and have less than a 12th-grade education, (3) smoke, and (4) had onset of sexual intercourse at younger than 18 years of age. These authors concluded that because the percentage of patients with adenocarcinoma seems to be increasing, researchers must identify the risk factors specific

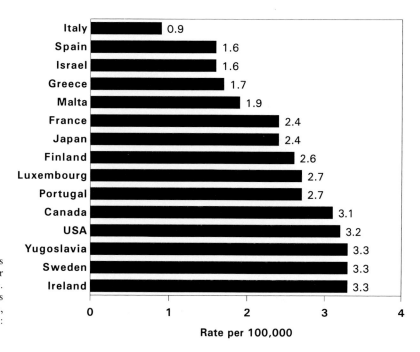

FIGURE 1-3. Fifteen countries with the lowest mortality rates for cancer of the cervix, 1984–1986. (Data from Boring CC, Squires TS, Tong T. Cancer statistics, 1991. CA Cancer J Clin 1991;41: 19)

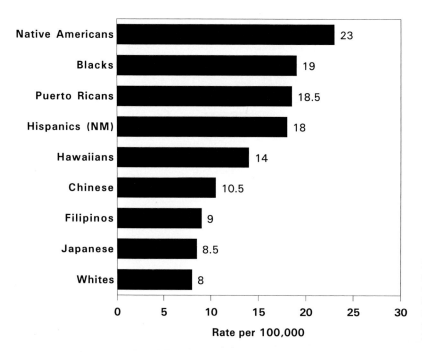

FIGURE 1-4. Incidence of cancer of the cervix in populations within the United States. (Modified from Freeman HP. Cancer in the socioeconomically disadvantaged. CA Cancer Clin 1989;39: 266, with permission)

to this particular histology. In their opinion and in our own experience, patients with adenocarcinoma tend to be better educated, and more affluent, and may have been less sexually active as adolescents.

Peters and colleagues (1986) called attention to an increased frequency of adenocarcinoma of the cervix in young women in Los Angeles County in the years between 1972 and 1982. Others have hypothesized that oral contraceptives might have a carcinogenic effect when used during periods of active metaplasia (for instance, during adolescence). Of interest, therefore, are young women who were in their teenage years when oral contraceptives were introduced. Using the Los Angeles County population-

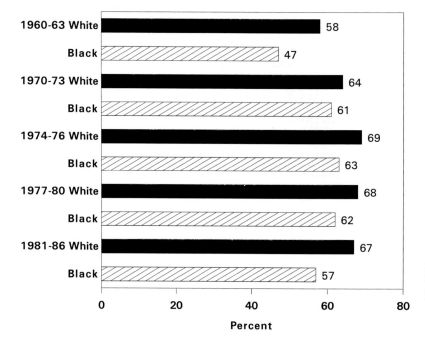

FIGURE 1-5. Trends in survival by race and year (United States). (Data from Boring CC, Squires TS, Tong T. Cancer statistics, 1991. CA Cancer J Clin 1991;41: 19)

based tumor registry, the frequency of invasive cervical adenocarcinoma in women younger than 35 years of age was found to have increased at an average rate of 8% per year during this time, a statistically significant ($p < .01$) observation. This trend was not present in women older than 35, whereas squamous cell carcinomas decreased at a rate of about 3% a year in the younger women and even more rapidly in older women. The increase in adenocarcinoma was most striking among those residing in middle- to upper-class neighborhoods; in this subgroup, the average rate of increase was 16% per year ($p < .05$). Clearly, the association of adenocarcinoma of the cervix with oral contraceptive use warrants further study.

References

Armstrong B, Jensen OM, et al. Human papilloma virus and cervical cancer. Lancet 1988;I:756.

Astruc. A treatise on the diseases of women. Translated from the French original and printed in London for J. Nocuse. 1762.

Baird PJ. Serological evidence for the association of papilloma-virus and cervical neoplasia. Lancet 1983;I:17.

Beral V, Hannaford P, Kay C: Oral contraceptive use and malignancies of the genital tract. Lancet 1988;I:1331.

Blomfield PI. Wart virus and cervical cancer. Current Obstet Gynaecol 1991;1:130.

Bonney V. The treatment of carcinoma of the cervix by Wertheim's operation. Am J Obstet Gynecol 1935;30:815.

Boring CC, Squires TS, Tong T. Cancer statistics, 1991. CA Cancer J Clin 1991;41:19.

Brinton LA, Huggins GR, Lehman HF, et al. Long term use of oral contraceptives and risk of invasive cervical cancer. Int J Cancer 1986;38:339.

Brunschwig A. Complete excision of pelvic viscera for advanced carcinoma. Cancer 1948;1:177.

Butterworth CE, Hatch KD, Macaluso M. Folate deficiency and cervical dysplasia. JAMA 1992;267:528.

Carenza L, Corrado V. Schauta radical vaginal hysterectomy. Clin Obstet Gynecol 1982;25:913.

Castello G, Esposito E, Stellato G, Mora LD, Abate G, Germano A. Immunological abnormalities in patients with cervical carcinoma. Gynecol Oncol 1986;25:61.

Clark JG. The radical abdominal operation for cancer of the uterus. Surg Gynecol Obstet 1913;16:255.

Cleaves MA. Radium: with a preliminary note on radium rays in the treatment of cancer. Med Rec 1903;64:601.

Crum CP, Levine RU. Cervical condyloma and CIN: how are they related? Contemporary Ob/Gyn 1983;September:116.

Dallenbach-Hellweg G. On the origin and histological structure of adenocarcinoma of the endocervix in women under 50 years of age. Pathol Res Pract 1984;179:38.

de Villiers E, Schneider A, Gross G, zur Hausen H. Analysis of benign and malignant urogenital tumors of human papillomavirus infection by labeling cellular DNA. Med Microb Immunol 1986;174:281.

de Villiers EM. Heterogeneity of the human papillomavirus group. J Virol 1989;63:4898.

Farnsworth A, Laverty C, Stoler M. Human papillomavirus messenger RNS expression in adenocarcinoma in situ of the uterine cervix. Int J Gynecol Pathol 1989;8:321.

Freeman HP. Cancer in the socioeconomically disadvantaged. CA Cancer J Clin 1989;39(5):266.

Freund WA. Eine neue Methode der Exstirpation des ganzen Uterus. Leipzig, Sammlung Klinischen Vortrage, 1878; 133 (Gynak No. 41:911).

Fukushima M, Okagaki T, Twiggs LB, et al. Histological types of carcinoma of the uterine cervix and the detectability of human papillomavirus DNA. Cancer Res 1985;45:3252.

Gagnon F. Contributions to the study of the etiology and prevention of cervical cancer. Am J Obstet Gynecol 1950;60:516.

Gissman L, Boshart M, Durst M, Ikenberg H, Wagner D, zur Hausen H. Presence of human papillomavirus in genital tumors. J Invest Dermatol 1984;83:26s.

Gissmann L. Linking HPV to cancer. Clin Obstet Gynecol 1989;32:141.

Graham JB, Sotto LSJ, Paloucek F. Carcinoma of the cervix. Philadelphia: WB Saunders, 1962.

Gram IT, Austin H, Stalsberg H. Cigarette smoking and the incidence of cervical intraepithelial neoplasia grade III (CINIII) and cancer of the cervix uteri. Am J Epidemiol 1992;135:341. In press.

Grunebaum AN, Sedlis A, Sillman F, Fruchter R, Stanek A, Boyce J. Association of human papillomavirus infection with cervical intraepithelial neoplasia. Obstet Gynecol 1983;62:448.

Hare MJ, Taylor-Robinson D, Cooper P. Evidence for an association between *Chlamydia trachomatis* and cervical intraepithelial neoplasia. Br J Obstet Gynaecol 1982; 89:489.

Harris RWC, Brinton LA, Cowdell RH, et al. Characteristics of women with dysplasia or carcinoma in situ of the cervix uteri. Br J Cancer 1980;42:359.

Hatch KD, Gelder MS, Soong S-J, Baker VV, Shingleton HM. Pelvic exenteration with low rectal anastamosis: survival, complications and prognostic factors. Gynecol Oncol 1991;38:462.

Hellberg D, Nilsson S, Haley NJ, et al. Smoking and cervical intraepithelial neoplasia: nicotine and cotinine in serum and cervical mucus in smokers and nonsmokers. Am J Obstet Gynecol 1988;158:910.

Horowitz IR, Jacobson LP, Zucker PK, Currie JL, Rosenshein NB. Epidemiology of adenocarcinoma of the cervix. Gynecol Oncol 1988;31:25.

Howley PM. Role of the human papillomavirus in human cancer. Cancer Res 1991;51:5019S.

Jameson E (ed). Clio medica. Gynecology and obstetrics. New York, Paul B. Heober, 1936.

Jones RE, Wegrzyn RJ, Patrick DR, et al. Identification of the HPV16-E7 peptides that are potent antagonists of E7 binding to the Rb suppressor protein. J Biol Chem 1990;265:12782.

Kessler II: Epidemiological aspects of uterine cervix cancer. In Lurain JR, Sciarra JJ, eds. Gynecology and Obstetrics 1990, vol 4. Philadelphia: JB Lippincott 1990:1.

Kessler II: Human cervical cancer as a venereal disease. Cancer Res 1976;36:783.

Kyriakos M, Kemoson RL, Konikov NF. A clinical and pathologic study of endocervical lesions associated with oral contraceptives. Cancer 1968;22:99.

Logan WPD. Marriage and childbearing in relation to cancer of the breast and uterus. Lancet 1953;I:1199.

Lorincz AT, Temple GF, Kyrman RJ, et al. Oncogenic association of specific human papillomavirus types with cervical neoplasia. J Natl Cancer Inst 1987;79:671.

Lyon JL, Gardner JW, West DW, et al. Smoking and carcinoma in situ of the uterine cervix. Am J Public Health 1983;73:558.

Macnab JCM: Herpes simplex virus and human cytomegalovirus: their role in morphological transformation and genital cancers. J Gen Virol 1987;68:2525.

Maiman M, Fruchter RG, Serur E, Remy JC, Feuer G, Boyce J. Human immunodeficiency virus infection and cervical neoplasia. Gynecol Oncol 1990;38:377.

Mann MA. System of gynecology. Philadelphia: Lea Bros, 1887.

Martzloff KH. Cancer of the cervix uteri: recognition of early manifestations. JAMA 1938;111:1921.

Massi G, Savino L, Susini T. Schauta-Amreich vaginal hysterectomy and Wertheim-Meigs abdominal hysterectomy in the treatment of cervical cancer: a retrospective analysis. Am J Obstet Gynecol 1993;168:928.

Mazur MT, Hsueh S, Gersell DJ. Metastases to the female genital tract. Analysis of 325 cases. Cancer 1984; 53:1978.

McGraw TA. Cases of operations for cancer of the womb. Mich Med News 1879;2:98.

Meanwell CA. The epidemiology and etiology of cervical cancer. In Blackledge GRP, Jordan JA, Shingleton HM, eds. Textbook of gynecologic oncology. Philadelphia: WB Saunders, 1991:250.

Meigs CD. Carcinoma of the womb. In Women: her diseases and remedies. Philadelphia: Blanchard & Lea, 1854:307.

Meigs JV. Radical hysterectomy with bilateral pelvic Iymph node dissections. A report of one hundred patients operated on five or more years ago. Am J Obstet Gynecol 1951;63:854.

Meigs JV. Carcinoma of the cervix: the Wertheim operation. Surg Gynecol Obstet 1944;78:195.

Mettler C. History of medicine. Philadelphia: Blakiston, 1947.

Novak E. Gynecological and obstetrical pathology; with clinical and endocrine relations. Philadelphia: WB Saunders, 1940.

O'Connell D, Howard N, Joslin CA, Ramsey NW, Liversage WE. A new remotely controlled unit for the treatment of uterine carcinoma. Lancet 1965;2:570.

Okagaki T. Female genital tumors associated with human papillomavirus infection and the concept of genital neoplasm-papilloma syndrome (GENPS). Pathol Annu 1984;19:31.

Parazzini F, LaVecchia C. Epidemiology of adenocarcinoma of the cervix. Gynecol Oncol 1990;39:40.

Pemberton FA, Smith GVS. The early diagnosis and prevention of carcinoma of the cervix. A clinical pathologic study of borderline cases treated at the Free Hospital for Women. Am J Obstet Gynecol 1929;17:165.

Peters RK, Chao A, Mack TM, Thomas D, Bernstein L, Henderson BE. Increased frequency of adenocarcinoma of the uterine cervix in young women in Los Angeles County. J Natl Cancer Inst 1986;76:423.

Reeves WC, Brenes MM, de Britton RC, Valdes PF, Joplin CF. Cervical cancer in the Republic of Panama. Am J Epidemiol 1984;119:714.

Ricci JV. The development of gynaecological surgery and instruments. San Francisco: Norman Publishing, 1990.

Ricci JV. The genealogy of gynaecology. Philadelphia: Blakiston, 1950.

Ricci JV. 100 years of gynaecology. Philadelphia: Blakiston, 1945.

Ries E. Eine neue Operation: Methode des Uterus carcinoma. Z Geburtshilfe Gynakol 1895;32:266.

Rigoni-Stern D. Environmental variables related to cervical cancer. Am J Obstet Gynecol 1842;83:720.

Rowland B (trans). Medieval woman's guide to health. London: Croom Helm, 1981.

Sasieni P. Trends in cervical cancer mortality. Lancet 1991;338:818. Letter.

Schachter J, Hill EC, King EB, et al. *Chlamydia trachomatis* and cervical neoplasia. JAMA 1982;248:2134.

Schäfer A, Friedman W, Miekle M, et al. The increased frequency of cervical dysplasia-neoplasia in women infected with the human immunodeficiency virus is related to the degree of immunosuppression. Am J Obstet Gynecol 1991;164:593.

Schauta F. Die Operation des Gebarmutterkrebes mittels des Schuchardt'schen Paravaginatschmittes. Monatsschr Geburtshilfe Gynakol 1902;15:133.

Scheffner M, Werness BA, Huibregtse JM, Levine AJ, Howley PM. The E6 protein encoded by human papillomavirus types 16 and 18 promotes the degradation of p53. Cell 1990;63:1129.

Schmitz HG. Lest we forget. Am J Obstet Gynecol 1955;69:467.

Schneider V, Kay S, Lee HM. Immunosuppression as a high-risk factor in the development of condyloma acuminatum and squamous neoplasia of the cervix. Acta Cytologica 1983;27:220.

Shingleton HM, Jones WB, Russell AH. American College of Surgeons invasive cervical cancer patterns of care study. 1995. In preparation.

Sievert RM. Two arrangements for inducing irradiation dangers in teleradium treatment. Acta Radiol 1937;18:157.

Sillman F, Stanek A, Sedlis A, et al. The relationship between human papillomavirus and lower genital intraepithelial neoplasia in immunosuppressed women. Am J Obstet Gynecol 1984;150:300.

Skegg DCG, Corwin PA, Paul C: Importance of the male factor in cancer of the cervix. Lancet 1982;II:581.

Skrabanek P. Cervical cancer in nuns and prostitutes: a plea for scientific continence. J Clin Epidemiol 1988; 41:577.

Smotkin D, Berek JS, Fu YS, Hacker NF, et al. Human papillomavirus deoxyribonucleic acid in adenosquamous carcinoma of the uterine cervix. Obstet Gynecol 1986; 68:241.

Stitt JA. High-dose-rate intracavitary brachytherapy for gynecologic malignancies. Oncology 1992;6:59.

Stubblefield PG. Oral contraceptives and neoplasia. J Reprod Med 1984;29(Suppl):524.

Syrjanen KV, Kataja V, Vyliskoski M, Chang F, Syrjänen S, Saarikoski S. Natural history of cervical human papillomavirus lesions does not substantiate the biologic relevance of the Bethesda system. Obstet Gynecol 1992; 79:675.

Tabbara S, Saleh ADM, et al. The Bethesda classification for squamous intraepithelial lesions: histologic, cytologic, and viral correlates. Obstet Gynecol 1992;79:338.

Tase T, Okagaki T, Clark B, et al. Human papillomavirus DNA in adenocarcinoma in situ, microinvasive adenocarcinoma of the uterine cervix, and coexisting cervical squamous intraepithelial neoplasia. Int J Gynecol Pathol 1989;8:8.

Taussig FJ. Iliac lymphadenectomy for group II cancer of the cervix. Am J Obstet Gynecol 1943;45:733.

Tsunokawa Y, Nakebe N, Nozawa S, et al. Presence of human papillomavirus type-16 and type-18 DNA sequences and their expression in cervical cancers and cell lines from Japanese patients. Int J Cancer 1986;37:499.

Valente PT, Hanjani P. Endocervical neoplasia in long-term users of oral contraceptives: clinical and pathologic observations. Obstet Gynecol 1986;67:695.

van den Brule A, Claas ECJ, du Maine M, et al. Use of anti-contamination primers in the polymerase chain reaction for the detection of human papillomavirus genomes in cervical scrapes and biopsies. J Med Virol 1989;29:20.

Vineberg HN. The etiology of cancer of the pelvic organs. Am J Obstet 1906;53:410.

Wagner D, Ikenberg H, Boehm N, Gissman L. Identification of human papillomavirus in cervical swabs by deoxyribonucleic acid in situ hybridization. Obstet Gynecol 1984;64:767.

Wertheim E; Grad H (trans). The extended abdominal operation for carcinoma uteri. American Journal of Obstetrics and Diseases of Women and Children 1912;66:169.

Whelan SL, Parkin DM, Masuyer E (eds). Patterns of cancer in five continents. Lyon: International Agency for Research on Cancer, 1990.

Wilczynski SP, Walker J, Liao S, et al. Adenocarcinoma of the cervix associated with human papillomavirus. Cancer 1988;62:1331.

Winkelstein W, Shillitoe EJ, Brand R, Johnson KK. Further comments on cancer of the uterine cervix, smoking and herpes virus infection. Am J Epidemiol 1984;119:1.

Yoshikawa H, Matsukura T, Yamamoto E, et al. Occurrence of human papillomavirus types 16 and 18 DNA in cervical carcinomas from Japan: age of patients and histological type of carcinomas. Jpn J Cancer Res 1985;76:667.

zur Hausen H. Viruses in human cancers. Science 1991; 254:1167.

Cancer of the Cervix by Hugh M. Shingleton and James W. Orr, Jr.
J. B. Lippincott Company, Philadelphia, © 1995.

2

Screening

A cancer-screening program theoretically provides a cost-effective public health measure, when designed to evaluate a disease that constitutes a significant health problem to individuals and society. To be most effective, the natural history of the disease to be screened should be known. Successful treatment should be available and readily accepted. A sufficiently sensitive, acceptable screening that detects the disease in a precursor or early stage test should be available to prevent or significantly reduce the occurrence of advanced or late-stage disease. Screening costs should be reasonable, both in proportion to health benefit and total expenditure of healthcare resources.

Cancer of the cervix represents a true success story for screening, early detection, and treatment. In 1945, the American Cancer Society endorsed the use of the vaginal smear for cervical cancer screening (Koss 1993). Although the actual incidence of invasive cervical cancer began to decline before the introduction of widespread Papanicolaou (Pap) testing (Table 2-1), the incidence of cervical cancer deaths have declined 3% to 4% per year for the past 30 years. Cytologic screening apparently allocates newly diagnosed patients to a more favorable stage (Arneson et al 1987). In the United States, these two factors have reduced the mortality rate for cervical cancer by more than 70% over the last 40 years. The yearly incidence of cervical cancer has fallen to 13,000 cases during 1991 (compared with 20,000 cases in 1960) and represents only 19% of female genital tract cancers. During this same period, the lifetime risk of a woman dying from cancer of the cervix has decreased from 41 in 10,000 to 5 in 10,000 (Koss 1993).

The lifetime risk of invasive squamous cell carcinoma (SCC) of the cervix for American women has been estimated at 0.7%. Without screening, a 20-year-old average-risk asymptomatic woman has a 250 in 10,000 risk (2.5%) of developing cervical cancer. Her mortality risk is 188 in 10,000 (1.8%; Eddy 1990). It should be remembered that despite screening, some patients still develop invasive cancer (Bearman et al 1987) and specific symptoms should not be ignored despite results of cytology.

Van Ballegooijen and coworkers (1992) evaluated savings on treatment and care of advanced cervical cancer resulting from cervical cancer screening. It was their conclusion that mass screening for cervical cancer resulted in reduction of both advanced disease and mortality. The potential savings compensate about 10% of the costs of screening.

THE PROBLEM

Although the number of deaths related to cervical cancer in the United States has fallen to about 3500 per year, the risk or incidence in other nations, particularly developing countries, remains high. Estimates from the National Cancer Institute suggest that there are about 50 million Pap smears performed each year in the United States, and about 4 million of these are abnormal. High-grade squamous intraepithelial lesions (SILs) are identified in 100,000 to 200,000 women and low-grade lesions in more than 1 million (Krumholz 1994). Even where screening is readily available, it is estimated that as many as 27% of women aged 18 or older have not had a Pap smear in the last 2 years (Table 2-1). Eight percent of women aged 45 or older and 15% of women aged 65 or older have never had a Pap test. A newer Technical Bulletin of the American College of Obstetricians and Gynecologists indicated only 60% of women have been screened within the past 5 years. Nearly 50% of cervical cancers in the United States occur in women who have never been screened, and more than 60% occur in women who have not had a smear in at least 5 years.

TABLE 2-1

Use of the Papanicolaou Test Among Women 18 and Older in the United States

	EVER TESTED (%)	W% RECENT TEST*	
		Age 18–44	45 or Older
Median	92.5	85.7	70.7
Range†	86.8–95.9	78.5–90.7	57.4–82.9

*Recent Pap test: within last 2 years (women who have not had hysterectomy).
†By state: Illinois lowest, Colorado highest.

Behavioral Risk Factor Surveillance System, 1991, Atlanta, GA: US Dept. of Health & Human Services, Centers for Disease Control and Prevention.

The relation of Pap testing and physician visits to stage at diagnosis has been evaluated. When compared with those who have carcinoma in situ, a significantly smaller percentage of women having invasive cancer had at least one Pap test in the last 3 years. The rate of Pap testing decreased with increasing age for women having carcinoma in situ or invasion. There was no difference, however, in the number of physician visits during this time. Although 65% of patients with invasive cancer who were older than 65 had not had a Pap test until diagnosis, 88% had seen a physician in the preceding 3 years. More than 70% of unscreened women received ambulatory care, and 16% were hospitalized, in the 5-year period preceding the diagnosis of cervical cancer. This information emphasizes that strategies for early cervical cancer detection must eliminate missed screening opportunities and somehow incorporate those who are not under surveillance into the existing system (Norman et al 1991). Hospitalization represents an important situation for opportunistic screening, and hospitalized women may benefit from a routine cervical smear because the frequency of abnormalities may be as high as 2% (Hudson et al 1983).

Cervical cancer remains one of the most common female malignancies (Devesa 1984, Lunt 1984). Worldwide, an estimated 500,000 women are diagnosed with this malignancy each year. Associated mortality is exceeded only by that of breast cancer. In some countries (Nigeria, Liberia, Algeria), cervical cancer represents about 30% of all female malignancies. This rate increases to more than 50% in India and Korea. Additionally, the risk or incidence of cervical intraepithelial neoplasia (CIN) or SIL may be increasing, even in developed countries (Boyes 1983, Alawa Hegama 1984). Some believe that this increase in precancerous cervical lesions suggests a future increase in the incidence of invasive SCC.

The average ages of women having carcinoma in situ (38 years) and dysplasia (34 years) have become progressively younger. As alarming are the age groups affected: the incidence of SIL lesions in younger women reportedly ranges from 0.78% (Diller et al 1983) to 2.9% (Alawa Hegama 1984, Sadeghi 1984). Benedet and associates (1992) reported a retrospective analysis of cytologic results of all patients examined providentially in 1988. Forty percent of all women older than 15 in this population (490,985) were screened. Abnormal smears were present in 9.2% of those screened. A total of 79% of women screened were younger than 50, and abnormal results from this age group comprised 86% of all abnormal smears. Actually, women younger than 35 were more likely than older women to have high-grade squamous intraepithelial lesions. The investigators concluded that intensive comprehensive cytology and colposcopic programs reduced not only the incidence of mortality of cervical carcinoma but also the rates of in situ disease and other precursors (Benedet et al 1992). Unfortunately, just more than 50% of teenage women in the United States are aware of the Pap smear but only about 10% recognize the preventive nature of cervical cytology or have had a smear (Charlton 1983).

The only areas worldwide where cervical mortality has significantly decreased are those that have comprehensive screening programs. As a corollary, the risk of developing invasive cancer is three- to tenfold or more in selected unscreened populations (Johannesson 1982, Aristizabal et al 1983, Stenkvist et al 1984, Eddy 1990). Most authors report a 50% to 75% decrease in cancer-related mortality in participating women (Christopherson et al 1970, Bjerre et al 1983, Bourne et al 1983, Boyes 1983, Draper et al 1983). Regular cervical cytology detects premalignant lesions, allowing evaluation and possible conservative therapy, but it also detects invasive cancer at an earlier stage (Carmichael et al 1984). This effect is readily demonstrated in the Scandinavian countries (Draper et al 1983). Dramatically decreased risks of cervical cancer have been reported in Iceland (where nearly 100% of patients participate) and in Finland and Sweden (where about 40% of patients participate). In Norway, however (where only 5% of women participate), there has been a slight increase in the risk of developing cervical cancer. Although many variables exist, estimates suggest that cervical cancer risks may drop to less than 5 in 100,000 cases in a completely screened population (Stenkvist 1984). Although women are fearful of developing an abnormal smear, participation in the testing procedure—even with abnormal findings—results in no serious psychologic sequelae (Reelick et al 1984). Schapira and colleagues (1993) indicated that when physicians recommend specific cancer screening tests, patient compliance is high.

CERVICAL CYTOLOGY

Dramatic changes in population screening methods have occurred since the introduction of the Pap smear in 1943. The efficacy of Pap testing is shown in historical surveys, cross-cultural correlation studies, case control studies, and analysis of data from large-scale screening programs. The evidence of benefit is sufficiently compelling that a prospective randomized trial of Pap testing at this time may be precluded by ethical considerations (Dewar et al 1992).

Cytologic detection of precancerous lesions and small, curable, occult invasive carcinoma of the cervix is based on a complex system of clinical and laboratory procedures. Optimal system performance only occurs when all the links in this chain function well (Koss 1989).

False-Negative Tests

The most serious problem, false-negative Pap tests, may result from failure (1) by clinicians to obtain abnormal cells in the cytology specimen (sampling error); (2) by cytotechnologists to recognize abnormal cells during screening (screening error); and (3) by pathologists to accurately identify abnormal cells in reviewing the slides (interpretive error). The success of any screening program depends on appropriate clinical follow-up or evaluation of abnormal smears.

Consensus suggests that screening and interpretive errors are responsible for about a third of false-negative cervical smears. The remaining two thirds of false-negative Pap smears are a result of sampling errors, primarily related to the inability of clinicians to obtain an adequate sample of cells from the squamocolumnar junction and transformation zone (Eddy 1990, Kristensen et al 1991). The proportion of errors may change as they relate to specific laboratories and the interpretation of the individual smear may show significant variation. In controlled conditions, under-called smears of CIN III or invasive SCC occur in 25% and 18% of respective smears (Morgan 1982).

Pairwuti (1991) evaluated false-negative Pap smears in 4781 cases of malignant and premalignant cervical lesions. Seventy cases (1.5%) had false-negative smears—represented by screening errors in 58.5%, interpretation errors in 2.9%, and sampling errors in 38.6%.

Van der Graaf and coworkers (1987) rescreened 555 cervical smears that were previously reported negative or mildly atypical in Dutch women who within 3 years had smears suggesting high-grade or invasive squamous lesions. Review indicated that 12% of the previous negative smears were actually inadequate. Screening errors (undercall) were present in 17% of the cases.

Controversy continues regarding the potential benefit of endocervical cells as they relate to an increased detection of abnormalities. Actually, endocervical cells may not be obtained in 10% of premenopausal and 50% of postmenopausal women, even on repeated smears (Richart et al 1992). Although the medicolegal implications of finding endocervical cells has become important, there exists little evidence that their presence is associated with fewer false-negative smears.

The cytopathologist should be hesitant to declare a smear inadequate. Retrospective reviews (Rylander 1977, Berkowitz et al 1979, Fetherston 1983, Walker et al 1983, Patterson et al 1984) suggest that about 25% of patients having invasive cervical cancer and recent "normal" smears actually had inadequate cervical cytology.

Although the precise source of the metaplastic squamous cells at the squamocolumnar junction is still uncertain, the cervical sample should contain cells from the squamous epithelium of the vaginal portion of the cervix and from the endocervical epithelium. Ideally, a sampling instrument should be selected that is most appropriate for the patient's anatomy. It generally is assumed that gynecologists perform most smears and that obtaining a cervical smear is an easily executed, clinically simple procedure. Neither assumption is entirely correct. Almost 50% of the Pap smears in the United States are performed by other primary care physicians, who may have a lesser degree of experience. To obtain an optimal smear, the cervix must be visualized without the use of lubricants. The examination can be performed painlessly when appropriately sized speculums are used.

Technique of Obtaining Cervical Smears

Since the initial description of the Pap smear, vaginal pool cytology has been abandoned because of consistently high (40%) false-negative rates. Neoplastic cells are less cohesive than normal epithelial cells, and a surface exocervical scrape and endocervical sample represent the best method of obtaining cervical cytology with low false-negative rates (Richart and Vaillant 1965, Garite et al 1978, Shen et al 1984). Theoretically, the detection of the abnormality is directly proportional to the timing and adequacy of the sample. Although a menstrual smear is not necessarily an unsatisfactory smear, blood may obscure specific abnormalities and increase screening errors. Therefore, the middle of the menstrual cycle represents the optimal time to take a Pap smear.

Obtaining the appropriate exocervical and endocervical sample is important but it is not the only part of the process (King et al 1992). Dysplastic cells are less cohesive than normal cells, thus cleaning off or wiping the cervix before obtaining the smear in addition to inadequate scraping may result in fewer cells in the sample and a less than optimal smear (Richart et al 1992). Despite rigid adherence to collection technique, other pitfalls (Table 2-2) may contribute to the variation in reported false-negative rates of 5% to 50%. Inadequate fixation, allowing the slides to air dry, or the use of obscuring or lubricating substances make interpretation difficult. Preparation of the smear requires that both sides of the sampling instrument be carefully and rapidly pressed to clean glass slides and that air drying be prevented by immediate fixation. Appropriate patient identification is paramount (Koss 1989).

TABLE 2-2
Pitfalls in Cervical Cytology

PATIENT

Recent douching or heavy discharge
Blood or vaginal preparations

PROVIDER

Inappropriate sampling techniques
Inadequate endocervical cells
Failure to spread cells appropriately
Improper fixation
Improper labeling
Failure to submit clinical data

LABORATORY

Errors in processing slides
Screening errors due to overtired or poorly trained cytotechnicians
Poor quality control measures
Failure to identify abnormal or inadequate smears

INTERPRETATION

Confusing terminology
Use of imcomplete or inexact definitions including "atypia" or HPV

CLINICAL JUDGMENT

Misinterpretation of cytology report
Inadequate follow-up or evaluation of clinical signs (cervical lesion) or symptoms (vaginal bleeding) regardless of cytology

COMMUNICATION

Inability to reach patient with smear results
Difficulty in communicating significance of "mildly abnormal" smear results

Modified from Boyce JG, Fruchter RG. Lengthening the interval between Pap smears. Contemp OB/GYN 1992;37(a):82.

A thick cervical smear with an abundance of red cells or inflammatory exudate is less than optimal and makes interpretation difficult or even impossible. The screening physician should not assume that an inflammatory smear is negative because the necrosis associated with invasive cancer may mask a malignancy. Appropriate evaluation of abnormal symptoms or signs may further decrease the risk of a false-negative evaluation.

False-Negative Smears

There is a marked decrease in false-negative rates when smears contain at least 40,000 cells (Bartels et al 1979). The degree of abnormality (particularly as it relates to atypical immature squamous metaplastic cells or other abnormalities) may relate to the actual number of abnormal cells in the cytologic specimen (Hatein et al 1992). Rubio and associates (1980) demonstrated that the highest diagnostic yield is obtained when the specimen is placed on a slide using a clockwise circular motion.

False-negative rates are increased when an exocervical scrape (Garite et al 1978) or endocervical swab (Garite et al 1978, Shen et al 1984) is used alone. Some (Beilby et al 1982) suggest that paired simultaneous sampling decreases the false-negative rate. One slide is considered satisfactory but two slides are acceptable. The use of two slides may decrease drying artifact but doubles screening time and costs. Unfortunately, some physicians still fail to combine the exocervical and endocervical samples and use only one or the other (Garite et al 1978, Benoit et al 1984). It has been argued that cotton-tipped endocervical swabs trap cells and that the type of spatula (wooden, plastic) may alter results; however, it appears that cytologic results are rarely affected when the physicians or other healthcare providers are attentive to good collection techniques (Germain et al 1994).

Automated Cytology

Automated interpretive techniques have been described (Mukawa et al 1983) but have not been widely accepted. Much of the difficulty associated with automated technology is related to the necessity of preparing a monolayer slide to allow computerized interpretation. This process may alter the slide-associated tumor diathesis or result in significant cell loss (Rutenberg 1994). A promising "semi-automated" system relies on a computer neural network that searches cytology slides for the most abnormal cellular areas and digitally displays them for visual analysis. This system relies on cellular morphology being the most sensitive indicator of abnormality. Papnet evaluation of the 300,000 or more epithelial cells on each smear eliminates or minimizes the more tedious aspects of the cytologist's task of searching for a "needle" (atypical cells) "in a haystack." This is particularly important because most Pap smears do not contain atypical cells. The published results of rescreening using this system are promising and suggest that precursors may be detected by automated screening 5 to 7 years before their clinical discovery (Rosenthal et al 1993, Boon et al 1993, Sherman et al 1994); pending Food and Drug Administration approval, this system may be invaluable in rescreening smears and reducing the incidence of false-negative smears. The introduction of self-collection techniques (Noguchi et al 1982) may assist in overcoming the cultural or educational bias that may prevent women from participation in screening programs; however, using these techniques will surely increase sampling errors and unsatisfactory samples.

In the laboratory, the smears must be logged into a recording system and given identifying numbers. Improper labeling does not allow identification of the individual having the abnormal smear. Importantly, smears treated with spray fixative must be processed and washed before staining (Koss 1989).

Notification of the patient of her smear results is important. Unfortunately, many women assume "no news is good news" and fail to inquire about the results of the smear. It seems prudent that in each screening situation, the physician, institution, or program should have a formal method (e.g., mail, phone) of patient notification.

Every physician should develop some interoffice method to follow-up cytologic abnormalities in order to avoid delays in excess of 6 months (Carmichael et al 1984). When a repeat smear is necessary because of inadequate sample of minimal epithelial atypia, a repeat interval of at least 6 weeks should be used. This time allows the previously scraped cervical surface to regenerate and decreases the risk of a repeat false-negative or inadequate smear (Morgan 1982, Koss 1993).

Kost and colleagues (1993) reported the results of early versus late repeat cervical cytology for women having less than optimal cervical cytology. The rates of dysplasia or combined abnormalities were significantly lower in women undergoing early (fewer than 4 weeks) repeat smear. Although less than optimal cervical cytology occurred more frequently (two times) in obstetric patients, these results indicated that early repeat smears of gynecologic patients was a low-yield situation.

ABRASIVE CYTOLOGY

In an attempt to improve endocervical sampling, several new cell collection devices have been developed. Taylor and coworkers (1987) reported smear results in

510 patients, comparing the use of a spatula that was combined with a cotton-tipped swab with an endocervical brush (Cytobrush). The Cytobrush reduced the incidence of suboptimal smears (those without endocervical cells) from 12% to 1.7%. These findings have been subsequently confirmed in both pregnant (Orr 1991, Rivlin 1993) and nonpregnant women (Germain et al 1994).

Many variants (sleeves, different brush heads) have been developed in an attempt to increase sensitivity and specificity. Germain and colleagues (1994) compared the results of cervical smears taken when using a cotton-tipped swab and spatula, a Cytobrush and spatula, or the cervibrush alone. Although associated with more bleeding, the Cytobrush yielded the greatest number of endocervical cells and the fewest number of inadequate smears (4%).

In a cost evaluation, Harrison and associates (1993) noted that a cervical Cytobrush was about 100 times more expensive than a cotton swab (brush, $29 per 100; cotton swabs, $0.30 per 100). The cost of nursing time ($3) for follow-up of inadequate or less than optimal smears, the cost of a short office visit for repeat smear ($23), and the pathology department technical and professional fees ($28) for Pap smears were evaluated over a 2-month period. This report indicated that routine use of the endocervical brush was associated with significant ($22,000) net yearly savings. Therefore, regardless of the screening strategy used, the Cytobrush appears to be cost-effective because fewer repeat smears were needed.

The Cytobrush may be useful for endocervical evaluation. Anderson and colleagues (1988) evaluated 87 consecutive conization specimens to determine the accuracy of endocervical curettage for the detection of endocervical canal dysplasia and to investigate the role of the endocervical brush for outpatient management of patients having atypical Pap smears. The observed false-negative rate was 45% for endocervical curettage (reduced to 16.7% if an abundant volume of endocervical material was required) and 9.4% for the Cytobrush. Despite a higher false-positive rate for endocervical dysplasia associated with the endocervical brush, the published results of most studies confirm a potentially important cost-effective benefit of Cytobrush screening cytology.

THE BETHESDA SYSTEM

In response to the variability in reporting and classifying cervical intraepithelial lesions, the Bethesda system was developed in 1988 (Lundberg 1989). The initial Bethesda system format included potentially important clinical statements regarding specimen adequacy, general groupings of abnormal cytology, and descriptive

TABLE 2-3
The 1991 Bethesda System

Adequacy of the specimen
  Satisfactory for evaluation
  Satisfactory for evaluation but limited by (specify reason)
  Unsatisfactory for evaluation (specify reason)
General categorization (optional)
  Within normal limits
  Benign cellular changes: see descriptive diagnosis
  Epithelial cell abnormality: see descriptive diagnosis
Descriptive diagnoses
  Benign cellular changes
    Infection
      Trichomonas vaginalis
      Fungal organisms morphologically consistent with
        Candida spp
      Predominance of coccobacilli consistent with shift in
        vaginal flora
      Bacteria morphologically consistent with *Actinomyces*
        spp
      Cellular changes associated with herpes simplex virus
      Other
    Reactive changes
      Reactive cellular changes associated with:
        Inflammation (includes typical repair)
        Atrophy with inflammation (atrophic vaginitis)
        Radiation
        Intrauterine contraceptive device (IUD)
        Other

Epithelial cell abnormalities
  Squamous cell
    Atypical squamous cells of undetermined significance:
      qualify*
    Low-grade squamous intraepithelial lesion encompass-
      ing HPV†, mild dysplasia/CIN I
    High-grade squamous intraepithelial lesion encom
      passing moderate and severe dysplasia, CIS/CIN II,
      and CIN III
    Squamous cell carcinoma
  Glandular cell
    Endometrial cells, cytologically benign, in a post-
      menopausal woman
    Atypical glandular cells of undetermined significance:
      qualify*
    Endocervical adenocarcinoma
    Endometrial adenocarcinoma
    Extrauterine adenocarcinoma
    Adenocarcinoma, NOS
Other malignant neoplasms: specify
Hormonal evaluation (applies to vaginal smears only)
  Hormonal pattern compatible with age and history
  Hormonal pattern incompatible with age and history:
    specify
  Hormonal evaluation not possible because of (specify)

---

*Atypical squamous or glandular cells of undetermined significance should be further qualified as
to whether a reactive or a premalignant/malignant process is favored.
†Cellular changes of HPV—previously termed koilocytosis, koilocytotic atypia, or condylomatous
atypia—are included in the category of low-grade squamous intraepithelial lesion.
HPV, human papillomavirus; *CIN*, cervical intraepithelial neoplasia; *NOS*, not otherwise specified.

Modified from Broders S. Report of the 1991 Bethesda workshop, JAMA 1992;267:1892.

---

diagnoses (Table 2-3). The Bethesda system created significant controversy and clinical concern regarding the grouping terminology (low-grade and high-grade SILs) in addition to concerns regarding specimen adequacy (Bottles et al 1991). Unfortunately, the term "unsatisfactory" smear was not defined by the Bethesda system I but was required by the Clinical Laboratory Improvement Act. Until recently, it was determined by each individual laboratory. Published guidelines, however, are available (Kurman et al 1994).

It was apparent from the outset that changes related to this system would require periodic reevaluation and revision. The second meeting, Bethesda system II (1991), also resulted in three main classifications (the adequacy of specimen, general categorization, and descriptive diagnosis [Richart et al 1993,

Luff 1992, Sherman et al 1992b]), but attempts have been made to streamline and simplify them (Table 2-4). This report, however, attempts to improve diagnostic and sample adequacy criteria. One pictorial publication (Kurman et al 1994b) attempts to minimize these problems. The Bethesda system II indicated that pathology recommendations should focus on the pathology problem to be clarified and not attempt to direct therapeutic management.

It has been estimated that changes in the Bethesda system are probably responsible for at least doubling the number of abnormal Pap smears (Julian 1993). A third Bethesda system conference was held in June 1992 in response to the marked increase in the number of cytologic abnormalities that were reported using the new system.

The specific clinical problem of grouping low-

TABLE 2-4
Selected Cervical Cytology Nomenclature Systems

PAP SYSTEM	WHO SYSTEM	CIN SYSTEM	BETHESDA SYSTEM
Class I	Normal	Normal	Normal
Class II	Atypical		Other
			Infection
			Reparative
Class III	Dysplasia		SIL
	Mild	CIN I	Low-grade SIL
	Moderate	CIN II	High-grade SIL
	Severe	CIN III	High-grade SIL
Class IV	CIS	CIS	High-grade SIL
Class V	ICC	ICC	Squamous cell carcinoma
Class V	Adenocarcinoma	Adenocarcinoma	Glandular cell abnormality
			Adenocarcinoma
			Nonepithelial malignant neoplasm

WHO, world health organization; *CIN,* cervical intraepithelial neoplasia; *CIS,* carcinoma in situ; *ICC,* invasive squamous carcinoma; *SIL,* squamous intraepithelial lesion.

Modified from Dewar MA, Hall K, Perchalski J. Cervical cancer screening. Past success and future challenge. Prim Care 1992;19(3):589.

grade and high-grade cervical lesions was retrospectively evaluated by Robertson and coworkers (1994). Their findings in 62 women who developed squamous cell cervical cancer (with up to 18 years of previous smears) suggested little role for the progression of mild abnormalities. Others (Kivati 1993) also suggest little role for progression of low-grade intraepithelial lesion to cancer but believe that these lesions serve as a marker for more severe changes.

Within the Bethesda system, reports of cellular atypia of undetermined significance should always be accompanied by a recommendation for follow-up to avoid confusion regarding the importance of the abnormality (Averette et al 1993, Kurman 1994a). The Atypical Squamous Cells of Undetermined Significance (ASCUS) classification is an attempt to collect that category of cells previously overused and described as inflammatory atypia under the previous terminology. This classification is not an attempt to confuse the clinician but to force the cytopathologist to be more specific and recognize the frequent diagnostic dilemma (Kurman 1992b). Generally, ASCUS rates of 3% are reasonable; however, rates of 5% to 10% are not (Richart et al 1993). In cases wherein this terminology is overused, it is the responsibility of the screener to determine laboratory adequacy. Although this may be difficult, some guidelines exist (Table 2-5). A significant proportion (20% to 30%) of patients having ASCUS smears have dysplasia (Montz 1991, Julian 1993). This risk may be lower in the older population (Kaminski et al 1989). Only recently have manage-

ment guidelines for ASCUS smears and low-grade abnormalities been published (Kurman et al 1994a).

Reid and associates (1991) suggested that women who have ASCUS or low-grade SIL Pap smears who test negative for human papillomavirus (HPV) DNA can be safely returned to routine cytologic surveillance rather than undergoing colposcopic biopsy. The interim management guidelines point out the limitations of this approach (Kurman et al 1994a).

The presence of atypical glandular cells is an abnormality that requires colposcopy and evaluation. The presence of glandular atypia should be considered to be serious because when definite glandular atypia is seen in a Pap smear, some 30% to 40% of patients have a high-grade lesion on conization.

INTERPRETATION

Unfortunately, cytopathology has not always been considered to be an important part of surgical pathology training. Ng (1978) reported that fewer than 2% of American pathology residents devoted at least 12 weeks to cytopathology training during their residencies. This problem is associated with the large volume of smears in a given laboratory and may contribute to the difficulty in maintaining sufficient quality control.

The process of screening smears is a time-consuming task, even for the most talented cytotechnologist. Considering that each smear contains as many as 300,000 epithelial cells, the number of necessary ob-

TABLE 2-5
Criteria for Selecting a Cytology Laboratory

1. The laboratory should process a minimum 10,000 Papanicolaou smears per year.
2. There should be a minimum of one certified cytotechnologist (FTE) for every 12,000 cases screened per year.
3. The laboratory should have at least one physician who is certified in pathology with additional training in cytopathology. All cytotechnologists should be licensed.
4. No single technologist should read more than 190 slides/24-hour period.
5. There should be 1:3 ratio of supervisors; senior cytotech. Five percent to 10% of smears should need review.
6. The lab should have a system for cytopathologist review, 1/16 cytotechnologists (including four senior cytotechnologists). If no senior cytotechnologists are present, no more than a 4:1 tech:MD ratio should exist.
7. There should be statistics for each cytotechnologist and for the laboratory regarding:
   A. Unsatisfactory specimens (1–10% acceptable)
   B. No endocervical component (suspect if under 2%)
   C. Normal specimens
   D. Abnormal by degree (expect 2–5% dysplasia)
8. There should be an 80% agreement between cytotechnologists within one grade of abnormality.
9. There should be a computerized recording and follow-up system.
10. Cost per slide should not be too low.
11. Normal slides should be kept at least 5 years. Abnormal slides should be kept permanently.
12. Turnaround time should be less than 3 days from the receipt of the slide to receipt of the report by the sending clinic. Slides shoud be **read on site,** not sent out.
13. Laboratory staff should be regularly available by phone for consultation.
14. Report should include:
    A. Satisfactory/unsatisfactory comment
    B. Presence or absence of endocervical material
    C. Infections present
    D. Abnormal histopathology described, not by class by findings
    E. The lab must have a quality assurance program in place.

Modified from Julian T. The minimally abnormal pap smear and cervical cancer screening. Colposcopist 1993;XXV:1.

servations per slide is appreciable. Careful screening of a Pap smear requires a minimum of 5 minutes per slide. Thus, even under optimal circumstances (assuming no fatigue), no cytotechnologist can adequately screen more than 12 smears in an hour, 90 smears in a $7\frac{1}{2}$ hour day, or 450 smears in a $37\frac{1}{2}$ hour week. Assuming a 48-week year, one cytotechnologist could screen a maximum of 21,600 smears annually. In reality, however, screening of 90 smears a day is a target that only a few technologists can attain (Koss 1993).

Even with fewer slides evaluated, specific interpretive problems exist. Available information suggests that trained cytopathologists "miss" subtle cytologic abnormalities during screening, even when aware of their presence (Bosch et al 1993).

In 1988, the Clinical Laboratory Improvement Act mandated rescreening of 10% of all negative smears as a means of quality control for labs licensed for interstate commerce (Koss 1993). Although other potential methods of quality control include comparison of cytologic and histologic findings, the most accepted method of quality control involves random rescreening of previously negative smears.

Another method of screening quality control involves review of the previous material from women who develop abnormalities after several consecutive normal smears (Koss 1989).

Targeted Rescreening

Some authors have suggested the use of targeted rescreening (Koss 1993). The effectiveness of targeted rescreening requires the clinician to convey to the laboratory the information that triggers a rescreening process. Although clinical information may allow better use of smear review, even targeted rescreening will not eliminate all errors of omission and commission. This methodology, however, may reduce the error rate. Unfortunately, rescreening with this method may have a negative impact on interpretive turnaround time and will not alleviate the shortage of cytotechnologists. Koss (1993) reported his results of targeted rescreening of 10,374 smears. Prospective targeted rescreening uncovered an average false-negative primary screening rate of 3.9%.

HIGH-RISK GROUPS

That unscreened women are at greatest risk for developing cervical cancer suggests that all women should participate in cervical cancer–screening programs. Patient compliance in obtaining a smear and follow-up of abnormalities may be related to a lack of understanding, which can potentially be corrected (Stewart et al 1994, Lerman et al 1992). Many methods (mail, phone, printed material, educational tapes) are available and it is important to incorporate these materials in large screening programs as well as in individual routine care (Free 1991).

Numerous publications relate the known risk factors (Chou 1991, Dewar et al 1992, Eddy 1990). Factors associated with a higher risk of developing cervical cancer include:

- Early intercourse (younger than 17 years old)
- Multiple sexual partners
- Early pregnancy

- HPV (oncogenic subtype)
- Urban population
- Low socioeconomic status
- Immunocompromised state
- Nicotine abuse
- Previous abnormal smear
- Failure to participate in screening
- Nutritional deficits
- Infertility (tubal damage)
- Use of oral contraceptives
- High-risk male partners
- Diethylstilbestrol (DES) exposure

Although complex and intertwined, the important risk factors suggest some venereal causation. Although sexual history becomes a less important factor when corrected for HPV infection, reports from developed countries suggest that sexual activity in young women is increasing. Starreveld and colleagues (1983) reported that 32.4% of all teenagers were sexually active. Seventeen percent of 13-year-olds were sexually active and 67% of 19-year-olds had experienced intercourse. Newer data suggest that this number may be an underestimate. Surveys in the United States indicate that more than 70% of teenagers have had sexual intercourse, and earlier sexual distinctions by socioeconomic status have decreased (Boyce et al 1992). Sadeghi (1984) indicated that at least 50% of sexually active teenagers have multiple partners. Clearly, an increasing number of young women are subjecting themselves to the risk of developing cervical cancer.

Wright and Riopelle (1982) suggested that a screening program based on the number of years of intercourse may be more uniform and efficient than one based on chronologic age for screening intervals. It is suggested that cytologic examinations should be concentrated during the time when most cases develop, 6 to 30 years after the time of first intercourse. Unfortunately, selective screening has only a limited applicability because the average interval for developing cervical cancer from the time of first coitus may be as long as 28 years (Chou 1991).

Unquestionably, young women seek gynecologic care more frequently for issues relating to reproduction, contraception, or pain. In the Cardiff screening project (1980), 92% of women in the 25- to 28-year-old group had been screened. The cessation of reproductive function, however, is associated with a decreased participation in screening programs. Boon and associates (1982) indicated that only 26% of women in the 65- to 69-year-old group had participated in screening, despite a significant risk of developing cervical cancer and death (Boon et al 1982) in this age group. United States data confirm that young women are more likely to have had a recent Pap smear (see Table 2-1).

Although teenage pregnancy probably increases risk, some reports suggest that oral contraceptive use (Vessy et al 1983, WHO 1994) or intrauterine device use (Blenkinsopp et al 1982) is also associated with increased risk. Whether these factors are related to sexual activity at an age when the prevalent epithelial metaplasia makes the cervix vulnerable to carcinogens or to local or systemic alteration in immunocompetence (Grant 1983) remains to be determined.

The interrelation and effect of socioeconomic status, urban location, and sexual attitudes is difficult to unravel but this effect becomes less important when corrected for race. Regardless, urban women have an increased risk and should be encouraged to participate in screening programs (Beral 1974, Chung et al 1982).

The risk of developing SIL appears to be increased by as much as tenfold in patients receiving immunosuppressant drug therapy (Balachandran et al 1984). The documentation of an increased risk in HIV-positive women represents another aspect of this problem (Maiman et al 1991, 1993; Conti et al 1991). It appears that a careful, regular surveillance program should be instituted in these subpopulations. Moreover, the increased risk of SIL in those women having vulvar intraepithelial or invasive disease (Hammond 1983) may be indicative of a natural immune-deficit phenomenon or infection with HPV.

The multifocal predisposition for the development of lower genital tract intraepithelial neoplasia has been detailed. Patients with premalignant or malignant vulvar or vaginal lesions have a 20% risk of having a synchronous or metachronous carcinoma in situ of the cervix (Friedrich 1983). This emphasizes not only the need for screening but also the importance of careful evaluation of the entire lower genital tract before the treatment of an isolated lesion.

The incidence of HPV infections involving the female genital tract is reported to have risen. This risk may have tripled in the United States in the past decade, and some reports suggest that since 1945, the incidence of HPV infections has risen 1000-fold. This problem, however, may not have been previously recognized. Bernstein and colleagues (1985) reevaluated 1264 consecutive cervical biopsies performed in 1972. Their findings suggested that HPV infection was not a new but a previously overlooked entity. It is estimated that 1% of unselected men and women 15 to 49 years of age and as many as 13% of adults with sexually transmitted disease have evidence of condyloma (Krowchuk et al 1992). Initial consultation with private practitioners for the diagnosis and treatment of genital warts increased considerably, 4.5-fold between 1966 and 1984. Newer information (Koutsky et al 1992) suggests that in some populations, the risk of developing SIL is increased tenfold in women who acquire HPV. These studies suggest this risk to be an apparent early manifestation of HPV infection.

The amplification of molecular biology techniques (Table 2-6) has added additional evidence to support a causal association of HPV, CIN, and cervical cancer (Bornstein et al 1993). Failure to detect HPV DNA in genital SCCs by conventional hybridization techniques (i.e., Southern blot, dot blot, in situ) may reflect a sampling error (missing the lesion), the presence of small amounts of virus that may not be detected by methods used, the presence of a virus type unrelated to the probes, or the absence of HPV in the tumor (Beckmann et al 1991).

The diagnosis of koilocytosis occurs in 2% to 3% of Pap smears in women of reproductive age. Any clinician who receives reports of koilocytosis in more than 5% of Pap smears (and particularly more than 10%) should contact the laboratory to ensure that koilocytosis is not being overdiagnosed (Crum 1993). In Crum's experience, about 50% of smears containing koilocytosis are associated with a low-grade intraepithelial lesion on biopsy. More importantly, about 20% of these smears are associated with cervical biopsies that contain a high-grade lesion.

Human Papillomavirus Typing

The potential role of HPV DNA typing has interested many practitioners. Because HPV types 16, 18, 31, and 33 are commonly found in preinvasive and invasive cancers, it has been suggested that HPV typing may lead to early identification of high-risk patients among those having intraepithelial lesions or atypia. Evidence fails to support universal HPV typing. As many as 25% who test positive for HPV may be nega-tive for HPV 5 to 7 days later when screened by polymerase chain reaction. In addition to method variation, it is estimated that only 3% of patients who are infected with HPV eventually develop invasive cervical cancers (Averette et al 1993).

Cox and coworkers (1992) evaluated the effectiveness of HPV testing as a triage method for predicting the risk of a biopsy-confirmed SIL in a cohort of 482 women referred for colposcopy. Their conclusions suggested that HPV testing may increase the sensitivity for screening in this group of women but indicated that the eventual usefulness or role of HPV testing relates to costs, availability, and accuracy of specific cytologic and colposcopic evaluation.

Borst and associates (1991) evaluated the use of HPV DNA screening and colposcopy in the management of women whose Pap smears demonstrated atypia less than dysplasia. Human papillomavirus 16 DNA screening did not predict which patients with atypical smears had underlying CIN. They believed that colposcopically directed biopsy remains the evaluation method of choice. Hatch (1994) indicated that the use of hybrid capture evaluation of intermediate or high-risk HPV typing did not significantly add to the sensitivity or specificity of cervical cytology. Based on available information, it appears that HPV testing contributes little to the routine use of cervical cytology or the clinical evaluation of abnormal smears.

Evidence suggests that women who smoke are at increased risk for the development of cervical cancer (Berggren et al 1983, Clarke et al 1983, Trevathan et al 1983, Dewar et al 1992). Although the data are not always controlled for sexual activity, the risk appears real and women who use nicotine should be encour-

TABLE 2-6
Comparison of the Various Laboratory Tests for Diagnosis of HPV Infection

TEST	SENSITIVITY	SPECIFICITY	ADVANTAGE	DISADVANTAGES
Southern blot	High	High	Nearly all positives are true positives	Labor intensive (research tool)
Dot blot	High	Medium	Quick	False positives
FISH	Medium	Low	Simple	False positives
In situ				
DNA-DNA	Medium	Medium	Morphology available	False positives, false negatives
RNA-DNA	High	High	Morphology available	False positives, false negatives
PCR	High	Unknown	Very sensitive	False positives, unknown clinical relevance

HPV, human papillomavirus; *FISH,* in situ filter; *PCR,* polymerase chain reaction.

Modified from Garland SM, Faulkner–Jones BE, Fortune DW, Quinn MA. Cervical cancer—what role for human papillomavirus? Med J Aus 1992;156:204.

aged to participate regularly in screening programs. This problem may be a partial explanation of the reason that patients treated for cervical cancer have a higher risk of later developing lung cancer (see Chap. 11).

Once a woman has had an abnormal cervical smear, regardless of treatment, she remains at risk for later developing invasive cervical cancer. Richart (1980) reported 3000 women (with all degrees of dysplasia) who were successfully treated and who were followed for up to 15 years. Patients who had normal colposcopic and cytologic findings at 4 and 12 months had a low risk of later developing cervical cancer. Women with a previous abnormality are at risk. McIndoe and colleagues (1984) reported that a patient who has continuing abnormal cytology after initial management of carcinoma in situ in the cervix is 24.8 times more likely to develop invasive carcinoma than a woman who has normal results after cytologic follow-up. That 1% to 2% of women surgically treated for CIN III later develop invasive vaginal cancer underscores this increased risk when compared with the expected incidence of invasive cancer in 10 of 100,000 women in a screened population. Patients undergoing conservative or extirpative procedures must understand the risk, and they should remain under surveillance after treatment.

Women who have had a hysterectomy for benign disease, with removal of all cervical tissue, constitute a low-risk group for the incidence of invasive cancer. Nonetheless, history alone does not suffice to guide screening interval in these women for the detection of vaginal cancer (Eddy 1990). Mandelblatt and Fahs (1988), however, found that a third of 280 women with a history of prior hysterectomy had an intact cervix on examination; therefore, history is not invariably reliable.

Nutrition and Cervical Cancer

Nutritional alterations have been linked to cancers at other sites; however, the evidence relative to cervical cancer is only now being collected. Some reports suggest an increased risk of dysplasia when women have low levels of vitamin A (Bernstein et al 1984) or vitamin C (Romney 1985). Our data (Orr 1985) demonstrated a significantly lower level of vitamin A precursors (beta carotene) and vitamin C in patients having invasive cervical cancer. Folic aid levels are also low in patients having cervical cancer, and folate replacement has been reported to reverse premalignant cervical changes (Butterworth et al 1982). Although most reports are preliminary, women who are malnourished should be considered to be at increased risk and encouraged to participate in screening programs. Further evaluation is necessary to determine the association of

nutritional deficits and other risk factors, such as urban living and low socioeconomic status.

Reports of a role for the "high-risk" male, which further delineated the venereal etiology of cervical cancer, surfaced in the 1970s (Beral 1974, Singer et al 1976). Women whose husbands have had multiple sexual partners were said to be at increased risk (Buckley et al 1981) and second wives of men whose first wives had cervical cancer may also be at increased risk (Singer et al 1976). Newer studies to substantiate these theories are lacking.

Our early report (Orr et al 1981) suggested that women having in utero DES exposure are at increased risk for the development of cervical squamous atypias. The association of DES exposure with clear cell adenocarcinoma has been established (Herbst et al 1981), and the predisposition of these women to develop squamous precursor lesions was confirmed in large prospective trials (Robboy et al 1984). Women having in utero DES exposure who have widespread metaplasia should be screened as a high-risk population for squamous abnormalities and adenocarcinoma.

SCREENING COMMENCEMENT, FREQUENCY, AND TERMINATION

Because cervical cancer likely has a sexually transmitted factor or cofactor, there is little rationale for beginning screening before the initiation of sexual activity. Because many American teenagers are sexually active by age 18, most recommend initiating Pap testing by this age, even in the absence of an individual history of commencement of sexual activity (Eddy 1990). In the United Kingdom, the initiation of cervical cancer screening at a later age (35 years) was associated with a dramatic increase in cervical cancer in younger women (Draper et al 1983).

The concept of a yearly Pap smear has been widely accepted yet occurred without prospective studies to determine optimal frequency. Newer recommendations (Table 2-7) suggest implementation of a less than yearly screening interval. The initial recommendation by Boyes was proposed in an attempt to solve the economic problems associated with yearly examinations (Boyes 1983). Although progression from a premalignant to an invasive lesion is thought to take years, this process may occur more rapidly (Peterson 1956, Richart 1980). Many reports have appeared concerning women who developed invasive cancer after recent normal examinations (Morrel et al 1982, Bain et al 1983, Bamford et al 1983).

A single negative Pap smear may decrease the risk of developing cervical cancer by 45% and nine negative

TABLE 2-7
Selected Papanicolaou Smear Screening Guidelines

GROUP	RECOMMENDATION
American Cancer Society National Cancer Institute American College of Obstetricians and Gynecologists American Academy of Family Physicians American Medical Association	Pap smears annually beginning at age 18, or with the onset of sexual activity; after three consecutive normal examinations, testing may be performed less frequently at the discretion of the physician
U.S. Preventive Services Task Force	Pap smears every 1–3 years beginning with the onset of sexual activity; testing may be discontinued at age 65 if consistently normal
1982 Canadian Task Force	Pap smears every 1–3 years beginning at age 18 or with the onset of sexual activity; screening interval may be extended to every 5 years at age 35 and discontinued at age 60 if consistently normal

Modified from Dewar MA, Hall K, Perchalski J. Cervical cancer screening. Past success and future challenge. Prim Care 1992;19(3):589.

TABLE 2-8
Reduction in Cumulative Rate of Invasive Cervical Cancer

INTERVAL BETWEEN SCREENINGS (YEARS)	REDUCTION IN CUMULATIVE INCIDENCE (%)	TESTS (N)
1	93.5	30
2	92.5	15
3	90.8	10
5	83.6	6
10	64.1	3

Percentage is in women aged 35 to 64 with different frequencies of screening

Modified from Boyce JG, Fruchter RG. Lengthening the interval between Pap smears. Contemp OB/GYN 1992;37(a):82.

smears during a lifetime decrease risk by as much as 99%. Eddy (1990), using a mathematic model, indicated that in women 35 to 64 years of age, screening intervals of 10, 5, and 3 years reduced the incidence of invasive cancer by 64%, 84%, and 91%, respectively (Table 2-8). Decreasing the interval to every year produced only an additional 3% risk reduction but significantly increased the necessary number and resultant costs of smears.

Regardless, the optimal frequency and timing remain controversial (see Table 2-7). In Walton and coworkers' initial report (1980), the Canadian government suggested that smears should be performed at the start of sexual activity. After two yearly negative smears, repeat examination should be performed in low-risk individuals every 3 years. In view of increasing numbers of women at high risk, Morgan (1982) from the Canadian Task Force revised these guidelines to yearly smears during the ages of 18 to 35 and further stated that annual examination should not be discouraged in women older than 35 years of age. This report indicates that the only low-risk women are those who (1) reach the age of 60 with all prior smears negative, (2) have had a hysterectomy with a confirmed well-studied benign cervix, and (3) are virgins. The Canadian Task Force on Cervical Cancer Screening continues to recommend an upper age limit but in 1991

extended that limit from 60 to 70 years of age. It also added the provision that women should have a history of two recent satisfactory normal smears and no abnormal smears within the last 9 years before the cessation of screening.

The recommended age to discontinue Pap tests is somewhat problematic. In Canada, cytology is discontinued in women older than 69 who have had at least two satisfactory normal smears, no significant epithelial abnormality in the last 9 years, and never had biopsy-proven CIN III (Miller 1992). Older women from minority and low-income groups are more likely than nonminority and nonpoor older women to have inadequate screening histories (Fahs et al 1992). Although a quarter of invasive cervical cancer deaths and more than 40% of cervical cancer deaths occur in women older than 65, the de novo development of carcinoma in situ and invasive carcinoma of the cervix in older women is rare. Several studies, however, have demonstrated that many older women have not undergone regular Pap testing. Mandelblatt and Fahs (1988) evaluated more than 1300 women older than 65 and reported that a quarter had never had a Pap smear, and only 26% had such smears at least every 5 years (Eddy 1990).

In 1988, the American Cancer Society, the National Cancer Institute, the American College of Obstetricians and Gynecologists, and American Medical Association issued a consensus statement that called for cervical Pap smear screening throughout a woman's lifetime without specifying an age of discontinuation (Fahs et al 1992). The U.S. Preventive Services Task Force recommends discontinuing screening at age 65 "but only if the physician can document previous Pap screening in which smears have been consistently normal." The most recent U.S. Preventive Services Task Force recommends regular cervical cytology for all sexually active women. Screening should commence with the onset of sexual activity and be repeated at least every 3 years, with the optimal interval determined by the physician, based on the patient's risk factors. Women who have had regular consistently normal smears can discontinue smears at age 65.

Fahs and associates (1992) analyzed the cost and benefit of alternative cervical cancer screening schedules among older women. A hypothetical cohort of 1 million 65-year-old women were evaluated. Triennial screening reduced mortality from cervical cancer among the older women by 74% at a cost of $2,254 per year of life saved. Annual screening increased cost to $7,345 per year of life saved. These results were more related to the quality of the Pap smear than to the characteristics of the women being screened. If the sensitivity of the Pap smear is reduced from a baseline estimate of 75% to 50% and the specificity is decreased from 95% to 87%, the cost-effectiveness ratio increases by nearly $7,000 per year of life saved. Screening women who have been screened regularly, however, is considerably less efficient, increasing costs to $32,572 per year of life saved. In their evaluation, mammography screening for the older woman costs about $12,000 per year of life saved. In contrast, the cost of a common medical therapy, hypertension monotherapy, in a non–older patient ranges from $16,000 to $72,000 per year of life saved.

Despite published guidelines, one newer survey (Dewar et al 1992) found that 95% of physicians report the use of Pap tests in asymptomatic women, and more than 80% advocated more frequent screening than recommended by national guidelines.

COLPOSCOPY AND CERVICOGRAPHY

Colposcopy is more sensitive than Pap smears in detecting cervical epithelial abnormalities (Breitenecker et al 1992); however, the lack of quality control (Benedet et al 1991) and relatively high false-positive rate of colposcopy and the time and expense involved in performing colposcopic evaluation make colposcopy less effective than cytology for cervical cancer screening (Eddy 1990).

Cervicography (a modified less-expensive form of colposcopy) was introduced in the 1970s. This photographic screening technique, in which a 35-mm photo is taken of the cervix after staining with 3% or 5% acetic acid, has potential as a screening test. Abnormal details can be identified from a series of photographic enlargements. In a limited trial, cervicography has

been found to be more sensitive but significantly less specific than cytologic screening. The sensitivity of cervicography is reported to be as high as 94% (Averette et al 1993).

One study (Tawa et al 1988), comparing screening with cervicography and Pap testing in 3271 women between 18 and 50 years of age, indicated that the total cost of cervicography screening exceeded that of Pap testing. The cost per case of intraepithelial neoplasia detection was less (3.7:1) with cervicography, however. Reid and coworkers (1991) screened 1012 women aged 18 to 35 by cytologic testing, cervicography, and HPV hybridization, followed by colposcopic confirmation. Although cytology screening alone detected only 52% of squamous cell intraepithelial lesions, a combination of all three modalities increased the detection rate to 83%. The added cost of combined screening, however, must be weighed against the value of increasing the detection rate of the Pap test.

August (1991) reported 681 consecutive patients who were referred to the Denver General Hospital colposcopy clinic for smears demonstrating atypical nuclear or cytoplasmic changes insufficient to justify a cytologic diagnosis of dysplasia. Interestingly, his findings suggested that from 1984 to 1988, the percentage of abnormal Pap smears reported as atypical nearly doubled at the Denver General Hospital, rising from just more than 9% to more than 17% of all gynecologic cytologic smears. Fourteen percent of patients demonstrated CIN and 29% had condyloma without CIN. August's rate of defective cervicograms was 9% (compared with a published range of 18% to 42%), which was thought to result from the newer instructional techniques available from national testing laboratories. Neither cervicography nor the colposcopic impression was ideal but both were superior to repeat smear, HPV typing, or both (Table 2-9).

The cost per patient and case of detected SIL was determined by averaging a sampling of current charges by private practitioners, university-affiliated physicians, and various local laboratories. The cost per case of CIN detected was $3,728 for patients who were evaluated with repeat smears, $3,713 for patients evaluated by colposcopy and $2,005 for patients undergoing cervicogram with selected colposcopy.

TUMOR MARKERS

In an early study, Holloway and associates (1989) reported the measurement of squamous cell antigen (SCA) as a nonsensitive screening method for cervical cancer (sensitivity, 53.3%). Many other studies have confirmed these findings.

Borras and colleagues (1991) also evaluated the

TABLE 2-9
Comparison of Specific Cervix Screening Methods With Histology

METHOD	SENSITIVITY (%)	SPECIFICITY (%)	POSITIVE PREDICTIVE VALUE (%)	NEGATIVE PREDICTIVE VALUE (%)
Cervicography (586 patients)	82	62	60	84
Colposcopic impression (586 patients)	84	62	61	84
Repeat cytology (428 patients)	26	97	85	71
Human papillomavirus typing (333 patients)	42	85	72	63

Modified from August N. Cervicography for evaluating the "atypical" Papanicolaou smear. J Reprod Med 1991;36:89.

role of serum SCC in 68 cervical cancer patients. Although a stage-related increase in this tumor marker was reported, only 56% of patients who had cervical cancer had an elevated marker.

Serum levels of squamous SCC, CA-125, and tissue polypeptide antigen were evaluated in 142 women having primary cervical cancer (Åvall-Lundqvist et al 1992). Specificity of any elevated tumor marker ranged from 94.6% to 97.7%; however, sensitivity was highest (44.4%) for SCC, and a stage-related increase was noted. Interestingly, in patients having stage IB disease, squamous cell serum marker levels increased according to tumor volume and were significantly related to patient survival in addition to stage. In cervical SCC, the risk of a fatal outcome increased 16 times when SCC was greater than 4.5 ng/mL when compared with SCCs of less than 1.3 ng/mL.

ONCOGENES

Several oncogenes have been implicated in the pathogenesis of cervical cancer. The amplification and overexpression of the C-*myc* oncogene in rapidly progressive and advanced cervical cancer has been reported. There is also a reported close correlation between C-*myc* overexpression with node metastasis and relapse. Estimates suggest that C-*myc* overexpression increases the risk of distant metastasis by a factor of six (Averette et al 1993). There is little information to provide a role for routine oncogene screening.

SUMMARY RECOMMENDATIONS

In 1975, the American College of Obstetricians and Gynecologists recommended annual cervical cytology as the standard of practice (Boyce et al 1992). In

1980, the American Cancer Society recommended routine cytology every 3 years for women who have had two previous consecutive normal smears. This recommendation was based on two sources of data: (1) mass screening programs, and (2) case control studies from Denmark, Iceland, Finland, Sweden, Scotland, Italy, and Canada. In each of these mass screening programs, cytology services were standardized and centrally organized. Laboratory procedures were monitored and reviewed. The populations screened were well-defined and stable by census and other official data. The health delivery systems in which the mass screening programs operated were structured and organized. Patient identification allowed effective follow-up and continuity, and the direct costs of screening to the patient were usually minimal.

In contrast, the population in the United States at greatest risk of developing cervical cancer is highly mobile. The 1980 census reported that 25% of United States residents had changed residence within the previous 5 years. The most mobile group was adults aged 20 to 44.

Additionally, the United States medical care system includes a multiplicity of primary care providers who lack ready access to all previous medical records. Many patients use multiple providers. Therefore, any assessment of patient screening history in this country usually relies heavily on the patient's memory. Unfortunately, important patient information on screening intervals and results of Pap smears is often inaccurate because most studies consistently indicate that women are more likely to report more frequent and more recent smears than can be documented. Additionally, women are likely to report abnormal smears as having been normal or negative, whereas record review indicates some degree of abnormality that may have warranted a repeat follow-up or even a biopsy. In Boyce and colleagues' (1990) study of 174 women having invasive cervical cancer, 28 had smears taken within 36 months before developing cervical cancer symptoms. Seventeen of these women (61%) had believed that their smears were normal. Among 41 women who were screened within 3 years of developing cancer symptoms, 39% had normal smear histories and 61% had abnormal histories. These difficulties suggest that if clinicians were to use a 3-year interval for screening, 10% to 20% of patients who needed screening would not be screened appropriately if self-reporting rather than documentation were used.

Unlike machine-processed complete blood counts, Pap smears have an inherently low sensitivity. Cytology results depend highly on humans at every level. Even with optimal training of laboratory personnel, errors occur and there may be as high as a 20% to 30% false-negative rate for a single Pap smear. In the United States, unlike other countries having organized mass screenings, a multiplicity of laboratories have standards and licensing criteria that vary from state to state. The 1988 Clinical Laboratory Improvement Act may raise standards but such improvement has not yet been documented.

In using discretion in deciding whether to perform a Pap smear, the clinician must address the following questions:

1. Is there an adequately documented history of normal annual smears?
2. What was the quality of the clinician and laboratory taking and interpreting the previous smears?
3. Is the patient at high risk for cervical neoplasia?
4. Will the patient comply with recommendations for future care?

Although the exact frequency of smears can only be determined by economic resources and individual attitudes, all women should be encouraged to participate in a cervical cancer screening program at least once; it appears to be unwise to encourage prolonged intervals between examination because this may discourage the use of screening and allow progression to invasive cancer. Asymptomatic women should be encouraged to participate in regular screening and symptomatic women should seek immediate physician consultation. It seems to be appropriate to attempt to increase the number of women receiving a smear because most invasive cancers occur in the unscreened portion of the population.

More patients need to be screened; furthermore, newer data suggest that patient compliance is high when tests are recommended by the primary care physician (Schapira et al 1993). Additionally, Pap smear screening may serve as a sentinel test because women who have cervical cytology are more likely to have received other potentially beneficial screening tests (Hueston et al 1994). For these reasons, physi-

cians and healthcare professionals should encourage Pap smear screening at every opportunity.

References

Alawa Hegama AB. Screening for cervical intraepithelial neoplasia and cancer in the Sheffield STD clinic. Br J Venereal Dis 1984;60:117.

Anderson W, Frierson H, Barber S, et al. Sensitivity and specificity of endocervical curettage and the endocervical brush for the evaluation of the endocervical canal. Am J Obstet Gynecol 1988;159:702.

Aristizabal SA, Surwit E, Valencia A, Havezi J. Treatment of locally advanced cancer of the cervix with transperineal interstitial irradiation. Report on 106 cases. Am J Clin Oncol 1983;6:645.

Arneson AN, Kao MS. Long term observations of cervical cancer. Am J Obstet Gynecol 1987;156:614.

August N. Cervicography for evaluating the "atypical" Papanicolaou smear. J Reprod Med 1991;36:89.

Åvall-Lundqvist, EH, Sjövall K, Nilsson BR, Eneroth PHE. Prognostic significance of pretreatment serum levels of squamous cell carcinoma antigen and CA125 in cervical carcinoma. Eur J Cancer 1992;28A(10):1695.

Bain RW, Crocker DW. Rapid onset of cervical cancer in an upper socioeconomic group. Am J Obstet Gynecol 1983;146:366.

Balachandran I, Galagan KS. Cervical carcinoma in situ associated with azathioprine therapy. A case report and literature review. Acta Cytol 1984;28:166.

Bamford PN, Beilby JD, Steele SJ, Vlies R. The natural history of cervical intraepithelial neoplasia as determined by cytology and colposcopic biopsy. Acta Cytol 1983;27:482.

Bartels PH, Bibbo M, Wied GL. Estimation of proportion of the patients with a very low number of tumor cells from carcinoma in situ in the cervical smear. Anal Quant Cytol 1979;1:136.

Bearman DM, MacMillan J, Creasman WT. Papanicolaou smear history of patients developing cervical cancer: an assessment of screening protocols. Obstet Gynecol 1987;69:151.

Beckmann AM, Acker R, Christiansen AE, Sherman KJ. Human papillomavirus infection in women with multicentric squamous cell neoplasia. Am J Obstet Gynecol 1991;165:1431.

Beilby JO, Bourne R, Guillebaud J, Steele ST. Paired cervical smears: a method of reducing the false negative rate in population screening. Obstet Gynecol 1982;60:46.

Benedet JL, Anderson GH, Matisic JP. A comprehensive program for cervical cancer detection and management. Am J Obstet Gynecol 1992;166:1254.

Benedet JL, Anderson GH, Matisic JP, Miller DM. A quality control program for colposcopic practice. Obstet Gynecol 1991;78:872.

Benoit AG, Krepart GV, Lotocki RJ. Results of prior cytologic screening in patients with a diagnosis of stage I carcinoma of the cervix. Am J Obstet Gynecol 1984; 148:690.

Beral V. Cancer of the cervix: a sexually transmitted infection! Lancet May 1974;25:1037.

Berggren G, Sjostedt S. Preinvasive carcinoma of the cervix uteri and smoking. Acta Obstet Gynecol Scand 1983; 62:593.

Berkowitz RS, Ehrmann RL, Lavizzo-Mourey R, Knapp RC. Invasive cervical carcinoma in young women. Gynecol Oncol 1979;8:311.

Bernstein A, Harris B. The relationship of dietary and serum vitamin A to the occurrence of cervical intraepithelial neoplasia in sexually active women. Am J Obstet Gynecol 1984;148:309.

Bernstein SG, Voet RL, Guzick DS, et al. Prevalence of papillomavirus infection in colposcopically directed cervical biopsy specimens in 1972 and 1982. Am J Obstet Gynecol 1985;151(5):577.

Bjerre B, Johansson S. Invasive cervical cancer in a cytologically screened population. Acta Obstet Gynecol Scand 1983;62:569.

Blenkinsopp WK, Chapman P. Prevalence of cervical neoplasia and infection in women using intrauterine contraceptive devices. J Reprod Med 1982;27:709.

Boon ME, Rietveld WJ, Kirk RS. Investigation of possible changes in the detection of cervical carcinoma in patients of Dutch general practitioners. Tumori 1982; 68:299.

Boon ME, Kok LP. Neural network processing can provide means to catch errors that slip through human screening of Pap smears. Diagn Cytopathol 1993;9(4):411.

Bornstein J, Ben-David Y, Atad J, et al. Treatment of cervical intraepithelial neoplasia and invasive squamous cell carcinoma by interferon. Obstet Gynecol Survey 1993; 48(4):251.

Borras G, Molina R, Ballesta A, et al. SCC in cervical cancer. Eur J Gynaecol Oncol 1991;XII:123.

Borst M, Butterworth CE, Baker V, et al. Human papillomavirus screening for women with atypical Papanicolaou smears. J Reprod Med 1991;36:95.

Bosch MM, Rietveld-Scheffers PE, Boon ME. Characteristics of false-negative smears tested in the normal screening situation. Acta Cytol 1992;36(5):711.

Bottles K, Reiter RC, Steiner AL, et al. Problems encountered with the Bethesda system: the University of Iowa experience. Obstet Gynecol 1991;78:410.

Bourne RG, Grove WD. Invasive carcinoma of the cervix in Queensland. Change in incidence and mortality, 1959–1980. Med J Aust 1983;1:156.

Boyce JG, Fruchter RG, Romanzi L, et al. The fallacy of the screening interval for cervical smears. Obstet Gynecol 1990;76:627.

Boyce JG, Fruchter RG. Lengthening the interval between Pap smears. Contemp OB/GYN 1992;37a:82.

Boyes DA. The current status of screening for uterine cancer. Prog Clin Biol Res 1983;132E:483.

Breitenecker G, Gitsch G. What's new in diagnosis and treatment of HPV associated cervical lesions. Pathol Res Pract 1992;188:242.

Broder S. Report of the 1991 Bethesda workshop. JAMA 1992;267:1892.

Buckley JC, Harris RW, Doll R. Case control study of the husbands of women with dysplasia and carcinoma of the cervix uteri. Lancet 1981;ii:1010.

Butterworth CE, Hatch KD, Gore H, et al. Improvement in cervical dysplasia associated with folic acid therapy in users of oral contraceptives. Am J Clin Nutr 1982; 35:73.

Cardiff Study. J Epidemiol Community Health 1980;34:9.

Carmichael JA, Jeffrey JF, Steele HD, Ohlke ID. The cytologic history of 245 patients developing invasive cervical carcinoma. Am J Obstet Gynecol 1984;148:685.

Charlton A. Young people's knowledge of the cervical smear test. Soc Sci Med 1983;17:235.

Chou P. Review on cervical cancer screening. Chin Med J (Taipei) 1991;48:1.

Christopherson WM, Parker JE, Mendez WM, Lundin FE. Cervix cancer death rates and mass cytologic screening. Cancer 1970;26:808.

Chung RH, Ruccio JA, Gerstung RA, et al. Discovery rate of dysplasia and carcinoma of the uterine cervix in an urban medical center serving patients at high risk. Int J Gynaecol Obstet 1982;20:449.

Clarke EA, Hilditch S. Problems in determining the incidence of cervical cancer. Can Med Assoc J 1983; 129:1271.

Conti M, Muggiasca ML, Agarossi A, Casolati E. Study and followup of HIV positive women with HPV infection and CIN. Eur J Gynaecol Oncol 1991;XII:22.

Cox JT, Schiffman MH, Winzelberg AJ, Patterson JM. An evaluation of human papillomavirus testing as part of referral to colposcopy clinics. Obstet Gynecol 1992; 80(3):389.

Crum CP. Koilocytosis in Pap smears: how useful a finding? Contemp OB/GYN 1993;38:66.

Devesa SS. Descriptive epidemiology of cancer of the uterine cervix. Obstet Gynecol 1984;63:605.

Dewar MA, Hall K, Perchalski J. Cervical cancer screening. Past success and future challenge. Prim Care 1992; 19(3):589.

Diller C, Murphy G, Lauchlan SC. Cervicovaginal cytology in patients 16 years of age and younger. Acta Cytol 1983;27:426.

Draper GJ, Cook GA. Changing patterns of cervical cancer rates. Br Med J 1983;287:510.

Eddy GL. Screening for cervical cancer. Ann Int Med 1990;113:214.

Fahs MC, Mandelblatt J, Schechter C, Muller C. Cost effectiveness of cervical cancer screening for the elderly. Ann Intern Med 1992;117:520.

Fetherston WC. False negative cytology in invasive cancer of the cervix. Clin Obstet Gynecol 1983;26:929.

Free K, Roberts S, Bourne R, et al. Cancer of the cervix—old and young, now and then. Gynecol Oncol 1991; 43:129.

Friedrich EG. Vulvar disease, 2nd ed. Philadelphia: WB Saunders, 1983:93.

Garite TJ, Feldman MJ. An evaluation of cytologic sampling techniques: a comparative study. Acta Cytol 1978; 22:883.

Germain M, Heaton R, Erickson D, et al. A comparison of the three most common Papanicolaou smear collection techniques. Obstet Gynecol 1994;84:168.

Grant EC. Cervical cancer and oral contraceptives. Lancet 1:528, 1983. Letter.

Hammond IG, Monaghan JM. Multicentric carcinoma of the female lower genital tract. Br J Obstet Gynaecol 1983; 90:557.

Harrison DD, Hernandez E, Dunton CJ. Endocervical brush versus cotton swab for obtaining cervical smears at a clinic: a cost comparison. J Reprod Med 1993;38:285.

Hatch KD. The role of hybrid capture for evaluation of HPV (abstract). Meeting of the American Gynecologic Obstetric Society, Homestead, Virginia, September 1994.

Hatim F, Wilbur D. High grade cervical lesions following negative cytologic examinations: false negatives or rapid progression? Mod Pathol 1993;6:30a. Abstract.

Herbst AL, Bern HA. Developmental effects of diethylstilbestrol (DES) in pregnancy. New York: Thieme Stratton, 1981.

Holloway RW, To A, Moradi M, et al. Monitoring the course of cervical carcinoma with the squamous cell carcinoma serum radio-immunoassay. Obstet Gynecol 1989;74:944.

Hudson, E, Kewertson S, Jansz C, Gordon H. Screening hospital patients for uterine cervical cancer. J Clin Pathol 1983;36:611.

Hueston WJ, Stiles MA. The Papanicolaou smear as a sentinel screening test for health screening in women. Arch Intern Med 1994;154:1473.

Johannesson G, Geirrson G, Day N, Tulinius H. Screening for cancer of the uterine cervix in Iceland 1965-78. Acta Obstet Gynecol Scand 1982;61:199.

Julian T. The minimally abnormal pap smear and cervical cancer screening. Colposcopist 1993;XXV(3).

Kaminski PF, Stevens CW Jr, Wheelock JB. Squamous atypic on cytology. The influence of age. J Reprod Med 1989;34(9):617.

King A, Clay K, Felmar E, et al. The Papanicolaou smear. West J Med 1992;156:202.

Kivati A. The role of premalignant changes in the cervix. Presented at Pathogenesis, detection and management of cervical neoplasia: A multidisciplinary perspective, Arthur L. Herbst, Chairman; Hotel del Coronado, San Diego, CA, August 1994.

Koss LG. The Papanicolaou test for cervical cancer detection. A triumph and a tragedy. JAMA 1989;261:737.

Koss LG. Cervical (Pap) smear. New directions. Cancer 1993;71:1406.

Kost ER, Snyder RR, Schwartz LE, Hankins GDV. The "less than optimal" cytology: importance in obstetric patients and in a routine gynecologic population. Obstet Gynecol 1993;81:127.

Koutsky LA, Holmes KK, Critchlow CW, et al. A cohort study of the risk of cervical intraepithelial neoplasia grade 2 or 3 in relation to papillomavirus infection. N Engl J Med 1992;327(18):1272.

Kristensen GB, Skyggebjerg KD, Holund B, Holm K, Hansen MK. Analysis of cervical smears obtained within three years of the diagnosis of invasive cervical cancer. Acta Cytol 1991;35:47.

Krowchuk DP, Anglin TM. Genital human papillomavirus infections in adolescents: implications for evaluation and management. Semin Dermatol 1992;11:24.

Krumholz BA. Presidential address. Amer Soc for Colposcopy and Cervical Pathology Biennial Meeting, March 25, 1994, Orlando, Florida. Colposcopist 1994;XXVI(2):1.

Kurman RJ, Henson DE, Herbst AL, et al. Interim guidelines for management of abnormal cervical cytology. JAMA 1994;271(23):1866.

Lapaquette TK, Dinh TV, Hannigan EV, et al. Management of patients with positive margins after cervical conization. Obstet Gynecol 1993;82:440.

Lerman C, Hanjani P, Caputo C, et al. Telephone counseling improves adherence to colposcopy among lower income minority women. J Clin Oncol 1992;10:330.

Luff R, Kurman R, Solomon D. The Bethesda system for reporting cervical/vaginal cytologic diagnoses. Report of the 1991 Bethesda workshop. Am J Surg Pathol 1992;16(9):914.

Lundberg GD. The 1988 Bethesda System for reporting cervical/vaginal cytological diagnoses. JAMA 1989;262 (7):931.

Lunt R. Worldwide early detection of cervical cancer. Obstet Gynecol 1984;63:808.

McIndoe WA, McLean MR, Jones RW, Mullins PR. The invasive potential of carcinoma in situ of the cervix. Obstet Gynecol 1984;64:451.

Maiman M, Fruchter RG, Guy L, et al. Human immunodeficiency virus infection and invasive cervical carcinoma. Cancer 1993;71:402.

Maiman M, Tarricone N, Vieira J, et al. Colposcopic evaluation of human immunodeficiency virus seropositive women. Obstet Gynecol 1991;78:94.

Mandelblatt J, Fahs MC. The cost effectiveness of cervical cancer screening for low income elderly women. JAMA 1988;259:2409.

Miller AB. The cost effectiveness of cervical cancer screening. Ann Intern Med 1992;117(6):529.

Morgan PP. Challenges in screening for cancer of the cervix: delivery, technology and evaluation of programs. Can Med Assoc J 1982;127:571. Editorial.

Montz FJ, Monk BJ, Fowler JM, Nguyen L. Natural history of the minimally abnormal Pap smear. Obstet Gynecol 1992;80:385.

Morrel ND, Taylor JR, Snyder RN, et al. False negative cytology rates in patients in whom invasive cervical cancer subsequently developed. Obstet Gynecol 1982; 60:41.

Mukawa A, Kamitsuma Y, Jisaki F, et al. Progress report on experimental use of CYBEST model 2 for practical gynecologic mass screening. Alterations of the specimen rejection threshold and specimen preparation. Anal Quant Cytol 1983;5:31.

Ng ABP. Presidential address. The American Society of Clinical Pathologists. Acta Cytol 1978;22:121.

Noguchi M, Nakanishi M, Kato K. Appraisal of a newly developed self collection device for obtaining cervical specimens. Acta Cytol 1982;26:633.

Norman SA, Talbott EO, Kuller LH, et al. The relationship of Papanicolaou testing and contacts with the medical care system to stage at diagnosis of cervical cancer. Arch Intern Med 1991;151:58.

Orr JW Jr, Shingleton HM, Gore H, et al. Cervical intraepithelial neoplasia associated with exposure to diethylstilbestrol in utero: a clinical and pathologic study. Obstet Gynecol 1981;58:75.

Orr JW, Wilson KW, Bodiford C, Cornwell A, Soong SJ, Honea KL, et al. Pretreatment comparison of nutritional parameters in patients with cervix and corpus cancer. Trans Am Gynecol Obstet Soc 1985;111:159.

Pairwuti S. False-negative Papanicolaou smears from women

with cancerous and precancerous lesions of the uterine cervix. Acta Cytol 1991;35:40.

Patterson ME, Peel KR, Joslin CA. Cervical smear histories of 500 women with invasive cervical cancer in Yorkshire. Br Med J 1984;289:896.

Peterson O. Spontaneous course of cervical precancerous conditions. Am J Obstet Gynecol 1956;72:1063.

Reelick NF, de Haes WF, Schuurman JH. Psychological side effects of the mass screening on cervical cancer. Soc Sci Med 1984;18:1089.

Reid R, Greenberg MD, Lorincz A, et al. Should cervical cytologic testing be augmented by cervicography or human papillomavirus deoxyribonucleic acid detection? Am J Obstet Gynecol 1991;164:1461.

Richart RM, Fu US, Winkler B. Pathology of cervical squamous and glandular neoplasia. In Coppleson M, ed. Gynecologic oncology, 2nd ed. London: Churchill Livingstone, 1992:557.

Richart RM. Have Pap screening tests outlived their usefulness? Continuing Obstet Gynecol 1980;15:142.

Richart RM. Moderator, symposium. Interpreting the new Bethesda classification system, Contemp OB/GYN 1993;38:86.

Richart RM, Vaillant HW. Influence of cell collection techniques upon cytological diagnosis. Cancer 1965; 18:1474.

Richart RM, Wright TC Jr. Controversies in the management of low-grade cervical intraepithelial neoplasia. Cancer 1993;71:1413.

Richart RM, Wright TC Jr. Pathology of the cervix. Curr Opin Obstet Gynecol 1991;3:561.

Rivlin ME, Woodliff JM, Bowlin RB, et al. Comparison of Cytobrush and cotton swab for Papanicolaou smears in pregnancy. J Reprod Med 1993;38(2):147.

Robboy SJ, Noller KL, O'Brien P, et al. Increased incidence of cervical and vaginal dysplasia in 2980 diethylstilbestrol exposed young women. Experience of the national collaborative diethylstilbestrol adenosis project. JAMA 1984;252:2979.

Robertson JH, Woodend B, Elliott H. Cytological changes preceding cervical cancer. J Clin Pathol 1994;47(3): 17809.

Romney SL, Basu J, Vermund S, Palan PR, Duttagupta C. Plasma reduced and total ascorbic acid in human uterine cervix dysplasias and cancer. Ann NY Acad Sci 1987;498:132.

Rosenthal DL, Mango L, Acosta DA, Peters RD. "Negative" Pap smears preceding carcinoma of the cervix: rescreening with the Papnet system. 1993. Abstract.

Rubio CA, Kock Y, Berglund K. Studies on the distribution of abnormal cells in cytological preparations I. Making the smear with a wooden spatula. Acta Cytol 1980;24:49.

Rutenberg MR. Improving screening accuracy: technological developments. Presented at Pathogenesis, detection and management of cervical neoplsia: A multidisciplinary perspective, Arthur L. Herbst, Chairman; Hotel del Coronado, San Diego, CA, August 1994.

Rylander E. Negative smears in women developing invasive cervical cancer. Acta Obstet Gynecol Scand 1977; 56:115.

Sadeghi SB, Hsieh EW, Gunn SW. Prevalence of cervical intraepithelial neoplasia in sexually active teenagers and young adults. Am J Obstet Gynecol 1984;148(6):726.

Schapira DV, Pamies RJ, Kumar NB, et al. Cancer screening. Knowledge, recommendations, and practices of physicians. Cancer 1993;71:839.

Shen JT, Nalick RH, Schlaerth JB, Morrow CP. Efficacy of cotton tipped applicators for obtaining cells from the uterine cervix for Papanicolaou smears. Acta Cytologica 1984;28:541.

Sherman ME, Kelly D. High grade squamous intraepithelial lesions and invasive carcinoma following the report of three negative Papanicolaou smears: screening failures or rapid progression? Mod Pathol 1992a;5(3):337.

Sherman ME, Mango LJ, Kelly D, et al. PAPNET analysis of reportedly negative smears preceding the diagnosis of a high-grade squamous intraepithelial lesion or carcinoma. Mod Pathol 1994;7(5):578.

Sherman ME, Schiffman MH, Erozan YS, et al. The Bethesda system. A proposal for reporting abnormal cervical smears based on the reproducibility of cytopathologic diagnoses. Arch Pathol Lab Med 1992b;116(11):1155.

Singer A, Reid BL, Coppleson M. The role of the high risk male in the etiology of cervical cancer—a correlation of epidemiology and molecular biology. Am J Obstet Gynecol 1976;126:110.

Starreveld AA, Romanowski B, Hill GB, et al. The latency period of carcinoma in situ of the cervix. Obstet Gynecol 1983;62:348.

Stenkvist B, Bergstrom R, Eklund G, Fox CH. Papanicolaou smear screening and cervical cancer. What can you expect? JAMA 1984;252:1423.

Stewart DE, Buchegger PM, Lickrish GM, Sierra S. The effect of educational brochures on follow-up compliance in women with abnormal Papanicolaou smears. Obstet Gynecol 1994;83:583.

Tawa K, Forsythe A, Cove KJ, et al. A comparison of the Papanicolaou smear and the cervicogram: sensitivity, specificity, and cost analysis. Obstet Gynecol 1988; 71:229.

Taylor PT, Anderson WA, Barber SR, et al. The screening Papanicolaou smear: contribution of the endocervical brush. Obstet Gynecol 1987;70:734.

Trevathan E, Layde P, Webster LA, et al. Cigarette smoking and dysplasia and carcinoma in situ of the uterine cervix. JAMA 1983;250:499.

van Ballegooijen M, Koopmanschap MA, Subandono Tjokrowardojo AJ, van Oortmarssen GJ. Care and costs for advanced cervical cancer. Eur J Cancer 1992; 28A(10):1703.

van der Graaf Y, Vooijs GP, Gaillard HL, Go DM. Screening errors in cervical cytologic screening. Acta Cytol 1987;31:434.

Vessey MP, Lawless M, McPherson K, Years D. Neoplasia of the cervix uteri and contraception: a possible adverse effect of the pill. Lancet 1983;II:930.

Walker EM, Hare MJ, Cooper P. A retrospective review of cervical cytology in women developing invasive squamous cell carcinoma. Br J Obstet Gynaecol 1983; 90:1087.

Walton LA, Edelman DA, Fowler WC Jr, Photopulos GH.

Cryosurgery for the treatment of cervical intraepithelial neoplasia during the reproductive years. Obstet Gynecol 1980;55:353.

World Health Organization Task Force for Epidemiological Research on Reproductive Health. Progestogen–only contraceptives during lactation: I. Infant growth. Contraception 1994;50:35.

Wright VC, Riopelle MA. Age at time of first intercourse v. chronologic age as a basis for Pap smear screening. Can Med Assoc J 1982;127:127.

Cancer of the Cervix by Hugh M. Shingleton and James W. Orr, Jr.
J. B. Lippincott Company, Philadelphia, © 1995.

3

Diagnosis of Intraepithelial Lesions and Microinvasive Tumors

SQUAMOUS LESIONS

Investigations of the biologic behavior of squamous intraepithelial precursor lesions of cervical cancer that are followed cytologically are fraught with many problems (Anderson 1991). Most studies suffer from inconsistent criteria for entry, inconsistent establishment of diagnosis, loss of patient follow-up, and inadequate (too short) follow-up. Studies using a biopsy diagnosis may be biased because biopsy of cervical lesions probably completely removes some small lesions and incites a local inflammatory (immune) response that likely changes the natural history of the premalignant cervical disease. Considering the contemporary medicolegal climate, investigators are justifiably reluctant to observe progression of precursors to in situ or invasive disease. It is easy to understand why almost all available data regarding progression and regression within the intraepithelial phase and progression to invasive carcinoma must be considered unreliable. Review of pertinent data, however, allows some conclusions to be drawn: some lesions progress, some regress, some can be removed by biopsy or by the effects of adjacent tissue damage, and some lesions remain unchanged. Most authorities agree that invasive squamous cell carcinoma is preceded by an intraepithelial phase. Rather than attempt to follow-up many of these women without treatment once cytologic evidence of an intraepithelial lesion is found, most clinicians elect to evaluate the patient by colposcopic examination, to biopsy the cervix if indicated, and to then treat the patient or to follow her carefully.

A review of the natural history of cervical intraepithelial neoplasia, as reflected in the voluminous literature on the subject, has been completed by Östör (1993a). After considering the relevant literature since 1950, he concluded that (1) the probability of squamous intraepithelial lesions (SIL) becoming invasive increases with the severity of the atypia, (2) progression to invasion does not always occur, and (3) even the higher degrees of atypia may regress. After considering many series with varying degrees of follow-up, he quotes approximate rates of regression as being 57% for cervical intraepithelial neoplasia (CIN) I, 43% for CIN II, and 32% for CIN III. The rates of progression to invasive cancer are thought to be 1%, 5%, and 12%, respectively.

Squamous Intraepithelial Lesions

HISTOLOGIC FEATURES

Atypical premalignant and malignant SILs develop primarily within maturing metaplastic epithelium in the transformation zone of the cervix. Metaplastic epithelium initially develops beneath endocervical columnar epithelium, either on the surface of the endocervix or lining clefts. Nuclei of metaplastic cells are regular and centrally placed. Near the surface, some maturation may occur, yet an immature squamous epithelium persists.

Sometimes in immature squamous metaplasia, nuclear atypia may be present; thus the term "atypical immature metaplasia." In this form, nuclei are only slightly enlarged and are less atypical than in SIL. It may be difficult to differentiate these lesions from SIL but only rarely does the surface mucinous epithelium persist with cervical intraepithelial neoplasia. When atypical immature metaplasia is associated with marked inflammation of stroma, it appears to be an inflammatory effect.

Human papillomavirus (HPV) infections of the cervix are common. Although exophytic or spiked condylomas may occur, condylomas are more commonly flat, appearing colposcopically as slightly raised plaques in which there is superficial koilocytosis, with varying degrees of atypia (Fig. 3-1).

Abnormal maturation patterns with cellular atypia in proliferative intraepithelial squamous lesions are designated as dysplasia or carcinoma in situ in the World Health Organization classification and as CIN (Richart 1973) and low- and high-grade intraepithelial lesions (National Cancer Institute Workshop 1989, 1992). Subdivisions are made within these groups according to the extent of abnormal proliferating cells and the degree of nuclear atypia and mitotic activity.

In mild dysplasia, the proliferative activity is confined to the lower third of the epithelium. In the upper two thirds, cells are mature but may be abnormal. This is the pattern later classified as CIN I and included in the Bethesda low-grade SIL group (see Fig. 3-1). In these lesions, varying degrees of koilocytosis with cytoplasmic vacuolization and nuclear atypia may be present, apparently related to HPV infection.

In moderate dysplasia, proliferative activity extends into the lower two thirds of the epithelium. Marked nuclear pleomorphism in an otherwise mild dysplasia pattern may warrant its classification as moderate dysplasia. Moderate dysplasia is essentially CIN II (Fig. 3-2) and is included in the Bethesda high-grade SIL group.

In severe dysplasia, the proliferative activity and marked nuclear pleomorphism extend beyond the lower two thirds of the epithelium and yet there is some surface differentiation. In squamous cell carcinoma in situ there is no surface differentiation, and nuclei of the atypical immature cells tend to be arranged in a vertical pattern (Fig. 3-3). The simplest description of squamous cell carcinoma in situ is a strip of malignant squamous epithelium that is not invading. When there is severe dysplasia with minimal surface differentiation, it may be difficult to decide whether this is a well-differentiated carcinoma in situ. Problems in distinguishing between these two subsequently led to grouping the lesions together as CIN III. The Bethesda classification includes both of these lesions in the high-grade SIL category, together with moderate dysplasia.

The Bethesda classification is said to be useful in identifying the high-grade lesions that require therapy. It is likely that pathologists will use combinations of old and new terminology to convey as accurate a histologic picture as possible to the clinician until the new terminology is accepted and understood. This is advocated in the guidelines for conversion to the Bethesda classification.

Squamous intraepithelial lesions may develop in surface epithelium, in endocervical clefts, or in both simultaneously. Anderson and Hartley (1980) were the first to study cleft involvement by SILs in a quantitative evaluation. The mean depth of involved clefts was 1.24 mm, whereas the mean depth of uninvolved clefts was 3.38 mm. They noted that CIN could be eradicated in 95% of cases by destroying tissue to a

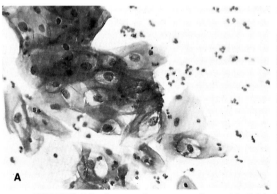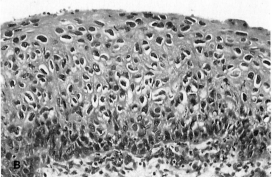

FIGURE 3-1. Low-grade squamous intraepithelial lesion. (**A**) Pap smear including intermediate and superficial squamous epithelial cells with enlarged atypical nuclei, hyperchromatic, with coarse chromatin. There is perinuclear clearing surrounded by a dense zone of cytoplasm. Nucleus is usually towards the periphery. This is the cytologic pattern of human papillomavirus (HPV) effect. (**B**) In this section of cervix, there are large squamous cells with enlarged atypical nuclei surrounded by a clear perinuclear zone, koilocytosis (or koilocytotic atypia), HPV effect. Only rare cells are binucleate. The appearance of the exfoliated cells may be correlated with the histologic pattern. See Color Figure 3-1.

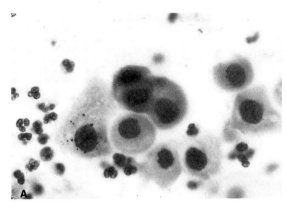
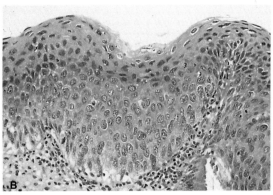

FIGURE 3-2. High-grade squamous intraepithelial lesion (moderate dysplasia). (**A**) Cells in the Pap smear have nuclei of varying size, well-demarcated and hyperchromatic. There is increased nuclear-cytoplasmic ratio, with the nucleus occupying half of the cell area to about three quarters. The cytologic pattern is that of moderate dysplasia. (**B**) In this section of cervix, proliferative activity with atypical cells, increased nuclear-cytoplasmic ratio, and loss of polarity involves the lower two thirds of the epithelium. There is some surface differentiation. This pattern of moderate dysplasia correlates with the Pap smear. See Color Figure 3-2.

depth of 2.9 mm, whereas destruction to a depth of 3.8 mm would eradicate 99.7% of CIN. Their work is generally accepted as the standard for ablative therapy.

CYTOLOGIC FEATURES

Atypical cells were noted in vaginal smears by numerous observers and in the 1890s had been illustrated in line drawings; however, the 1943 publication of *Diagnosis of Uterine Cancer by the Vaginal Smear* by Papanicolaou (an anatomist) and Traut (a gynecologist) began a new era in cancer detection in the female patient. Although initially vaginal pool specimens were studied, it was not long before cervical scrapings,

endocervical swabbings, and aspirations were included. Generally, the gynecologists were enthusiastic about the technique and often were responsible for setting up laboratories. It took some time to convince many pathologists of the value of the new procedure.

Classification of cytologic findings has been developed in parallel with histologic patterns up to the present Bethesda classification. This development and the correlation with histologic findings were parallel with the further understanding of so-called preinvasive lesions (Table 3-1).

As noted, histologically low-grade SIL includes changes consistent with the effect of HPV infection, mild dysplasia, or both (see Fig. 3-1*A*).

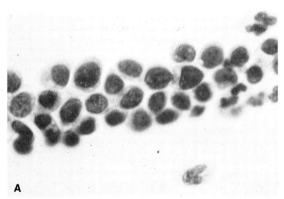
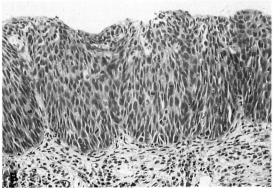

FIGURE 3-3. High-grade squamous intraepithelial lesion (squamous carcinoma in situ). (**A**) Strands of malignant squamous cells, with well-demarcated hyperchromatic nucleus surrounded by a thin rim of cytoplasm in a Pap smear with "clean" background consistent with origin from squamous cell carcinoma in situ. (**B**) Cells in the surface squamous epithelium in this biopsy are all atypical, with loss of polarity. Nuclei are at right angles to the basal layer, and only rarely is there a suggestion of surface differentiation. This pattern of squamous cell carcinoma in situ correlates with cells in the Pap smear. See Color Figure 3-3.

TABLE 3-1
Nomenclature in Cervical Cytology

| | CLASSIFICATION | |
Papanicolaou	World Health Organization	Bethesda System
Class I: Absence of atypical or abnormal cells	Normal	Negative, within normal limits
Class II: Atypical cytology but no evidence of malignancy	Atypical	Reactive or reparative changes
		Atypical squamous cells of undetermined significance (ASCUS)
		Atypical glandular cells of undetermined significance (AGCUS)
Class III: Cytology suggestive of but not conclusive for malignancy	Dysplasia	Squamous intraepithelial lesion (SIL)
	Mild dysplasia	Low-grade squamous intraepithelial lesion (LGSIL)
	Moderate dysplasia ⎫ Severe dysplasia ⎬	High-grade squamous intraepithelial lesion (HGSIL)
Class IV: Cytology strongly suggestive of malignancy	Carcinoma in situ	High-grade squamous intraepithelial lesion (HGSIL)
Class V: Cytology conclusive for malignancy	Squamous cell carcinoma	Suspicious or positive for malignancy Squamous cell carcinoma
	Adenocarcinoma	Adenocarcinoma

Adapted from Wright TC, Richart RM. Pathogenesis and diagnosis of preinvasive lesions of the lower genital tract. In Hoskins WJ, Perez CA, Young RC (eds). Principles and practice of gynecologic oncology. Philadelphia, JB Lippincott, 1992:528.

The characteristic cell in HPV infection is the koilocyte, named by Koss and Durfee (1956). Koilocytes are usually distinguished by a large perinuclear (or paranuclear) halo. Nuclear changes in these cells may be difficult to distinguish from dysplasia. Mildly dysplastic cells are usually of intermediate or superficial type, having only slightly hyperchromatic nuclei and occupying less than a third of the cell.

High-grade SIL includes the old terms "moderate dysplasia," "severe dysplasia," and "carcinoma in situ" (see Figs. 3-2A and 3-3A). The size of the moderately dysplastic cells is variable; the nucleus is enlarged and slightly to moderately hyperchromatic. The increased nuclear-cytoplasmic ratio of such cells results in the nucleus usually occupying about half the total cell area. Severely dysplastic cells are more likely to be parabasal in type, have a scanty cytoplasmic rim, and have hyperchromatic nuclei with a coarse granular chromatin pattern. Cells in high-grade SIL may occur singly or in groups, particularly in those that are closest to being classic carcinoma in situ, which occurs as a syncytium. Severe dysplasia and carcinoma in situ are often difficult to distinguish cytologically. This is one of the problems that led to the new SIL classification. It should be noted that some groups of poorly differentiated cells may cause difficulty in distinguishing between squamous cell carcinoma in situ and atypical glandular cells.

Microinvasive Carcinoma

HISTOLOGIC FEATURES

Microinvasive carcinoma was said to constitute only 2% to 8% of invasive cervical cancers in series published 15 to 20 years ago (Creasman et al 1973, Fennell 1978). With increased cytologic screening increasing the frequency of early diagnosis of invasive carcinoma, microinvasive carcinoma (Fédération Internationale de Gynécologie et Obstetrique [FIGO] stage IA1) and microcarcinoma FIGO stage IA2 are seen more frequently (Kurman et al 1992). For instance, Copeland and coworkers (1992) reported a 13% incidence in their study. A National Patterns of Care Study of the American College of Surgeons (Shingleton 1994) reports an incidence of 25.7% of FIGO stage IA in a series of 6186 patients diagnosed with cervical cancer in the years 1984 and 1990, although this large multi-hospital data set reflects pathology reports rather than pathology review and consensus. The data lend support to the concept that microinvasive carcinoma comprises an increasing segment of the disease.

Mestwerdt (1947) introduced the term "microcarcinoma" to describe a lesion with both depth and width. This was further defined by Lohe (1978) as having width or length up to 10 mm and depth up to

5 mm; the definition of FIGO stage IA has evolved from this (Table 3-2). In FIGO staging, stage IA is preclinical carcinoma that is diagnosed only by microscopic examination. This is subdivided into stage IA1, in which there is invasion of stroma no greater than 3 mm in depth and no wider than 7 mm, and stage IA2, in which there is measured invasion of stroma greater than 3 mm, but not greater than 5 mm nor wider than 7 mm. The epithelium from which the invasion originates may be on the surface or in a cleft; vascular space involvement, either venous or lymphatic, should not alter the staging. Measurement and interpretation may vary among pathologists.

The Society of Gynecologic Oncologists in 1974 defined microinvasion as invasion of the stroma from the point of origin to a depth of 3 mm but without evidence of lymphvascular space (LVS) involvement (Seski 1977; see Table 3-2). This may be difficult to evaluate uniformly because it is not always clear from exactly what point an invasive focus developed. More

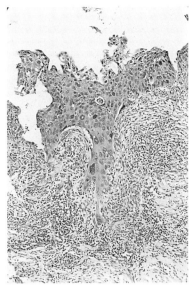

FIGURE 3-4. Microinvasive squamous cell carcinoma. A prong of malignant cells with large irregular nuclei and minimal differentiation is extending from the surface malignant epithelium into the underlying cytoplasm and is surrounded by inflammatory cells. This is the classic pattern of early microinvasive squamous cell carcinoma. See Color Figure 3-4.

TABLE 3-2
Cervical Cancer Staging

INTERNATIONAL FEDERATION OF GYNECOLOGY AND OBSTETRICS (FIGO) 1995*

Stage I: The carcinoma is strictly confined to the cervix.
Stage IA: Invasive cancer identified only microscopically. All gross lesions even with superficial invasion are stage IB cancers.
Invasion is limited to measured stromal invasion with maximum depth of 5 mm and no wider than 7 mm.**
Stage IA1: Measured invasion of stroma no greater than 3 mm in depth and no wider than 7 mm.
Stage IA2: Measured invasion of stroma greater than 3 mm and no greater than 5 mm in depth, and no wider than 7 mm.
Stage IB: Clinical lesions confined to the cervix or preclinical lesions greater than stage IA.
Stage IB1: Clinical lesions no greater than 4 cm in size.
Stage IB2: Clinical lesions greater than 4 cm in size.

SOCIETY OF GYNECOLOGIC ONCOLOGISTS (SGO) 1974†

A microinvasive lesion is one in which neoplastic epithelium invades the stroma in one or more places to a depth of 3 mm or less below the base of the epithelium and in which lymphatic or blood vessel involvement is not demonstrated.

Staging Announcement; Cancer Committee FIGO, 1995 Society of Gynecologic Oncologists.
**The depth of invasion should not be more than 5 mm taken from the base of the epithelium, either surface or glandular, from which it originates. Vascular space involvement, either venous or lymphatic, should not alter the staging.*
†*From Seski JC, Murray RA, Morley G. Microinvasive squamous carcinoma of the cervix. Definition, histologic analysis, late results of treatment. Obstet Gynecol 1977;50:410.*

commonly, a depth of invasion is given from either the base of the overlying epithelium or from its surface to the point of deepest invasion, stating how the measurement is made. The SGO definition has been preferred over the FIGO definition by most U.S. gynecologic oncologists, but the new staging should remedy that.

In the earliest form of invasion, often termed early stromal invasion, irregularly shaped epithelial strands extend from the base of the surface epithelium or from involved clefts, typically with cellular differentiation at the point of invasion and with variable stromal response and inflammatory infiltrate (Fig. 3-4) and subsequently with small tumor nests in the stroma (Fig. 3-5).

In Östör's 1993 study of 200 cases of early squamous cell carcinoma, he found that this lesion invaded no more than 0.5 mm in 78% of those with early stromal invasion and no more than 3 mm in 65% of patients with microcarcinomas. He concluded from his study that width (or length) of microcarcinoma (FIGO stage IA2) should not be part of its definition. He also noted that early stromal invasion (FIGO stage IA1) behaves in the same manner as CIN (presumably CIN III, although not stated) and can be treated by conization alone when the cone is properly sectioned and the margins are clear.

Tumor volume, using three dimensions, is more complicated and impractical for routine application. Burghardt (1979), using a sophisticated measurement technique, reported that microcarcinoma with a volume less than 400 mm^3 does not metastasize to lymph

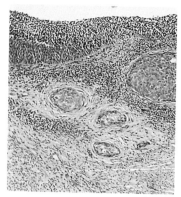

FIGURE 3-5. Small foci of invasive squamous cell carcinoma invading stroma, deep to surface squamous cell carcinoma of the cervix, and compressing adjacent stroma. The focus just beneath the surface epithelium has split away from the adjacent stroma. A few flattened cells remain attached to the stroma. These may be split-off cancer cells, but this is the type of focus wherein the possibility of lymphvascular space extension might be considered and further investigated. The small space at the edge of the next focus appears to be shrinkage artifact, and the other focus is just stromal invasion. Although this is consistent with microinvasive carcinoma, such a diagnosis could not be made without knowledge of what is elsewhere in the cervix. See Color Figure 3-5.

nodes. The number of patients with these lesions was small, even in Burghardt's study. Östör (1993b) reports 5 women who had tumor volume ranging from 21 mm^3 to 108 mm^3 and in whom tumor recurred. Although one study considered possible lymph node metastases and the other considered tumor recurrence, the relevance of measuring volume is questionable.

Significance of various patterns of invasion is worthy of mention. Although "confluence" would seem more likely in more deeply invasive or higher volume tumors (Ruch et al 1976, Sedlis 1979, Duncan 1982), as an isolated factor it is not valuable in establishing risk of node metastasis or recurrence (Hasumi et al 1980, Simon et al 1986, Östör 1993b).

Node Metastases in Microscopically Invasive Lesions. Within the group of microinvasive lesions, a range of risk for lymph node metastases exists—of less than 1% in those with early stromal invasion (Table 3-3) to 5% in microcarcinoma (Table 3-4).

Significance of Lymphvascular Space Involvement. Lymphvascular space involvement has concerned pathologists and clinicians alike for many years. Tissue shrinkage may give the impression of tumor lying in a space, but to diagnose LVS involvement, an endothelial lining of the space should be identified. Lymphvascular space involvement (see Fig. 3-5) does not necessarily exclude a diagnosis of microinvasive

carcinoma by FIGO definition, although such a finding rules out the diagnosis by the SGO definition.

Interest has centered on LVS involvement because increased recurrence rates are thought to be more likely with this finding (Table 3-5). Maiman and associates (1988) reported a trend toward increasing incidence of pelvic node metastasis with the presence of LVS invasion. Duncan (1991) observed that 10% of

TABLE 3-3
Node Metastases in FIGO* Stage IA1
(Early Stromal Invasion)

			METASTASES	
STUDY	YEAR	PATIENTS (N)	(n)	(%)
Averette, et al	1976	162	0	0
Lohe	1978	159	1	0.6
Hasumi, et al	1980	61	1	1.6
Simon, et al	1986	25	0	0
Maiman, et al	1988	24	0	0
Kolstad	1989	68	0	0
TOTAL		499	2	0.4

*International Federation of Gynecology and Obstetrics.

Modified from Shingleton HM, Orr JW Jr. Cancer of the cervix: diagnosis and treatment. New York, Churchill Livingstone, 1987:32.

TABLE 3-4
Node Metastases in Microcarcinoma*
(FIGO Stage IA2)

			METASTASES	
STUDY	YEAR	PATIENTS (N)	(n)	(%)
Hasumi, et al	1980	29	4	13.8
Boyce, et al	1981	47	2	4.3
van Nagell, et al	1983	32	3	9.4
Simon, et al†	1986	69	1	1.5
Maiman, et al	1988	117	6	5.1
Delgado, et al	1989	177	6	3.3
Greer, et al	1990	50	2	4.0
Copeland, et al‡	1992	28	1	3.6
TOTAL		549	25	5.0

*Microscopic lesions invading no more than 5 mm in depth, with patterns other than focal (early stromal) invasion.
†Authors' data.
‡Depth >3 mm, <5 mm invasion.

Modified from Shingleton HM, Orr JW Jr. Cancer of the cervix: diagnosis and treatment. New York, Churchill Livingstone, 1987:34.

TABLE 3-5
Significance of Lymphvascular Space Involvement in Microcarcinoma
having ≤5 mm depth

STUDY	YEAR	PATIENTS (N)	RECURRENCE	DEATHS
Foushee, et al	1969	7	1	1
Mussey, et al	1969	19	2	1
Boyes, et al	1970	12	1	1
Leman, et al	1976	12	0	0
Burghardt	1979	53	2	1
Coppleson	1979	39	0	0
Iversen, et al	1979	8	5	NS
Boyce, et al	1981	10	3	1
Simon, et al*	1986	7	0	0
Copeland, et al	1992	11	1	NS
TOTAL		178	15 (8.4%)	5 (2.8%)

*University of Alabama at Birmingham data.
NS, not specified.

Modified from Shingleton HM, Orr JW Jr. Cancer of the cervix: diagnosis and treatment. New York, Churchill Livingstone, 1987:36.

patients with LVS involvement have positive nodes when the stromal invasion is 3 to 5 mm deep. Copeland and coworkers (1992), summarizing the literature and including his own patients, reported a 4.4-fold risk of recurrence in lesions invading to 3 mm with LVS invasion, compared with those without LVS invasion. With invasion between 3 and 5 mm, he reported a 9.1-fold risk of recurrence in the same comparison. Curiously, the chance of pelvic node metastases did not increase with LVS invasion in the 3- to 5-mm invasive group, even though recurrences were observed. This may relate to the diminished accuracy of detecting and reporting of micrometastases in pelvic nodes in routine examination. Östör (1993b) was not able to show that LVS invasion affects prognosis in microscopically invasive cancer.

CYTOLOGIC FEATURES

Cytologic features of microinvasive carcinoma are difficult to interpret. Some experienced cytopathologists claim good correlation, although others are less confident. Adequate uniformly stained smears are necessary and all findings should be confirmed histologically. Ng and Reagan (1969,1988) indicated that diagnosis could be made prospectively and on review with great accuracy. Johnston and colleagues (1982) stated that cytology was 81% predictive. Nguyen (1984) suggested that overall, cytology predicts microinvasion in about 60% of cases. Generally, the greater the invasive depth, the greater the cytologic accuracy (i.e., microinvasion with a depth between 1 and

3 mm was said to be predictable in 78% to 80% of cases).

Bibbo (1991) finds some cytologic features typical of early invasion. Findings are basically similar to those of invasive carcinoma but the changes are less prominent and there is little associated necrosis. Cells are often arranged in syncytial aggregates, although in microinvasion the average number of abnormal cells is lower than in invasive cancer. Nuclear chromatin is more often uniformly granular and less often irregularly distributed than in invasive carcinoma.

GLANDULAR LESIONS

Adenocarcinoma In Situ

HISTOLOGIC FEATURES

Adenocarcinoma in situ (AIS) is defined as architecturally and cytologically atypical glands without obvious invasion. The glands are lined by cytologically malignant cells and similar epithelium may extend on the surface of the endocervix, often in continuity with atypical glandular epithelium but without extension into the stroma. Often, glands are only partly involved, with a sharp line of demarcation between neoplastic and normal epithelium. Superficial glands are more likely to be involved, and single atypical glands or small clusters lie amid normal glands. Distribution of the atypical glands may be focal (a single field with separate foci involving different parts of the mucosa) or of a somewhat more diffuse distribution. Atypical glands are confined to the glandular zone but sometimes extend beyond the deepest normal endocervical cleft (Fig. 3-6). Depth of AIS reported by Östör and associates (1984) ranged from 0.5 to 4.0 mm (mean, 2.6 mm), with length of extent from 0.5 to 30 mm (mean, 7 mm) and width from 0.5 to 25 mm (mean, 12 mm).

Usually, the histologic pattern is the endocervical mucinous type, although intestinal and endometrioid patterns have been described, with rare examples of adenosquamous carcinoma in situ and clear cell carcinoma in situ.

A high proportion of cases of AIS are associated with SILs or even invasive lesions. Among 21 cases of AIS, Östör and coworkers (1984) found 15 patients with associated lesions—two microinvasive squamous cell carcinomas, one microinvasive mucoepidermoid carcinoma, and 12 SILs. They found only about 160 AIS cases in the literature and speculated that others probably had been included with invasive lesions. Among 72 cases of AIS, Jaworski and associates (1988) found 45 cases with various degrees of SILs and six with microinvasive or invasive squamous cell carcinoma.

It is difficult to determine what proportion of patients with adenocarcinoma of the cervix have only an in situ lesion. Hopkins and coworkers (1988) reported that 18 patients with AIS represented 9.2% of all adenocarcinomas seen during the study period. Although a pattern consistent with AIS may be noted in a biopsy, such a specific diagnosis cannot be made without further tissue evaluation. Such might include a

cervical conization specimen with margins well clear of any lesions or the complete cervix. Either of these specimens should be completely examined after cutting them into blocks 2 mm in thickness, with additional levels of tissue cut from a block when indicated.

CYTOLOGIC FEATURES

Cells of endocervical AIS are usually scraped or brushed from the endocervical canal for preparation of a Papanicolaou (Pap) smear. This results in large sheets of overlapping, crowded cell strips, rosettes, or syncytium-like sheets with indistinct cell borders. Partial separation of cells at the edge produces a feathery appearance. Individual cells are large, with abundant cytoplasm but a high nuclear-cytoplasmic ratio. The nuclei are oval or round, and hyperchromatic nucleoli are inconspicuous or absent. The cytoplasm is finely granular and usually lacks evidence of mucin secretion. The necrosis and "messy" background found with invasive tumors is absent (Ramzy et al 1991).

Microinvasive Adenocarcinoma

HISTOLOGIC FEATURES

Although the entity microinvasive adenocarcinoma probably exists, defining it in a way so that is has clinical relevance is difficult. There is no accepted definition for this entity, nor is it reported with any degree of uniformity. Kolstad (1989) referred to it in his large study of women having microinvasive cervical cancer. In his review of 679 patients, 26 women were identified with microinvasive adenocarcinoma, 7 with microinvasive adenosquamous carcinoma, and 3 with microinvasive clear cell carcinoma. Unfortunately, the histologic criteria for these particular diagnoses were not included.

Adenocarcinoma with early invasion includes irregularly infiltrating glands lacking the lobular glandular pattern of AIS. A budding papillary pattern or small nests of tumor in the stroma associated with a stromal response are other early features of early invasion.

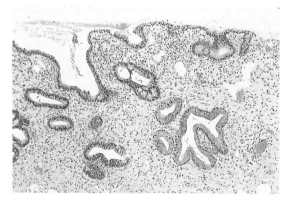

FIGURE 3-6. Atypical columnar epithelium with minimal nuclear pseudostratification is on the surface to the left; there are some glands lined by similar epithelium, including two clusters. Immediately beneath one atypical group and to the right of some single atypical glands is a group of physiologic endocervical glands (clefts). The hyperchromatic glands are adenocarcinoma in situ. See Color Figure 3-6.

CYTOLOGIC FEATURES

Microinvasive adenocarcinoma is essentially impossible to diagnose cytologically because there is no clear-cut histologic pattern for correlation. Features said to be associated with microinvasion include abnormal chromatin clearing, nucleoli, and some background necrosis. If the smear otherwise suggests AIS, these features raise the likelihood of stromal invasion.

EVALUATION METHODS

Colposcopy

Colposcopy, introduced by Hinselmann in 1925, has been used extensively in the United States in the last quarter century, and the technique is taught in all residency programs in obstetrics and gynecology. The method is available in most communities to women who have atypical Pap smears.

Colposcopically directed biopsies constitute the proper method of evaluation for the woman with an atypical Pap smear. This technique is cost-effective and allows selected (rather than routine) use of outpatient loop diathermy conization or inpatient cold knife conization in diagnosis and treatment. Colposcopic expertise is gained only with adequate training in the technique, frequent use, and careful correlation of the visual and biopsy findings; even in the best hands, conization is required to establish a definitive diagnosis in some women, especially when cytologic and biopsy results suggest but do not prove early invasive disease.

The major abnormal visual patterns of colposcopy are acetowhite epithelium, punctation, mosaicism, and atypical vessels (Table 3-6; Figs. 3-7 through 3-13). With 3% acetic acid application to the cervix, a transient coagulation of protein in the superficial cells oc-

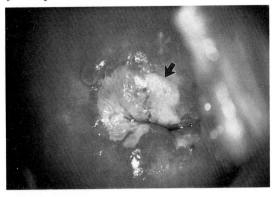

FIGURE 3-7. Low-grade squamous intraepithelial lesion. Epithelium with well-demarcated borders extends from the 7 o'clock position around (and covering) much of the anterior lip. The surface changes (*arrow*) in one area suggest a flat condyloma. (Courtesy of Kenneth D. Hatch, MD, University of Arizona, Tucson, AZ.) See Color Figure 3-7.

curs due to an altered nuclear-cytoplasmic ratio and immaturity of metaplastic, dysplastic, or neoplastic cells, causing them to reflect light differently and appear whiter than surrounding mature squamous epithelium. Punctation patterns result from vertically penetrating vessels in the thickened epithelium, which when seen from the surface appear as red dots in a white field (see Figs. 3-9 through 3-12). Mosaic pat-

TABLE 3-6
Categories of Colposcopic Findings

NORMAL	ABNORMAL	UNSATISFACTORY	MISCELLANEOUS
1. Original squamous epithelium undisturbed	An atypical TZ that suggests neoplasia	TZ cannot be entirely visualized	1. Vaginitis/cervicitis—regular, diffuse punctation
2. Columnar epithelium with long papillae and deep clefts; grape-like after acetic acid	Hyper- and parakeratosis—elevated white plaques seen before acetic acid		2. Erosion—focally denuded area (superficial)
3. TZ—an area of relatively orderly transition from squamous, through squamous-metaplastic, to columnar epithelium but no evidence of SIL	White epithelium—focal, transient phenomenon seen after acetic acid		3. Atrophy—thin epithelium, with clear vascular pattern
	Punctation—focal lesion with stippled capillary pattern		4. Condyloma, papilloma, polyps—exophytic and flat lesions
	Mosaicism—epithelial compartmentalization by vascular papillae (fine vs coarse)		
	Abnormal vessels—irregular vessels with comma, corkscrew, or spaghetti forms; surface contour changes, including deep ulcers, exophytic areas		

SIL, squamous intraepithelial lesion; *TZ,* transformation zone.

Modified from Schmidt WA. Cytologic and histologic correlations in colposcopy. Cancer Bull 1983;35:184.

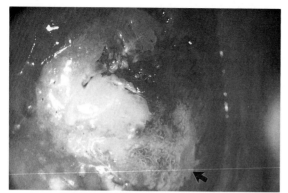

FIGURE 3-8. Low-grade squamous intraepithelial lesion. Lesion occupies most of the transformation zone. On the posterior lip (*arrow*), a fine mosaic is present. (Courtesy of Kenneth D. Hatch, MD, University of Arizona, Tucson, AZ.) See Color Figure 3-8.

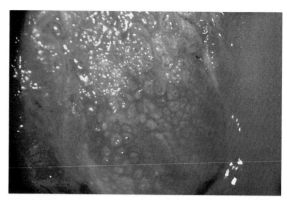

FIGURE 3-10. High-grade squamous intraepithelial lesion. A coarse mosaic pattern is present, with some punctation. (Courtesy of Kenneth D. Hatch, MD, University of Arizona, Tucson, AZ.) See Color Figure 3-10.

terns occur when deepening rete pegs of the epithelium are surrounded by the vessel-rich stroma; from the surface, the rete pegs appear white and the surrounding vascular stroma (nearer the surface) appears red, producing a mosaic pattern (see Figs. 3-8 through 3-11 and Fig. 3-13). Bizarre comma- or corkscrew-shaped vessels running horizontal to the surface suggest microscopic invasion, whereas deeply ulcerated areas or proliferative lesions causing changes in the surface contour may represent invasive cancer (Table 3-7). Immature squamous metaplasia mimics the colposcopic patterns of SIL; however, the finer, less distinct mosaic patterns and acetowhite changes in metaplasia can usually be distinguished by the experienced colposcopist from the coarser patterns in high-grade SIL (see Table 3-7).

When using colposcopy and target biopsies, physicians must guard against relying on inadequate or unrepresentative biopsies. The clinician must communicate with the pathologist on a case-by-case basis to ensure proper correlation of the cytologic, colposcopic, and histologic findings. In the absence of this communication, some women are underdiagnosed and may receive inadequate treatment.

In experienced hands, outpatient evaluation using a combination of cytology, colposcopic evaluation, adequate colposcopically directed biopsies, and endocervical curettage (ECC) is quite accurate. Under ideal

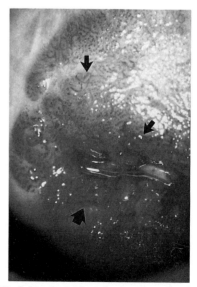

FIGURE 3-11. Probable microinvasion. Atypical vessels (*arrows*) of various shapes run parallel to the surface in a transformation zone that also contains coarse punctation. Such vessels suggest superficial invasive disease. (Courtesy of Kenneth D. Hatch, MD, University of Arizona, Tucson, AZ.) See Color Figure 3-11.

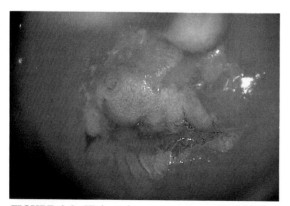

FIGURE 3-9. High-grade squamous intraepithelial lesion. The lesion on the anterior lip contains extensive punctuation and mosaic patterns. (Courtesy of Kenneth D. Hatch, MD, University of Arizona, Tucson, AZ.) See Color Figure 3-9.

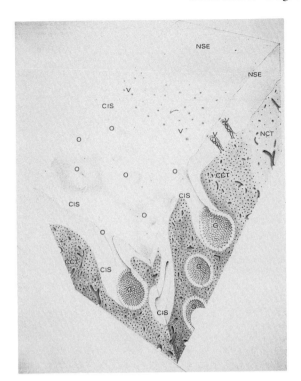

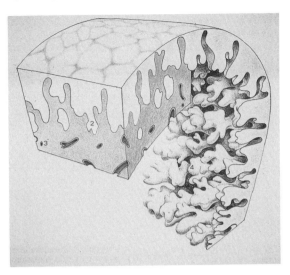

FIGURE 3-13. (*1*) Cobbles of mosaic, unequal and separated by a red interval, which corresponds to the areas where the epithelium is very thin. (*2*) Epithelial buds dip in and become ramified in the connective tissue. (*3*) Connective tissue. (*4*) Deep surface of the epithelium without connective tissue. Note the shape of the digital processes of the squamous epithelium and their ramifications. (Cartier R [ed]. Practical colposcopy, 3rd ed. Lausanne: IRL Imprimenies Reunies, 1993;129, with permission of Dr. Rene Cartier and Dr. Isabelle Cartier.)

FIGURE 3-12. Normal squamous epithelium (*NSE*) remains translucent after application of acetic acid. It covers a normally vascularized connective tissue (*NCT*). This part of the cervix has a rose color. The carcinoma in situ (*CIS*), coagulated by acetic acid, has whitened. It penetrates into the duct of the glands (*G*). The connective tissue is congested (*CCT*); the vessels are numerous and dilated. There is a dense leukocyte infiltration (*black points*). Around the openings of the glands (*O*), the thick carcinomatous epithelium completely masks congestion and forms a white ring. At the point where the epithelium is thinner, congestion is visible, the cervix is red. At the summit of the stromal papillae, the vessels (*V*) appear in the form of red dots. (Cartier R [ed]. Practical colposcopy, 3rd ed. Lausanne: IRL Imprimenies Reunies, 1993;136, with permission of Dr. Rene Cartier and Dr. Isabelle Cartier.)

circumstances, when such an outpatient diagnosis is compared with the final pathologic diagnosis, based on therapeutic conization or hysterectomy, there can be correlation within one grade of intraepithelial neoplasia in 99% of women (Shingleton et al 1983). Most women are found to have intraepithelial neoplasia, not invasive cancer (Table 3-8).

COLPOSCOPY IN RECOGNIZING HUMAN PAPILLOMAVIRUS INFECTION

Papillomavirus infections of the cervix are common. Recognizing and distinguishing such infections from CIN is difficult for the inexperienced colposcopist. Attempts to grade lesions by the prominence of the acetowhite epithelial reaction or by the presence of

prominent surface capillaries (secondary to inflammation) may fail. Differences in color tone, vascular atypia, and iodine-staining characteristics are said to be more predictive than such things as lesion thickness or surface contour (Reid 1984). In another publication (1985), Reid and Scalzi emphasized that the sharpness of the peripheral margin of the colposcopic lesion may be useful in differentiating papilloma virus infections from high-grade SIL (sharply defined margins).

COLPOSCOPY IN EVALUATION OF POSTMENOPAUSAL WOMEN

The evaluation of postmenopausal women with abnormal cytologic smears is more of a problem than the evaluation of young women. Vaginal atrophy or stenosis may impair colposcopic examination. The percentage of adequate examinations fall because more significant abnormalities are situated in the anatomic endocervical canal rather than in the portio of the cervix. Atrophic cytologic changes due to lack of estrogen may be misinterpreted and reported as atypia. It is often advisable to ask postmenopausal women to use vaginal estrogen for 4 to 6 weeks before a reexamination. This regimen may restore a more normal appearance to the cervical and upper vaginal epithelium and aid the colposcopist in locating neoplastic areas.

TABLE 3-7
Colposcopic/Histologic Correlates

COLPOSCOPIC		Histologic
Finding	Appearance	
Hyperkeratosis or condylomata	Raised, irregular surface; sharp borders visible before acetic acid	
White epithelium	Sharp-bordered white area after acetic acid	SIL
Punctation	Sharp-bordered area of red dots; epithelium whitens after acetic acid	SIL
Mosaicism	Sharp-bordered area with tile-like pattern; epithelium whitens after acetic acid	Fine pattern: metaplasia Coarse pattern: high-grade SIL
Abnormal vessels	Irregular vascular pattern, usually focal comma, corkscrew forms	High-grade SIL or microinvasive cancer
Deep ulcers, major surface contour changes	"Peaks, valleys" craters associated with abnormal vessels	Invasive cancer

SIL, squamous intraepithelial lesion.

Modified from Schmidt WA. Cytologic and histologic correlations in colposcopy. Cancer Bull 1983;35:184.

COLPOSCOPY OF MICROINVASIVE OR INVASIVE LESIONS

The capability of colposcopists to correctly diagnose microinvasive cancer is not great. Benedet and colleagues (1985) reported in his study of 180 patients with microinvasive or occult invasive squamous cell carcinoma that 42% of those with microinvasion and 28% with occult invasion had unsatisfactory colposcopic examinations. A small but definite group of patients have lesions in which the colposcopic appearance is not sufficiently distinct or characteristic to permit a diagnosis of early invasion. Kolstad (1989), reporting 125 women with FIGO stage IA1 lesions and 197 with FIGO stage IA2 lesions, found the colposcopic diagnosis to be accurate in only 30.4% and 34.0% of these groups, respectively. In most patients, lesser diagnoses were entertained. Sugimori (1991) reported that only about 50% of stage IA lesions were correctly predicted colposcopically, whereas 89% of cases with stage IB lesions were correctly predicted.

TABLE 3-8
Outpatient Evaluation of Atypical Papanicolaou Smears in Reproductive-Aged Women*

HISTOLOGIC DIAGNOSIS	PATIENTS	
	(n)	(%)
Invasive cancer	78	4
Microinvasion	41	2
CIN III	946	45
CIN I, II	1048	49
TOTAL	2113	100

*University of Alabama at Birmingham, 1970–1980; Public Health Department patients.

From Shingleton HM, Orr JW Jr. Cancer of the cervix: diagnosis and treatment. New York, Churchill Livingstone, 1987:77.

USE OF ENDOCERVICAL CURETTAGE

Endocervical curettage has been proposed as a necessary routine part of colposcopic examination (DiSaia et al 1989). The technique generally has been taught in postgraduate courses and residency programs because it has the potential to yield important diagnostic information. When endocervical curettings contain neoplastic epithelium, a group of potentially high-risk patients who require conization is identified; when an adequate negative curettage is obtained, it makes the inexperienced colposcopist more secure in basing a therapeutic decision on the colposcopic appearance of the portio lesion and on the target biopsies. As many as 17% of patients have a positive curettage (i.e., curettings containing dysplastic or neoplastic tissue; Grainger et al 1987). In women with neoplasia and an adequate colposcopic examination, Drescher and associates (1983) reported that 48.7% had positive endocervical curettage.

Invasive carcinoma is seldom encountered in an endocervical curettage specimen in a patient in whom invasion is not otherwise suspected or apparent (Shingleton et al 1976). Grainger and coworkers (1987) reported 2 patients with unsuspected endocervical cancers (of 712 patients) who had diagnostic conizations performed because of a positive endocervical curettage. Clinically invasive lesions of the ectocervix and occult invasive lesions situated in the anatomic endocervical canal invariably have neoplastic epithelium demonstrable by curettage (Shingleton et al 1976, Drescher et al 1983).

Endocervical curettage is particularly important in postmenopausal women, who are more likely to have endocervical canal involvement by the neoplasm because of the physiologic inversion of the cervical canal in old age. It has also been suggested (Kaufman et al 1973) as a yearly screening procedure for patients who have had cryosurgery or cautery treatment for SIL, especially when the canal was originally involved by SIL, when the squamocolumnar junction is located in the canal, or when stenosis of the external os interferes with colposcopic evaluation of the lower canal.

Provided that there is adequate material and proper handling of the tissue fragments by the surgical pathologist, most samples are adequate for pathologic interpretation. In young women, the inadequate rate should not exceed 10%, but a fifth of those at the age of 50 years and a third after the age of 60 have inadequate specimens (Shingleton et al 1976). There is no convincing evidence that prior endocervical curettage interferes with the interpretation of later conization specimens, although some disagree (Lovecchio and Gal 1992).

In patients with an adequate colposcopic examination, the endocervical curettage specimen is frequently contaminated when the curette hits the edge of the portio lesion. Although the predictive value for invasive cancer in women with a *positive* endocervical curettage is only 2%, the predictive value of a *negative* endocervical curettage in women with a satisfactory or adequate colposcopic examinations is 100%.

Many experienced colposcopists, particularly in Europe, find endocervical curettage to be unnecessary (especially in young women) with adequate colposcopic examination in which all margins of the intraepithelial lesion are seen. Involvement of the anatomic endocervical canal increases with increasing grade of SIL (Grainger et al 1987).

ALTERNATIVES TO ENDOCERVICAL CURETTAGE

Hald and coworkers (1988) suggested using a Vabra aspirator rather than a curette for sampling the endocervical canal and reported that this was not only more accurate (80% versus 49% for standard endocervical curettage) but that the pain experienced by the patient was considerably less. Andersen (1988) compared Cytobrush specimens to endocervical curettage and found that although more sensitive (92% versus 55%), the Cytobrush was less specific (38% versus 75%). The false-negative rate for the Cytobrush was lower (8% versus 45%) but the false-positive rate was higher (63% versus 25%).

Conization of the Cervix

Cervical conizations were first performed in the 1860s to debulk clinical cancers of the cervix. In 1930, Hyams proposed excisional cervical conizations performed with electrosurgical loops. Graham, in his 1962 book, *Carcinoma of the Cervix*, suggested that cone biopsies were better taken with a knife than with a diathermy because the diathermy distorted the cells and interfered with histologic interpretation. For a time thereafter, cervical cold knife conization was the principal technique for investigation of abnormal Pap smears. By the 1970s, colposcopy became the gold standard in diagnosis, with cold knife conization being used only selectively.

Inpatient diagnostic conization is seldom required when colposcopic evaluation is used. This varies by age group: in a teenage group, less than 2% require conization, whereas women older than 60 may require conization a fourth to a third of the time. The eversion of the cervix in premenopausal parous women allows adequate colposcopic evaluation and conservative outpatient treatment in 87% of cases (Shingleton et al 1983). The inversion or retraction of the endocervical canal during the postmenopausal years leads more often to inadequate colposcopic examination and thus more often to conization.

INDICATIONS FOR COLD KNIFE CONIZATIONS

There are specific indications for traditional inpatient surgical conization of the cervix (Table 3-9). When cervical biopsies suggest but are not diagnostic for invasive carcinoma, conization is mandatory, whereas endocervical curettage specimens containing severely dysplastic or neoplastic epithelium require it. Atrophy of the cervix and upper vagina, stenosis of the endocervical canal, or anatomic situations that prevent the cervix from being completely visualized during colposcopy are circumstances that may also require anesthesia and evaluation by surgical conization. When cytologic smears suggest the presence of high-grade SIL or invasion not confirmed by colposcopic examination, directed biopsies, and endocervical curettage, a conization should be performed. Unfortunately, even

TABLE 3-9
Indications for Cold Knife Conization

- Cervical biopsies suggestive of (but not diagnostic for) invasive cancer
- Inadequate colposcopic study of the cervix
  Cervical/vaginal atrophy
  Vaginal strictures
  Stenosis of endocervical canal
  Displacements of the cervix due to other disease
- Positive endocervical curettage specimens, suggesting high-grade SIL or invasion
- High-grade SIL smears *not* explained by target biopsies or endocervical curettage

SIL, squamous intraepithelial lesion.

microinvasion on biopsy specimens was not considered sufficient indication for conization in 47% of a group of 187 women thought to fall in the 3- to 5-mm depth of invasion category in a study reported by Creasman and colleagues (1994). The 87 women in this group who had surgery that was not preceded by conization were found to have lymph node metastases (7%) and ultimately recurrence (13%). Without the interval conization, however, one does not have accurate information about how many had invasion exceeding 5 mm.

IMPORTANCE OF CONIZATION MARGINS

Many authors have addressed the subject of cone margins and the relation to prediction of persistent neoplasia of the uterus. Special handling of the specimen is required to allow optimal study of margins (Fig. 3-14). In Abdul-Karim and Nunez's series (1985), only 2% of patients with clear cone margins had persistent or recurrent disease, whereas those with involved margins had a 55% relapse rate. Ostergard (1980) noted that older patients and patients with high-grade SIL have a significantly greater chance of having non–clear cone margins, which is probably related to the fact that these lesions involve larger areas of the portio of the cervix as well as (at times) the lower endocervical canal. Dietl and associates (1983) stated that with increasing age, the incidence of non–clear cone margins doubles. Although involved portio (exocervical) margins are less likely when the conization is performed under colposcopic guidance or with Lugol's solution staining, involved or unclear endocervical margins are sometimes unavoidable, especially in older women. The purpose (and thus the size) of the conization procedure is relevant; Kolstad (1989) noted a 27.7% incidence of involved margins in *diagnostic* cones, compared with a 4.9% incidence in

cones performed specifically with *therapy* as the intent. Watson and colleagues (1993) reported that in 738 cone biopsies, residual CIN was documented in 42.9% of women whose conizations involved endocervical margins. Demopoulos and coworkers (1991) reported that deep gland (cleft) involvement on conization specimens is also a significant predictor of residual or recurrent disease. It is apparent that positive cone margins do not invariably indicate the presence of persistent SIL in the subsequent hysterectomy specimen; in fact, most of these patients have a negative hysterectomy specimen or no recurrence. Although one can follow-up those patients with positive ectocervical margins, it is prudent to further investigate those who have positive endocervical margins (Watson et al 1993, Lapaquette et al 1993).

To accept a diagnosis of microinvasive cancer on a conization specimen, clear cone margins must be present. Unless the entire area of invasion is present and available for depth measurements, one cannot be certain that the worst area has been studied or that the patient has been properly staged. Greer and associates (1990) reported follow-up of 33 women whose cone biopsies had positive margins; 21 had residual invasive disease at the time of radical hysterectomy, 6 had carcinoma in situ, and 6 had no residual disease.

LASER CONIZATION

Several reports have promoted the use of laser conization. Delmore and colleagues (1992) compared cold knife and laser excision cones in a residency program. No difference in operating time, length of anesthesia, or success of treatment was noted, although fewer complications were seen in the laser-excision group. Grundsell and coworkers (1983) stated that the procedure could be safely performed on an outpatient basis. Meandzija and associates (1984) stated that laser conization, in comparison with conventional knife conization, provides greater visibility of the squamocolumnar junction after healing. Baggish and Dorsey (1985) reported that the volume of tissue removed by laser conization was less than half that of the conventional surgical cone, thus fewer complications resulted.

Fowler and coworkers (1992) studied the effect of CO_2 laser cone on the pathologic interpretation of premalignant lesions. They believed that in 50% of the patients, thermal damage was severe enough to preclude accurate diagnosis. Howell and colleagues (1991) noted extensive epithelial denudation in 36% of laser cones, whereas an additional 24% had coagulation artifacts that made recognition of CIN difficult or impossible and assessment of margins unreliable. The prolonged handling of laser cone specimens with hooks and forceps during the procedure causes addi-

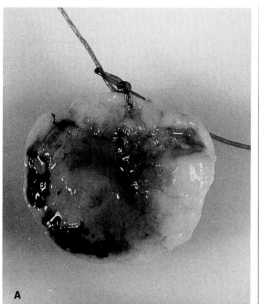

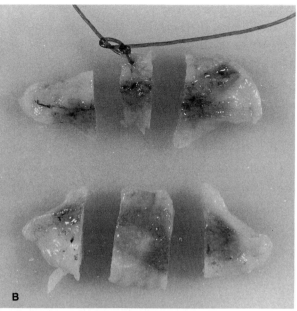

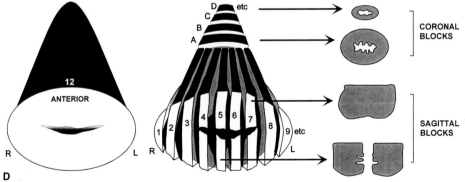

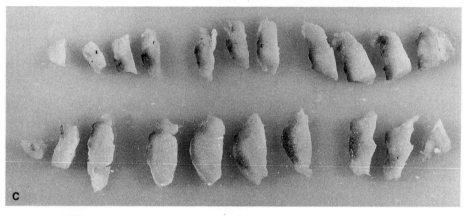

FIGURE 3-14. (**A–C**) Handling of conization specimen for optimal study (technique of Hazel Gore). The tie indicates the 12 o'clock position. Cone is opened at the 3 and 9 o'clock positions. The central segment from each lip is complete from endocervix to portio margin. Each of these segments is divided into blocks, taking care to preserve the lines of surgical excision. The lateral segments are also divided into blocks, realizing that only the portio margin is a line of surgical excision. (Shingleton HM, Orr JW Jr. Cancer of the cervix: diagnosis and treatment. Edinburgh: Churchill Livingstone, 1987:83 with permission.) (**D**) Another technique for examination of a cervical cone as suggested by Östör. This presumes a perfectly symmetric cone; from a practical observation, most cones do not fall into this category. Furthermore, the cost of processing this number of sections would be great, and it is doubtful whether there would be any real benefit. (Redrawn from Östör AG. Studies on 200 cases of early squamous cell carcinoma of the cervix. Int J Gynecol Pathol 1993;12:193, with permission.)

tional artifact and mechanical distortion. Greer and coworkers (1990) stated that the coagulation artifact of laser conization obscures margins and depth of invasion. For these reasons, laser conization has not gained general use in gynecologic practice and is not recommended by the authors.

LOOP DIATHERMY CONIZATION

The technique of large loop diathermy excision of the transformation zone has gained popularity and may replace cold knife and laser conization in most physicians' practices. Loop cone excision offers the ability to manage patients in an outpatient setting with low morbidity. A great advantage is that the entire transformation zone may be excised easily in one piece (Fig. 3-15). Byrne and associates (1991) suggest that this technique should be used only in patients for whom local destructive therapy is contraindicated. There is concern that the universal application of loop cone excision will return us to an era (before the introduction of colposcopy) in which abnormal Pap smears are mostly evaluated by (inpatient) conization. When used indiscriminately, a high percentage of the patients have negative specimens. For example, Luesley (1990) and Alvarez and colleagues (1994) encountered 27% and 32%, respectively, of patients with no evidence of SIL on outpatient loop cone excision, reminiscent of the 44% negative cones in the precolposcopy era (Mc-Cann et al 1969). That patients can be seen in a single visit and a loop cone excision can be performed for both diagnosis and treatment offers such a clear advantage over other evaluation schemes that it almost ensures overuse of the technique. Each physician must judge whether a procedure of this type should be overapplied simply because it has little morbidity. A more conservative approach is to use it in conjunction with colposcopic evaluation; patients with suspected higher grade lesions (based on the cytologic and col-poscopic findings) can undergo loop conization, whereas those with low-grade SIL (and particularly women younger than age 25) can be evaluated colposcopically and managed with minor destructive therapy, such as cryotherapy or trichloroacetic acid applications (Demars et al 1992) to prevent potential damage to the cervix by the loop cone excision procedure.

Cervicography

Blythe (1985), and Tawa (1988), Szarewski (1991) and their associates advocate cervicography as a method of evaluating women with abnormal Pap smears, a concept originally proposed by Stafl (1981). Although the idea of primary care providers photographing the cervix of women with abnormal smears and having these photographs reviewed by an expert has some merit, the cost of providing the equipment and the networking of a referral system to make this practical suggest that the method will not gain general use.

DNA Subtyping to Evaluate Human Papillomavirus–Associated Lesions

Although HPV typing has been advocated as a screening tool to augment the sensitivity and specificity of cervical cytology, evidence supporting typing as being cost-effective and efficacious is lacking. Although cervical HPV infection is the highest known risk factor for the subsequent development of cervical neoplasia (Reeves et al 1989), most individuals with HPV infection never develop significant cervical disease. As many as 30% of a population of women with normal cervical cytology test positive for HPV with a single evaluation (Stone 1989). In a prospective study of 241 patients reported by Koutsky and coworkers (1992), 28% of

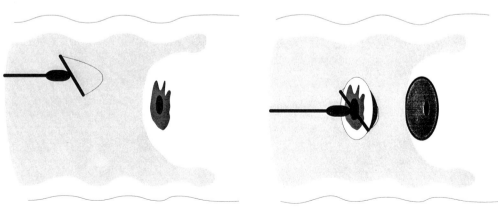

FIGURE 3-15. Loop diathermy conization, showing the removal of the entire transformation zone in one piece.

FIGURE 3-16. (**A**) Endocervical curetting sample on histowrap. (This may also be placed on a square of paper towel or Telfa). After it adheres (a few seconds), it is placed gently in fixative; after fixation, it is removed as a globule for processing. (**B**) Colposcopically directed cervical biopsy on Telfa (this may also be placed on a square of paper towel or histowrap). After it adheres, it is placed gently in fixative; after fixation, it is removed for processing. See Color Figure 3-16.

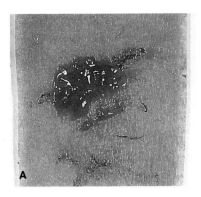
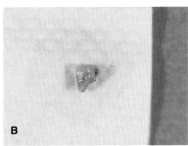

women who were determined to be positive for HPV by molecular hybridization methods developed high-grade SIL within 24 months of testing, compared with 3% of women testing negative for HPV. In the study, however, 45% (110) of the 241 women tested positive for HPV at some point during the 24-month study period. A test whereby almost half of the population are positive and considered to be at risk lacks the necessary specificity to be clinically helpful. In a German study (Schneider et al 1992), 21 women were evaluated for HPV-16 infection every 5 weeks for 1 year after 5 previous years of negative Pap smears. The cumulative prevalence of HPV-16 was 66.7% for this cytologically normal population. Only 1 patient in the HPV-positive group developed SIL over the subsequent 5-year period. Therefore, large-scale screening of populations for HPV DNA is not recommended as a part of the evaluation, treatment, or prevention of cervical cancer.

Examination of Tissue Specimens

A true complete cone specimen is halved and pinned out for fixation, after fixation, parallel slices are made with the central slices from the two halves, including proximal and distal margins (see Fig. 3-14). The complete slices are identified and all tissue is sectioned. With cold knife conization, some pathologists prefer to ink surgical margins. This is not the only method to section and examine a cervical cone. Östör (1993b) has described a somewhat more complicated method. It should be left to the pathologist to determine the technique that is most acceptable. With loop cone excision, the coagulated tissue identifies margins, and such specimens are usually already affixed when received. If the loop cone specimen is received in several pieces, it may be difficult to determine which coagulated margin is the last portion removed from the patient.

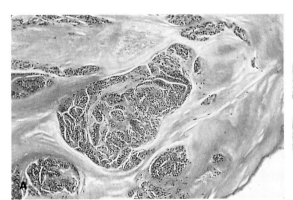
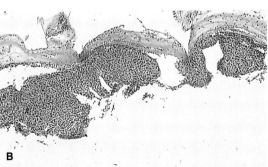

FIGURE 3-17. (**A**) A good example of a "negative" endocervical curettage. The specimen is adequate and there are numerous strips of unremarkable endocervical columnar epithelium amid mucus. (**B**) A good example of a "positive" endocervical curettage. Partly attached to a strand of mucus with inflammatory cells is an irregular strip of atypical epithelium, dysplastic/?neoplastic. This is at least high-grade squamous intraepithelial lesion, but from this singular focus, the possibility of invasive carcinoma cannot be ruled out. See Color Figure 3-17.

Handling of the curetted material is also important. A small curette is used to scrape the endocervical canal circumferentially. The curettings, including the blood clot in the canal, may be picked up with forceps and placed as a single aggregate on a piece of dry paper towel, on a piece of histowrap or on a piece of Telfa and then fixed in formalin (Fig. 3-16*A*). We have not found sponges satisfactory, although they may work well in some laboratories. Any material floating free in the container may be filtered through histowrap, although this is a time-consuming procedure; the more adherent the specimen is to the histowrap or Telfa, the better. The pathologist can process the material as a unit wrapped in histowrap. Tissue obtained with biopsy forceps can be oriented on paper towel or on Telfa in a similar fashion (see Fig. 3-16*B*). Examples of negative and positive curettings are shown in Figure 3-17*A* and *B*.

References

Abdul-Karim FW, Nunez C. Cervical intraepithelial neoplasia after conization: a study of 522 consecutive cervical cones. Obstet Gynecol 1985;65:77.

Alvarez RD, Helm CW, Edwards RP, Naumann RW, Partridge EE, Shingleton HM, et al. Prospective randomized trial of LLETZ versus laser ablation in patients with cervical intraepithelial neoplasia. Gynecol Oncol 1994; 52:175.

Anderson MC, Hartley RB. Cervical crypt involvement by intraepithelial neoplasia. Obstet Gynecol 1980;55:546.

Anderson MC. The natural history of cervical intraepithelial neoplasia. Curr Obstet Gynaecol 1991;1:124.

Averette HE, Nelson JH Jr, Ng ABP, Hoskins WJ, Boyce JG, Ford JH Jr. Diagnosis and management of microinvasive (stage IA) carcinoma of the uterine cervix. Cancer 1976;38:414.

Baggish MS, Dorsey JH. Carbon dioxide laser for combination excisional—vaporization conization. Am J Obstet Gynecol 1985;15:23.

Benedet JL, Andersen GH, Boyes DA. Colposcopic accuracy in the diagnosis of micro-invasive and occult invasive carcinoma of the cervix. Obstet Gynecol 1985;65:557.

Bibbo M, ed. Comprehensive cytopathology. Philadelphia: WB Saunders, 1991.

Blythe GJ. Cervicography: a preliminary report. Am J Obstet Gynecol 1985;152:192.

Boyce J, Fruchter RG, Nicastri AD, Ambinvagar EC, Reinis MS, Nelson JH Jr. Prognostic factors in stage I carcinoma of the cervix. Gynecol Oncol 1981;12:154.

Boyes DA, Worth AJ, Fidler HK. The results of treatment of 4389 cases of preclinical cervical squamous carcinoma. Br J Obstet Gynaecol 1970;77:769.

Broder S. The Bethesda system for reporting cervical/vaginal cytologic diagnoses. JAMA 1992; 267:1892.

Burghardt E. Microinvasive carcinoma. Obstet Gynecol Surv 1979;34:836.

Byrne P, Ogueh O, Sant-Cassia LJ. Outpatient loop diathermy conisation (letter). Lancet 1991;337:917.

Cancer Committee FIGO. Staging announcement. Gynecol Oncol 1986;25:383.

Copeland LJ, Silva EG, Gershenson DM, Morris M, Young DC, Wharton JT. Superficially invasive cell carcinoma of the cervix. Gynecol Oncol 1992;45:307.

Coppleson M. Microinvasive cervical cancer. Obstet Gynecol Surv 1979;34:840.

Creasman W, Bundy B, Zaino R, Homesley H, Majors F. Early invasive carcinoma of the cervix with 3–5mm of invasion—risk factors and prognosis (abstract). 25th Annual Meeting, Society of Gynecologic Oncologists, Orlando, Florida, February 6–9, 1994.

Creasman WT, Parker RT. Microinvasive cervical cancer. Obstet Gynecol 1973;16:261.

Delgado G, Bundy BN, Fowler WC Jr, et al. A prospective surgical pathological study of stage I squamous carcinoma of the cervix: a Gynecologic Oncology Group study. Gynecol Oncol 1989;35:314.

Delmore J, Horbelt DV, Kallail KJ. Cervical conization: cold knife and laser excision in residency training. Obstet Gynecol 1992;79:1016.

Demars L, Vlaea F, Fowler WC Jr, Walton L. Trichloroacetic acid as first line treatment in HPV-associated low-grade dysplasia (abstract). 23rd Annual Meeting, Society of Gynecologic Oncologists, San Antonio, Texas, March 15–18, 1992.

Demopoulos RI, Horowitz LF, Vamvakas EC. Endocervical gland involvement by cervical intraepithelial neoplasia grade III. Cancer 1991;68:1932.

Dietl J, Semm K, Hedderich J, Bucholz F. CIN and preclinical cervical carcinoma. A study of morbidity trends over a 10-year period. Int J Gynaecol Obstet 1983;21:283.

DiSaia PJ, Creasman WT, eds. Clinical gynecologic oncology. St Louis: CV Mosby, 1989.

Drescher CW, Peters WA III, Roberts JA. Contribution of endocervical curettage in evaluating abnormal cervical cytology. Obstet Gynecol 1983;62:343.

Duncan ID. The management of microinvasive carcinoma of the cervix. Curr Obstet Gynecol 1991;1:143.

Duncan ID. Microinvasive and occult invasive carcinoma: the British experience in the management of microinvasive carcinoma of the cervix. In Jordon JA, Sharp F, Singer A, eds. Pre-clinical neoplasia of the cervix. London: Royal College of Obstetricians and Gynaecologists, 1982.

Fennell RH Jr. Microinvasive carcinoma of the uterine cervix. Obstet Gynecol Surv 1978;33:406.

Foushee JHS, Greiss FC, Lock FR. Stage IA squamous cell carcinoma of the uterine cervix. Am J Obstet Gynecol 1969;105:46.

Fowler JF, Davos I, Leuchter RS, Lagasse LD. Effect of CO_2 laser conization of the uterine cervix on pathologic interpretation of cervical intraepithelial neoplasia. Obstet Gynecol 1992;79:693.

Graham JB, Sotto LSJ, Paloucek FP. Carcinoma of the cervix. Philadelphia: WB Saunders, 1962.

Grainger DA, Roberts DR, Wells MM, Horbelt DV. The value of endocervical currettage in the management of the patient with abnormal cytologic findings. Am J Obstet Gynecol 1987;156:625.

Greer BE, Figge DC, Tamimi HK, Cain JM, Lee RB. Stage IA2 squamous carcinoma of the cervix: difficult diagnosis and therapeutic dilemma. Am J Obstet Gynecol 1990;162:1406.

Grundsell H, Alm P, Larsson G. Cure rates after laser conization for early cervical neoplasia. Ann Chir Gynaecol Fenniae 1983;2:218.

Hald F, Kristoffersen SE, Hairi J, Hansen MK. Diagnostic accuracy of outpatient endocervical curettage using conventional and Vabra curettage of the cervix. Acta Obstet Gynecol Scand 1988;67:71.

Hasumi K, Sakamoto A, Sugano H. Microinvasive carcinoma of the uterine cervix. Cancer 1980;45:928.

Hopkins MP, Roberts JA, Schmidt RW. Cervical adenocarcinoma in situ. Obstet Gynecol 1988;71:842.

Howell R, Hammond R, Pryse-Davies. The histologic reliability of laser cone biopsy of the cervix. Obstet Gynecol 1991;77:905.

Hyams MN. High frequency current in the treatment of chronic endocervicitis. Arch Phys Ther 1930;11:171.

Iversen T, Abeler V, Kjorstad KE. Factors influencing the treatment of patients with stage IA carcinoma of the cervix. Br J Obstet Gynaecol 1979;86:593.

Jaworski RD, Pacey NF, Greenberg ML, Osborn RA. The histologic diagnosis of adeno-carcinoma in situ and related lesions of the cervix uteri: adeno-carcinoma in situ. Cancer 1988;61:1171.

Johnston WW, Myers B, Creasman WT, Owens SM. Cytopathology and the management of early invasive cancer of the uterine cervix. Obstet Gynecol 1982;60:350.

Kaufman RH, Strama T, Norton PK, et al. Cryosurgical treatment of cervical intraepithelial neoplasia. Obstet Gynecol 1973;42:881.

Kolstad P. Follow-up study of 232 patients with stage IA1 and 411 patients with stage IA2 squamous cell carcinoma of the cervix (microinvasive carcinoma). Gynecol Oncol 1989;33:265.

Koss LG, Durfee GR. Unusual patterns of squamous epithelium of uterine cervix: cytologic and pathologic study of koilocytotic atypia. Ann NY Acad Sci 1956;63:1245.

Koutsky LA, Holmes KK, Critchlow CW, et al. A cohort study of the risk of cervical intraepithelial grade 2 and 3 in relation to papillomavirus infection. N Engl J Med 1992;327:1272.

Kurman RJ, Norris HJ, Wilkinson E. Atlas of tumor pathology. Tumors of the cervix, vagina and vulva. Washington DC, Armed Forces Institute of Pathology, 1992.

Lapaquette TK, Dinh TV, Hannigan EV, Doherty MG, Yandell RB, Buchanan VS. Management of patients with positive margins after cervical conization. Obstet Gynecol 1993;82:440.

Leman MH, Benson WL, Kurman RJ, Park RC. Microinvasive carcinoma of the cervix. Obstet Gynecol 1976;48:571.

Lohe KJ. Early squamous cell carcinoma of the uterine cervix. I. Definition and histology. Gynecol Oncol 1978;6:10.

Lovecchio JL, Gal D. Diagnostic techniques in gynecologic oncology. In Hoskins WJ, Perez CA, Young RC, eds.

Principles and practice of gynecologic oncology. Philadelphia: JB Lippincott, 1992:434.

Luesley DM, Cullimore J, Redman CWE, Lawton FG, Emens JM, Rollason TP, et al. Loop diathermy excision of the cervical transformation zone in patients with abnormal cervical smears. Br Med J 1990;300:1690.

Luesley DM, McCrum A, Teng PB, et al. Complications of cone biopsy related to the dimensions of the cone and the influence of prior colposcopic assessment. Br J Obstet Gynaecol 1985;92:158.

Maiman MA, Fruchter RG, DiMaio TM, Boyce JG. Superficial invasive squamous cell carcinoma of the cervix. Obstet Gynecol 1988;72:399.

McCann SW, Mickal SW, Crapanzano JR. Sharp conization of the cervix. Obstet Gynecol 1969;33:470.

Meandzija MP, Locher G, Jackson JD. CO_2 laser conization versus conventional conization: a clinico-pathologic appraisal. Lasers Surg Med 1984;4:139.

Mestwerdt G. Die fruhdiagnose des kollumkarzinoms. Zentralbl Gynakol 1947;69:198.

Mussey E, Soule EH, Welch JC. Microinvasive carcinoma of the cervix. Am J Obstet Gynecol 1969;104:738.

National Cancer Institute Workshop. The 1988 Bethesda system for reporting cervical/vaginal cytological diagnoses. JAMA 1989;262:931.

Ng ABP, Reagan JW. Microinvasive carcinoma of the uterine cervix. Am J Clin Pathol 1969;52:511.

Ng ABP, Reagan JW. Pathology and cytopathology of microinvasive squamous cell carcinoma of the uterine cervix. In Weid GL, Keebler CM, Koss LG, Reagan JW, eds. Chicago: Tutorials of Cytology. A publication of the International Academy of Cytology, Chicago: 1988:114.

Nguyen GK. Exfoliative cytology of microinvasive squamous-cell carcinoma of the uterine cervix. A retrospective study of 42 cases. Acta Cytol 1984;28:457.

Ostergard DR. Prediction of clearance of cervical intraepithelial neoplasia by conization. Obstet Gynecol 1980; 56:77.

Östör AG, Pagano R, Davoren RA, Fortune DW, Chanen W, Rome R. Adenocarcinoma in situ of the cervix. Int J Gynecol Pathol 1984;3:179.

Östör AG. Natural history of cervical intraepithelial neoplasia. A critical review. Int J Gynecol Pathol 1993a;12:186.

Östör AG. Studies of 200 cases of early squamous cell carcinoma of the cervix. Int J Gynecol Pathol 1993b; 12:193.

Papanicolaou GN, Traut HF. Diagnosis of uterine cancer by the vaginal smear. Cambridge, MA: Harvard University Press, 1943.

Ramzy L, Mody DR. Gynecologic cytology. Practical considerations and limitations. Clin Lab Med 1991:271.

Reeves WC, Brinton L, Garcia M, et al. Human papillomavirus infection and cervical cancer in Latin America. N Engl J Med 1989;320:1437.

Reid R. Genital warts and cervical cancer. IV. A colposcopic index for differentiating subclinical papillomaviral infection from cervical intraepithelial neoplasia. Am J Obstet Gynecol 1984;149:815.

Reid R, Fu YS, Herschman BR, et al. Genital warts and cervical cancer. VI. The relationship between aneuploid and polyploid cervical lesions. Am J Obstet Gynecol 1984;150:189.

Reid R, Scalzi P. Genital warts and cervical cancer. VII. An improved colposcopic index for differentiating benign papilloma-viral infections from high-grade cervical intraepithelial neoplasia. Am J Obstet Gynecol 1985; 153:611.

Richart RM. Cervical intraepithelial neoplasia. In Sommers SC (ed). Pathology annual. New York: Appleton-Crofts, 1973.

Richart RM. Influence of diagnostic and therapeutic procedures on the distribution of cervical intraepithelial neoplasia. Cancer 1966;19:1635.

Ruch RM, Pitcock JA, Ruch WA Jr. Microinvasive carcinoma of the cervix. Am J Obstet Gynecol 1976;125:87.

Schmidt WA. Cytologic and histologic correlations in colposcopy. Cancer Bulletin 1983;35:184.

Schneider A, Kirchkoff T, Meinhardt G, Gissmann L. Repeated evaluation of human papillomavirus 16 status in cervical swabs of young women with a history of normal Papanicolaou smears. Obstet Gynecol 1992;79:683.

Sedlis A, Sall S, Tsukada Y, et al. Microinvasive carcinoma of the uterine cervix: a clinical—pathologic study. Am J Obstet Gynecol 1979;133:64.

Shingleton HM, Gore H, Austin JM. Outpatient evaluation of patients with atypical Papanicolaou smears: contribution of endocervical curettage. Am J Obstet Gynecol 1976;126:122.

Shingleton HM, Hatch KD, Orr JW Jr, Gore H, Soong S-J. Diagnosis and treatment of preinvasive and microscopically invasive squamous cell carcinoma of the cervix: including comments on surveillance of DES-exposed patients with cytologic atypias. Cancer Bulletin of the University of Texas M. D. Anderson Hospital and Tumor Institute 1983;35:172.

Shingleton HM. American College of Surgeons national patterns of care study. 1995. In preparation.

Simon NL, Gore H, Shingleton HM, Soong S-J, Orr JW Jr, Hatch KD. A study of superficially invasive carcinoma of the cervix. Obstet Gynecol 1986;68:19.

Stafl A. Cervicography: a new method for cervical cancer detection. Am J Obstet Gynecol 1981;139:815.

Stone KM. Epidemiologic aspects of genital HPV infection. Clin Obstet Gynecol 1989;32:112.

Sugimori H, Kawarabayashi T, Iwasaka T, Fukada K, Hachisuga T, Hayash Y. Colposcopic assessment of Stage I cervical cancer. Int J Gynecol Cancer 1991;1: 179.

Szarewski A, Cuzick J, Edwards R, Butler B, Singer A. The use of cervicography in a primary screening service. Br J Obstet Gynecol 1991;98:313 (Obstet Gynecol Surv 1991;46(9):632).

Tawa K, Forsythe A, Coye K, et al. A comparison of the Papanicolaou smear and the cervigram: sensitivity, specificity, and cost analysis. Obstet Gynecol 1988;71:229.

van Nagell JR Jr, Greenwell N, Powell DF, Donaldson ES, Hanson MG, Gay EC. Microinvasive carcinoma of the cervix. Am J Obstet Gynecol 1983;145:981.

Watson AJS, Tuffnell DJ, Lowe JW, Rand RJ, Wilkinson RK. The incomplete cone biopsy: a comparison of conservative and surgical management. Eur J Obstet Gynecol Reprod Biol 1993;51:119.

Cancer of the Cervix by Hugh M. Shingleton and James W. Orr, Jr.
J. B. Lippincott Company, Philadelphia, © 1995.

4

Treatment of Intraepithelial Lesions and Microinvasive Tumors

OBSERVATION ONLY

Several prospective studies provide data concerning the risks of no treatment in women with mild dysplasia (low-grade squamous intraepithelial lesions [SIL]). Nashiell (1986) observed 555 women, with a mean follow-up of 39 months. Sixty-two percent of these lesions regressed to normal, whereas 16% progressed, including two (0.4%) that progressed to invasive carcinoma. Importantly, many patients with low-grade SIL do not return for therapy (Laedtke and Dignan 1992). Women with mild dysplasia had a five to six times greater risk of developing high-grade SIL when compared to women without a diagnosis of mild dysplasia. Nashiell calculated the risk of progression from mild dysplasia to a higher grade lesion as being 250 to 800 per 100,000 woman-years.

Östör (1993), in a collected series of 4504 women with low-grade SIL, reported a 57% rate of regression. Although the quoted risk of progression to carcinoma in situ and invasive cancer is small (11% and 1% respectively; Table 4-1), it varies with the method of diagnosis and duration of follow up. An added factor is that as many as 32% of women diagnosed with SIL do not return for therapy. Therefore, many physicians advocate simple and inexpensive local treatment of the cervix for most patients having documented SIL, particularly for women judged to be noncompliant for long-term observation.

Observation has the least risk of cervical distortion and impact on future reproductive potential. Cytologic observation of biopsy-proved low-grade SIL can be used in certain reliable and well-informed women. It is imperative, however, that the physician, in addition to performing cytology, exclude the pres-

ence of high-grade colposcopic lesions. The treating physician should also have a clear understanding and open communication with the cytopathologist who evaluates the cytologic samples to ensure that repeat colposcopic evaluation can be performed if warranted, based on cytologic progression.

Generally, there is no role for observing high-grade SIL because they have a higher and more rapid rate of progression to invasive disease (5%–12%) than do low-grade lesions (see Table 4-1). Depending on the interval, as many as 25% to 78% of patients with high-grade SIL develop invasive cancer when followed-up without treatment (Piringer-Kuchinka et al 1956, Noda 1966, Gad 1976, Fu et al 1981, McIndoe and colleagues 1984). Although short periods of observation (e.g., in pregnancy) are justified, it is reported that as many as 4% of high-grade SIL transit to invasion during 1 year.

CONIZATION OF THE CERVIX

Conization has been in use for many years for the treatment of premalignant cervical disease (Table 4-2), especially in countries other than the United States. Hysterectomy generally has been the preferred treatment by American gynecologists for high-grade SIL; low-grade lesions have been conventionally treated with local ablative techniques, including cryosurgery, laser evaporation, or diathermy. The more recently described loop diathermy excision techniques offer potential advantages over destructive methods because the entire transformation zone (including the disease) can be removed and studied histologically. Although the use of the outpatient loop conization procedure

TABLE 4-1
Summary of the Natural History of Cervical Intraepithelial Neoplasia

	PATIENTS (N)	REGRESSION (%)	PERSISTENCE (%)	PROGRESSION TO CIS (%)	PROGRESSION TO INVASION (%)
CIN I	4504	57	32	11	1
CIN II	2247	43	35	22	5
CIN III	767	32	<56	—	>12

CIN, cervical intraepithelial neoplasia; *CIS*, carcinoma in situ.

Östör AG. Natural history of cervical intraepithelial neoplasia: a critical review. Int J Gynecol Pathol 1993;12:186.

has the potential for overuse on patients having minor or insignificant lesions, the general movement in the United States is away from radical surgical treatment (hysterectomy) to more conservative outpatient treatment using conization (albeit that performed with loop excision). Although postconization recurrence is relatively rare (2% to 10%), these patients remain at risk for later developing invasive cancer; their risk of developing invasive disease may be 100-fold higher than that for women without cervical intraepithelial neoplasia (CIN). Brown and associates (1991) reported a mean interval of 6.7 years in those women developing invasive cancer after conization. If coniza-

tion is the selected treatment, these women should be informed of the need for lifelong cytologic surveillance. Routine endometrial curettage at the time of conization potentially increases costs and risks (Pearl and Beretta 1993). In contrast, endometrial sampling should be considered during treatment in any woman with historical or physical criteria for evaluation. In those women electing or requiring a more definitive surgical therapy (i.e., hysterectomy), a pretreatment conization may be necessary to preclude invasive disease. In this situation, frozen-section conization is associated with a degree of accuracy that allows the surgeon to make appropriate decisions regarding the

TABLE 4-2
Conization Compared With Hysterectomy as a Treatment for Squamous Intraepithelial Lesions (CIN)

STUDY	Year	Original Diagnosis	RECURRENCE AFTER CONIZATION			RECURRENCE AFTER HYSTERECTOMY		
			Patients (n)	CIN (%)	Invasive (%)	Patients (n)	CIN (%)	Invasive (%)
Boyes, et al	1970	CIS	808	3.5	0.4	2849	0.7	0.1
Creasman, et al	1972	CIS	65	7.7	NS	642	2.4	NS
Gad	1976	CIS	101	10.0	0	226	0.9	NS
Kolstad and Klem	1976	CIS	795	2.1	0.9	238	1.2	2.1
Jones and Buller	1980	CIN	114	3.5	1.8	61	1.6	1.6
Andersch and Moinian	1982	CIN	414	5.3	0	—	—	—
Mettlin, et al	1982	CIS	1692	3.1	NS	7066	0.5	NS
Baggish, et al*	1989	CIN	954	3.0	NS	—	—	—
Hellberg and Nilsson	1990	CIN III	635	—	—	154		
Tabor and Berget[†]	1990	CIN	425	6.4	0	—	—	—

[†]53% cases laser conization, 47% CKC.
*Laser conization.
CIN, cervical intraepithelial neoplasia; *CIS*, carcinoma in situ; *NS*, not stated.

Modified from Shingleton HM and Orr JW Jr. Cancer of the cervix: diagnosis and treatment. New York, Churchill Livingstone, 1987:85.

TABLE 4-3
Electrocautery as Treatment of Squamous Intraepithelial Lesions (CIN)

STUDY	YEAR	PATIENTS (N)	DIAGNOSIS	FAILURE (%)	OVERALL SUCCESS (%)
Richart and Sciana	1968	170	CIN	11	98.8
Ortiz, et al	1973	148	Dysplasia (96)	11	92
			CIS (52)	15	
Chanen and Rome	1983	1864	CIN	2.7	NS
Schuurmans, et al	1984	426	CIN	14	96.6
Deigan, et al	1986	726	CIN	10–11	100
Chanen	1989	181	CIN	5	98

CIN, cervical intraepithelial neoplasia; *CIS*, carcinoma in situ; *NS*, not stated.

Modified from Shingleton HM, Orr JW Jr. Cancer of the cervix: diagnosis and treatment. New York: Churchill Livingstone, 1987:90.

extent of therapy (Hoffman and colleagues 1993, Hannigan and coworkers 1986). In Hoffman and associates' report, all invasive lesions were detected. Frozen-section conization for a positive endocervical curettage (ECC), unsatisfactory colposcopy, or discordant cytology did not contribute to the diagnosis of invasive cancer.

ELECTROCAUTERY

Chanen (1983, 1989) has long advocated electrocoagulation diathermy as treatment for CIN and in 1983 reported a 15-year experience on 1864 patients managed with this method. Two thirds of patients had CIN III, some with lesions involving multiple quadrants of the cervix and some with endocervical canal involvement. He successfully treated CIN in 97.3% of patients in a single sitting. Importantly, he did not observe progression to invasive cancer in any patient. Schuurmans and colleagues (1984) and Deigan and coworkers (1986) reported a single-treatment control rate of 86% and 89%, respectively, increasing to 97% and 100% with retreatment of the failures. Some American investigators have reported good success rates using this technique (Table 4-3); however, although electrocautery was used in the United States before the advent of cryosurgical and laser vaporization equipment, the technique enjoys little popularity today, perhaps because of the need for anesthesia or the better patient and physician acceptance of the newer outpatient therapies.

CRYOSURGERY

Cryosurgery is an effective treatment for precancerous squamous lesions (Table 4-4). Relapse rates after a single treatment vary between 7% and 16%. The overall cure rate can be improved by retreating those who relapse. The risk of recurrent or persistent SIL varies according to the grade, size, and location of the original lesion. Townsend (1979), in a series of 874 patients, reported recurrence rates of 7%, 10%, and 16% in CIN grades I to III, respectively. He reported a 7.5% recurrence rate in lesions 1 cm or less in size, 14% in those 1 to 2 cm, and a 42% recurrence rate when the lesion involved most of the cervix. Kaufman and coworkers (1973), reporting on a series of 395 patients, observed that 64% of recurrent (persistent) SIL were detected within 6 months and 77% were detected within 12 months. They reported a 6% failure rate in patients with pretreatment-negative endocervical curettage; 21% of patients failed cryotherapy when the pretreatment endocervical curettage suggested endocervical involvement. The presence of CIN in cervical clefts is also identified as a factor that predicts an increased relapse rate (Anderson and Hartley 1980, Abdul-Karim and associates 1982, Savage and coworkers 1982). Anderson and Hartley (1980) measured the depth to which CIN involves cervical clefts. They reported that tissue excision (or destruction) to a depth of 3.8 mm eradicated involved crypts in 99.7% of patients. Therefore, it appears that the number of quadrants involved, the size of the lesion, the location of the lesion, and deep involvement of cervical clefts are all important factors to be considered before the selection of cryosurgery as treatment for SIL.

The actual technique of performing cryosurgery affects cure rates. Schantz and Thormann (1984) reported that the double-freeze technique is significantly more effective than the single-freeze technique, with respective recurrence rates of 6.2% and 16.3%. Cryosurgery has been used extensively at the University of Alabama at Birmingham, especially for treatment of low-grade SIL. More than three quarters of the patients with CIN I and CIN II were treated with

TABLE 4-4
Cryosurgery as Treatment of Precancerous Squamous Intraepithelial Lesions (CIN)

STUDY	YEAR	PATIENTS (N)	DIAGNOSIS	RELAPSE RATE (%)	OVERALL SUCCESS (%)*
Coney, et al	1983	240	CIN I	13	97
van Lent, et al	1983	102	CIN III	7	NS
Arof, et al	1984	393	CIN	16	NS
Creasman, et al	1984	770	CIN	10.1	96
Bryson, et al	1985	453	CIN III	7	98
Benedet, et al	1987	1675	CIN	NS	94
Hellberg and Nilsson	1990	104	CIN II, III	NS	87
Draeby-Kristiansen, et al	1991	96	CIN II, III	9	98
Gordon and Duncan	1991	1628	CIN III	NS	92
Andersen and Husth	1992	261	CIN	NS	83.5

*Usually involved retreatment with cryosurgery.
CIN, cervical intraepithelial neoplasia; *NS,* not stated.

Modified from Shingleton HM, Orr JW Jr. Cancer of the cervix: diagnosis and treatment. New York: Churchill Livingstone, 1987:85.

cryotherapy at this institution during 1970 to 1980; however, only a third of patients with CIN III (severe dysplasia [CIS]) were treated with these methods (Table 4-5). At the University of Alabama at Birmingham, the necessity for diagnostic conization after cryosurgery failure was about 5%. One invasive carcinoma occurred after cryosurgery in a series of 1834 treated patients. The occurrence of a high-grade SIL smear after cryotherapy demands careful evaluation. Conization should be considered because the risk of coexisting or eventual development of invasive cancer is appreciable. A review of three reports suggests the

risk of invasive cancer in this population of women to be as high as 40% (Schmidt and associates 1992).

Several technical problems may be encountered when using cryosurgery as treatment. Equipment malfunction may lower the probe temperature, rendering it inadequate for successfully eradicating the cervical disease. Some advocate that instead of actually timing the freeze, therapy should be continued until the iceball extends at least 0.5 cm from the border of the probe to encompass both the entire exocervical component and the depth of the involved cervical clefts. In those situations in which the cervical or vaginal

TABLE 4-5
Cryosurgery for Squamous Intraepithelial Lesions (CIN) (University of Alabama at Birmingham 1970–1980[1])

DIAGNOSIS	PATIENTS (N)	CRYOTHERAPY		EVALUATED AFTER CRYOTHERAPY*		CONIZATION/ HYSTERECTOMY AFTER CRYOTHERAPY		INVASIVE DISEASE AFTER CRYOTHERAPY	
		(n)	(%)	(n)	(%)	(n)	(%)	(n)	(%)
CIN I, II	957	722	(75.4)	99	(13.7)	25	(3.5)	0	(0)
CIN III	877	246	(28.1)	46	(18.7)	22	(8.9)	1	(0.4)
TOTAL	1834	968	(52.8)	145	(15.0)	47	(4.9)	1	(0.1)

[1]K.D. Hatch 1981
*For cytologic atypias after initial treatment.
CIN, cervical intraepithelial neoplasia.

Modified from Shingleton HM, Orr JW Jr. Cancer of the cervix: diagnosis and treatment. New York: Churchill Livingstone, 1987:86.

anatomy prohibits adequate application of the cryoprobe over the lesion or in the situation wherein a large transformation zone or cervical lesion extends beyond the probe, cryosurgery may be a poor treatment choice (Towsend 1979).

Delayed bleeding, infection, or cervical stenosis are sometimes reported as complications of cryosurgery. Ferenczy (1985) noted these complications in fewer than 1% of his patients; however, Benedet and colleagues (1991) reported a 4.8% risk of delayed cervical bleeding. Our experience (Hatch et al 1981) more closely resembles that of Ferenczy in that significant bleeding has not been observed except in very rare instances. Although it alters the position of the squamocolumnar junction, a popular concern that cryosurgery produces cervical stenosis and interferes with subsequent pregnancy has not been realized. Gordon and Duncan (1991), in a series of 1628 women, reported no effect on fertility or on rates of miscarriage or preterm or operative delivery. Overall, cryotherapy can be successfully used in many patients who have SIL. The ease of treatment, relative lack of expense for treatment and equipment, and overall success rates makes it a useful tool.

LASER VAPORIZATION

Laser vaporization of SIL has been used extensively, with a success rate equal to that of cryosurgery (Table 4-6). Watchler (1984) compared treatment by laser vaporization and cryosurgery. Cryosurgery was reported to be less expensive, require less training, and use more reliable, less expensive, and less cumbersome equipment. When compared with cryotherapy, laser allows more precise tissue destruction (Fig. 4-1), leaves less necrotic tissue, heals faster, and may result in a healed cervix in which the transformation zone less frequently moves cephalad. Laser vaporization can also be used for large intraepithelial lesions that the cryosurgery probe does not cover, particularly for those involving the vaginal cuff or lateral vaginal fornices. Fortunately, laser treatment results in minimal structural cervical deformity and has little apparent effect on future fertility (Baggish and coworkers 1989). Evans and Monaghan (1983) indicated that laser failures are not related to age, parity, or lesion size. Popkin (1983), who used laser vaporization without anesthesia or analgesia, reported no major complications with this technique. Many physicians use a local 1% xylocaine paracervical infiltration anesthetic at the time of treatment.

Delayed bleeding after therapy appears to be the most often reported complication of laser vaporization (Table 4-7). This is usually managed with packing or suturing and rarely requires hospitalization or transfusion. Although it is a more precise therapy method, the use of laser vaporization has a learning curve. Success rates increase as operator experience increases (Baggish and coworkers 1989). Additionally, successful treatment correlates in inverse proportion to the size of the intraepithelial lesion (Baggish and coworkers 1989). Importantly, the risk of accidental patient or personal injury during laser treatment is higher than with cryotherapy. As with any conservative treatment, a few cases of posttreatment invasive cervical cancer occur (Pearson and coworkers 1989).

TABLE 4-6
Laser Vaporization as Treatment of Squamous Intraepithelial Lesions (CIN)

STUDY	YEAR	PATIENTS (N)	DIAGNOSIS	PERSISTENCE (%)	OVERALL SUCESS* (%)
Burke	1982	131	CIN	NS	87
Bellina, et al	1983	292	CIN	7	96
Evans and Monaghan	1983	408	CIN	7.1	96
Popkin	1983	138	CIN	9.4	—
Stanhope, et al	1983	99	CIN III	9	100
Wright	1984	545	CIN	3	99.5
Baggish, et al	1989	3070	CIN	6.2	—
Higgins, et al	1990	253	CIN	11	100
Pearson, et al	1989	3738	CIN	9	99.7
Paraskevaidis, et al	1991	2130	CIN	5.6	NS

*Usually involved retreatment with laser vaporization.
CIN, cervical intraepithelial neoplasia; *NS,* not stated.

Modified from Shingleton HM, Orr JW Jr. Cancer of the cervix: diagnosis and treatment. New York: Churchill Livingstone, 1987:87.

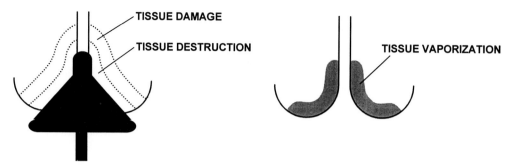

FIGURE 4-1. Tissue vaporization by laser causes minimal damage to immediately adjacent tissue, whereas graded damage occurs adjacent to cryoprobe. This results in an infected cervix after cryosurgery, but the cervix heals more rapidly and cleanly after laser vaporization. (Modified from Shingleton HM, Orr JW Jr. Cancer of the cervix: diagnosis and treatment. New York: Churchill Livingstone 1987:87.)

LASER CONIZATION

Several authors have promoted the use of laser coniza-tion for treatment of SIL. Bekassy and associates (1983), reporting on a series of 151 patients, indicated that removal of a 5-mm disk of the cervix allows the pathologist to examine the entire transformation zone histologically. They also believe that laser conization is associated with a decreased risk of postoperative bleed-ing, when compared with laser vaporization. Grundsell and colleagues (1983) reported cure rates equal to those of laser vaporization and further state that the procedure could be safely performed on an outpatient basis. Meandzija and coworkers (1984) stated that laser conization, when compared with conventional surgical (cold knife) conization, provides greater visi-bility of the healed squamocolumnar junction.

Although laser conization compares favorably with other therapies (Table 4-8), it has not become popular for general use. Such expensive equipment for office treatment is not available to many physicians.

Additionally, laser conization results in a surgical spec-imen that has a high percentage of artifact, frequently making the histologic interpretation difficult (Howell and associates 1991, Fowler and colleagues 1992). Laser conization has been superseded by loop diathermy conization in the United States. Although the actual extent of tissue thermal injury (in microns) does not differ between laser and loop conization, ex-tensive areas of carbonization and epithelial distortion are more common after laser conization (Wright et al 1992b).

LOOP DIATHERMY CONIZATION

Cartier (1984) has long advocated the use of loop diathermy excision in the investigation and manage-ment of SIL. This treatment is performed on outpa-tients, using local anesthesia, and offers the advantage of allowing histologic examination of an adequate specimen (see Fig. 3-15 in Chap. 3). With proper use,

TABLE 4-7
Complications of Laser Vaporization

STUDY	YEAR	PATIENTS (N)	BLEEDING (%)	STENOSIS (%)	INFECTION (%)	COMMENT
Burke	1982	131	3.5	NS	NS	—
Wright	1984	787	11	NS	NS	2% admitted for bleed-ing
Ferenczy	1985	147	NS	NS	NS	7.4% had bleeding and/or infection
Baggish, et al	1989	3070	NS	1.1	0.05	—
Higgins, et al	1990	253	0	NS	0	—
Benedet, et al	1991	1786	4.8	NS	NS	Bleeding mostly treated by packing; 2 patients required suturing

NS, not stated.

TABLE 4-8
Laser Conization as Treatment for Squamous Intraepithelial Lesions (CIN)

STUDY	YEAR	PATIENTS (N)	DIAGNOSIS	SUCCESS (%)
Baggish, et al	1989	954	CIN	97
Tabor and Berget	1990	224	CIN	95

CIN, cervical intraepithelial neoplasia.

the histologic specimen has minimal artifact and can be examined easily. The importance of determining the presence of invasive cancer is obvious; however, the capability of determining margin involvement (in the absence of invasive disease) is suspect, especially when the specimen is removed in multiple pieces. Clinically, the procedure is used to excise the entire transformation zone (as outlined with acetic acid and Lugol's solution). Colposcopic evaluation of the lower endocervix allows additional tissue excision with small loops until the entire canal lesion (white epithelium) is removed. As with other techniques, loop excision failure rates are related to lesion size. Wright (1992a) reported a 6% failure rate with single-quadrant involvement and a 26% failure rate when four quadrants were involved.

Conization margins (in the absence of invasive disease) have only a small predictive effect on the risk of persistent SIL. With involved margins, persistent or recurrent SIL occurs in 34%, compared with 16% of women who have negative margins (Ostergard 1980). In the clinical situation of SIL in the margin, an observation protocol can be used, and there is no immediate need for repeat conization or hysterectomy (unless other coexisting indications exist). The information obtained from an ECC at the end of the loop excision is not predictive of recurrence (Wright 1992a).

Reported success rates for loop diathermy coniza-

tion as treatment are about 95% (Table 4-9), almost identical to those for other outpatient therapies. Microinvasive lesions are found in 1% to 2% of specimens (Anderson 1991).

The relatively inexpensive equipment (when combined with the ease of performance of outpatient loop diathermy conization), the high patient acceptance of diagnosis and treatment in one visit, and the low complication rates make this procedure worthwhile. However, one-visit treatment has a negative feature, that is, overtreatment of insignificant lesions by this technique. In reporting 616 loop diathermy conization procedures, Luesley and coworkers (1990) found 27% of patients to have insignificant (mostly koilocytic) lesions and 5% to have negative findings. This experience is similar to that at the University of Alabama at Birmingham (Alvarez and coworkers 1993); in a prospective study comparing laser ablation and loop diathermy conization, 26% of women randomized to loop conization had no SIL. This occurred even when "white" lesions were colposcopically evident before treatment. This information suggests that patients with low-grade SIL may not be the best candidates for this treatment.

The treating physician must make decisions regarding reliability of follow-up before using less invasive treatment regimens. Byrne and coworkers (1991) suggested that outpatient cone biopsy using a loop

TABLE 4-9
Diathermy Loop Conization as Treatment for Squamous
Intraepithelial Lesions (CIN)

STUDY	YEAR	PATIENTS (N)	DIAGNOSIS	SUCCESS (%)
Bigrigg, et al	1990	1000	CIN	95.9
Gunasekera, et al	1990	199	CIN II, III	94.7–95*
Luesley, et al	1990	557	CIN	95.6
Keijser, et al	1992	424	CIN	91
Wright	1992	432	CIN	94†

*6- to 12–month follow-up.
†6-month follow-up only.
CIN, cervical intraepithelial neoplasia.

electrode be used only for patients in whom other local destructive therapy is contraindicated, rather than applying it to any and all individuals with atypical or abnormal Pap smears. Such a treatment protocol may be cost-effective and safe.

SPECIAL TREATMENT CONSIDERATIONS

Treatment of Extensive Squamous Intraepithelial Lesions

Perhaps because of the lessened efficacy of cryosurgery in the treatment of women with large transformation zones, it has become a common practice of many physicians to use or recommend laser vaporization for patients not considered to be good candidates for cryosurgery. Prendiville and Turner (1991), however, noted that loop diathermy may be used to excise widespread SIL. A large transformation zone can be removed in multiple segments. Rollerball diathermy coagulation also can supplement the loop excision and decreases bleeding. Gunasekera and coworkers (1990), comparing laser evaporation with loop diathermy conization, stated that the latter causes less delayed hemorrhage and less patient discomfort, significantly decreases operative time, is associated with less capital expenditure, and presents no hazard to the eyesight of the surgeon. Loop conization procedures are not associated with interference with fertility or with pregnancy outcome (Keijser and associates 1992, Bigrigg and coworkers 1991). It is probable that loop excision conization will replace the CO_2 laser in the treatment of most women who have SIL.

Delayed hemorrhage is rare with loop conization and may relate to the presence of local infection and in some degree to the size of the excised specimen. The local use of postexcision ferric subsulfate paste decreases the role of immediate bleeding. Wright (1992a) reported delayed bleeding in fewer than 2% of patients and cervical stenosis in fewer than 1%, figures similar to those observed in the colposcopy clinic at the University of Alabama at Birmingham.

TRACHELECTOMY IN ELDERLY PATIENTS

Krebs and colleagues (1985) addressed the subject of diagnosis and treatment of higher grade SIL in elderly women. They indicate that with advancing age and atrophy, not only is colposcopy more difficult but traditional conization can be extremely difficult. They suggest that partial trachelectomy might be the treatment method of choice in elderly women who have a small, atrophic cervix. This procedure can be performed on an outpatient basis or during a short hospital stay, provides a sufficiently large specimen to reduce the incidence or risk of positive cervical margins, and decreases the need for additional therapy. In this clinical situation, the cervix is usually stenotic and short and does not easily accept a tandem for brachytherapy. Therefore, performing a trachelectomy, with a resulting diagnosis of early invasive cancer, does not necessarily compromise a chance for cure, even if additional therapy is necessary.

Treatment of Adenocarcinoma In Situ

Hopkins and associates (1988) reviewed the clinical findings and pathologic data of 18 women having adenocarcinoma in situ (AIS). Cone biopsy margins accurately predicted the presence or absence of disease in 10 of 12 subsequent hysterectomy specimens. There was a recurrence in one patient, who died of the cancer 16 years after the original diagnosis. Muntz and coworkers (1992) reported 46 women with AIS. All individuals had previous abnormal Papanicolaou smears, although AIS or adenocarcinoma cells were recognized in only 12 (26%); half (23 women) had coexistent SIL (21 patients) or squamous microinvasive (MIV) (two patients). Although 13% of those with reports of negative cone margins had residual AIS in the hysterectomy specimens, 18 other women (39%) were treated exclusively by conization; all remained relapse-free after a median follow-up of 2.5 years.

When the diagnosis of AIS is confirmed by consultation with an experienced gynecologic pathologist, conization (with negative margins) or total hysterectomy represents adequate therapy. If any cervical stromal invasion is present, more aggressive treatment (possibly including radical hysterectomy and pelvic lymphadenectomy, or alternatively, radiation therapy) should be considered.

Treatment of Microinvasive Squamous Lesions

HYSTERECTOMY VERSUS CONIZATION AS TREATMENT

The proposed operative treatment of early microinvasion (FIGO stage IA1, in which invasive nests of tumor are in continuity with an in situ lesion or separated by no more than 1 mm from the surface or crypt basement membrane) is conventional (total) hysterectomy. In selected patients who desire conservation of fertility, conization of the cervix may be recommended. Kolstad (1989) reported 232 patients with early microinvasion; only 3 developed local recurrence and none died from cancer. He concludes that conization alone is adequate therapy for these lesions if the cone margins are negative. He believes that lesions invading up to 3 mm can be safely and successfully treated in the same manner (conization with free margins or hysterectomy), although he acknowledges that most clinicians prefer to perform a total hysterectomy, even when conization margins are negative. He bases his recommendation on follow-up data from 224 patients who had tumor infiltration from 1 to 2.9 mm. Only 1 of these patients (0.4%) died of cancer. This patient, who had a 2-mm invasive lesion, had a free cone margin but had vessel invasion on the cone; she had a recurrence in the pelvis at 5 years and died a year later.

Burghardt and colleagues (1991) addressed the use of conization as treatment of microinvasive carcinoma of the cervix (according to the FIGO definitions). Ninety-three women who underwent conization for stage IA1 (early stromal invasion—protrusions of tongues of invasion from the base of a carcinoma in situ) were followed for a minimum of 5 years. Disease recurred in 1 patient, who died (1.1%). In contrast, when conization was used as the sole therapy in 18 women having stage IA2 (microcarcinoma—invasion to a depth of 5 mm, with a horizontal width measurement not to exceed 7 mm), disease recurred in 3 women (16.7%) and 1 (5.6%) died of disease. An increased risk of recurrence or death from disease after conservative treatment of lesions invading 3 to 5 mm in depth is suggested by Burghardt and associates' report.

The Society of Gynecologic Oncologists' (SGO) 1974 definition of microinvasion (invasion below the basement membrane ≤3 mm without lymphvascular space [LVS] involvement) is used in the United States in preference to the FIGO definition (see Table 3-2 in Chap. 3). Women whose cancers conform to this definition are commonly treated with abdominal hysterectomy, which also allows pelvic node sampling if enlarged nodes are encountered. If tumor is found to involve any pelvic node, the surgical procedure may be extended to conform to the class II hysterectomy (Piver and coworkers 1974) with complete pelvic lymphadenectomy. If the nodes are not suspicious, a total hysterectomy should be adequate as treatment. We recommend that conization as treatment should be used selectively in women with lesions invading no more than 3 mm (SGO definition). The potential role for laparoscopically assisted hysterectomy and lymph node assessment in this clinical situation remains to be determined.

The 1985 FIGO definition of stage IA2 cervical cancer specifies that microscopically measurable lesions should not exceed 7 mm in width or 5 mm in depth of invasion. Copeland and associates (1992) summarized the data from the literature and performed a retrospective review of 180 patients having superficially invasive

(0 to 5 mm) squamous cell carcinoma. They reported a 0.3% risk of pelvic node metastasis in individuals without LVS invasion whose lesions invaded 3 mm or less. In a summary of the literature (Table 4-10), they reported that LVS invasion increased the risk of node metastases (2.6%) and recurrence (4%); it was not a significant factor in overall outcome in some series in which no patients died from recurrent disease. Copeland and colleagues concluded that lesions invading no more than 3 mm without LVS invasion (SGO definition) should be treated by total hysterectomy because the risk of recurrence and of pelvic node metastasis with these lesions is less than 1% for both. With informed consent, patients with superficial tumors that fall within the SGO definition might be treated by conization alone if they desire to retain fertility, provided the cone margins are negative. Morris and coworkers (1993) also reported the safety of conization as treatment for selected patients with invasive lesions 0.5 to 2.8 mm. A modified radical hysterectomy and pelvic lymphadenectomy is recommended for the other patients in the IA2 category, in which the SGO definition is exceeded by depth of invasion or LVS involvement.

Tsukamoto and associates (1989) addressed the problem of the FIGO definition of stage IA and attempted to retrospectively reclassify 118 of their patients using the FIGO definition. They concluded that the FIGO definition is vague and that the border between stages IA1 and IA2 is confusing. They proposed that lesions having 3 mm or less stromal invasion with-

TABLE 4-10
Cumulative Data Comparing Recurrences and Pelvic Node Metastases

PATHOLOGIC GROUPS	RECURRENCES		PELVIC NODE METASTASES	
	(n)	(%)	(n)	(%)
≤3 mm				
VS−	4/453	(0.9)*	1/339	(0.3)†
VS+	4/99	(4)	1/63	(2.6)
>3, ≤5 mm				
VS−	0/88	(0)‡	7/106	(6.6)§
VS+	3/33	(9.1)	2/51	(3.9)

*P>.05, ns.
†P>.05, ns.
‡P<.05.
§P>.05, ns.
VS+, with vascular space involvement; *VS−*, without vascular space involvement.

Copeland LJ, Silva EG, Gershenson DM, Morris M, Young DC, Wharton JT. Superficially invasive squamous cell carcinoma of the cervix. Gynecol Oncol 1992;45:307.

TABLE 4-11
Choice of Operative Procedure for Cervical Squamous Neoplasms Diagnosed
by Conization

HISTOLOGIC FINDINGS	TERMINOLOGY	RECOMMENDED PROCEDURE
Stromal invasion: to 1 mm as isolated projections arising at base of CIS or dysplasia	Focal microinvasion (early stromal invasion)	Total hysterectomy (abdominal or vaginal) or Therapeutic conization (selected patients)*
Stromal invasion: to 3 mm	Microinvasion	Abdominal, hysterectomy† Node assessment (optional)
Stromal invasion: 3–5 mm	Microcarcinoma	Class II (modified) radical hysterectomy Pelvic node dissection
Stromal invasion: >5 mm	Invasive carcinoma	Class III (standard) radical hysterectomy Aortic node assessment Pelvic node dissection

*Implies free margins on conization specimen.
†If lymphvascular spaces are involved by tumor, class II (modified) radical hysterectomy recommended.
CIS, carcinoma in situ.

Modified from Shingleton HM, Orr JW Jr. Cancer of the cervix: diagnosis and treatment. New York: Churchill Livingstone, 1987:135.

out LVS involvement and confluency be identified within FIGO stage IA1 and be treated by conservative means.

Because of the clinical problems associated with the FIGO definition, we believe that it will undergo further refinement. Because the SGO definition has stood the test of time and protects the patient, we propose a treatment schema (Table 4-11) for the selection of the proper operative procedure for women who have superficial cervical cancers. We recognize that in some instances, however, patient treatment and selection must be individualized.

Treatment of Microinvasive Adenocarcinoma

This clinical entity is not well defined and there are essentially no data available to suggest the use, safety, or efficacy of less than radical treatment. If surgery is the selected treatment, a modified radical hysterectomy and pelvic lymphadenectomy should be performed. In older women or those who are not deemed good surgical candidates, cervical irradiation might be used, with or without external radiotherapy to the pelvic lymph nodes.

In the event that adenocarcinoma with definite stromal invasion is encountered on a total hysterectomy specimen, further treatment of the pelvic nodes and the parametrial tissues should be considered. This may be achieved by reoperation, removal of the medial parametrium, and dissection of the pelvic lymph nodes (Orr and colleagues 1986) or by the delivery of postoperative radiotherapy to the central and lateral pelvis.

PSYCHOLOGICAL IMPACT OF ABNORMAL PAPANICOLAOU SMEARS

McDonald and associates (1989) discussed the psychological effect of abnormal Papanicolaou smears, which is usually overlooked by most authors. When informed of an abnormal pap smear, most women believe that they have cancer. This belief and the attendant fear of future suffering and death often influences their acceptance of medical care. These investigators followed 20 patients (ranging in age from 15 to 40 years) through diagnosis and treatment; self-esteem was low and anxiety was high during both diagnosis and therapy. Anxiety about the medical condition of the women was shared by their sexual partners. The treating physician should assume that this process occurs in all women who have SIL and should always take time to address patient concerns and allay anxiety.

References

Abdul-Karim FW, Fu YS, Reagan JW, Wentz WB. Morphometric study of intraepithelial neoplasia of the uterine cervix. Obstet Gynecol 1982;60:210.

Alvarez RD, Helm CW, Edwards RP, et al. Prospective randomized trial of LLETZ versus laser ablation in patients with cervical intraepithelial neoplasia. Gynecol Oncol 1994;52:175.

Andersch B, Moinian M. Diagnostic and therapeutic viewpoints on cervical intraepithelial neoplasia. 10-year follow-up of a conization material. Gynecol Obstet Invest 1982;13:193.

Andersen ES, Husth M. Cryosurgery for cervical intraepithelial neoplasia: 10-year follow-up. Gynecol Oncol 1992; 45:240.

Anderson MC, Hartley RB. Cervical crypt involvement by intraepithelial neoplasia. Obstet Gynecol 1980;55:546.

Anderson MC. Should conization by hot loop or laser replace cervical biopsy? J Gynecol Surg 1991;7:191.

Arof HM, Gerbie MV, Smeltzer J. Cryosurgical treatment of cervical intraepithelial neoplasia: four-year experience. Am J Obstet Gynecol 1984;150:865.

Baggish MS, Dorsey JH, Adelson M. A ten-year experience treating cervical intra-epithelial neoplasia with the CO_2 laser. Am J Obstet Gynecol 1989;161:60.

Bekassy Z, Alm P, Grundsell H, Larsson G, Aastedt B. Laser miniconization in mild and moderate dysplasia of the uterine cervix. Gynecol Oncol 1983;15:357.

Bellina JH, Ross LF, Voros JI. Colposcopy and the CO_2 laser for treatment of cervical intraepithelial neoplasia. An analysis of seven years' experience. J Reprod Med 1983;28:147.

Benedet JL, Miller DM, Nickerson KG, Anderson GH. The results of cryosurgical treatment of cervical intraepithelial neoplasia at one, five and ten years. Am J Obstet Gynecol 1987;157:268.

Benedet JL, Miller DM, Nickerson KG. Conservative treatment for cervical intra-epithelial neoplasia (CIN) (abstract). 7th International Meeting Gynecol Oncol, Venice, Italy, April 14–18, 1991. Eur J Gynaecol Oncol 1991;XII(Suppl):90.

Bigrigg MA, Codling BW, Pearson P, Read MD, Swingler GR. Colposcopic diagnosis and treatment of cervical dysplasia at a single clinic visit. Experience of low-voltage diathermy loop in 1000 patients. Lancet 1990; 336:229.

Boyes DA, Worth AJ, Fidler HK. The results of treatment of 4389 cases of preclinical cervical squamous carcinoma. J Obstet Gynaecol Br Commonw 1970;77:769.

Brown JV, Peters WA, Corwin DJ. Invasive carcinoma after cone biopsy for cervical intraepithelial neoplasia. Gynecol Oncol 1991;40:25.

Bryson SCP, Lenehan P, Lickrish GM. The treatment of grade 3 cervical intraepithelial neoplasia with cryotherapy: an 11-year experience. Am J Obstet Gynecol 1985;151:201.

Burghardt E, Girardi F, Lahousen, Pickel H, Tamussino K. Microinvasive carcinoma of the uterine cervix (International Federation of Gynecology and Obstetrics Stage IA). Cancer 1991;67:1037.

Burke L. The use of the carbon dioxide laser in the therapy of cervical intraepithelial neoplasia. Am J Obstet Gynecol 1982;144:337.

Byrne P, Ogueh O, Wilson J, Sant-Cassia LJ. Outpatient loop diathermy cone biopsy (abstract). 7th Int'l Mtg Gynecol Oncol, Venice, Italy, April 14–18, 1991. Eur J Gynaecol Oncol 1991;XII:95.

Cartier R (ed). Practical colposcopy. Lausanne: IRL Imprimenies Reunies, 1984:100.

Chanen W, Rome RM. 1983 electrocoagulation diathermy for cervical dysplasia and carcinoma in situ: a 15-year survey. Obstet Gynecol 1983;61:673.

Chanen W. The efficacy of electrocoagulation diathermy performed under local anaesthesia for the eradication of precancerous lesions of the cervix. Aust NZ J Obstet Gynaecol 1989;29:189.

Coney P, Walton LA, Edelman DA, Fowler WC Jr. Cryosurgical treatment of early cervical intraepithelial neoplasia. Obstet Gynecol 1983;62:463.

Copeland LJ, Silva EG, Gershenson DM, Morris M, Young DC, Wharton JT. Superficially invasive cell carcinoma of the cervix. Gynecol Oncol 1992;45:307.

Creasman WT, Hinshaw WM, Clarke-Pearson DL. Cryosurgery in the management of cervical intraepithelial neoplasia. Obstet Gynecol 1984;63:145.

Creasman WT, Rutledge F. Preoperative evaluation of patients with recurrent carcinoma of the cervix. Gynecol Oncol 1972;1:111.

Deigan EA, Carmichael JA, Ohlke ID, Karchmar J. Treatment of cervical intraepithelial neoplasia with electrocautery: a report of 776 cases. Am J Obstet Gynecol 1986;154:255.

Draeby-Kristiansen J, Garsaae M, Bruun M, Hansen K. Ten years after cryosurgical treatment of cervical intraepithelial neoplasia. Am J Obstet Gynecol 1991;165:43.

Evans AS, Monaghan JM. The treatment of cervical intraepithelial neoplasia using the carbon dioxide laser. Br J Obstet Gynaecol 1983;90:553.

Ferenczy A. Comparison of cryo and carbon dioxide laser therapy for cervical intraepithelial neoplasia. Obstet Gynecol 1985;66:793.

Fowler JF, Davos I, Leuchter RS, Lagasse LD. Effect of CO_2 laser conization of the uterine cervix on pathologic interpretation of cervical intraepithelial neoplasia. Obstet Gynecol 1992;79:693.

Fu YS, Reagan JW, Richart RM. Definition of precursors. Gynecol Oncol 1981;12:220.

Gad C. The management and natural history of severe dysplasia and carcinoma in situ of the uterine cervix. Br J Obstet Gynaecol 1976;83:554.

Gordon HK, Duncan ID. Effective destruction of cervical intraepithelial neoplasia (CIN) 3 at 100 using the SEMM cold coagulator: 14 years experience. Br J Obstet Gynaecol 1991;98:140.

Grundsell H, Alm P, Larsson G. 1983 cure rates after laser conization for early cervical neoplasia. Ann Chir Gynaecol Fenn 1983;72:218.

Gunasekera PC, Phipps JH, Lewis BV. Large loop excision of the trans-formation zone (LLETZ) compared to carbon dioxide laser in the treatment of CIN: a superior mode of treatment. Br J Obstet Gynaecol 1990;97:995.

Hannigan EV, Simpson JS, Dillard EA Jr, Dinh TV. Frozen section evaluation of cervical conization specimens. J Reprod Med 1986;31:11.

Hatch KD, Shingleton HM, Austin M, Soong S-J, Bradley DH. Cryosurgery of cervical intraepithelial neoplasia. Obstet Gynecol 1981;57:692.

Hellberg D, Nilsson S. 20-year experience of follow-up of the abnormal smear with colposcopy and histology and treatment by conization or cryosurgery. Gynecol Oncol 1990;38:166.

Higgins RV, van Nagell JR, Donaldson ES, et al. The efficacy of laser therapy in the treatment of cervical intraepithelial neoplasia. Gynecol Oncol 1990;36:79.

Hoffman MS, Collins E, Roberts WS, Fiorica JV, Gunasekaran S, Cavanagh D. Cervical conization with frozen section before planned hysterectomy. Obstet Gynecol 1993;82:394.

Hopkins MP, Roberts JA, Schmidt RW. Cervical adenocarcinoma in situ. Obstet Gynecol 1988;71:842.

Howell R, Hammond R, Pryse-Davies J. The histologic reliability of laser cone biopsy of the cervix. Obstet Gynecol 1991;77:905.

Jones HW III, Buller RE. The treatment of cervical intraepithelial neoplasia by cone biopsy. Am J Obstet Gynecol 1980;137:882.

Kaufman RH, Strama T, Norton PK, et al. Cryosurgical treatment of cervical intraepithelial neoplasia. Obstet Gynecol 1973;42:881.

Keijser KGG, Kenemans P, van der Zanden P. Diathermy loop excision in the management of cervical intraepithelial neoplasia: diagnosis and treatment in one procedure. Am J Obstet Gynecol 1992;166:1281.

Kolstad P. Follow-up study of 232 patients with stage Ia1 and 411 patients with stage Ia2 squamous cell carcinoma of the cervix (microinvasive carcinoma). Gynecol Oncol 1989;33:265.

Kolstad P, Klem V. Long term follow-up of 1121 cases of carcinoma-in-situ. Obstet Gynecol 1976;48:125.

Krebs H-B, Wilstrup MA, Wheelock JB. Partial trachelectomy in the elderly patient with abnormal cytology. Obstet Gynecol 1985;65:579.

Laedtke TW, Dignan M. Compliance with therapy for cervical dysplasia among women of low socioeconomic status. South Med J 1992;85:5.

Luesley DM, Redman CWE, Buxton EJ, Lawton FG, Williams DR. Prevention of post-cone biopsy cervical stenosis using a temporary cervical stent. Br J Obstet Gynaecol 1990;97:334.

McDonald TW, Neutens JJ, Fischer LM, Jessee D. Impact of cervical intraepithelial neoplasia diagnosis and treatment on self-esteem and body image. Gynecol Oncol 1989;34:345.

McIndoe WA, McLean MR, Jones RW, Mullins P. The invasive potential of carcinoma in situ of the cervix. Obstet Gynecol 1984;64:451.

Meandzija MP, Locher G, Jackson JD. CO_2 laser conization versus conventional conization: a clinico-pathologic appraisal. Lasers Surg Med 1984;4:139.

Mettlin C, Mikuta JJ, Natarajan N, Priore R, Murphy GP. Treatment and follow-up study of squamous cell carcinoma in situ of the cervix uteri. Surg Gynecol Obstet 1982;155:481.

Morris M, Mitchell MF, Silva EG, Copeland LJ, Gershenson DM. Cervical conization as definitive therapy for early invasive squamous carcinoma of the cervix. Gynecol Oncol 1993;51:193.

Muntz HG, Bell DA, Lage JM, Goff BA, Feldman S, Rice LW. Adenocarcinoma-in-situ of the uterine cervix. Obstet Gynecol 1992;80:935.

Nashiell K. Behavior of mild cervical dysplasia during long-term followup. Obstet Gynecol 1986;67:665.

Noda K. Follow-up study of cervical dysplasia. Nippon Sanka Fujinka Gakkai Zasshi 1966;18:875.

Orr JW Jr, Ball GC, Soong S-J, Hatch KD, Partridge EE, Austin JM. Surgical treatment of women found to have invasive cervix cancer at the time of total hysterectomy. Obstet Gynecol 1986;68:353.

Ortiz R, Newton M, Tsai A. Electrocautery treatment of cervical intraepithelial neoplasia. Obstet Gynecol 1973; 41:113.

Östör AG. Natural history of cervical intraepithelial neoplasia: a critical review. Int J Gynecol Pathol 1993;12:186.

Ostergard DR. Prediction of clearance of cervical intraepithelial neoplasia by conization. Obstet Gynecol 1980; 56:77.

Paraskevaidis E, Jandial L, Mann EM, Fisher PM, Kitchener HC. Pattern of treatment failure following laser for cervical intraepithelial neoplasia: implications for follow-up protocol. Obstet Gynecol 1991;78:80.

Pearl ML, Beretta S. Routine endometrial curettage is not indicated at the time of cervical cone biopsy. Surg Obstet Gynecol 1993;176:251.

Pearson SE, Whittaker J, Ireland D, Monaghan JM. Invasive cancer of the cervix after laser treatment. Br J Obstet Gynaecol 1989;96;486.

Piringer-Kuchinka Von A, Martin I, Kofler E. Zur Frage der biologischen wertigkeit und therapie des sogennanten präinvasive portiokarizinoms. Geburtshilfe Frauenheilkd 1956;16:971.

Piver MS, Rutledge F, Smith JP. Five classes of extended hysterectomy for women with cervical cancer. Obstet Gynecol 1974;44:265.

Popkin DR. Treatment of cervical intraepithelial neoplasia with the carbon dioxide laser. Am J Obstet Gynecol 1983;145:177.

Prendiville W, Turner M. Large loop excision of the transformation zone. Lancet 1991;337:618. Letter.

Richart RM, Sciana JJ. Treatment of cervical dysplasia by outpatient electrocauterization. Am J Obstet Gynecol 1968;101:200.

Savage EW, Matlock DL, Salem FA, Charles EH. The effect of endocervical gland involvement on the cure rates of patients with cervical intraepithelial neoplasia undergoing cryosurgery. Gynecol Oncol 1982;14:194.

Schantz A, Thormann L. Cryosurgery for dysplasia of the uterine ectocervix. A randomized study of the efficacy of the single- and double-freeze techniques. Acta Obstet Gynecol Scand 1984;63:417.

Schmidt C, Pretorius RG, Bonin M, Hanson L, Semrad N, Watring W. Invasive cervical cancer following cryotherapy for cervical intraepithelial neoplasia or human papillomavirus infection. Obstet Gynecol 1992;80:797.

Schuurmans SN, Ohlke ID, Carmichael JA. Treatment of cervical intraepithelial neoplasia with electrocautery: report of 426 cases. Am J Obstet Gynecol 1984;148:544.

Stanhope CR, Phibbs GD, Stuart GC, Reid R. Carbon dioxide laser surgery. Obstet Gynecol 1983;61:624.

Tabor A, Berget A. Cold knife and laser conization for cervical intraepithelial neoplasia. Obstet Gynecol 1990; 76:633.

Townsend DE. Cryosurgery for cervical intraepithelial neoplasia. Obstet Gynecol Surv 1979;34:838.

Tsukamoto N, Kaku T, Matsukuma K, et al. The problem of stage Ia (FIGO, 1985) carcinoma of the uterine cervix. Gynecol Oncol 1989;34:1.

van Lent M, Trimbos JB, Heintz AP, van Hall EV. Cryosurgical treatment of cervical intraepithelial neoplasia (CIN III) in 102 patients. Gynecol Oncol 1983;16:240.

Watchler SJ. Treatment of cervical intraepithelial neoplasia with the CO_2 laser: laser versus cryotherapy. A review of effectiveness and cost. Obstet Gynecol Surv 1984; 39:469.

Wright TC Jr, Gagnon S, Richart RM, Ferenczy A. Treatment of cervical intraepithelial neoplasia using the loop electrosurgical excision procedure. Obstet Gynecol 1992a;79:173.

Wright TC Jr, Richart RM, Ferenczy A, Koulos J. Comparison of specimens removed by CO_2 laser conization and the loop electrosurgical excision procedure. Obstet Gynecol 1992b;79:147.

Wright VC. Carbon dioxide laser surgery for cervical intraepithelial neoplasia. Lasers Surg Med 1984;4:145.

Cancer of the Cervix by Hugh M. Shingleton and James W. Orr, Jr.
J. B. Lippincott Company, Philadelphia, © 1995.

5

The Cytology and Histopathology of Cervical Cancer

Although identification of atypical cells that are exfoliated or scraped from malignant tumors is important as an indication for further evaluation of the gynecologic patient, an understanding of the histopathologic findings is necessary for optimal management of the patient with cancer. Most obstetric and gynecologic training programs include some exposure to gross and microscopic evaluation of surgical specimens. The ability to visualize what the pathologist has written and put it together with the clinical findings is most valuable, as is direct communication with the cytopathologist and surgical pathologist when reports are unclear or when the clinical picture differs from the pathologic findings. Although the material presented in this chapter represents only a summary of the most important features of the disease, it may act as a guide for decisions concerning individual patients.

NATURAL HISTORY

Henriksen, in his classic study (1960) detailing the distribution of the metastases in women dying of cancer of the cervix, stated that "cancer cells regardless of the site of the primary lesion, the histologic grade and the age and parity of the patient can spread in any direction. The direction and the degree of spread are not predictable. The anterior and posterior spread is almost as frequent as the lateral extension. Any attempt to remove all . . . . cancer bearing tissue must include these areas." Effective treatment strategies for cervical cancer can be developed only after an understanding is achieved of the various methods and routes of spread.

Paracervical and Parametrial Extension

The lateral spread of cervical cancer occurs through the cardinal ligament, and significant involvement of the medial portion of that ligament may result in ureteral obstruction and (if bilateral) uremia. Historically, uremia and hemorrhage have been the leading causes of death from the disease. In most cases, it is not likely that this results from direct contiguous extension of the tumor from the cervix through the cardinal ligament (Burghardt et al 1992). Tumor cells more commonly spread laterally by parametrial lymphatic vessels to expand and replace parametrial lymph nodes. Enlargement and confluence of these individual tumor masses in and adjacent to lymphatics and nodes results in shortening of the parametrial tissues, producing the palpable findings consistent with International Federation of Gynecology and Obstetrics [FIGO] stages IIB and IIIB disease (see Fig. 7-12 in Chap. 7).

Bladder and Rectal Involvement

The anterior or posterior spread of cervical cancer to the bladder and rectum in the absence of lateral parametrial disease is uncommon. As many as a third of patients with suspected parametrial involvement also have elevation of the bladder base, discovered by cystoscopy or computed tomography scans. One of 5 patients with clinical stage IIIB disease has biopsy-proven bladder invasion (Lifshitz et al 1990). A deep pouch of Douglas can represent an anatomic barrier to the direct posterior spread from the cervix to the rectum. Direct cervical tumor extension to the upper vagina, however, allows a more direct route for bladder and/or rectal involvement. Rectal involvement may also occur by posterolateral extension along the course of the uterosacral ligaments.

Vaginal Extension

As primary tumor volume increases and the cancer leaves the confines of the cervix, the upper vagina is frequently involved (50%). On rare occasions, noncontiguous vaginal extension occurs. In women undergoing radical hysterectomy, direct anterior extension through the vesicovaginal septum may be encountered and "clean" dissection of the bladder from the underlying tumor may be difficult or impossible. Tumor involvement of the posterior vagina less commonly interferes with surgical removal because the cul-de-sac is interposed between the upper third of the vagina and rectum. Microscopic involvement of the cul-de-sac peritoneum may explain positive washings from this area.

Endometrial Involvement

Endometrial involvement with cervical cancer occurs in 2% to 10% of cases (Perez et al 1977). Endometrial involvement is best appreciated in surgical patients when the entire uterus is available for study. Although ultrasonography or magnetic resonance imaging may be used to assess tumor volume and location in patients to be treated with radiation therapy, these studies have a low sensitivity rate; the difficulty of proving endometrial extension by curettage through a carcinomatous cervix is apparent in the absence of tumor within endometrial tissue. Therefore, the exact incidence and significance of tumor extension into the endometrial cavity is not known. Although some believe that endometrial extension has an adverse effect on prognosis (Noguchi et al 1983, Gonzales et al 1989), treatment is not altered with this finding. Most American gynecologists and radiotherapists make no attempt to determine endometrial extension as part of pretreatment evaluation, and it is not included in any of the contemporary staging systems.

Ovarian Metastasis

Ovarian involvement by cervical cancer is rare. Ovarian spread most likely occurs by way of the lymphatic connection between the uterus and the adnexal structures. In patients treated surgically (disease stage IB, IIA), ovarian metastases occur in fewer than 1% of women with squamous cell carcinoma and in slightly more than 1% with adenocarcinoma of the cervix (Reisinger 1991; see Table 7-7 in Chap. 7). Its rarity in women with FIGO stage I disease is such that routine removal

of the ovaries in young women is not advocated as part of surgical treatment. In women treated with radiation, the ovaries are usually within the treatment portals.

Peritoneal Involvement

Although Sotto and coworkers (1960) reported peritoneal involvement in a third of women who underwent autopsy after death from this disease, the risk of peritoneal involvement by cervical cancer at the time of initial treatment was not appreciated before the advent and use of surgical staging. Invasive tumor involving the endocervix, the posterior ectocervix, and/or posterior upper third of the vagina may directly extend to and through the peritoneum of the pouch of Douglas or uterine serosa. Malignant cells in peritoneal washings are reported in 0.3% to 12.6% of surgical patients (Hughes et al 1980, Kilgore 1984, Welander et al 1981, Abu-Ghazelah et al 1984, Imachi et al 1987, Delgado et al 1989). Peritoneal spread seems to be more a part of advanced (stages II and III) than of stage I disease (Imachi et al 1987). Most believe that positive cytology is associated with other poorrisk factors and is of little value as an independent prognostic factor.

Lymph Node Involvement

Lymph node involvement in squamous cell carcinoma or adenocarcinoma of the cervix follows an orderly and reasonably predictable pattern. The obturator, the external iliac, and the hypogastric nodes are commonly involved by the disease in descending order of incidence; the parametrial, inferior gluteal, and presacral nodes are less commonly involved. These groups, however, are rarely reported separately, and reports may not reflect the true incidence (Table 5-1). For reporting purposes, standard nomenclature is suggested in reference to lymph node drainage of cervical cancers (Fig. 5-1). The secondary nodes (common iliac, paraaortic) are rarely involved in the absence of involvement of the primary pelvic groups (Lifshitz et al 1990). The regional lymph nodes may serve as anatomic barriers to more distal spread of tumor cells. Cancer cells are captured in the subcapsular nodal sinuses, multiply, and may eventually replace the node (see Fig. 7-11 in Chap. 7), obstructing and leading to collateral or even retrograde lymph flow. Involvement of higher (secondary) nodes may occur by passage of tumor emboli by normal lymphatic flow or around the involved obstructed node through collateral lymph channels. Nodal involvement may also occur with retrograde lymphatic embolization. The inguinal nodes rarely contain metastatic tumor, attributable probably to no direct lymphatic drainage to them from the

TABLE 5-1
Incidence of Metastases to Pelvic Node Groups in Cancer of the Cervix

STUDY	YEAR	STAGE	PATIENTS (N)	COMMON ILIAC (%)	EXTERNAL ILIAC (%)	OBTURATOR (%)	HYPOGASTRIC (%)	PRESACRAL (%)	PARAMETRIAL (%)
Cherry, et al	1953	I, II	213	14	47	20	7	NS	NS
Liu, et al	1955	I, II	104	47	20.1	50	3.8	NS	NS
Plentl, et al*	1971	*	744	13	23	19	17	3.7	NS
Martimbeau, et al	1982	IB	120	27	48	25	NS	NS	NS
Kjorstad, et al	1984	IB	293	23	42	31.3	6	NS	NS
Burghardt, et al	1987	IB–II	565	NS	30	31	36	1.8	NS
Noguchi, et al	1987	IB–IIIB	627	NS	4.4	5	7	3.4	25
Ferraris, et al	1988	NS	402	3.6	17.9	35.7	7.1	1.8	NS

*Collected series, stage not specified.
NS, not stated.

cervix. With increasing cervical tumor growth, malignant cells gain access to adjacent cervical and parametrial lymphatic vessels; therefore, it is not surprising that as tumor volume increases, so does the percentage of involved regional nodes (see Fig. 7-10 in Chap. 7). Some (Berek 1985) believe that adenocarcinomas and mixed tumors metastasize earlier and at a higher rate and follow a more virulent course. Indeed, there is a trend toward higher recurrence rates in adenocarcinoma, compared with squamous cell carcinoma (see Table 7-17 in Chap. 7). Korhonen and Stenback (1984) and Berek and associates (1985) reported similar pelvic node metastasis rates in stage IB (4% and 6%, respectively; not different from matched squamous cell carcinoma patients) but their reported metastasis rates of 71% and 40%, respectively, for stage II adenocarcinomas suggest a higher risk of nodal metastases for that stage. Unfortunately, because of the small number of patients in most adenocarcinoma series, the question is unresolved. Berek and coworkers further observed a higher mortality rate (90%) for patients with adenocarcinoma metastatic to pelvic nodes when compared with squamous cell carcinoma patients with nodal metastases. We also have observed a high death rate for adenocarcinoma patients with nodal metastases and can offer no explanation for this apparent difference in curability of node-positive adenocarcinoma compared with squamous cell carcinoma, unless adjunctive pelvic radiation therapy is more effective in those with squamous cell lesions.

Paraaortic lymph node involvement varies also with clinical stage (Table 5-2). The percentage involvement within any one stage varies, perhaps because of comprehensiveness of node dissection and of lymph node examination by the pathologist. Once tumor has spread to the aortic nodes, further extension to the thoracic or scalene nodes in the left supraclavicular fossa may occur. Malignant nodes in the left neck are not uncommon in patients with clinically advanced or recurrent disease. The importance of evaluation of lymph nodes at this level before undertaking a radical operation is apparent.

Hematogenous Spread

Malignant cells are present in the circulatory system of most cancer patients and thought to be far more common than clinical metastases (Melamed 1992). Blood vessel invasion by tumor appears to occur almost exclusively through the venous system (Kindermann et al 1972). Cancer cells are also thought to enter the bloodstream by lymphatics through the thoracic ducts or by smaller lymphaticovenous communications (Fuchs 1965, Fisher et al 1968). Although metastases to virtually every area of the body have been reported and although one cannot be certain that older references quoting data from autopsy series refer exclusively to untreated patients, the most common areas for hematogenous spread may be the lung, liver, and bone (Table 5-3). The fate of most circulating tumor cells may be determined by the host immune response.

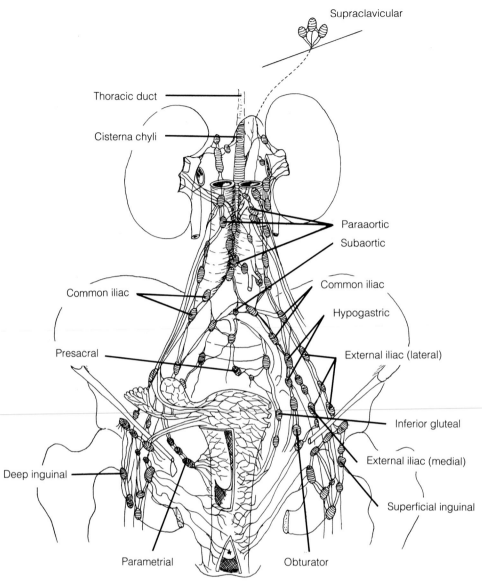

FIGURE 5-1. The lymphatic system of the female genital organs. (Adapted from Meigs JV [ed]. Surgical treatment of cancer of the cervix. New York: Grune & Stratton 1954:90, with permission.)

CYTOPATHOLOGY OF CERVICAL CANCER

Microscopic study of exfoliated cells and those scraped or brushed from the ectocervix or aspirated from the endocervical canal constitutes the basis of the Papanicolaou (Pap) smear. A technically good sample (appropriately spread on the slide, promptly fixed, well-stained, and carefully examined by a well-trained cytotechnologist–cytopathologist team) should be an integral part of every woman's health care. When abnormal cells are recognized, an attempt is made to classify them and the significance of those considered to be from high-grade squamous intraepithelial lesions or from malignant lesions should be determined by tissue evaluation (management of lesser degrees of atypia is discussed in Chap. 3).

The appearance of malignant cells, usually with a background of necrotic debris, blood, and inflammatory cells, suggests the diagnosis of carcinoma (Fig. 5-2). Identification of specific cell type (i.e., squamous cell or adenocarcinoma) is possible in well- and moderately well-differentiated lesions but often becomes more difficult in poorly differentiated tumors. Cyto-

TABLE 5-2
Incidence of Paraaortic Node Metastases by Stage

Study	Year	Stage IB Patients (n)	Stage IB Positive (%)	Stage IIA Patients (n)	Stage IIA Positive (%)	Stage IIB Patients (n)	Stage IIB Positive (%)	Stage III Patients (n)	Stage III Positive (%)	Stage IVA Patients (n)	Stage IVA Positive (%)
Nelson, et al	1977	—	—	16	12.5	47	14.9	39	38.0	—	—
Wharton, et al	1977	21	0	10	0	47	21.2	34*	32.3	8†	37.5
Sudarsanam, et al	1978	153	7.0	21	14.0	22	18.0	19	26.3	—	—
Buchsbaum	1979	16	25.0	4	0	15	6.7	104	32.7	10	40.0
Bonanno, et al	1980	—	—	23	4.0	73	12.0	52	31.0	3	33.0
Hughes, et al	1980	140	4.3	35	8.5	45	24.4	96	23.9	23	43.5
Lagasse, et al	1980	143	5.6	22	18.2	58	32.8	63	30.2	3	33.0
Ballon, et al	1981	22	23.0	16	19.0	32	19.0	24	16.7	—	—
Chung, et al	1981	110	4.5	15	6.7	17	17.6	14	42.9	3	66.6
Welander, et al	1981	14	28.6	22	22.7	41	19.5	38	26.3	12	33.3
Berman, et al	1984	158	5.1	25	12.0	240	16.7	135	25.0	—	—
Totals		777	7.2	209	12.0	637	18.5	618	28.5	62	40.3

*IIIA only
†IIIB and IV

Modified from Shingleton HM, Orr JW Jr. Cancer of the cervix: diagnosis and treatment. New York, Churchill Livingstone, 1987:121.

TABLE 5-3
Hematogenous Metastases in Cervical Carcinoma*

SITE	(%)
Lung	26.5
Liver	15.8
Bone	14.2
Bowel	8.2
Adrenal	3.8
Spleen	2.3
Brain	1.4

*Based on autopsy of 1093 patients

From Lifshitz S, Buchsbaum HJ. The spread of cervical carcinoma. In Lurain JR, Sciarra JJ (eds). Gynecology and obstetrics, vol 4. Philadelphia, JB Lippincott, 1990; with permission.

logic pattern indicates whether the cervix is the likely primary site. With a thorough clinical history and physical examination, invasive cervical carcinoma is diagnosed (or strongly suspected) before receipt of a cytology report. Thus, whereas some occult invasive cervical carcinomas are detected cytologically, the major value of cytology is for the detection of preinvasive or early invasive lesions and for surveillance of patients after treatment.

Relevant clinical data should accompany a Pap smear submitted for evaluation; for optimal patient management, it is essential that biopsy material be submitted to the same laboratory for smear–tissue correlation. Such correlation provides the pathologist with a check on the accuracy of his or her evaluation. It is important that the histologic and cytologic diagnoses agree. In most laboratories, follow-up of women

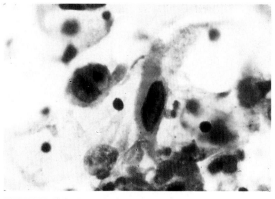

FIGURE 5-2. Papanicolaou smear from patient with invasive squamous cell carcinoma. Malignant squamous cells have a large irregular nucleus, increased nuclear cytoplasmic ratio, and either basophilic or eosinophilic cytoplasm. A normal superficial squamous epithelial cell is at the left. See Color Figure 5-2.

reported as having abnormal Pap smears is part of quality control. Rescreening and restudying any "false-negative" smears to determine the reason for a lack of correlation of smears and biopsies should be an integral part of good laboratory procedure.

HISTOPATHOLOGY OF CERVICAL CANCER

Malignant tumors usually arise from tissues found normally within the cervix, although there are some exceptions (Table 5-4).

Epithelial Tumors

SQUAMOUS CELL CARCINOMA

Squamous cell carcinoma is the most common cervical cancer, occurring in 85% to 90% of cases in most series (Table 5-5). Although most lesions are clinically evident, some occult carcinomas are not visible on routine examination. In early invasive tumors, only minimal superficial ulceration or induration may be evident (Fig. 5-3). Larger lesions may produce large ulcers, may distort the cervical portio by their expansion, or may extend into (and sometimes expand) the anatomic endocervix, producing the so-called "barrel-shaped" cervix (see Fig. 9-1B in Chap. 9). A few carcinomas are polypoid, with masses of various sizes extending from the cervical os.

Many invasive carcinomas retain elements of carcinoma in situ. Groups and strands of malignant squamous cells, with variable stromal and inflammatory response, extend into the cervical stroma, sometimes infiltrating as solid masses. The neoplastic squamous cells vary in their maturity; nuclei may be fairly uniform or pleomorphic, with variable mitotic activity (Fig. 5-4).

Traditionally, squamous cell carcinomas are divided into three grades. Grade 1 includes well-differentiated tumors with mature squamous cells, often keratinized, and with "pearl" formation (groups of malignant squamous cells surrounding a central accumulation of keratin; Fig. 5-5). Mitotic activity is low. Moderately well-differentiated carcinomas (grade 2) have higher mitotic activity and less well-differentiated cells, with more nuclear pleomorphism. Poorly differentiated carcinomas (grade 3) are composed of smaller cells with less cytoplasm and have higher mitotic activity, often with bizarre nuclei. Whether the grade of tumor can be correlated with prognosis is controversial (this is discussed further in Chaps. 7 and 8).

Other descriptive evaluations have been made in an effort to predict outcome by morphologic pattern. The best known is that of Wentz and Reagan (1959),

TABLE 5-4
Histologic Classification of Malignant Tumors
of the Cervix

EPITHELIAL TUMORS

Squamous cell carcinoma
  Keratinizing and nonkeratinizing
    carcinoma
  Verrucous carcinoma
  Papillary squamous cell carcinoma
Adenocarcinoma
  Mucinous (endocervical)
  Endometrioid
  Clear cell
  Papillary serous
  Mesonephric
  Minimal deviation adenocarcinoma
    (adenoma malignum)
Other malignant epithelial tumors
  Adenosquamous carcinoma
  Mixed epithelial tumors
  Glassy cell carcinoma
  Mucoepidermoid carcinoma
  Adenoid cystic carcinoma
  Adenoid basal carcinoma
Neuroendocrine
  Carcinoid
  Small cell carcinoma

MESENCHYMAL TUMORS

Leiomyosarcoma
Rhabdomyosarcoma
Chondrosarcoma
Osteosarcoma
Alveolar soft-part sarcoma
Angiosarcoma
Sarcoma botryoides

**MIXED EPITHELIAL AND MESENCHYMAL
TUMORS**

Adenosarcoma
Malignant mixed Müllerian tumor

**MISCELLANEOUS MALIGNANT
TUMORS**

Malignant melanoma
Lymphoma and leukemia
Endodermal sinus tumor
Primary cervical choriocarcinoma

SECONDARY TUMORS

Direct spread, e.g. endometrial metastatic,
  e.g. breast

Classification of Hazel Gore, MB, BS

who divided squamous cell carcinomas into large cell keratinizing, large cell nonkeratinizing, and small cell types. In the large cell keratinizing type, the groups of squamous cells form epithelial pearls. Mitotic activity tends to be low. Large cell nonkeratinizing squamous cell carcinomas are formed by groups of malignant squamous cells, often with individual cell keratinization but without pearl formation. Cells tend to be uniform, with prominent mitotic activity. Squamous cell carcinomas of the small cell type (said to comprise about 5% of tumors; Wentz et al 1959) are composed of groups of small squamous cells, sometimes with keratinization and without pearl formation and with high mitotic activity (Fig. 5-6). Because these tumors must be distinguished from the small cell carcinomas of neuroendocrine type, use of the term "small cell," applied to a subdivision of squamous cell carcinoma, leads to confusion. Although small cell tumors generally are thought to be associated with reduced survival rates (van Nagell et al 1971, Silva et al 1984, Yoshida et al 1984, Randall et al 1986, Miller et al 1991), the categorization of the large cell tumors by keratin status is clinically irrelevant because there is no universal agreement on the prognostic significance of the Wentz-Reagan classification and therapeutic decisions do not require its use (Beecham et al 1978, Will'en et al 1982, Shingleton et al 1987, Delgado et al 1990).

Verrucous carcinoma. Verrucous carcinoma (Fig. 5-7) is a rare warty fungating tumor, composed of well-differentiated papillary squamous strands, without the central stromal core usually found in a condyloma. The tumors are often hyperkeratotic. There is little nuclear variation, mitotic activity is low, and there is no obvious stromal invasion at the base; should definite nests of invasive carcinoma be found in the stroma, such a tumor should not be classified as verrucous carcinoma. Although verrucous carcinomas often are clinically bulky tumors, superficial biopsies can appear histologically benign and may be easily confused with condyloma acuminatum. For this reason, it is important that the surgical pathologist be adequately appraised of the suspicious clinical nature of such lesions. Partridge and colleagues (1980) noted that these tumors cause local destruction but rarely metastasize. Okagaki (1984), using DNA hybridization techniques, confirmed that verrucous carcinomas are associated with human papillomavirus (HPV) infection. Tiltman and Atad (1982) and Raheja and coworkers (1983) reported cases involving the endometrial cavity; Raheja's case is further noteworthy because there was no visible exophytic lesion on the cervix, the entire lesion being confined within the endocervix and endometrium.

The treatment of choice for verrucous carcinoma is surgical, with wide excision in the form of hysterectomy or extended hysterectomy considered sufficient

TABLE 5-5
Percentage of Adenocarcinomas or Mixed Tumors

STUDY	YEAR	PATIENTS WITH INVASIVE CANCER OF CERVIX	ADENOCARCINOMA OR MIXED TUMORS (%)
Anderson, et al	1976	661	4.0
Kjorstad	1977	2002	5.4
Beecham, et al	1978	245	15.0
van Nagell, et al	1979	526	8.4
Benedet, et al	1980	241	18.1
Volteranni, et al	1980	417	9.1
Tamimi, et al	1982	520	12.7
Milsom, et al	1983	1081	6.2
Berek, et al	1985	560	18.2
Ireland, et al	1985	901	8.1
Shingleton, et al	1985	2211	9.9
TOTAL		9365	8.8%
Lee, et al	1989	954	8.7
Eifel, et al	1990	3176	10.6*
Ng, et al	1992	701	8.9
Favalli, et al	1993	819	8.3
Shingleton	1994	11,000	17.0
TOTAL		16,650	14.5%

*1965–1975, 8.6%; 1976–1984, 14.6%.

Modified from Shingleton HM, Orr JW Jr. Cancer of the cervix: diagnosis and treatment. New York, Churchill Livingstone, 1987:50.

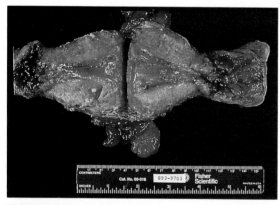

FIGURE 5-3. Squamous cell carcinoma involves both anterior and posterior endocervix and extends from lower segment/endocervical junction outward to the portio. There is some exophytic tumor in the proximal part but most is superficially ulcerated and appears to be largely endophytic. See Color Figure 5-3.

in most cases, depending on stage and volume of tumor. Primary treatment with radiation therapy has been questioned because of reports of radioresistance and malignant transformation by the irradiation (Kraus et al 1966, Gallousis 1972, Demian et al 1973, Vayrynen et al 1981). Some patients, however, have been treated successfully with radiation, and the validity of the observation regarding malignant transformation is in question (de Jesus et al 1990).

Papillary Squamous Cell Carcinoma. Papillary squamous cell carcinoma (PSCC) is composed of papillary folds, with central stromal core covered by poorly differentiated malignant squamous epithelium, histologically resembling bands of squamous cell carcinoma in situ. This malignant epithelium may invade the stroma of the core or the base of the tumor. If no invasion is identified, such a lesion is classified as papillary squamous cell carcinoma in situ. Note that in each of these papillary lesions, complete examination of the base of such lesions is most important in determining invasion. Therapy for PSCC is the same as for other squamous carcinomas of equivalent clinical stage (Ran-

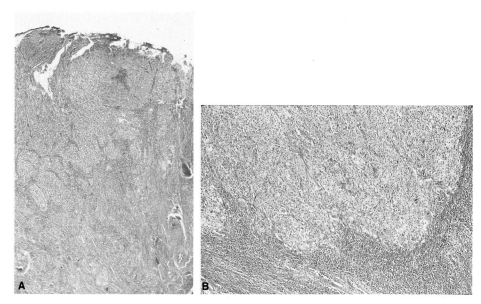

FIGURE 5-4. (**A**) In this invasive squamous cell carcinoma, groups of malignant squamous cells are extending into the cervical stroma. (**B**) An inflammatory response is evident at the infiltrating margin. See Color Figure 5-4.

dall et al 1986). The importance in making the diagnosis is to distinguish it from verrucous carcinoma.

ADENOCARCINOMA

Adenocarcinoma is a neoplasm of the endocervical epithelium, although vestigial remnants of the mesonephric duct are thought to produce a few of these tumors. The incidence of adenocarcinoma is less than that of squamous cell carcinoma (see Table 5-5), yet it may be increasing in incidence. A variety of histologic patterns has been described.

Mucinous Adenocarcinoma. Mucinous adenocarcinoma is the most common pattern, usually resembling endocervical epithelium, with all degrees of differentiation (Fig. 5-8). The glandular pattern may be complex or even papillary. Some mucinous carcinomas

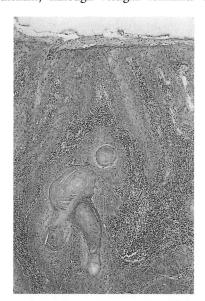

FIGURE 5-5. Within the invasive squamous cell carcinoma is a large lobulated mass of keratinizing squamous cells with central keratinization, a so-called epithelial pearl. See Color Figure 5-5.

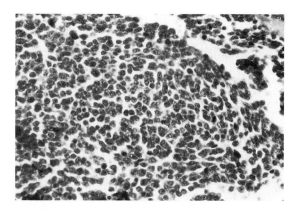

FIGURE 5-6. Classic small cell carcinoma, formed by fairly uniform small cells with high nucleus-cytoplasm ratio, histologically similar to small cell carcinoma of the lung. See Color Figure 5-6.

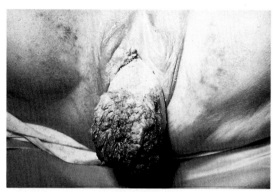

FIGURE 5-7. Verrucous carcinoma (occurring with uterine procidentia) with a fungating warty appearance. See Color Figure 5-7.

resemble intestinal epithelium and include goblet cells and (in less well-differentiated tumors) signet ring cells; such tumors may be difficult to distinguish from gastrointestinal tumors metastatic to the cervix.

Endometrioid Carcinoma. Endometrioid carcinoma is histologically indistinguishable from endometrial adenocarcinoma. Whether tumors of this pattern are derived from ectopic endometrial glands in the cervix, from endometriosis, or from a metaplastic change in endocervical mucosa is unclear. Endometrioid carcinoma should be distinguished from endometrial adenocarcinoma extending to endocervix if possible.

Clear Cell Adenocarcinoma. Clear cell adenocarcinoma may have a papillary, microcystic, tubular, or solid pattern in which cells have clear or finely granular eosinophilic cytoplasm, sometimes with hobnail

appearance (Fig. 5-9). The pattern is similar to such tumors in the endometrium, ovary, and vagina.

Papillary Serous Carcinoma. Papillary serous carcinoma is another histologic pattern, with stromal cores in papillary processes covered by a layer of atypical cells, sometimes resembling those in borderline serous tumors of the ovary and serous tumors of the endometrium and sometimes approaching a "hobnail" type.

Mesonephric Adenocarcinoma. Mesonephric adenocarcinoma is extremely rare. When such a tumor is considered, the most important problem is distinguishing it from florid mesonephric hyperplasia; such a distinction may not be made until the entire cervix has been evaluated after hysterectomy.

Adenoma Malignum. Adenoma malignum (or minimal deviation adenocarcinoma) of the uterine cervix is a rare variant of well-differentiated adenocarcinoma, with a deceptively benign-appearing histologic pattern. It is reported to represent 1% of cervical adenocarcinomas (Kaminski et al 1983). In such tumors, the cervix may have intact surface epithelium. Microscopically, irregular glands lined by mucin-containing cells having basal nuclei are scattered through the stroma, usually with a stromal inflammatory response. Mitoses are present but rare. There may be vascular or perineural invasion, and the malignant glands may extend to the uterine serosa or into the parametrial tissue (Gilks et al 1989). Because most of the patients reported were diagnosed with advanced stage disease (Kaku et al 1983, Kaminski et al 1983, Podczaski et al 1991), determination of the clinical behavior of these tumors is difficult. Women with this diagnosis are treated stage for stage, as with any other adenocarcinoma.

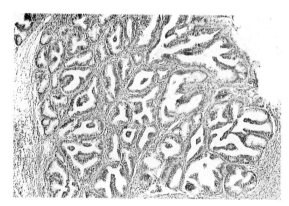

FIGURE 5-8. Well-differentiated adenocarcinoma of mucinous (endocervical) type. See Color Figure 5-8.

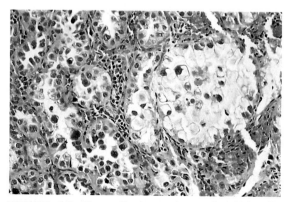

FIGURE 5-9. Clear cell adenocarcinoma, in which cells have clear or finely granular cytoplasm; some cells are of hobnail type, in which hyperchromatic nuclei surrounded by very scanty cytoplasm push into the gland lumen. See Color Figure 5-9.

SIGNIFICANCE OF HISTOLOGIC PATTERNS IN ADENOCARCINOMA

In our original review (Shingleton et al 1981) and follow-up publication (Kilgore et al 1988), we concluded that the varied patterns of adenocarcinoma had little prognostic significance. Tumor volume and to a lesser degree, tumor grade, correlated best with survival. These studies, which used matched squamous cell carcinoma controls, failed to demonstrate a difference in survival between surgically treated women with either stage IB adenocarcinoma or stage IB squamous cell carcinoma. The rates of pelvic node metastases for the two tissue types were identical.

OTHER MALIGNANT EPITHELIAL TUMORS

Adenosquamous Carcinoma. Adenosquamous carcinoma refers to a primary carcinoma with malignant-appearing glandular and squamous cell elements. Adenocarcinoma with histologically benign squamous differentiation is *not* adenosquamous carcinoma.

Mixed Epithelial Tumors. In situ or invasive squamous cell carcinoma and adenocarcinoma may coexist as separate lesions or may collide, resulting in a combined lesion with persisting distinct adenocarcinomatous and squamous cell components. This is better considered as two tumors and when "colliding" is better considered as a collision tumor (Fig. 5-10).

Maier and Norris (1980), reviewing 389 primary adenocarcinomas of the cervix at the Armed Forces Institute of Pathology, reported a 43% association of cervical intraepithelial neoplasia and cervical adenocarcinomas (Fig. 5-11A). A third of the patients in our series of cervical adenocarcinoma had a clearly recognizable squamous cell carcinoma (Shingleton et al 1981), the same incidence reported by Yajima and associates (1984) for adenosquamous carcinoma (see Fig. 5-11B).

Glassy Cell Carcinoma. Glassy cell carcinoma was first described by Glucksmann and Cherry (1956), and they initially considered it to be a variant of poorly differentiated adenosquamous carcinoma. In this rare tumor (perhaps representing 2% to 3% of adenocarcinomas), cells are large and contain a distinctive "ground glass" or granular cytoplasm, a distinct nuclear membrane, and a large nucleus with one or more prominent nucleoli. The surrounding cervical stroma may be densely infiltrated by inflammatory cells, usually including numerous eosinophils and plasma cells. Not all pathologists agree that these are characteristic diagnostic features. Poor fixation of nonkeratinizing squamous cell carcinoma and pale staining of the tissues may obscure classic findings and such tumors may then resemble "glassy cell" tumors. Whether the prognosis of glassy cell tumors is different from other poorly differentiated carcinomas is debatable because of the diagnostic difficulties and its rarity.

Mucoepidermoid Carcinoma. Mucoepidermoid carcinoma, a form of adenosquamous cancer, is squamous cell carcinoma that contains foci of pale mucin-containing cells, demonstrated by mucin stains. Yajima and coworkers (1984) observed a positive mucin reaction without glandular structure in a third of their reported adenosquamous carcinomas. They recommended that invasive lesions having less than 5% glandular structure and a negative mucin reaction be classified as squamous cell carcinoma, that those with more than 80% glandular structure be classified as adenocarcinoma, and that the remainder be called "mixed." It is unclear whether mucoepidermoid cancers have a worse prognosis than do pure squamous cell tumors; thus, the need to report it as a separate entity is in doubt.

CLINICAL BEHAVIOR OF ADENOSQUAMOUS CARCINOMA

The clinical behavior of these tumors is controversial. Wheeless and colleagues (1970) and Julian and associates (1977) observed that stage by stage, adenosquamous carcinomas of the cervix carry a poorer 5-year survival than SCC. We have not confirmed this in the Alabama material. Kilgore and coworkers (1988), in a surgical series of the Alabama experience, and Randall and associates (1988), in a radiation therapy series, actually reported better survival for this histologic subtype as compared to SCC or pure adenocarcinoma.

Adenoid Cystic Carcinoma. Adenoid cystic carcinoma has a cribriform or cylindromatous pattern and

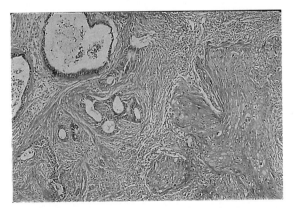

FIGURE 5-10. Adenocarcinoma and invasive squamous cell carcinoma, growing as two separate tumors. See Color Figure 5-10.

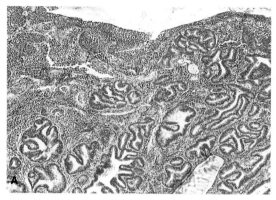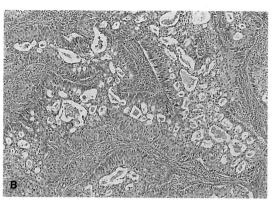

FIGURE 5-11. (A) Well-differentiated adenocarcinoma of endometrioid type is invading the endocervical stroma, whereas on the surface there is carcinoma in situ, which also involves some relatively superficial clefts. These are two separate tumors. **(B)** Adenosquamous carcinoma with small glandular spaces and malignant squamous epithelial component. See Color Figure 5-11.

small basaloid cells with scanty cytoplasm. Within solid nests of these cells are cystic spaces of varying size, often containing hyaline eosinophilic material (Fig. 5-12). Association of this pattern with ordinary adenocarcinoma, confirmed by immunohistochemical findings; the less frequent finding of myoepithelial elements, compared with adenoid cystic tumors in other sites; and ultrastructural studies (Shingleton et al 1981) indicate that these are adenocarcinomas with adenoid cystic differentiation and different from primary tumors of similar appearance occurring in the head and neck. Such tumors are thought to behave more aggressively than classic adenocarcinoma (Fowler et al 1978, Hoskins et al 1979), perhaps because of early lymphvascular space extension. Fowler and associates indicated that such tumors are aggressive; for instance, lung metastases were reported in almost half of the 29 patients accumulated from the literature. The increased rate of metastasis is possibly best explained by this pattern occurring as a component of poorly differentiated adenosquamous carcinomas.

Adenoid Basal Carcinoma. Adenoid basal carcinoma is composed of round to oval branching nests of small regular cells resembling those of basal cell carcinoma of the skin. There are only rare gland-like spaces, the hyaline material of the adenoid cystic carcinoma is not present, and there are rare mitoses. Tumors with a pure adenoid basal pattern are thought to be slow-growing and only simple hysterectomy is required as treatment (van Dinh et al 1985). Rare aggressive adenoid basal carcinomas with myxomatous stromal response have been described.

NEUROENDOCRINE TUMORS

Carcinoid Tumor of the Cervix. Carcinoid tumor of the cervix (adenocarcinoma with features of carcinoid tumor) differs from typical carcinoids of the gastrointestinal tract, and it is not clear whether a pure carcinoid exists. These tumors are composed of sheets of small cells, sometimes including gland lumina. None of the cases have been associated with carcinoid syndrome, although a variety of immunoreactive substances have been identified. Mitoses are numerous. There may be vascular invasion (such tumors are thought to be resistant to traditional modes of therapy).

Small Cell Carcinoma. Small cell carcinoma is composed of a uniform population of small cells resembling small cell carcinoma (oat cell carcinoma of the lung). About half to a third react to markers for neuroendocrine granules. Differential diagnosis may be difficult. Squamous or glandular differentiation should be minor or inconspicuous.

FIGURE 5-12. Adenoid cystic carcinoma with large groups of fairly uniform cells, in which are small round lumens. See Color Figure 5-12.

Mesenchymal Tumors

Stromal tumors similar to those occurring in the uterus may be found in the cervix. Criteria for diagnosis of leiomyosarcoma are similar to those in the myometrium. Rhabdomyosarcoma, chondrosarcoma, osteosarcoma, alveolar soft-part sarcoma, and angiosarcoma have been reported. Another type, the so-called endocervical stromal sarcoma, is thought to be histologically similar to endometrial stromal sarcoma. Such tumors, when noted in the cervix, may have extended from the endometrium.

Sarcoma botryoides is a type of embryonal rhabdomyosarcoma arising in the cervix of children and young women, forming multiple grape-like structures or polyps with a myxoid stroma.

Mixed Epithelial and Mesenchymal Tumors

ADENOSARCOMA

Adenosarcoma is comparable with the similar tumor arising in the endometrium. The tumor stroma is sarcomatous and there is a histologically benign epithelial component, although it appears to be an intrinsic part of the tumor.

MALIGNANT MIXED MÜLLERIAN TUMOR

When found in the cervix, mixed müllerian (mesodermal) tumor (carcinosarcoma) usually extends from an endometrial tumor. Rare examples of primary tumors of both homologous and heterologous types have been reported, and these tumors are said to have a poor prognosis.

Miscellaneous Malignant Tumors

PRIMARY MALIGNANT MELANOMA

Primary malignant melanoma of the cervix is extremely rare. The lesion usually contains dark brown pigment and is morphologically identical to melanoma elsewhere. Its pathogenesis is unclear, although various theories have been suggested.

LYMPHOMA

This entity may have its origin in the cervix, although such a lesion in the cervix is usually part of systemic spread.

PRIMARY CERVICAL CHORIOCARCINOMA

Primary cervical choriocarinoma is rare, most probably developing from a low implantation intrauterine pregnancy, a cervical pregnancy, or extension of molar trophoblast. Although it may occur primarily in the cervix, it does not arise from tissue intrinsic to the cervix. The histologic pattern is the same as that of choriocarcinoma elsewhere.

GERM CELL TUMORS

Germ cell tumors, including mature teratoma (Hanai et al 1981) and endodermal sinus tumor (Copeland et al 1985), have been described but rarely.

Metastatic Tumors

Most commonly, the cervix is involved by direct extension of tumor from an adjacent site such as endometrium, rectum, or bladder. Adenocarcinoma involving both endometrium and endocervix can present a problem in determining the primary site. A larger endometrial component, an endometrioid pattern, and coexistent endometrial hyperplasia support endometrial origin, whereas adenocarcinoma in situ of the cervix and cervical intraepithelial neoplasia favor a primary endocervical tumor. Lymphvascular spread may occur but is less common than direct extension. Metastases from distant foci are rare, most commonly from gastrointestinal tract, ovary, or breast (Mazur et al 1984). Metastatic tumor from an unrecognized primary breast carcinoma may present a diagnostic problem. Secondary lymphomatous involvement of the cervix and leukemic infiltration may also occur.

Korhonen and Stenback (1984), studying 208 patients with adenocarcinoma in the cervix, found in 45 of these patients that the adenocarcinoma was metastatic. The primary lesion location was endometrial (31), ovarian (6), fallopian tube (2), colon (5), or breast (1). Dollar and coworkers (1987) reported the Alabama experience of 40 patients with adenocarcinoma metastatic to the cervix and Lemoine and Hall (1986) reported 33 such cases.

PROCESSING THE PATHOLOGIC SPECIMENS

There are various reasons to evaluate the surgical specimen: to establish histologic tumor type, determine tumor extent, and document the presence or absence of involved surgical margins (Fig. 5-13A and B). If each of these is addressed, the method by which the specimen is examined cannot be criticized.

After excision, the surgical specimen should be delivered promptly to the pathologist for evaluation. Should the surgeon desire or need to see the specimen intraoperatively, the pathologist should be asked to open the specimen or there should be a prior under-

(text continues on page 86)

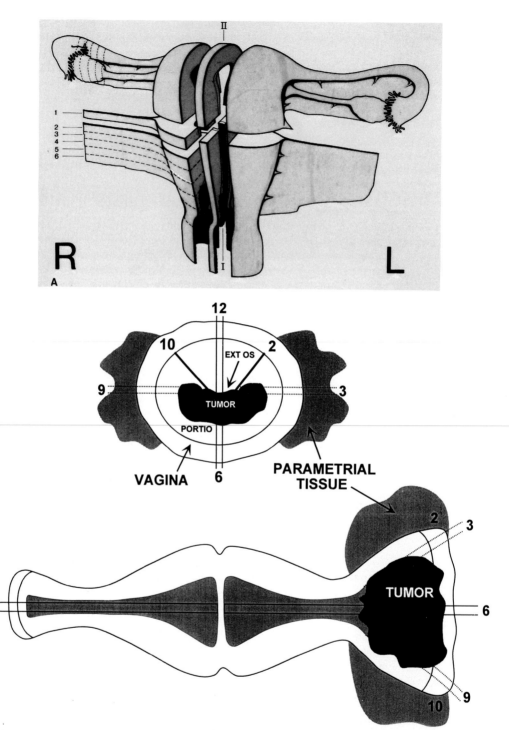

FIGURE 5-13. (**A**) Technique for examining surgical specimen suggested by Baltzer, which does not stress the importance of modifying the method depending on the site of the tumor. Gross evaluation by an experienced pathologist before taking sections is probably the most important factor. (Baltzer J, Koepcke W. Tumor size and lymph node metastases in squamous cell carcinoma of the uterine cervix. Arch Gynecol 1979;227:271, with permission) (**B**) An example of selective planning. Tumor grossly at 2:30 to 9:30 clock position shown above. Open cervix beginning at 2 and 10 o'clock position in the vagina, attempted to miss the tumor or cut through edge, veered toward 3 and 9 o'clock at lower segment/upper endocervical junction, then bivalve. Sections: vagina to fundus at 12 o'clock; vagina to fundus at 6 o'clock; endocervix (through tumor to parametrial tissue) at 9 and 3 o'clock.

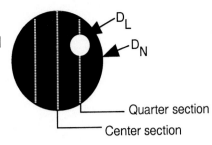

Model node sectioned in the center and in the quarter sections with lesion D_L

D_L

D_N

Quarter section

Center section

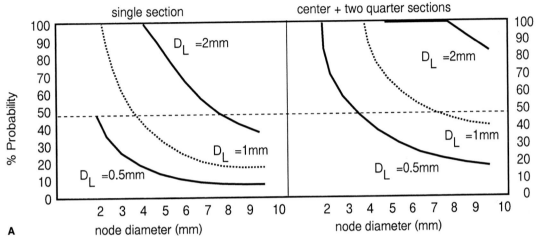

single section

center + two quarter sections

% Probability

D_L =2mm

D_L =1mm

D_L =0.5mm

D_L =2mm

D_L =1mm

D_L =0.5mm

% Probability

node diameter (mm)

node diameter (mm)

A

CONVENTIONAL LYMPH NODE BISECTION VERSUS
MULTI-SAMPLING STEP DISSECTION

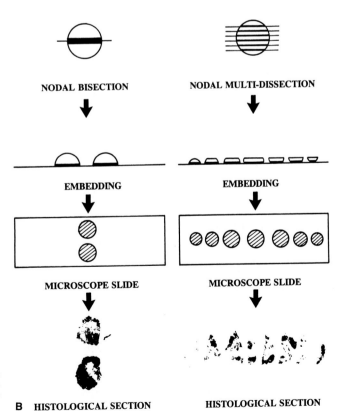

NODAL BISECTION

NODAL MULTI-DISSECTION

EMBEDDING

EMBEDDING

MICROSCOPE SLIDE

MICROSCOPE SLIDE

FIGURE 5-14. (A) Representation of a model lymph node sectioned in the center and in quarter sections. Percentage probability of identifying a randomly distributed lesion on a single section and two quarter sections. D_L, lesion; D_N, lymph node. (Wilkinson EJ, Hause L. Probability in lymph node sectioning. Cancer 1974;33:1269, with permission) (B) Representation of conventional lymph node bisection versus multinode sampling step dissection. (To ACW, Gore H, Shingleton HM, Wilkerson JA, Soong S-J, Hatch KD. Lymph node metastasis in cancer of the cervix: a preliminary report. Am J Obstet Gynecol 1986;155:388.)

B   HISTOLOGICAL SECTION

HISTOLOGICAL SECTION

standing of how the specimen is to be opened to ensure that accurate evaluation is not jeopardized.

In a radical hysterectomy specimen, the vagina, cervix, and corpus should be bivalved but the precise site of the incisions depends on the plan of examination. Exactly where the cervix is incised may depend on the position of visible cervical tumor, with the understanding that the best sections will be taken after fixation. At the lower segment, incisions are extended along the lateral wall of corpus to cornu. The specimen is then fixed flat overnight for best results.

Sections may be varied, depending on the gross appearance, while always planning to have one full-thickness section through the largest area of tumor. Large sections may be divided into suitable segments and adequately labeled, so that the original section may be reconstructed.

The purpose of the sectioning is to outline tumor extent. The need for additional tissue examination is usually apparent after review of the initial evaluation. Importantly, distal left and right parametrium and the distal vaginal surgical margins are shaved and submitted for examination. Parametrium, fallopian tubes, and ovaries (when included) are examined to exclude metastases or other significant pathology.

All lymph node tissue is examined carefully for individual nodes. Depending on size, all of the node (if small) is submitted; a mid-slice if the node is somewhat larger (removing a sliver from each of two surfaces to make a flat slice); and either half or both halves of a larger node. Matted nodes may present a problem but these usually are not found with cervical cancer radical specimens. Several idealistic methods for nodal evaluation have been reported (Fig. 5-14*A* and *B*; Girardi et al 1993). Individual lymph nodes are often too small to apply some of these techniques. The number of sections made from each node may be debated; cost has to be balanced against the importance and likelihood of increasing the detection of micrometastases and whether these findings are important.

HISTOPATHOLOGIC GRADING SYSTEMS AND OTHER STUDIES FOR PREDICTING PROGNOSIS

Several authors (Stendahl et al 1979, Pagnini et al 1980, Noguchi et al 1983, Crissman et al 1985, Bichel et al 1985, Ng et al 1992, Himmelmann et al 1992) have developed scoring systems to assist the clinician in determining a patient's prognosis with cervical cancer. Although these authors are well-meaning, the small biopsy sample available to a pathologist from a patient treated with radiation therapy is inadequate as the sole method of studying prognostic significance,

especially when one considers tumor heterogeneity. For instance, information on tumor volume, depth of stromal invasion of the cervix, documentation of parametrial extension and metastases to pelvic or aortic lymph nodes is only available from surgically treated or surgically staged patients. Histologic parameters such as keratinization status of cells; polymorphism of nuclei; mitotic counts; mode of the invasive front (pushing, diffuse); plasmolymphocytic cellular response; and lymphvascular space invasion, as noted in biopsy samples, have not been demonstrated to be significant or independent variables on multivariate analysis (see Tables 7-14 and 7-15 in Chap. 7). Their use as part of a pathologic grading system, therefore, only introduces bias. For this reason, histopathologic scoring systems do not have a place in the routine management of patients with cervical cancer, independent of tissue type.

DNA CONTENT AND CELL-CYCLE CYTOKINETICS

Abnormal cellular DNA content, as derived from flow cytometry, has been reported to correlate with prognosis in carcinoma of the cervix (Jakobsen 1984, Rutgers et al 1986, Leminen 1990). The degree of aneuploidy is thought to be associated with more advanced clinical stages of disease, an increased frequency of nodal metastases, and the rate of local treatment failure. The fraction of cells in the s-phase of the cell cycle can be determined from flow cytometry; several studies have suggested that the s-phase fraction (SPF) is an independent prognostic factor (Strang et al 1986, Strang 1989, Leminen 1990). The SPF is thought to correlate with the rate of relapse and the incidence of distant metastases (Strang et al 1987). Some investigators advocate measurement of DNA content and SPF and their use along with morphologic grading as prognostic indicators (Adelson et al 1987, Johnson et al 1987, Naus et al 1991), whereas others (Kenter et al 1990, Jakobsen 1991) note that there is no general agreement to the prognostic importance of flow-cytometric DNA analysis of human tumors. To resolve the disagreement, such measurements may be incorporated into future prospective clinical trials of cooperative groups.

ONCOGENES AND TUMOR-SUPPRESSOR GENES IN CERVICAL CANCER

Studies of the expression of oncogenes in cervical cancer are underway as part of the overall study of the molecular biology of cancer. Baker (1989) summa-

TABLE 5-6
Oncogene Expression in Squamous Cell Carcinoma

STUDY	YEAR	PATIENTS (N)	ONCOGENE	CONCLUSION
Riou, et al	1987	72	C-*myc*	Reduced lapse-free survival if C-*myc* expressed
Hayashi, et al	1991	52	RAS oncogene product 21	Expression associated with biologically aggressive tumors
Pinion, et al	1991	24 CIN III 10 SCC	HA-*ras*, C-*myc*, ERB-2	All amplified, compared with CIN I
Crook, et al	1992	28	p53	All HPV DNA-negative SCC contained p53 mutations and had a worse prognosis

CIN, cervical intraepithelial neoplasia; *HPV,* human papillomavirus; *SCC,* squamous cell carcinoma.

rized the status of these studies in relation to gynecologic tumors. Some authors (Table 5-6) have provided information on C-*myc* and HA-*ras* oncogene expression in squamous cell carcinoma of the cervix. Expression of either C-*myc* or HA-*ras* oncogene product 21 is thought to be associated with decreased survival and to identify biologically aggressive tumors.

Antioncogenes or tumor-suppressor genes may be more important than oncogenes in cervical carcinogenesis. Human papillomavirus mediates its carcinogenic activity by deactivating p53 and the retinoblastoma protein, two important antioncogenes. Primary p53 mutations have been associated with HPV-negative cervical cancers, that behave in a clinically aggressive fashion (Campo 1992, Crook et al 1992). Further studies evaluating oncogene and tumor-suppressor gene expression, perhaps combined with flow-cytometric analysis, may provide a needed mechanism for distinguishing tumors of low and high malignant potential.

HUMAN PAPILLOMAVIRUS DNA STUDIES IN CERVICAL CANCER

With the interest in HPVs regarding cervical carcinogenesis, many investigators have studied the presence of HPV DNA within tumors of both major tissue

TABLE 5-7
Human Papillomavirus RNA Studies in Cervical Cancer

STUDY	YEAR	PATIENTS (N)	HISTOLOGY	CONCLUSIONS
Barnes, et al	1988	30	Squamous, adenocarcinoma, mixed	HPV 16, 18 most commonly found; HPV 18 associated with aggressive tumors
King, et al	1989	85	Squamous, adenocarcinoma, mixed	HPV DNA (16, 18) did not correlate with survival or high-risk factors
Riou, et al	1990	106	Squamous, adenocarcinoma, mixed	HPV types 16, 18, 33, 35 detected in 84% of patients; HPV-negative tumors had worse prognosis
Kenter, et al	1991	69	Not stated*	Presence of HPV16 was of no prognostic value
Higgins, et al	1991	212	Squamous, adenocarcinoma, mixed	Younger HPV-positive patients, better prognosis; older HPV-negative patients, worse prognosis

*Probably mixed-tissue types, squamous cell carcinoma predominant.
HPV, human papillomavirus.

types (and in mixed tumors; Table 5-7). The presence of HPV has not been helpful in defining prognosis in invasive cervical cancer. Techniques to measure the transcriptional activity (messenger RNA) of HPV genes, such as the viral oncogenes E6 and E7, may find use in predicting aggressive tumors in the near future (zur Hausen 1991). Screening for HPV DNA in cervical cancer is not recommended for clinical management, however.

ESTROGEN AND PROGESTERONE RECEPTORS

Potish and associates (1986) reported that in surgically treated premenopausal women, clinical stage, surgical stage, and hormone-receptor levels independently predicted survival. Many studies since that time (Martin et al 1986, Hunter et al 1987, Mosny et al 1989, Darne et al 1990) failed to relate estrogen- and/or progesterone-receptors to survival. Although it is true that these receptors are demonstrable in most cases in the normal and neoplastic cervix, there seems to be no relevance to testing for them, at least for prognostic or therapeutic purposes.

References

Abu-Ghazaleh S, Johnston W, Creasman WT. The significance of peritoneal cytology in patients with carcinoma of the cervix. Gynecol Oncol 1984;17:139.

Adelson MD, Johnson TS, Sneige N, Williamson KD, Freedman RS, Peters LJ. Cervical carcinoma DNA content, S-fraction and malignancy grading. II. Comparison with clinical staging. Gynecol Oncol 1987;26:57.

Anderson MC, Fraser AC. Adenocarcinoma of the uterine cervix: a clinical and pathological appraisal. Br J Obstet Gynaecol 1976;83:320.

Baker VV: Oncogenes in gynecologic cancer. In Lurain JR, Sciarra JJ, eds. Gynecology and obstetrics, vol 4. Philadelphia: JB Lippincott, 1989.

Ballon SC, Berman ML, Lagasse LD, Petrilli ES, Castaldo TW. Survival after extraperitoneal pelvic and paraaortic lymphadenectomy and radiation therapy in cervical carcinoma. Obstet Gynecol 1981;57:90.

Baltzer J, Koepcke W. Tumor size and lymph node metastases in squamous cell carcinoma of the uterine cervix. Arch Gynecol 1979;227:271.

Barnes W, Delgado G, Kurman RJ, et al. Possible prognostic significance of HPV type in cervical cancer. Gynecol Oncol 1988;29:267.

Beecham JB, Halvorsen T, Kolbenstvedt A. Histologic classification, lymph node metastases and patient survival in stage IB cervical carcinoma. Gynecol Oncol 1978;6:95.

Benedet JL, Turko M, Boyes DA, Nickerson KG, Bienkowska BT. Radical hysterectomy in the treatment of cervical cancer. Am J Obstet Gynecol 1980;137:254.

Berek JS, Hacker NF, Fu Y-S, Sokale JR, Leuchter RC, Lagasse LD. Adenocarcinoma of the uterine cervix: histologic variables associated with lymph node metastasis and survival. Obstet Gynecol 1985;65:46.

Berman ML, Keys H, Creasman W, DiSaia P, Bundy B, Blessing J. Survival and patterns of recurrence in cervical cancer metastatic to periaortic lymph nodes (a gynecologic oncology group study). Gynecol Oncol 1984; 19:8.

Bichel P, Jakobsen A. Histopathologic grading and prognosis of uterine cervical carcinoma. Am J Clin Oncol 1985; 8:247.

Bonanno JP, Boyce J, Fruchter R, Khulpateea N, Macasaet M, Remy JC. Involvement of para-aortic lymph nodes in carcinoma of the cervix. J Am Osteopath Assoc 1980;79:567.

Buchsbaum HJ. Extrapelvic lymph node metastases in cervical carcinoma. Am J Obstet Gynecol 1979;133:814.

Burghardt E, Baltzer J, Tulusan AH, Haas J. Results of surgical treatment of 1028 cervical cancers studied with volumetry. Cancer 1992;70:648.

Burghardt E, Pickel H, Haas J, Lahousen M. Prognostic factors and operative treatment of stage IB and IIB cervical cancer. Am J Obstet Gynecol 1987;156:988.

Campo MS. Cell transformation by animal papillomaviruses. J Gen Virol 1992;73:217.

Cherry CP, Glucksmann A. Observations on lymph node involvement in carcinoma of the cervix. J Obstet Gynaecol Br Empire 1953;60:368.

Chung CK, Nahhas WA, Zaino R, Stryker JA, Mortel R. Histologic grade and lymph node metastasis in squamous cell carcinoma of the cervix. Gynecol Oncol 1981; 12:348.

Copeland LJ, Sneige N, Ordonez NG. Endodermal sinus tumor of the vagina and cervix. Cancer 1985;55:2558.

Crissman JD, Makuch R, Budhraja M. Histopathologic grading of squamous cell carcinoma of the uterine cervix: an evaluation of 70 stage IB patients. Cancer 1985;55: 1590.

Crook T, Wrede D, Tidy JA, Mason WP, Evans DJ, Vousden KH. Clonal p53 mutation in primary cervical cancer: association with human-papillomavirus-negative tumours. Lancet 1992;339:1070.

Darne J, Soutter WP, Ginsberg R, Sharp F. Nuclear and "cytoplasmic" estrogen and progesterone receptors in squamous cell carcinoma of the cervix. Gynecol Oncol 1990;38:216.

de Jesus M, Tang W, Sadjadi M, Belmonte AH, Poon TP. Carcinoma of the cervix with extensive endometrial and myometrial involvement. Gynecol Oncol 1990;36:263.

Delgado G, Bundy B, Zaino R, Sevin B-U, Creasman WT, Major F. A prospective surgical pathological study of disease-free interval in patients with stage IB squamous cell carcinoma of the cervix. A gynecologic oncology group study. Gynecol Oncol 1990;38:352.

Delgado G, Bundy BN, Fowler WC Jr, et al. A prospective surgical pathological study of stage I squamous carcinoma of the cervix. A gynecologic oncology group study. Gynecol Oncol 1989;35: 314.

Demian SD, Bushkin FL, Echervarrian R. Perineural invasion and anaplastic transformation of verrucous carcinoma. Cancer 1973;32:395.

Dollar JR, Orr JW Jr, Shingleton HM, et al. Metastatic tumors mimicking gynecologic cancer. Obstet Gynecol 1987;69:865.

Eifel P, Morris M, Oswald M, et al. Adenocarcinoma of the uterine cervix: prognosis and patterns of failure of 367 cases. Cancer 1990;65:2507.

Favalli G, Garbelli R, Ravelli V, Santin A, Pecorelli S, Bianchi UA. Adenocarcinoma of the uterine cervix: still a controversial issue (abstract). Int J Gynecol Cancer 1993; 3:15.

Ferraris G, Lanza A, Daddato F, et al. Techniques of pelvic and para-aortic lymphadenectomy in the surgical treatment of cervix carcinoma. Eur J Gynaecol Oncol 1988; 9:83.

Fisher B, Fisher ER. Role of the lymphatic system in dissemination of tumor. In Mayerson HS, ed. Lymph and the lymphatic system. Springfield, IL: Charles C Thomas, 1968.

Fowler WC Jr, Miles PA, Surwit EA, Edelman DA, Walton LA, Photopulos GJ. Adenoid cystic carcinoma of the cervix. Obstet Gynecol 1978;52:337.

Fuchs WA. Lymphographie and tumordiagnostik. Berlin: Springer-Verlag, 1965:75.

Gallousis S. Verrucous carcinoma. Report of three vulvar cases and review of the literature. Obstet Gynecol 1972;40:502.

Gilks CB, Young RH, Aguirre P, DeLellis RA, Scully RE. Adenoma malignum (minimal deviation adenocarcinoma) of the uterine cervix. A clinicopathological and immunohistological analysis of 26 cases. Am J Surg Pathol 1989;13:717.

Girardi F, Pickel H, Winter R. Pelvic and parametrial lymph nodes in the quality control of the surgical treatment of cervical cancer. Gynecol Oncol 1993;50:330.

Glucksmann A, Cherry CP. Incidence, histology and response to radiation of mixed carcinomas (adenoacanthomas) of the uterine cervix. Cancer 1956;9:971.

Gonzales DG, Kettin BW, van Bunningen, van Dijk JDP. Carcinoma of the uterine cervix stage IB and IIA: results of postoperative irradiation in the parametrium and/or lymph node metastasis. Int J Radiat Oncol Biol Phys 1989;16:389.

Hanai J, Tsuji M. Uterine teratoma with lymphoid hyperplasia. Acta Pathol Jpn 1981;31:153.

Hayashi Y, Hacisuga T, Iwasaka T, et al. Expression of *ras* oncogene product and EGF receptor in cervical squamous cell carcinomas and its relationship to lymph node involvement. Gynecol Oncol 1991;40:147.

Henriksen E. Distribution of metastases in stage I carcinoma of the cervix. Am J Obstet Gynecol 1960;80:919.

Higgins GD, Davy M, Roder D, Uzelin DM, Phillips GE, Burrell CJ. Increased age and mortality associated with cervical carcinomas negative for human papillomavirus RNA. Lancet 1991;338:910.

Himmelmann A, Will'en R, Josif R, Prien-Larsen J, Ranstam J, Astedt B. Prospective histopathologic malignancy grading to indicate the degree of postoperative treatment in early cervical carcinomas. Gynecol Oncol 1992;46:37.

Hoskins WJ, Averette HE, Ng ABP, Yon SL. Adenoid cystic carcinoma of the cervix uteri: report of six cases and review of the literature. Gynecol Oncol 1979;7:371.

Hughes RR, Brewington KC, Hanjani P, et al. Extended field irradiation for cervical cancer based on surgical staging. Gynecol Oncol 1980;9:153.

Hunter RE, Longcope C, Keough P. Steroid hormone receptors in carcinoma of the cervix. Cancer 1987;60:392.

Imachi M, Tsukamoto N, Matsuyama T, Nakano H. et al. Peritoneal cytology in patients with carcinoma of the uterine cervix. Gynecol Oncol 1987;26: 202.

Ireland D, Hardiman P, Monaghan JM. Adenocarcinoma of the uterine cervix: a study of 73 cases. Obstet Gynecol 1985;65:82.

Jakobsen A. Carcinoma of the uterine cervix: study of flow cytometric analysis (editorial). Gynecol Oncol 1991; 43:1.

Jakobsen A. Prognostic impact of ploidy level in carcinoma of the cervix. Am J Clin Oncol 1984;7:475.

Johnson TS, Adelson MD, Sneige N, Williamson KD, Lee AM, Katz R. Cervical carcinoma DNA content, S-fraction, and malignancy grading. I. Interrelationships. Gynecol Oncol 1987;26:41.

Julian CG, Daikoku NH, Gillespie A. Adenoepidermoid and adenosquamous carcinoma of the uterus. Am J Obstet Gynecol 1977;128:106.

Kaku T, Enjoji M. Extremely well differentiated adenocarcinoma ('adenoma malignum') of the cervix. Int J Gynecol Pathol 1983;2:28.

Kaminski PF, Norris HJ. Minimal deviation carcinoma (adenoma malignum) of the cervix. Int J Gynecol Pathol 1983;2:141.

Kenter CG, Carnelisse CJ, Aartsen EJ, Hermans WM, Heintz APM, Fleuren GJ. DNA ploidy level as prognostic factor in low stage carcinoma of the uterine cervix. Gynecol Oncol 1990;39:181.

Kenter GG, Cornelisse CJ, Jiwa NM, et al. HPV 16 in tumor tissue of low stage squamous carcinoma of the uterine cervix in relation to ploidy grade and prognosis. Eur J Gynaecol Oncol 1991;XII(Suppl):27.

Kilgore LE, Orr JW Jr, Hatch KD, Shingleton HM, Roberson J. Peritoneal cytology in patients with squamous cell carcinoma of the cervix. Gynecol Oncol 1984, 19:24.

Kilgore LC, Soong S-J, Gore H, Shingleton HM, Hatch KD, Partridge EE. Analysis of prognostic features in adenocarcinoma of the cervix. Gynecol Oncol 1988;31:137.

Kindermann G, Jabusch HP. The spread of squamous cell carcinoma of the uterine cervix into the blood vessels. Arch Gynaekol Obstet 1972;212:1.

King LA, Talledo OE, Gallup DG, Melhus O, Otken LB. Adenoid cystic carcinoma of the cervix in women under age 40. Gynecol Oncol 1989;32:26.

Kjorstad JE. Carcinoma of the cervix in the young patient. Obstet Gynecol 1977;50:28.

Kjorstad KE, Kolbenstvedt A, Strickert T. The value of complete lymphadenectomy in radical treatment of cancer of the cervix, stage IB. Cancer 1984;54:2215.

Korhonen M, Stenback F. Adenocarcinoma metastatic to the uterine cervix. Gynecol Obstet Invest 1984;17:57.

Kraus FT, Perez-Mesa C. Verrucous carcinoma: clinical and pathologic study of 105 cases involving oral cavity, larynx and genitalia. Cancer 1966;19:26.

Kurman RJ, ed. Blaustein's pathology of the female genital tract, 3rd ed. New York: Springer-Verlag, 1987.

Lagasse LD, Creasman WT, Shingleton HM, Ford JH, Blessing JA. Results and complications of operative staging in cervical cancer: experience of the gynecologic oncology group. Gynecol Oncol 1980;9:90.

Lee Y-N, Wang KL, Lin M-H, et al. Radical hysterectomy with pelvic lymph node dissection for treatment of cervical cancer: a clinical review of 954 cases. Gynecol Oncol 1989;32:135.

Leminen A. Tumor markers CA 125, carcinoembryonic antigen and tumor associated trypsin inhibitor in patients with cervical adenocarcinoma. Gynecol Oncol 1990;39:358.

Lemoine NR, Hall PA. Epithelial tumors metastatic to the uterine cervix: a study of 33 cases and review of the literature. Cancer 1986;57:2002.

Lifshitz S, Buchsbaum HJ. The spread of cervical carcinoma. In Lurain JR, Sciarra JJ, eds. Gynecology and obstetrics, vol 4. Philadelphia: JB Lippincott, 1990.

Liu W, Meigs JV. Radical hysterectomy and pelvic lymphadenectomy. Am J Obstet Gynecol 1955;69:1.

Maier RC, Norris HJ. Coexistence of cervical intraepithelial neoplasia with primary adenocarcinoma of the endocervix. Obstet Gynecol 1980;56:361.

Martimbeau PW, Kjorstad KE, Iversen T. Stage IB carcinoma of the cervix, the Norwegian Radium Hospital. Results of treatment and major complications. II. Results when pelvic nodes are involved. Obstet Gynecol 1982;60:215.

Martin JD, Hahnel R, McCartney AJ, DeKlerk N. The influence of estrogen and progesterone receptors on survival in patients with carcinoma of the uterine cervix. Gynecol Oncol 1986;23:329.

Mazur MT, Hsueh S, Gersell DJ. Metastases to the female genital tract. Analysis of 325 cases. Cancer 1984;53:1978.

Meigs JV, ed. Surgical treatment of cancer of the cervix. New York: Grune & Stratton, 1954:90.

Melamed MR. Circulating cancer cells. In Koss LG, ed. Diagnostic cytology and its histologic bases. Philadelphia: JB Lippincott, 1992:1403.

Miller B, Dockter M, El Torky M, Photopulos G. Small cell carcinoma of the cervix: a clinical and flow-cytometric study. Gynecol Oncol 1991;42:27.

Milsom I, Friberg LG. Primary adenocarcinoma of the uterine cervix. A clinical study. Cancer 1983;52:942.

Mosny DS, Herholtz J, Degen W, Bender HG. Immunohistochemical investigations of steroid receptors in normal and neoplastic squamous epithelium of the uterine cervix. Gynecol Oncol 1989;35:373.

Naus GJ, Zimmerman RL. Prognostic value of flow cytophotometric DNA content analysis in single treatment stage IB-IIA squamous cell carcinoma of the cervix. Gynecol Oncol 1991;43:149.

Nelson JH Jr, Boyce J, Macasaet M, et al. Incidence, significance and follow-up of para-aortic lymph node metastases in late invasive carcinoma of the cervix. Am J Obstet Gynecol 1977;128:336.

Ng GT, Shyu SK, Chen YK, Yuan CC, Chao KC, Kan YY. A scoring system for predicting recurrence of cervical cancer. Int J Gynaecol Cancer 1992;2:75.

Noguchi H, Shiozawa I, Sakai Y, Yamazaki T, Fukuta T. Pelvic lymph node metastasis of uterine cervical cancer. Gynecol Oncol 1987;27:150.

Noguchi H, Shiozawa K, Tsukamoto T, Tsukahara Y, Iwai S, Fukuta T. The postoperative classification for uterine cancer and its clinical evaluation. Gynecol Oncol 1983;16:219.

Okagaki T. Female genital tumors associated with human papillomavirus infection and the concept of genital neoplasm—papilloma syndrome (GENPS). Pathol Annu 1984;19:31.

Pagnini CA, Palma PD, DeLaurentiis G. Malignancy grading in squamous carcinoma of uterine cervix treated by surgery. Br J Cancer 1980;41:421.

Partridge EE, Murad T, Shingleton HM, Austin JM, Hatch KD. Verrucous lesions of the female genitalia. II. Verrucous carcinoma. Am J Obst Gynecol 1980;137:412.

Perez AC, Zivnuska F, Askin F, Camel HM, Ragan D, Powers WE. Mechanisms of failure in patients with carcinoma of the uterine cervix extending into the endometrium. Int J Radiat Oncol Biol Phys 1977;2:651.

Pinion SB, Kennedy JH, Miller RW, MacLean AB. Oncogene expression in cervical intraepithelial neoplasia and invasive cancer of cervix. Lancet 1991;8745:819.

Plentl AA, Friedman EA. Lymphatic system of the female genitalia. Philadelphia: WB Saunders, 1971.

Podczaski E, Kaminski PF, Pees RC, Singapuri K, Sorosky JI. Peutz-Jeghers syndrome with ovarian sex cord tumor with annular tubules and cervical adenoma malignum. Gynecol Oncol 1991;42:74.

Potish RA, Twiggs LB, Adcock LL, Prem KA, Savage JE, Leung BS. Prognostic importance of progesterone and estrogen receptors in cancer of the uterine cervix. Cancer 1986;58:1709.

Raheja A, Katz DA, Dermer MS. Verrucous carcinoma of the endocervix. Obstet Gynecol 1983;62:535.

Randall ME, Constable WC, Hahn SS, Kim J-A, Mills SE. Results of the radiotherapeutic management of carcinoma of the cervix with emphasis on the influence of histologic classification. Cancer 1988;62:48.

Randall ME, Kim J-A, Mills SE, Hahn SS, Constable WC. Uncommon variants of cervical carcinoma treated with radical irradiation: a clinoco-pathologic study of 66 cases. Cancer 1986;57:816.

Reisinger SA, Palazzo JP, Talerman A, Carlson J, Jahshan A. Stage IB glassy cell carcinoma of the cervix diagnosed during pregnancy and recurring in a transposed ovary. Gynecol Oncol 1991;42:86.

Riou G, Barrois M, Le MG, et al. C-*myc* proto-oncogene expression and prognosis in early carcinoma of the uterine cervix. Lancet 1987;1:71.

Riou G, Favre M, Jeannel D, Bourhis J, LeDoussal V, Orth G: Association between poor prognosis in early-stage invasive cervical carcinomas and non-detection of HPV DNA. Lancet 1990;335:1171.

Rutgers D, van der Linden P, van Peperseel H. DNA-flow cytometry of squamous cell carcinomas from the uterine cervix: identification of different subgroups. Radiother Oncol 1986;7:248.

Shingleton HM, Gore H, Soong S-J, Bradley D. Adenocarcinoma of the cervix: 1. Clinical evaluation and pathological features. Am J Obstet Gynecol 1981;138:799.

Shingleton HM, Orr Jw Jr. Cancer of the cervix: diagnosis and treatment. New York: Churchill Livingstone, 1987.

Shingleton HM. American College of Surgeons patterns of care study. 1995. In preparation.

Silva EG, Kott MM, Ordonez NG. Endocrine carcinoma intermediate cell type of the uterine cervix. Cancer 1984;54:1705.

Sotto LSJ, Graham JB, Pickren JW. Postmortem findings in cancer of the cervix. Am J Obstet Gynecol 1960;80: 791.

Stendahl U, Will'en H, Will'en R. Classification and grading of invasive squamous cell carcinoma of the uterine cervix. Acta Radiol 1979;18:481.

Strang P, Eklund G, Stendahl, Frankendal B. S-phase rate as a predictor of early recurrences in carcinoma of the uterine cervix. Anticancer Res 1987;7:807.

Strang P, Stendahl U, Frankendal B, Lindgren A. Flow cytometric DNA patterns in cervical carcinoma. Acta Radiol Oncol 1986;25:249.

Strang P. Cytogenetic and cytometric analysis in squamous cell carcinoma of the uterine cervix. Int J Gynecol Pathol 1989;8:54.

Sudarsanam A, Charyulu K, Belinson J, et al. Influence of exploratory celiotomy on the management of carcinoma of the cervix. Cancer 1978;41:1049.

Tamimi HK, Figge DC. Adenocarcinoma of the uterine cervix. Gynecol Oncol 1982;13:335.

Tiltman AJ, Atad J. Verrucous carcinoma of the cervix with endometrial involvement. Int J Gynecol Pathol 1982; 1:221.

To ACW, Gore H, Shingleton HM, Wilkerson JA, Soong S-J, Hatch KD. Lymph node metastasis in cancer of the cervix: a preliminary report. Am J Obstet Gynecol 1986;155:388.

van Dinh T, Woodruff JD. Adenoid cystic and adenoid basal carcinomas of the cervix. Obstet Gynecol 1985;65:705.

van Nagell JR Jr, Roddick JW Jr, Lowin DM. The staging of cervical cancer: inevitable discrepancies between clinical staging and pathologic findings. Am J Obstet Gynecol 1971;110:973.

van Nagell JR, Kielar R, Donaldson ES, et al. Correlation between retinal and pelvic vascular status: a determinant factor in patients undergoing pelvic irradiation for gynecologic malignancy. Am J Obstet Gynecol 1979;134: 551.

Vayrynen M, Romppanen T, Koskela E, et al. Verrucous squamous cell carcinoma of the female genital tract. Report of three cases and survey of the literature. Int J Gynecol Obstet 1981;19:351.

Volterrani F, Sigurta D, Gardani G, Milani A, Musumeci R. Role of lymphography in cancer of the uterine cervix (abstract). Radiol Med (Torino) 1980;66:611.

Welander CE, Pierce VK, Nori D, Hilaris BS, Kosloff C, Clark DGC. Pretreatment laparotomy in carcinoma of the cervix. Gynecol Oncol 1981;12:336.

Wentz WB, Reagan JW. Survival in cervical cancer with respect to cell type. Cancer 1959;12:384.

Wharton JT, Jones HW III, Day TG Jr, Rutledge FN, Fletcher GH. Preirradiation celiotomy and extended field irradiation for invasive carcinoma of the cervix. Obstet Gynecol 1977;49:333.

Wheeless CR Jr, Graham R, Graham JB. Prognosis and treatment of adenoepidermoid carcinoma of the cervix. Obstet Gynecol 1970;35:928.

Wilkinson EJ, Hause L. Probability in lymph node sectioning. Cancer 1974;33:1269.

Will'en H, Will'en R, Stendahl U. Invasive squamous cell carcinoma of the uterine cervix. VI. Prediction value of non-keratinizing, parakeratotic and orthokeratotic cell forms and clinical staging. Acta Radiol (Oncol) 1982;21:401.

Yajima A, Fukuda M, Noda K. Histopathological findings concerning the morphogenesis of mixed carcinoma of the uterine cervix. Gynecol Oncol 1984;18:157.

Yoshida A, Yoshida H, Fukunishi R, Inohara T. Carcinoid tumor of the uterine cervix. A light and electron microscopic study. Virchows Archives A Pathol Anat Histopathol 1984;402:331.

zur Hausen H. Viruses in human cancers. Science 1991;254: 1167.

Cancer of the Cervix by Hugh M. Shingleton and James W. Orr, Jr.
J. B. Lippincott Company, Philadelphia, © 1995.

6

Diagnosis, Staging, and Selection of Therapy for Invasive Tumors

DIAGNOSIS

Clinical cervical cancers present as exophytic, endophytic, ulcerative, or polypoid lesions (Figs. 6-1 through 6-5). Exophytic and ulcerative squamous cell carcinomas are more common than are endophytic and polypoid lesions. The clinical presentation of adenocarcinomas of the cervix does not differ appreciably, although there may be more endophytic and polypoid lesions. More adenocarcinomas are exophytic than are endophytic, which is perhaps related to the eversion of the lower endocervix in parous women. Because of the diversity of presentation of tumor regarding location, volume, histology, and growth patterns, we consider diagnosis in terms of symptoms, followed by methods of diagnosis such as colposcopic examinations and target biopsies, outpatient punch biopsy or diathermy loop excision, and endocervical curettage.

SYMPTOMS

Vaginal bleeding, the most common symptom in patients with invasive cancer of the cervix (Pretorius et al 1991), may occur as postcoital bleeding or as irregular bleeding, either of which may be mistaken by premenopausal women as a menstrual abnormality. In older women, postmenopausal bleeding may be the presenting symptom. Patients with large-volume International Federation of Gynecology and Obstetrics (FIGO) stages II through IV tumors often have a bloody, malodorous vaginal discharge. These patients are more likely to have associated nutritional deficits associated with a low performance status (Orr et al 1985).

COLPOSCOPIC FINDINGS IN EARLY INVASIVE CANCER

Colposcopic findings of area of ulceration, disturbance in surface contour, or presence of atypical blood vessels (Figs. 6-6 and 6-7) suggest invasive cancer. Sugimori and coworkers (1991) reported 89% accurate use of colposcopy in predicting invasion in patients with stage IB cancer but only 50% accuracy in predicting microinvasion (stage IA). If a colposcope is not available, the physician can still diagnose early cancer of the cervix in the office. Staining the cervix with Lugol's solution, taking multiple punch biopsies of the nonstaining areas, and performing endocervical curettage results in a diagnostic accuracy approaching that of colposcopy. Conization should be performed in follow-up of punch biopsy reports that suggest but are not diagnostic of invasive cancer.

BIOPSY OF VISIBLE OR PALPABLE CERVICAL LESIONS

Tissue confirmation of the diagnosis of invasive cervical cancer is accomplished by outpatient punch biopsy or diathermy loop excision of the cervical lesion. When biopsy of a superficial lesion produces an interpretation of "questionable invasion" or "microinvasion," conization of the cervix is in order.

A particular problem of diagnosis occurs when the physician's index of suspicion is low. All women with suspicious or symptomatic cervical lesions should undergo biopsy promptly, regardless of previous cytology. Visible or palpable cervical abnormalities during pregnancy or at the time of the postpartum examination should be evaluated and undergo biopsy if necessary to exclude invasion.

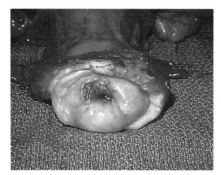

FIGURE 6-1. A one-quadrant superficial ulcerative carcinoma. Maximum depth of invasion in this tumor was 8 mm. (Shingleton HM, Orr JW Jr. Cancer of the cervix: diagnosis and treatment. New York: Churchill Livingstone, 1987:99.) See Color Figure 6-1.

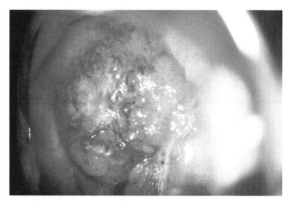

FIGURE 6-3. Adenocarcinoma of the cervix. The stage IB lesion, demonstrates disturbed surface contour and atypical surface blood vessels.

ENDOCERVICAL CURETTAGE

In addition to colposcopically directed biopsies, endocervical curettage is an important diagnostic tool to detect an occult lesion that may be present in the endocervical canal. (This is particularly true in symptomatic postmenopausal women.) Cervical conization is an essential part of the evaluation in women who have an abnormal endocervical curettage because the cone specimen provides the pathologist with adequate material to establish the location and extent of invasion. Loop diathermy outpatient conization may be performed rather than knife conization under general anesthesia (Phipps et al 1989, Fenton et al 1989). A partial trachelectomy is acceptable and perhaps easier to perform in evaluating the cervix in older women who have atrophic retracted cervices or in those who have had a previous supracervical hysterectomy (Krebs et al 1985).

Occult Carcinomas

Occult endophytic carcinomas that have not expanded the endocervix present problems and may result in diagnostic delays. These tumors inevitably cause irregular menses or postmenopausal bleeding or may be detected by cytologic screening. Endocervical curettage may result in an outpatient diagnosis of such tumors. Clinically, occult lesions usually behave in a manner similar to larger tumors; for example, Boronow (1977) reported pelvic node metastases in 20.7% of patients with stage IB occult tumors. In surgical data accumulated over 25 years at the University of Alabama at Birmingham, occult stage IB lesions have been associated with bilateral pelvic node metastases (15%) and aortic node metastases (8%). These findings may relate to increased access to lymphatic vessels as the tumor penetrates the cervical stroma high in the (anatomic) endocervical canal.

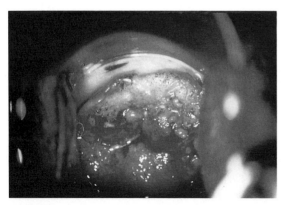

FIGURE 6-2. An exophytic squamous cell carcinoma involving the entire cervical circumference. (Shingleton HM, Orr JW Jr. Cancer of the cervix: diagnosis and treatment. New York: Churchill Livingstone, 1987.) See Color Figure 6-2.

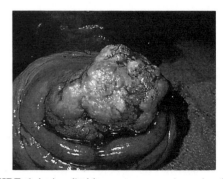

FIGURE 6-4. A radical hysterectomy specimen, in which a large polypoid adenosquamous carcinoma extends from the endocervical canal. (Courtesy of Dr. J. Max Austin Jr., Southern Gynecology Inc., Birmingham, Alabama) See Color Figure 6-4.

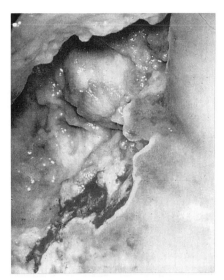

FIGURE 6-5. An advanced-stage ulcerative squamous cell carcinoma. Note the necrotic exudate replacing the cervix. (Giuntoli RL, Atkinson BF, Ernst CS, Rubin MM, Egan VS [eds]. Atkinson's correlative atlas of colposcopy, cytology, and histopathology. Philadelphia, JB Lippincott, 1987:175, with permission.) See Color Figure 6-5.

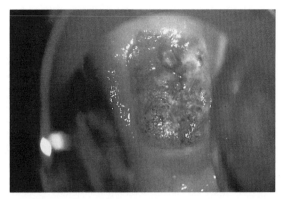

FIGURE 6-7. Atypical vessels in a squamous cell carcinoma of the posterior lip of the cervix. The surface contour is also altered. (Shingleton HM, Orr JW Jr. Cancer of the cervix: diagnosis and treatment. New York, Churchill Livingstone, 1987.) See Color Figure 6-7.

pecially important in women who have previously undergone cryosurgery for treatment of high-grade SIL, which has a potential for "burying" islands of neoplastic cells.

Large endophytic lesions that have distorted and expanded the endocervix to a "barrel" shape (Fig. 6-8) make clinical staging difficult and are associated with a poor prognosis (Gallion et al 1985). Regardless of treatment modality, these lesions are associated with an increased incidence of regional node metastases and a high central pelvic failure rate.

Rarely, nodular cervical carcinomas without a break in the overlying ectocervical epithelium are encountered. The cervix that is unusually large or abnormal to palpation should undergo biopsy. This is es-

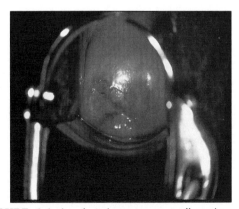

FIGURE 6-6. An ulcerating squamous cell carcinoma of the cervix in a 32-year-old pregnant woman. (Shingleton HM, Orr JW Jr. Cancer of the cervix: diagnosis and treatment. New York, Churchill Livingstone, 1987.) See Color Figure 6-6.

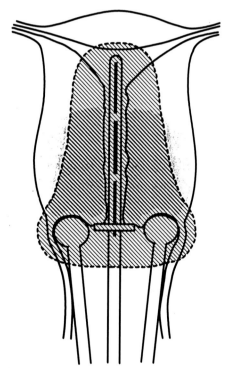

FIGURE 6-8. Diagram of an infiltrating endocervical tumor, causing expansion of the lower uterine segment, the so-called "barrel-shaped" tumor. (Redrawn from Gallion HH, van Nagell JR, Donaldson ES, et al. Combined radiation therapy and extrafascial hysterectomy in the treatment of stage IB barrel-shaped cervical cancer. Cancer 1985;56:262.)

Endometrial Extension

Although endometrial extension of cervical cancer has been reported to be a poor prognostic factor by some authors, it is difficult to determine the actual frequency of such extension because most patients with cancer of the cervix in FIGO stages II through IV do not undergo hysterectomy, which allows study of tumor distribution. In such women, it is difficult to collect a curettage specimen from the uterine cavity that is free of contamination from the primary cervical tumor, probably resulting in falsely elevated and inaccurate incidence figures. Perez and associates (1977) reported that 9% of their radiation therapy patients had direct extension to the lower uterine segment. Baltzer and colleagues (1981) reported that ovarian metastases are more likely if the tumor involves the endometrium. In a few (2% to 3%) patients undergoing radical hysterectomy (FIGO stages IB, IIA), endometrial involvement is demonstrated. Perhaps because of these factors, such extension is not a part of the FIGO staging system described in Table 6-1, and such extension is disregarded in treatment planning.

Cervical Stump Cancer

With few indications for subtotal hysterectomy today, carcinoma of the cervical stump is not commonly seen. Diagnostic and staging considerations are the same; however, these lesions sometimes present problems in treatment because of distorted anatomy and (presumed) adhesions of small bowel to the upper aspect of the remaining cervix as a consequence of the previous surgery. (See Chapter 8 for further discussion.)

STAGING

Clinical Staging

The FIGO staging system is detailed in Table 6-1 and depicted in Figure 6-9. Gal and Buchsbaum (1990), in a historical review, note that the only changes in FIGO staging since 1962 involved redefinition of stages IIIA and B (1971) and refinement of the definition of microinvasive carcinoma (1985). In 1995, a major change occurred with the subdivision of Stage IB into IB1 (lesions $\leq$ 4 cm) and IB2 (lesions > 4 cm) (Table 6-1). Regarding accuracy of clinical staging (all stages) compared with surgical staging, a 34% to 39% error rate is reported in the literature (Walsh et al 1981); when FIGO stages IB and II are considered alone, 20% to 22% of women in stage IB and 39% to 44% of women in stage II are understaged clinically (van Nagell et al 1971, Averette et al 1972). In five in-

ternational series totaling 7023 patients from several parts of the world (Table 6-2), slightly more than half of the patients were within stage I. In an American College of Surgeons Patterns of Care Study (Shingleton 1995) of 9336 women accrued in the United States in two study years (1984, 1990), 49.6% and 54.6% (respectively) were in clinical stages IA or IB.

Staging Studies

EXAMINATION UNDER ANESTHESIA

In addition to general physical assessment, speculum, and bimanual and rectovaginal pelvic examinations, the woman with cancer of the cervix requires other diagnostic studies to delineate the extent of disease and assist in selection of proper therapy (Table 6-3). The importance of an examination under anesthesia was stressed by van Nagell and associates (1971); they note that examination under anesthesia increased the accuracy of clinical staging by 25%. Examination under anesthesia allows a better inspection of the upper vagina and more precise palpation of the parametrial and lateral side wall tissues than that performed in the office. Opportunities for an examination under anesthesia occur either at the time of proposed surgical treatment or at the time of intracavitary radioisotope application. We rarely subject women to an anesthetic for examination under anesthesia alone unless primary therapy decisions cannot be made without clarification of the pelvic findings. In such circumstances, both the gynecologist and radiation oncologist should be present for the examination and cystoscopy and/or sigmoidoscopy may be performed at the same time.

CYSTOSCOPY AND PROCTOSIGMOIDOSCOPY

Cystoscopy and proctosigmoidoscopy are important studies when the primary lesion is bulky and particularly if it involves the anterior or posterior vagina. If the bladder or rectum are involved, the patient is assigned to FIGO stage IVA. The presence of bullous edema in the base of the bladder is an ominous finding because it ordinarily signifies tumor invasion of the bladder muscularis, which is associated with a poor prognosis.

CHEST FILMS

Chest films are an essential part of initial evaluation. If the chest x-ray is negative, there is little or no additional yield from the use of full lung tomography, which leads to more equivocal readings than do chest

TABLE 6-1
FIGO* Staging for Carcinoma of the Cervix Uteri (1995)

STAGE	DESCRIPTION	COMMENTS†
Stage 0	Carcinoma in situ, intraepithelial carcinoma	**Notes about the staging:**
Stage I	The carcinoma is strictly confined to the cervix.	Stage IA carcinoma should include minimal microscopically evident stromal invasion as well as small cancerous tumors of measurable size. Stage IA should be divided into those lesions with minute foci of invasion visible only microscopically as stage IA1 and macroscopically measurable microcarcinoma as stage IA2, in order to gain further knowledge of the clinical behavior of these lesions. The term "IB occult" should be omitted.
Stage IA	Invasive cancer identified only microscopically. All gross lesions even with superficial invasion are Stage IB cancers. Invasion is limited to measured stromal invasion with maximum depth of 5 mm and no wider than 7 mm.**	
Stage IA1	Measured invasion of stroma no greater than 3 mm in depth and no wider than 7 mm	The diagnosis of both stage IA1 and IA2 cases should be based on microscopic examination of removed tissue, preferably a cone, which must include the entire lesion. The lower limit of stage IA2 should be measurable macroscopically (even if dots need to be placed on the slide prior to measurement), and the upper limit of stage IA2 is given by measurement of the two largest dimensions in any given section. The depth of invasion should not be more than 5mm taken from the base of the epithelium, either surface or glandular, from which it originates. The second dimension, the horizontal spread, must not exceed 7mm. Vascular space involvement, either venous or lymphatic, should not alter the staging but should be specifically recorded, as it may affect treatment decisions in the future.
Stage IA2	Measured invasion of stroma greater than 3 mm and no greater than 5 mm in depth, and no wider than 7 mm	
Stage IB	Clinical lesions confined to the cervix or preclinical lesions greater than Stage IA	
Stage IB1	Clinical lesions no greater than 4 cm in size	
Stage IB2	Clinical lesions greater than 4 cm in size	
Stage II	The carcinoma extends beyond the cervix but has not extended to the pelvic wall. The carcinoma involves the vagina but not as far as the lower third.	Lesions of greater size should be classified as stage IB.
Stage IIA	No obvious parametrial involvement	As a rule, it is impossible to estimate clinically whether a cancer of the cervix has extended to the corpus or not. Extension to the corpus should therefore be disregarded.
Stage IIB	Obvious parametrial involvement	
Stage III	The carcinoma has extended to the pelvic wall. On rectal examination, there is no cancer-free space between the tumor and the pelvic wall. The tumor involves the lower third of the vagina. All cases with a hydronephrosis or nonfunctioning kidney are included unless they are known to be due to other causes.	A patient with a growth fixed to the pelvic wall by a short and indurated but not nodular parametrium should be allotted to stage IIB. It is impossible, at clinical examination, to decide whether a smooth and indurated parametrium is truly cancerous or only inflammatory. Therefore, the case should be placed in stage III only if the parametrium is nodular on the pelvic wall or if the growth itself extends to the pelvic wall.
Stage IIIA	No extension to the pelvic wall	The presence of hydronephrosis or nonfunctioning kidney due to stenosis of the ureter by cancer permits a case to be allotted to stage III even if, according to the other findings, the case should be allotted to stage I or stage II.
Stage IIIB	Extension to the pelvic wall and/or hydronephrosis or nonfunctioning kidney	
Stage IV	The carcinoma has extended beyond the true pelvis or has clinically involved the mucosa of the bladder or rectum. A bullous edema as such does not permit a case to be allotted to stage IV	The presence of bullous edema, as such, should not permit a case to be allotted to stage IV. Ridges and furrows in the bladder wall should be interpreted as signs of submucous involvement of the bladder if they remain fixed to the growth during palpation (ie, examination from the vagina or the rectum during cystoscopy). A finding of malignant cells in cytologic washings from the urinary bladder requires further examination and biopsy from the wall of the bladder.
Stage IVA	Spread of the growth to adjacent organs	
Stage IVB	Spread to distant organs	

*FIGO, International Federation of Gynecology and Obstetrics.
**The depth of invasion should not be more than 5 mm taken from the base of the epithelium, either surface or glandular, from which it originates. Vascular space involvement, either venous or lymphatic, should not alter the staging.
†Authors' note: FIGO modification (1995) of Stage I cancer occurred as this book went to press. The comments shown here were based on the 1988 staging for Stage I. The reader is advised to interpret some discussions in Chapters 3 and 6 with this modification in mind.

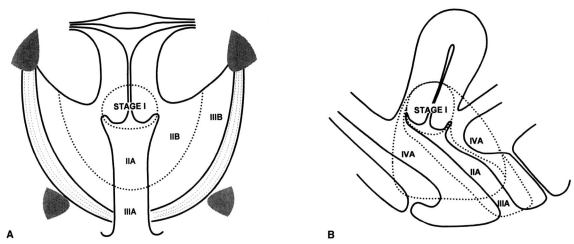

FIGURE 6-9. Representation of the clinical stages of cervical cancer. (**A**) Anterior projection. (**B**) Lateral projection. (Redrawn from Shingleton HM, Orr JW Jr. Cancer of the cervix: diagnosis and treatment. New York, Churchill Livingstone, 1987:103.)

films (Gordon et al 1983). Three to six percent of women with untreated clinical stage III or IVA disease have pulmonary metastases, whereas fewer than 0.5% of those with stage IB or II disease have such a finding (Gal et al 1990). If the chest x-ray demonstrates metastases (Fig. 6-10), treatment and prognosis of the patient are markedly altered. Full lung tomography is suggested as a follow-up of an abnormal chest x-ray.

INTRAVENOUS PYELOGRAM AND BARIUM ENEMA

The recognition that ureteral obstruction (Fig. 6-11) signified a poor prognosis produced a change in the FIGO staging system in 1971. Patients with findings of hydronephrosis or nonfunctional kidneys are assigned to FIGO stage III. Intravenous pyelograms (IVP) rarely reveal obstruction in patients with (by palpation) clinical stage I and II disease (6% and 15%, respectively; Gal et al 1990); however, 33% to 42% of patients with pelvic wall fixation in stages IIIB and IVA disease have abnormal pyelograms (Shingleton et al 1971, van Nagell et al 1975, Gal et al 1990). We do not believe that the IVP should be entirely replaced by computed tomography (CT) scans, as suggested by Hillman and coworkers (1984). The cost savings of IVP versus CAT scans in stage I and II disease are appreciable; however, it is recognized that additional information concerning metastases to paraaortic nodes and the paratracheal region may be gained by pelvic, abdominal, and chest CT scans in women with advanced disease. Intravenous pyelograms should not be routinely requested for women with stage IB disease who are scheduled to undergo radical surgery.

A barium enema is recommended in older women to identify intrinsic colon disease such as diverticulitis,

TABLE 6-2
Cancer of the Cervix: Percentage in Various Stages

STUDY	YEAR	PATIENTS (N)	CLINICAL STAGE			
			I	II	III	IV
Kjorstad	1977	2002	47	37	11	5
Jiminez, et al	1979	1227	31	55	12	2
Volterrani, et al	1980	417	45	24	30	1
Zander	1981	980	77.7	22.5	0.3	—
Shingleton*	1993	2397	58.4	26.1	10.8	4.7
TOTAL		7023	52.2	33.6	10.7	3.5

*University of Alabama at Birmingham data.

TABLE 6-3
Recommended Studies by Stage and Optional Studies in the Evaluation of Cervical Cancer Patients

RECOMMENDED STUDIES	IA	IB	IIA	IIB	III	IV	OPTIONAL STUDIES
Chest x-ray*	•	•	•	•	•	•	Coagulation studies
Examination under anesthesia*	•	•	•	•	•	•	Nutritional screen (serum albumin, transferrin)
CBC*, differential	•	•	•	•	•	•	Tumor markers (TA4)
BUN, creatinine,* electrolytes	•	•	•	•	•	•	Computerized axial tomography (chest)
Intravenous pyelogram		•	•	•			Ultrasonography (abdomen, pelvis)
Barium enema					•	•	Lymphangiography (abdomen, pelvis)
Abdomen/pelvic CT scan				•	•	•	Radioisotope scans (renal, liver, bone)
Cystoscopy			•	•	•	•	Retrograde pyelography
Proctoscopy					•	•	Bronchoscopy
							Skin testing
							Urodynamic testing
							Pulmonary function studies
							Electrocardiography

*Routine baseline studies.

---

ulcerative colitis, polyps, or other concurrent benign or malignant conditions that may modify the radiation treatment plan. Colorectal involvement by cervical cancer is almost always contiguous (i.e., a direct extension of tumor from the cervix to the adjacent rectosigmoid or rectum). This is better evaluated by proctoscopy than by barium enema. Neither procedure is cost-effective in women with clinical stage I or II disease, who are considered to be at low risk for tumor-associated intestinal abnormalities (5% and 7%, respectively; Gal et al 1990).

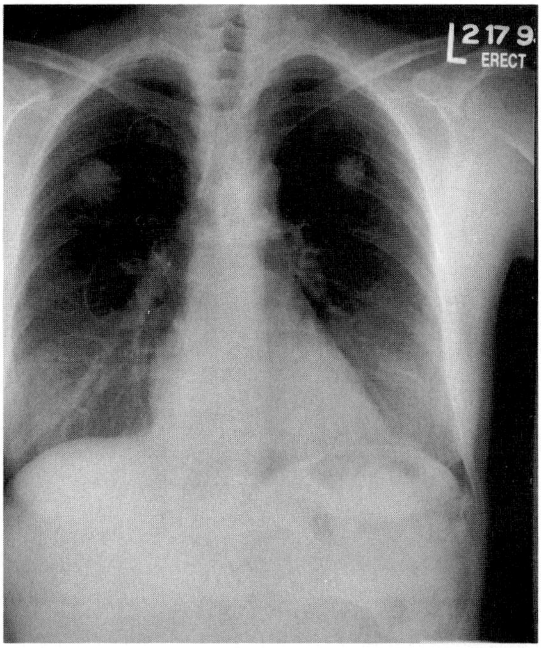

COMPUTED TOMOGRAPHY SCANS

Computed tomography scans of the abdomen, pelvis, and chest have been widely applied to the evaluation of patients with cancer of the cervix and can be of use in identification and measurement of enlarged retroperitoneal nodes, abdominopelvic masses or abscesses, or for clarification of chest findings (Figs. 6-12 through 6-14). These studies, however, are not mandatory in the evaluation of cervical cancer patients with small-volume (stages I and IIA) disease. Abdominopelvic CT scans can detect ureteral obstruction and liver metastases.

Radiologists have developed criteria for tumor invasion of the parametria (Vick et al 1984), although their radiologic interpretations can only be substantiated by surgical staging. In practice, CT scans are inaccurate for this purpose (Table 6-4). The main value of CT scanning in the untreated patient is in identifying enlarged nodes in the pelvis and especially in the paraaortic areas (Tables 6-5 and 6-6). Sensitivity rates are low, however. Bandy and colleagues (1985), reviewing published data on the correlation of paraaortic lymph node metastases and CT scan findings, observed that if one added extended-field irradiation to include paraaortic nodes based on the CT scan findings alone, numerous women would be undertreated

FIGURE 6-10. Chest film of metastatic disease in a 52-year-old patient. Right and left upper pulmonary lesions are present.

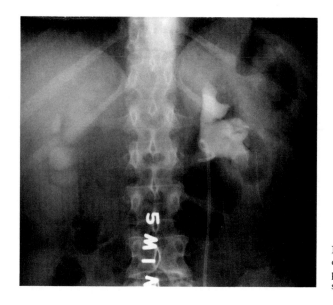

FIGURE 6-11. Intravenous pyelogram in a 49-year-old patient with advanced cervical cancer. There is complete obstruction of the right ureter and residual obstruction on the left after placement of stent.

or overtreated. Villasanta and coworkers (1983) and Bandy and associates (1985) showed that positive paraaortic lymph nodes can be detected 86% to 91% of the time when the nodes are enlarged to more than 1.0 to 1.5 cm in diameter. Because of the lack of sensitivity, CT scans cannot substitute for a pathologic diagnosis of metastases to nodes and should not be the basis for extending radiation therapy fields. Clinicians should be more discriminating in their requests for CT scans and for abdominal and pelvic ultrasound scanning procedures because in many cases, such scans are merely confirmatory (Kerr-Wilson et al 1984) and add little except expense to the evaluation. Computed tomography scans are not part of the FIGO staging systems.

MAGNETIC RESONANCE IMAGING SCANS

A newer technique, magnetic resonance imaging (MRI), is being applied to the evaluation of pelvic tumors. Criteria for the interpretation of MRI regarding

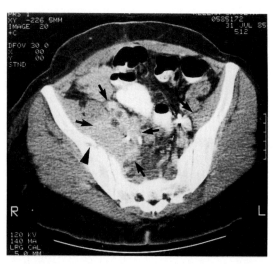

FIGURE 6-12. Pelvic CT scan of a patient with advanced cervical cancer. Pathologically enlarged nodes are present bilaterally (*arrows*). Incidentally noted is destruction of the iliac wing by metastatic disease (*arrowhead*). (Shingleton HM, Orr JW Jr. Cancer of the cervix: diagnosis and treatment. New York, Churchill Livingstone, 1987:111.)

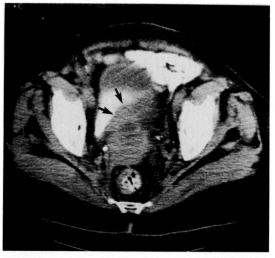

FIGURE 6-13. A pelvic CT scan in which a pelvic mass elevates the bladder base. The interface between the mass and the bladder is irregular (*arrows*), secondary to invasion of the bladder wall by carcinoma. (Shingleton HM, Orr JW Jr. Cancer of the cervix: diagnosis and treatment. New York, Churchill Livingstone, 1987:110.)

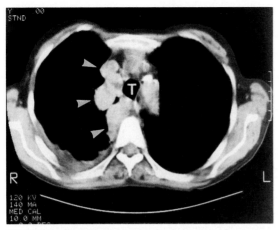

FIGURE 6-14. CT scan of the chest above the level of aortic arch, which shows enlarged mediastinal lymph nodes in the right paratracheal region. *T,* trachea; *arrows,* enlarged lymph nodes. (Shingleton HM, Orr JW Jr. Cancer of the cervix: diagnosis and treatment. New York, Churchill Livingstone, 1987:108.)

pelvic structures are less developed than those for CT scanning and judging by reports, MRI offers no unique contribution above that of CT scans, either in relation to assessment of parametrial disease or detection of node metastases (Tables 6-7 through 6-9). Hofmann and colleagues' (1988) 98% correlation coefficient for tumor volume in presurgical MRI scans

TABLE 6-4
Computed Tomography Scan Accuracy for Parametrial Extension: Surgically Confirmed Series

STUDY	YEAR	PATIENTS (N)	CONCLUSIONS
Walsh, et al	1981	75	50% false-positive
Vas, et al	1985	59	Little or no advantage over clinical staging (71% vs 66% accuracy)
King, et al	1986	25	Sensitivity, 100%; 36% false-positive; specificity, 36%
Newton, et al	1987	58	High false-positive; sensitivity, 53.6%; specificity, 86.7%
Vercamer, et al	1987	55	Overestimation of extent of disease is common
Parker, et al	1990	47	10.6% false-positive, provided no info that altered staging; not recommended in stage IB disease

has not been verified in other studies. Similar to CT scans, the value of MRI rises in proportion to the volume of pelvic disease and the presence of other disease, such as leiomyomata or adnexal masses (Fig. 6-15). Because MRI does not rely on ionizing irradiation, it may be considered in evaluation of pregnant patients who have invasive cervix cancer (Hricak et al 1991).

POSITRON EMISSION TOMOGRAPHY

Computed tomography and MRI imaging scans provide unparalleled morphologic detail but it is often difficult to reliably distinguish between reactive changes, sequelae of treatment, and active malignant tumor. Positron emission tomography (PET) is a new imaging technique that relies on the use of radionuclides, which decay with emission of positrons (positively charged particles). These positrons travel short distances in tissue before combining with a negatively charged electron, thus converting mass into energy. When the masses disintegrate, two photons (gamma rays) are produced, which are emitted at about 180° from each other. The simultaneous detection of two such photons by apposing detectors is used to reconstruct a three-dimensional representation of these events. Depending on the radionuclide used, different aspects of tissue metabolism and organ function can be measured (e.g., distribution of blood flow, oxygen utilization, protein synthesis, and glucose consumption). Cancer cells are avid for glucose. 2-[18F]Fluoro-2-deoxy-D-glucose, a radionuclide-labeled analogue of glucose, can thus be used to detect sites of malignancy. Positron emission images, especially when computer-combined with conventional section imaging such as CT and MRI, has the potential of more accurately delineating extent of disease at the primary site and more precisely localizing nodal disease. This can result in more accurate planning of treatment. Positron emission scans (Fig. 6-16) may demonstrate disease that is not identified by CT scans or MRI.

ULTRASONOGRAPHY

In vogue before development of CT scans and MRI, ultrasonography adds little to the evaluation of patients with cervical cancer, although occasionally this inexpensive, readily available technique can be of use because unlike CAT scans, longitudinal (sagittal) scans are possible (Fig. 6-17) and concurrent disease may be identified. Transrectal ultrasonography has been suggested as a method to assess parametrial involvement (Aoki et al 1990) but has not gained popularity among gynecologic oncologists in the United States.

TABLE 6-5
Detection of Pelvic Node Metastases by Computed Tomography Scans

STUDY	YEAR	PATIENTS (N)	SENSITIVITY (%)	SPECIFICITY (%)	ACCURACY (%)
Grumbine, et al	1981	24	0	94	72
Brenner, et al	1982	10	100	75	80
Whitley, et al	1982	7	100	83	66
Engelshoven, et al	1984	20	43	92	75
Vas, et al	1985	59	62	78	—
King, et al	1986	25	85	89	82
Newton, et al	1987	50	9.1	97.4	—
Vercamer, et al	1987	55	18	95	—
Camilien, et al	1988	51	25	97	80
Matsukuma, et al	1989	44	26.3	98.8	45

FINE-NEEDLE ASPIRATION

At the time of physical examination or during other screening studies, abdominal or pelvic masses or enlarged lymph nodes (paraaortic, inguinal, pelvic side wall, or supraclavicular) may be detected. Fine-needle aspiration may be performed under sonar or CT scan guidance (Table 6-10, Fig. 6-18). In experienced hands, the accuracy of this technique is high and it has been incorporated into modern diagnostic management. The technique is valuable in its ability to document tumor in extrapelvic nodes or masses, allowing modification of treatment plans (e.g., extending standard irradiation fields or canceling exploratory pelvic surgery). It is useful for aspiration of lung nodules, liver masses, abdominal wall masses, bone metastases, and other purposes. Regarding lung nodules, one should expect a 9% to 10% incidence of pneumothorax, requiring chest tube placement as a complication of the procedure (Fortier et al 1985).

LYMPHANGIOGRAPHY

Lymphangiography (Table 6-11, Fig. 6-19) has been advocated by some investigators for evaluation of pelvic and aortic nodes. The technique, however, lacks both sensitivity and specificity, especially in the evaluation of pelvic nodes. Heller and colleagues (1990), reporting a large study of the Gynecologic Oncology Group focusing on aortic nodes, concluded that a negative lymphangiogram may be adequate to eliminate surgical staging in subgroups at low risk for metastasis to aortic nodes and found lymphangiogram to be the most reliable (compared with CT scans and ultrasonography) "noninvasive" examination to evaluate spread to these nodes. In use, however, it is a painful procedure, with an associated febrile morbidity related to the injection sites on the dorsum of the feet. It also shares with CT and MRI scans the considerable problem of subjectivity of interpretation. For these reasons, we do not recommend it.

TABLE 6-6
Detection of Paraaortic Node Metastases by Computed Tomography Scans

STUDY	YEAR	PATIENTS (N)	SENSITIVITY (%)	SPECIFICITY (%)	ACCURACY (%)
Photopulos, et al	1979	17	60	100	76
Brenner, et al	1982	20	67	93	85
Whitley, et al	1982	16	80	92	88
Villasanta, et al	1983	42	77	86	83
Bandy, et al	1985	44	75	91	86
Vas, et al	1985	33	83	95	—
King, et al	1986	25	50	79	68
Newton, et al	1987	50	66.7	94	33
Camilien, et al	1988	61	67	100	—
Matsukuma, et al	1989	70	71.4	96.8	71
Heller, et al	1990	264	34	95.8	—

TABLE 6-7
Magnetic Resonance Imaging Assessment
of Tumor Volume: Surgically Confirmed

STUDY	YEAR	PATIENTS (N)	CONCLUSIONS
Worthington, et al	1986	22	More accurate than CT scans, yet a third of surgically verified lesions missed
Angel, et al	1987	10	Volume degree of stromal invasion correctly estimated in 90% of stage IB patients; superior to EUA
Hricak, et al	1988	57	Overall 81% accuracy
Rubens, et al	1988	27	90% accurate in tumor site and volume (stage IB disease), whereas clinical exam 30%
Burghardt, et al	1989	22	MRI correlates better (with tumor volume) than EUA accurate
Brodman, et al	1990	16	CT/MRI not collectively better than clinical staging
Oellinger	1991	13	84.6% accuracy of tumor dimension
Lichtenegger	1993	41	86% accuracy in tumor volume

CT, computed tomography; *EUA,* examination under anesthesia; *MRI,* magnetic resonance imaging.

TABLE 6-8
Magnetic Resonance Imaging Assessment
of Parametrial Disease: Surgically Confirmed

STUDY	YEAR	PATIENTS (N)	CONCLUSIONS
Togashi, et al	1986	12	Best in locally advanced 40% false-positive
Hricak, et al	1988	57	88% accuracy
Greco, et al	1989	46	85% accuracy
Sironi, et al	1991	25	Sensitivity, 100%; Specificity, 80%; Accuracy, 88%
Pellegrino, et al	1993	47	Sensitivity, 76.5%; specificity, 94.1%

TABLE 6-9
Magnetic Resonance Imaging Accuracy in Predicting
Metastases in Nodes: Surgically Confirmed

STUDY	YEAR	PATIENTS (N)	CONCLUSION
Togashi, et al	1986	12	25% false-positive
Waggonspeck, et al	1988	20	Probably equal to computed tomography
Greco, et al	1989	46	76% accuracy
Lichtenegger	1993	41	Lymph nodes difficult to detect

Other Studies

BLOOD CHEMISTRIES

Screening blood chemistries are important because they may predict or confirm other abnormal findings; for example, elevated serum blood urea nitrogen and creatinine levels are associated with ureteral obstruction or intrinsic renal disease, which may be demonstrated by an IVP or CT scan. Abnormal liver enzymes may accompany metastatic disease but are more likely to identify patients with nonmalignant liver disease. Elevated serum calcium values secondary to bone metastases or ectopic parahormone production may accompany advanced stages of disease. Additionally, routine evaluation of serum electrolytes may be important in treatment-related problems such as diarrhea.

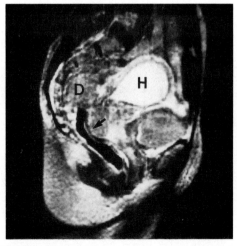

FIGURE 6-15. Sagittal magnetic resonance imaging scan. Note hydrometra (*H*) and cervical mass indenting the rectum (***arrow***). A dermoid cyst (*D*) is present in the presacral area. (Shingleton HM, Orr JW Jr. Cancer of the cervix: diagnosis and treatment. New York, Churchill Livingstone, 1987:113.)

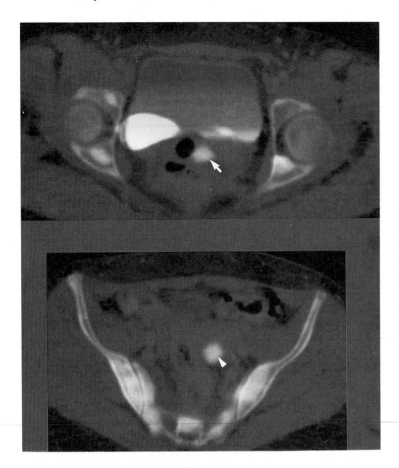

FIGURE 6-16. Patient referred for assessment of primary cervical carcinoma. Clinical evaluation included examination under anesthesia. Stage 1B CT scan demonstrated disease at the primary site but no pelvic node disease was identified. Registered CT-PET-FDG image showed clearly the primary disease and the isolated external iliac nodal spread. Histologic examinations after radical hysterectomy and lymphadenectomy confirmed the registered CT-PET-FDG findings. *CT,* computed tomography; *PET,* positron emission tomography; *FDG,* 2-[18F]fluoro-2-deoxy-D-glucose. (Courtesy of Dr. K.S. Raju and Dr. W.L. Wong, Department of Gynaecology and Radiology, United Medical and Dental Schools of Guy's and St. Thomas's Hospitals, University of London.) See Color Figure 6-16.

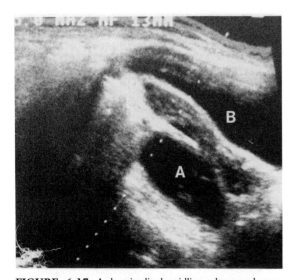

FIGURE 6-17. A longitudinal midline ultrasound scan, which reveals a large abscess in the cul-de-sac in a patient with squamous cell carcinoma of the cervix. *A,* abscess; *B,* bladder. (Shingleton HM, Orr Jr. Cancer of the cervix: diagnosis and treatment. New York, Churchill Livingstone, 1987:110.)

TUMOR MARKERS IN CERVICAL CANCER

Squamous Cell Carcinoma. Many investigators have performed tissue studies on squamous cell carcinoma (SCC) antigen, a tumor marker identified by rabbit antiserum raised against a purified extract of cervical squamous cell carcinoma (Table 6-12). It is likely to (1) be elevated in tumors of large volume (Maiman et al 1989, Yazigi et al 1991); (2) correlate with pathologic factors such as deep stromal invasion and nodal metastases (Duk et al 1990); and (3) correlate with exophytic tumors (Maiman et al 1989). Squamous cell carcinoma is thought to be expressed most frequently in large cell nonkeratinizing and keratinizing carcinomas and less frequently in the small cell type. Some believe that the tissue expression of SCC antigen is related to the differentiation of the tumor cells. Although there are some data correlating the tissue expression of SCC antigen and the disease course (Senekjian 1987), the marker has not gained widespread use in the routine management or follow-up of patients treated for cervical squamous cancers.

Tumor marker CA-125 has been tested as a prognostic indicator of women with squamous cell cancer.

TABLE 6-10
Accuracy of Fine-Needle Aspiration

STUDY	YEAR	PATIENTS (N)	SITE	ACCURACY (%)
Nordqvist, et al	1979	58	Abdominal/pelvic masses	95.0
Belinson, et al	1981	80	Abdominal/pelvic masses	96.5
Shepherd, et al	1981	50	Abdominal/pelvic masses	96.0
Zornoza, et al	1977	72	Abdominopelvic nodes	82.0
Dolan, et al	1981	51	Abdominopelvic nodes	86.0
Ewing, et al	1982	61	Abdominopelvic nodes	95.1
McDonald, et al	1983	50	Abdominopelvic nodes	74.0
Fortier, et al	1985	82	Abdominopelvic nodes	84.0
Cochand-Proillet, et al	1987	228	Abdominopelvic nodes	93.0
Sevin, et al	1979	124	Abdominal/pelvic masses; abdominopelvic nodes	94.5

Lehtovirta and coworkers (1990) found CA-125 to be elevated in only 26% of women with squamous cell tumors, compared with 75% of those with adenocarcinomas, and concluded that CA-125 was not of clinical value regarding squamous cell lesions. In contrast, Goldberg and associates (1991) reported 55 patients with squamous cell tumors, 51% of whom had elevated CA-125 levels; of 11 patients who had pre- and posttreatment levels exceeding 35 U/mL, 10 died of disease and 1 was alive with persistent disease. Of 20 women with elevated CA-125 levels at presentation who reverted to normal after treatment, 19 were without clinical evidence of disease at 14 to 46 months follow-up (mean, 27 months). There was no correlation between CA-125 levels and tumor grade or stage of disease. Although the marker may be of some clinical value, it has not been routinely used or recommended.

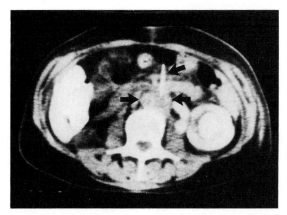

FIGURE 6-18. Computed tomography scan, demonstrating a needle (*upper arrow*) inserted into an enlarged paraaortic node (*lower arrow*). The path of the needle is only partially in the plane of the tomogram. (Courtesy of Dr. P.T. Taylor, in Shingleton HM, Orr JW Jr. Cancer of the cervix: diagnosis and treatment. New York, Churchill Livingstone, 1987:106.)

Kjorstad and colleagues (1982) reported that most cervical squamous cell carcinomas produce moderate amounts of carcinoembryonic antigen (CEA) and recommended its use clinically, although acknowledging it to be nonspecific and associated with significant numbers of false-positive values due to other associated medical disorders. te Velde and coworkers (1982) noted that CEA levels were elevated in 16% to 24% of patients in a stage-related manner. Pretreatment elevation of CEA levels was associated with a poor prognosis. Schwartz and associates (1987) found that CEA levels did not correlate with clinical status in cervical cancer, and it has not gained use.

Adenocarcinoma. Cohen and colleagues (1982), Ueda and associates (1983), and Meier and coworkers (1990) found CEA to be expressed in greater amounts and by a larger portion of the tumor cell population in endocervical compared with endometrial adenocarcinomas. Hurlimann (1984) studied the expression of CEA in both in situ and invasive cervical adenocarcinomas and found that the marker was expressed in both to varying extents. Contemporary reports focus on CA-125 and CEA (Table 6-13). Of the two, CA-125 appears to be more important because it is elevated in most patients before treatment and more commonly correlates with other high-risk factors. CA-125 may serve in some degree as a measure of tumor virulence and may be useful in follow-up of patients with cervical adenocarcinoma. Neither marker is in routine use in patient management, perhaps because of the rarity of cervical adenocarcinomas.

RENAL SCANS

Renal isotope scans provide superior information on renal function and are complementary to IVPs or CT scans, which primarily demonstrate renal anatomic change. Patricio and Baptista (1968) indicated that

TABLE 6-11
Lymphangiography for Detection of Node Metastases

STUDY	YEAR	NODE GROUP	PATIENTS (N)	SENSITIVITY (%)	SPECIFICITY (%)
Wallace, et al	1977	Pelvic	89	100	70
de Muylder, et al	1984		100	28	100
Feigan, et al	1987		36	25	82
Vercamer, et al	1987		43	29	86
Brown, et al	1979	Paraaortic	21	83	47
Lagasse, et al	1979		95	91	50
Ashraf, et al	1982		39	67	76
Heller, et al	1990		264	79	73
Averette, et al	1966	Paraaortic	83	77	90
Piver, et al	1971	and	103	77	98
Berman, et al	1977	Pelvic	65	56	86

more than half of patients with stages III and IV disease had abnormal renographic studies, and about a third of these changes improved after irradiation; however, renal scans are seldom indicated or employed in the routine management of cervical cancer patients.

LIVER AND BONE SCANS

Radionucleotide scans of the liver are only occasionally helpful and have been replaced by the more accurate CT scans. They provide an alternate method of evaluation of patients whose blood chemistries reveal abnormal liver function.

Nuclear isotope bone scans are rarely indicated unless the patient has bone pain and even then should be preceded by skeletal films of the affected area. Such scans have a low yield (1% stage I, 10% stage IV; Kamath et al 1983) and most of the studies are falsely positive (du Toit et al 1987). Routine pretreatment long bone x-ray studies are not indicated in asymptomatic women because they are rarely positive in the absence of bone pain. Pretreatment chest films and pyelograms offer an opportunity to survey the vertebral column, ribs, and pelvic bones (Figs. 6-20*A* and *B*).

MULTIPLE PRIMARY TUMORS

Axelrod and coworkers (1984) reported 78 second primary tumors among 2362 patients in the Downstate University Gynecologic Tumor Registry in Brooklyn, New York. Second primary tumors were

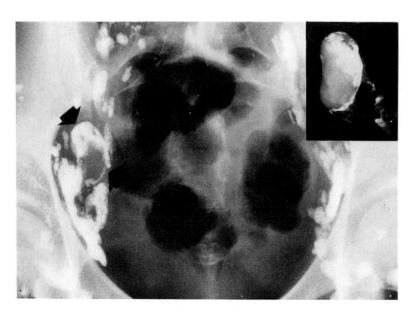

FIGURE 6-19. Details of a lymphangiographic study of pelvic lymph nodes. A large right pelvic node (*arrow*) has a filling defect secondary to invasion by squamous cell carcinoma. The *insert* shows the same node after removal. (Courtesy of Dr. P.T. Taylor, University of Virginia, Charlottesville, VA, in Shingleton HM, Orr JW Jr. Cancer of the cervix: diagnosis and treatment. New York, Churchill Livingstone, 1987:114.)

TABLE 6-12
Squamous Cell Carcinoma Antigen in Squamous Cell Cancers[†]

STUDY	YEAR	PATIENTS (N)	FIGO STAGE (%)					SENSITIVITY (%)	SPECIFITY (%)	COMMENTS
			I	II	III	IV	Overall			
Senekjian, et al	1987	24	—	—	—	—	67	—	—	Provides noninvasive means of monitoring
Crombach, et al	1989	—	—	—	—	—	—	61	—	WD, 78%; PD, 38%
Hsieh, et al	1989	78	50	53	78	100	54	—	—	
Patsner, et al	1989	65	—	—	—	—	—	68	91	Not accurate for prediction of node metastases
Duk, et al	1990	192	37	—	—	90	—	—	—	MVA, high levels with deep stromal invasion, +LN
Brioschi, et al	1991	125	54	86	97	—	—	—	—	—
Verlooy, et al	1991	50	—	—	—	—	50	—	—	Not useful for diagnosis
Yazigi, et al	1991	55	17	—	—	—	67	—	—	Levels↑ with ↑tumor volume
Avall-Lundquist, et al	1992	142	—	—	—	—	—	44	95	Elevated in 7/8 patients; +nodes $p = .005$
Borras, et al	1992	23	—	—	—	—	56	—	—	—
Lam, et al	1992	334	—	—	—	—	—	49	95	Rates ↑ with clinical stage
Bolli, et al	1994	911	—	—	—	—	—	—	98	Useful marker; values of 2.7 ng/mL have 95% positive predictive value

[†]Elevated levels >2.5 micrograms/mL.
*SCC or TA4.
FIGO, International Federation of Gynecology and Obstetrics; *PD*, poorly differentiated; *WD*, well differentiated; *MVA*, multivariate analysis; *LN*, lymph node.

found in 1.7% of patients with carcinoma in situ of the cervix (70% synchronous), whereas 3.9% of those with invasive cervical cancer had second primary tumors, synchronous in about a third of affected individuals. Significant synchronous tumor pairs included cervix–ovary, cervix– endometrial, and cervix–gastrointestinal tract. LiVolsi and associates (1983) reported several patients with endocervical adenocarcinoma who were also found to harbor synchronous mucinous neoplasms of the ovary. In each case, in situ components were found at both sites, lending credence to the idea that the lesions represented separate primaries rather than metastatic disease. Some synchronous tumors (ovary, endometrium, GI tract) and breast cancers are likely to be discovered at the time of initial evaluation for cervical cancer or may be detected in the follow-up years.

Nutritional Assessment

Orr (1985) performed a prospective nutritional assessment of 78 patients with untreated cervical cancer. Stage-related abnormal anthropometric measurements were present in 60% of patients; 67% had abnormal biochemical nutritional measurements. An appreciable number of patients (30%) were anergic to usual skin

TABLE 6-13
Tumor Markers in Adenocarcinoma of the Cervix

STUDY	YEAR	PATIENTS (N)	MARKERS	CONCLUSIONS
Leminen	1990	42	CA125, CEA, TATI*	CA125 and to lesser degree CEA + TATI useful in follow-up
Duk, et al	1990	77	CA125, CEA, SCC	CA125 important prognostic factor and indicator of tumor virulence
Tamimi, et al	1992	55	CEA	Patients whose tumors express CEA are at increased risk for recurrence

TATI, tumor-associated trypsin inhibitor.
CEA, carcinoembryonic antigen.

test antigens. The overall incidence of protein calorie malnutrition (also stage-related) was 12.5%. Surgical procedures tended to affect adversely the parameters under study. Vitamin assessment was also undertaken in the same group of patients; at least one abnormal vitamin level was present in two thirds of the patients, whereas individual levels were abnormal in as many as 38% of patients. Significantly lowered levels of plasma folate, vitamin A, and vitamin C were present. Although the prognostic effects on survival or treatment-related complications remain to be determined, the high incidence of nutritional abnormalities suggests the need for pretreatment assessment and replacement of specific deficiencies.

Surgical Staging

It is apparent, based on literature review, that clinical staging is highly inaccurate (Table 6-14). Overall errors range from 17.3% to 38.5% in patients with clinical stage I to 42.9% to 89.5% in patients with stage III disease. These inaccuracies prompted many early investigators (1970s and 1980s) to employ transperitoneal

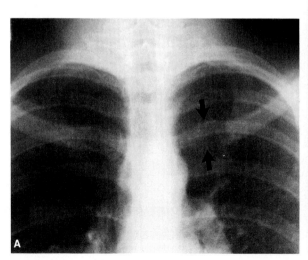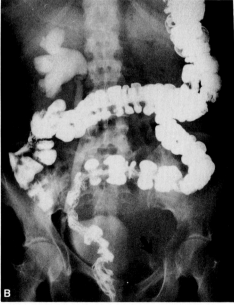

FIGURE 6-20. (**A**) Bony metastasis in a 27-year-old woman with squamous cell carcinoma. The medial portion of the left clavicle has been destroyed by tumor (*arrows*). (**B**) Bony invasion in the right pelvis in a 44-year-old woman with advanced squamous cell carcinoma of the cervix. (Shingleton HM, Orr JW Jr. Cancer of the cervix: diagnosis and treatment. New York, Churchill Livingstone, 1987:115.)

TABLE 6-14
Difference in Clinical and Surgical Staging

			INACCURACY (%)				
STUDY	YEAR	PATIENTS (N)	Stage I	Stage II	Stage III	Stage IV	Overall
van Nagell, et al	1971	125	—	—	—	—	33.0
Averette, et al	1972	82	—	—	—	—	38.6
Sudarsanam, et al	1978	220	28.0	48.8	89.5	0	36.8
Lagasse, et al	1979	95	—	—	—	—	33.6
Lagasse, et al*	1980	290	24.4	50.0	44.4	50.0	38.3
Chung, et al	1981	159	17.3	21.9	42.9	66.7	21.4
Rabin, et al	1984	92	38.5	71.5[†]	—	37.5	—

*Gynecologic Oncology Group data.
[†]Stage IIA.

surgical staging to identify tumor spread, determine the presence of extrapelvic disease, and offer adjunctive or extended field therapy. It soon became apparent, however, that transperitoneal surgical staging procedures followed by abdominopelvic irradiation were associated with appreciable complications and occasional deaths (Table 6-15). The more extensive the paraaortic nodal dissection, the more serious were the complications (Wharton et al 1977). Thirteen of Wharton and associates' 120 patients (10.8%) experienced major complications and 4 (3.3%) died as a result of the staging procedure.

Extraperitoneal Staging

Alternative methods of exploration have been devised. Schellhas (1975) suggested a vertical paraumbilical incision for an extraperitoneal approach, which allows

sampling or dissection of the aortic nodes. He noted that this procedure was associated with few complications. In our modification of Schellhas's operation, a small incision (Fig. 6-21) is made above the pelvic irradiation field. A small peritoneal window allows collection of peritoneal cytology and palpation of important pelvic structures. We have used this technique, even in obese patients, with little morbidity and little delay in initiation of radiation therapy. Previously, we had experienced many serious small bowel complications associated with transperitoneal aortic node sampling followed by paraaortic irradiation; we have not observed serious complications using the modified Schellhas surgical staging procedure.

Berman and colleagues (1977) reported significantly lower complication rates using an extraperitoneal approach through a low abdominal J-shaped incision. This incision allowed dissection of the pelvic

TABLE 6-15
Complications of Transperitoneal Surgical Procedures

STUDY	YEAR	PATIENTS (N)	COMPLICATIONS (%)	DEATHS (%)
Piver, et al*	1973	24	4.1	0
Berman, et al	1977	31	43.0	0
Nelson, et al	1977	104	18.3	1.9
Buchsbaum	1979	150	12.0	0.7
Bonanno, et al*	1980	150	12.6	0
Lagasse, et al	1980	245	15.5	0
Welander, et al	1981	127	1.6	0
LaPolla, et al	1986	44	14.0	2
Christopherson, et al	1987	30	10.0	3.3
Podczaski, et al	1989	51	14.0[†]	0

*Aortic dissection/biopsy.
[†]Overall percentage for 155 patients (trans- and extraperitoneal procedures).

TABLE 6-17
Incidence of Paraaortic Node Metastases by Stage

STUDY	YEAR	STAGE IB		STAGE IIA		STAGE IIB		STAGE III		STAGE IVA	
		Patients (n)	Positive (%)	Patients (n)	Positive (%)	Patients (n)	Positive (%)	Patients (n)	Positive (%)	Patients (n)	Positive (%)
Nelson, et al	1977	—	—	16	12.5	47	14.9	39	38.0	—	—
Wharton, et al	1977	21	0	10	0	47	21.2	34[1]	32.3	8[2]	37.5
Sudarsanam, et al	1978	153	7.0	21	14.0	22	18.0	19	26.3	—	—
Buchsbaum	1979	16	25.0	4	0	15	6.7	104	32.7	10	40.0
Bonanno, et al	1980	—	—	23	4.0	73	12.0	52	31.0	3	33.0
Hughes, et al	1980	140	4.3	35	8.5	45	24.4	96	23.9	23	43.5
Lagasse, et al	1980	143	5.6	22	18.2	58	32.8	63	30.2	3	33.0
Ballon, et al	1981	22	23.0	16	19.0	32	19.0	24	16.7	—	—
Chung, et al	1981	110	4.5	15	6.7	17	17.6	14	42.9	3	66.6
Welander, et al	1981	14	28.6	22	22.7	41	19.5	38	26.3	12	33.3
Berman, et al	1984	150	5.0	3[3]	3[3]	3[3]	3[3]	135	25.0	—	—

[1] IIIA only
[2] IIIB and IV
[3] Only combined figures for IIA and IIB were available: # pts = 222; % pos = 16
*University of Alabama at Birmingham data.

Scalene Nodes

Before beginning extended-field radiation therapy to the paraaortic nodes, it is important to determine that there is no spread beyond this treatment field. As many as a third of patients with metastases to paraaortic nodes may have involved scalene nodes (Table 6-18). One thus might elect to perform left supraclavicular lymph node biopsy under the same anesthetic when metastatic disease is found in paraaortic nodes. If they are positive, treatment is palliative. Before any biopsy procedure of the supraclavicular nodes, a chest CT scan should be performed to rule out chest metastases.

Conclusions Regarding the Place of Surgical Staging

What can one conclude regarding the value of surgical staging in the routine evaluation and treatment of patients with cervical cancer? Jones (1981) observed that whereas staging allows individualization of care by the knowledge gained, the extrapelvic disease that it uncovers has little likelihood of being managed successfully. Barber (1988), on review of the available literature, concluded that surgical staging could not be shown to benefit patients. Podczaski and colleagues (1989) estimated that less than 5% of patients undergoing a selective paraaortic lymphadenectomy derive benefit from it. Heaps and coworkers (1990) concluded that surgical staging has produced a modest boost in survival, most likely due to the high rate of systemic and pelvic failure in women with extrapelvic disease. Copeland (1991) and others believe that surgical staging should be limited to investigational settings. Christopherson (1992) concludes that because of the relative inability to effectively treat tumor in paraaortic nodes, surgical staging (if used) should be reserved for women with advanced stage disease who are good surgical risks. We only use surgical staging for protocol studies and particularly frown on revisiting biopsy or dissection of pelvic nodes by laparo-scopic techniques because such knowledge gained is not beneficial to patients with the disease.

CONSIDERATIONS IN SELECTION OF THERAPY

Several factors are important in the selection of treatment: the age of the woman, the tumor volume, the presence of parametrial extension, demonstrable extrapelvic disease, and the need for preservation of sexual function.

SURVIVAL AS A FACTOR OF AGE AT OCCURRENCE

Whether younger women have a lower survival rate than older women with the same stage cancer of the cervix is still controversial. Kjorstad (1977), studying a group of more than 2000 patients, reported that young patients had a more favorable stage distribution and a better prognosis than those older. Adcock and associates (1982) also reported better survival in young women (younger than 35) who have either squamous cell carcinoma or adenocarcinoma but a decreased survival rate for those with adenosquamous tumors. Baltzer and coworkers (1982) noted no difference in survival above and below the age of 35 in women with either squamous cell tumors or adenocarcinomas; he also reported a decrease in survival for those with adenosquamous tumors. In contrast, Cullhead (1978), Stanhope and associates (1980), Gynning and colleagues (1983), Hall and Monaghan (1983), Prempree and coworkers (1983), and Stehman and associates (1991) report that younger patients have lower 5-year survival rates. In most of these studies, there were no matched controls, no adjustment for volume of tumor within stage, and in most instances, few in the younger-aged treatment groups. Mann and coworkers (1980), reporting the University of Alabama experience (all treatments), found that young women with stage IB squamous cell cancer of the cervix did not differ in survival from older women, using an age cutoff of either 40 years or 30 years. O'Brien and Carmichael (1988) and Levrant and associates (1992), reporting surgical series of early stage disease, differed in their conclusions: in O'Brien and colleagues' series, women older than 50 did worse, whereas in Levrant and associates' study, there was not a significant difference in long-term survival. Baltzer and coworkers (1988), Spanos and associates (1989), and Gonzalez and colleagues (1989) concluded that age is not a prognostic factor. It is thus difficult to resolve this question, considering that the FIGO staging system is inaccurate because it allows great variation in tumor volume within a given stage and reliable assess-

TABLE 6-18
Scalene Node Metastases in Untreated Patients With Paraaortic Node Metastases

STUDY	YEAR	PATIENTS (N)	POSITIVE NODES (%)
Buchsbaum	1979	23	35
Brandt, et al	1981	25	28
Lee, et al	1981	10	30
TOTAL		58	31

ment of tumor volume and abdominopelvic spread is impossible, except in surgically treated or surgically staged patients.

Although some authors have stated that radical hysterectomy can be performed on women of almost any age, we have performed this surgery for women older than age 65 only when the patient is an excellent operative candidate. O'Leary and Symmonds (1966), discussing surgery as primary treatment, concluded that cardiovascular or renal impairment are more important considerations in selecting therapy than age alone. Levrant and associates (1992) found no difference in operative morbidity in women older or younger than 50. Kennedy and coworkers (1989), reporting on treatment for women 75 or older, concluded that older women can receive definitive therapy, including surgery, after careful preoperative medical evaluation and treatment.

Regarding radiated patients, Hanks and colleagues (1983), summarizing a national radiation therapy patterns-of-care study, concluded that young women actually have more irradiation complications than do older women, particularly those who have had previous pelvic disease (especially infectious disease) and that thin women (especially whites) did not tolerate the treatment well. Patients older than 75 may frequently require therapy modification but still have significant survival (Kennedy et al 1989).

TUMOR VOLUME

Tumor volume is the single most important factor in predicting survival in patients with cancer of the cervix, regardless of treatment. The presence of bulky tumors, especially those expanding the endocervical canal, may lead some to consider a combination of irradiation and surgery, based on the belief that central pelvic failure occurs in women with bulky lesions of the endocervix if irradiation is used as sole treatment. Such tumors actually recur frequently at distant sites, and it has not been established that routine adjunctive conservative hysterectomy alters survival rates, although it does decrease central pelvic recurrences (see Chap. 9).

PALPABLE PARAMETRIAL EXTENSION OF TUMOR

Palpable extension of presumed tumor into the parametrial tissues is given as the reason for choosing irradiation as the primary therapy of many women. For the past half century or more, American gynecologists and radiation therapists have arbitrarily excluded clinical stage IIB disease from surgical consideration, although surgical staging studies have shown that a high percentage of women with clinical stage IIB disease actually have no parametrial extension and thus are

surgical stage IB patients (see Table 6-14 and Table 7-13 in Chap. 7). European (especially German and Austrian) surgeons (Burghardt et al 1987, Winter et al 1988, Friedberg 1988, Tulusan et al 1988) and Asian surgeons (Matsuyama et al 1984, Inoue et al 1990, Cheng 1990) surgically stage and in most cases complete radical surgical removal of such tumors and the regional lymph nodes. Limiting surgical cases to women who have FIGO stage IB lesions 2 to 3 cm or less in size is also arbitrary, and an emerging literature (Creasman et al 1986, Alvarez et al 1993, Bloss et al 1993) suggests that bulky lesions up to or exceeding 6 cm in size are suitable for removal, with excellent survival results (see Chap. 7).

EXTRAPELVIC TUMOR

Finding extrapelvic tumor during the pretreatment evaluation invariably alters treatment. Chest (pulmonary) metastases relegate the patient to palliation treatment—usually palliative pelvic irradiation and systemic chemotherapy. Demonstration of microscopic tumor spread to the aortic nodes in the absence of spread to the lungs, the thoracic, or scalene nodes allows extension of the irradiation field to include the paraaortic area. Bortolozzi and colleagues (1983) reported a mean extension in survival of 15 months by performing adjunctive hysterectomy after pelvic irradiation in the presence of proved aortic node metastases; this has not been substantiated by other investigators, however. Most American gynecologic oncologists, ourselves included, leave the pelvic tumor in situ in such cases and complete therapy by pelvic irradiation and extended-field therapy to the aortic area in an attempt to eliminate the morbidity of the radical hysterectomy. The German–Austrian approach differs, however; radical excision of the cervical tumor occurs in conjunction with comprehensive radical aortic lymphadenectomy, even in the presence of paraaortic node metastases. To date, no clear advantage in survival has been reported using such an aggressive approach, and the surgical complications most likely exceed the complications of pelvic and paraaortic radiation therapy after surgical staging.

Distant metastases to bone, lung, liver, or other sites require consideration of systemic chemotherapy with or without palliative irradiation to the primary site. Metastases to the scalene nodes also change the goal of therapy to palliation, and chemotherapy may be offered as the sole therapy unless symptoms of the pelvic tumor (bleeding, pain) suggest the need for palliative irradiation.

SEXUAL FUNCTION

All therapy for cancer of the cervix has the potential to alter the woman's sexual function. If she has stage IB disease and radical surgery is selected, the vagina, although shortened, is not otherwise changed. Too often, physicians—adhering to the bias that older women have no interest in sexual activity—ignore this important feature of treatment planning. Abitbol and Davenport (1974) reported that radiation therapy, especially brachytherapy, markedly alters the vagina and sexual dysfunction occurs in 78% of patients, making intercourse impossible or less pleasurable. In contrast, only 6% of surgically treated (radical hysterectomy) patients experienced sexual dysfunction. Our experience is similar; we recommend vaginal dilators in the immediate postradiation period, followed by early resumption of sexual intercourse as a means of reducing strictures of the vagina. Women who are not sexually active after radiation therapy for cervical cancer experience stricturing and shortening of the vagina to the extent that posttreatment surveillance also is difficult or impossible. Because many women with locally advanced disease must be treated with pelvic/vaginal irradiation, every effort should be made (by proper selection of the vaginal applicator, skilled dosimetry, posttherapy vaginal dilation, and use of local vaginal estrogens) to minimize the damage to the vagina, so that the patient can have the potential for or can enjoy normal vaginal intercourse (see Chap. 14).

Adenocarcinoma and Mixed Tumors

For adenocarcinoma, the same factors (age, tumor volume, extracervical and extrapelvic extension, preservation of sexual function) are important; in most instances, selection of treatment should follow the same lines stage by stage, as for squamous cell lesions (Shingleton et al 1981, Berek et al 1985, Ireland et al 1985, Kleine et al 1989). Because of concern about the radiosensitivity of adenocarcinoma, Milsom and Friberg (1983) and Kjorstad and Orjasaester (1984) advocated a combined radiation therapy–surgical approach to remove the central lesion after intracavitary treatment. Prempree and associates (1985) could demonstrate no advantage of using combined therapy in stage I disease but reported higher survival rates in stage II patients treated by combined therapy. Kleine and coworkers (1989) believe that surgery is important for stage I and II adenocarcinomas because patients with those stages who were treated by irradiation alone had a poorer survival rates. Eifel and colleagues (1991) concluded that women with adenocarcinomas 3 cm or larger in diameter do better with combined therapy because those tumors treated by surgery alone recur more frequently (45% versus 11%). Some state that whereas pure adenocarcinomas may be treated the same as squamous tumors (stage for stage), adenosquamous carcinomas should be separated for combined treatment (irradiation and surgery, with or with-

out systemic chemotherapy). Korhonen and Stenback (1984), however, could not demonstrate any difference in survival between pure adenocarcinoma or adenosquamous carcinoma, even using combined irradiation and surgery. Helm and associates (1993), in a three-institutional matched control study of 43 women with stage IB adenosquamous tumors treated by radical hysterectomy and pelvic node dissection, did not report survival differences for the mixed tumors compared with either squamous cell or pure adenocarcinoma controls. Considering all treatment and all stages, adenocarcinoma patients seem to fare slightly worse than squamous cell cancer patients (Table 6-19), especially in FIGO stages II and III.

SURGERY OR RADIATION?

When cure rates of surgical and radiation treatment for FIGO stage IB cancer of the cervix are compared, the survival rates are almost identical. Delgado (1978), in a collected series, reported 83.4% 5-year survival after radical surgery (2600 patients) and 85.5% 5-year survival after radiation therapy (1995 patients). Apart from survival, there are other advantages of surgical treatment for healthy patients with FIGO stages I and IIA (Table 6-20). Although irradiation could be selected for all patients, major bladder and bowel damage occurs in 2% to 6% and chronic bladder dysfunction has been reported in 23% to 44% (Parkin 1989). Symptomatic irradiation cystitis or proctitis may occur months or years after treatment and persist for long periods of time. Bladder and rectal fistulas after irradi-

TABLE 6-19
Adenocarcinoma of the Cervix: 5-Year Survival by Stage —All Treatments

STUDY	YEAR	PATIENTS (N)	I	II	III and IV
Rutledge, et al	1975	107	84	48	28
Prempree, et al	1985	97	77	64	27
Kjorstad	1987	102	83	34	9
Kilgore, et al	1988	162	78	43	15
Goodman, et al	1989	70	82	90	38
Kleine, et al	1989	144	76	41	27
Lee, et al	1989	31	84	25	—
Hopkins, et al	1991	203	60	47	8
Tinga, et al	1992	33	72	—	—

TABLE 6-20
Selection of Treatment for Stage IB Cancer
of the Cervix

TREATMENT	ADVANTAGES	DISADVANTAGES
Radiation	Can apply to all patients Survival rates may equal those for surgery	Operative mortality, 0–1% (with intracavitary method) Serious bladder or bowel damage, 2–6% Destruction of ovary function Bulky centrally or in nodes, hard to irradiate Vaginal stenosis and sexual dysfunction common, especially in postmenopausal women Complications are delayed, difficult to correct
Surgery	Ovary conservation possible Establishes exact extent of tumor Complications early, correctable More functional vagina Psychological advantage of tumor removal	Long-term bladder dysfunction, 3–4% Urinary fistulas/strictures, 1–2% Operative mortality, 1% Not applicable for morbidly obese or older infirm women Post operative irradiation required 10–15% of time Vaginal shortening, resultant sexual dysfunction
Surgery and Irradiation	Debulking of large tumors, FIGO IB, or barrel-shaped tumors decreases pelvic recurrence	Risk of higher complications than with single-modality treatment; no proved survival advantage

ation are difficult to correct surgically because the endarteritis associated with the therapy reduces blood supply to the pelvic tissues and impedes healing after surgery. Although the rectal and bladder complications after irradiation (and surgery) have been emphasized in the literature, the vaginal complications and sexual problems associated with radiation therapy for cervical cancer have been largely ignored.

Another reason to select surgery for early disease is ovarian conservation. Metastases to the ovaries are rare (less than 1%) with early stage squamous tumors, although somewhat higher in adenocarcinoma patients (1.4%; Reisenger et al 1991; see Table 7-7 in Chap. 7), and the ovaries can be left in place. With a surgical approach, the extent of tumor can be established; the vagina is left without major changes in caliber or elasticity and the removal of the tumor offers a psychological advantage to the patient—the tumor is "out." The complications of surgical treatment occur early and usually are correctable, whereas those from irradiation may appear later and generally are more difficult to remedy. Operative deaths from surgery are rare (less than 1%; see Table 7-10 in Chap. 7).

Younger, healthier women are often offered surgery as primary treatment. The obese, the diabetic, and the woman with cardiac or other major health problems ordinarily receives primary radiation therapy. Postoperative radiation therapy is commonly given to 12% to 15% of surgically treated patients because of findings of pelvic node metastases or close surgical margins, although it is not established that such adjunctive irradiation improves survival.

Rutledge and coworkers (1979) stated that the issue is not how many radical surgical procedures should be employed but how best to select patients for a surgical approach. The likelihood of adequate resection, therefore, is a prime consideration before embarking on extended hysterectomy as primary treatment. Certainly, primary surgical treatment should not be attempted when the lesion is so large that it precludes tumor-free margins. Most patients with surgical margin involvement experience recurrence within 12 to 18 months of the operation, and the salvage rate is not impressive, even if early postoperative pelvic irradiation is administered. In such women, the normal anatomy is altered and adhesions may diminish the mobility of small bowel in the lower abdomen, resulting in increased numbers of bowel complications. The prudent surgeon should consider these risks, just as the radiotherapist should recommend a primary surgical approach for young women with resectable cervical lesions. An American College of Surgeons Patterns of Care Study involving 5817 women treated in the year 1990 revealed that 48.2% had total hysterectomy or radical hysterectomy. This rise in use of surgical treatment undoubtedly reflects earlier diagnosis (60% of the patients had stages IA, IB, IIA) and may relate to the influence of gynecologic oncologists, who perform most radical operations for this disease (Shingleton 1995), at least as reflected in this large national study encompassing about 45% of invasive cervical cancer occurring in the United States in 1990.

Rare Tumors

The therapy for such rare tumors as lymphoma, melanoma, or sarcoma of the cervix invariably involves combinations of surgery, irradiation, and chemotherapy. Descriptions of treatment occur primarily in the form of individual case reports and are discussed in Chapter 9.

References

Abitbol MM, Davenport JH. Sexual dysfunction after therapy for cervical carcinoma. Am J Obstet Gynecol 1974; 119:181.

Adcock LL, Julian TM, Okagaki T. Carcinoma of the uterine cervix FIGO stage I-B. Gynecol Oncol 1982;14:199.

Alvarez RD, Gelder MS, Gore H, Soong S-J, Partridge EE. Radical hysterectomy in the treatment of patients with bulky early stage carcinoma of the cervix uteri. Surg Gynecol Obstet 1993;176:539.

Angel C, Beecham JB, Rubins DJ. Magnetic resonance imaging and pathologic correlation in stage IB cervix cancers. Gynecol Oncol 1987;27:357.

Aoki S, Hata T, Senoh D, et al. Parametrial invasion of uterine cervical cancer assessed by transrectal ultrasonography: preliminary report. Gynecol Oncol 1990;36:82.

Ashraf M, Elyaderani MK, Gabrielle OF, Krall JM. Value of lymphangiography in the diagnosis of paraaortic lymph node metastases from carcinoma of the cervix. Gynecol Oncol 1982;14:96.

Avall-Lundqvist EH, Sjovall K, Nillson BR, Eneroth PH. Prognostic significance of pretreatment serum levels of squamous cell carcinoma antigen and CA 125 in cervical carcinoma. Eur J Cancer 1992;28A:1695.

Averette HE, Dudan RC, Ford JH Jr. Exploratory celiotomy for surgical staging of cervical cancer. Am J Obstet Gynecol 1972;113:1090.

Averette HE, LeMaire WJ, Lecart CJ, Ferguson JH. Lymphography in the preoperative detection of lymphatic metastases. Obstet Gynecol 1966;27:122.

Axelrod MM, Fruchter R, Boyce JG. Multiple primaries among gynecologic malignancies. Gynecol Oncol 1984; 18:359.

Ballon SC, Berman ML, Lagasse LD, Petrilli ES, Castaldo TW. Survival after extraperitoneal pelvic and paraaortic lymphadenectomy and radiation therapy in cervical carcinoma. Obstet Gynecol 1981;57:90.

Baltzer J, Lohe KJ, Koepcke W, Zander J. Formation of metastases in the ovaries in operated squamous cell carcinoma of the cervix uteri. Geburtshilfe Frauenheilkd 1981;41:673.

Baltzer J, Lohe KJ, Kopcke W, Zander J. Histological criteria for the prognosis in patients with operated squamous cell carcinoma of the cervix. Gynecol Oncol 1982; 13:184.

Baltzer J, Ober, Zander J. Adjuvant radiotherapy in patients undergoing surgical treatment for carcinoma of the cervix. Baillieres Clin Obstet Gynaecol 1988;2:999.

Bandy LC, Clarke-Pearson DL, Silverman PM, Creasman WT. Computed tomography in evaluation of extrapelvic lymphadenopathy in carcinoma of the cervix. Obstet Gynecol 1985;65:73.

Barber HRK. Cervical cancer: pelvic and para-aortic lymph node sampling and its consequences. Baillieres Clin Obstet Gynaecol 1988;2(4):768.

Belinson JL, Lynn JM, Papillo JL, Lee K, Korson R. Fine-needle aspiration cytology in the management of gynecologic cancer. Am J Obstet Gynecol 1981;138:148.

Berek JS, Hacker NF, Fu Y-S, Sokale JR, Leuchter RC, Lagasse LD. Adenocarcinoma of the uterine cervix: histologic variables associated with lymph node metastasis and survival. Obstet Gynecol 1985;65:46.

Berman ML, Keys H, Creasman W, DiSaia P, Bundy B, Blessing J. Survival and patterns of recurrence in cervical cancer metastatic to periaortic lymph nodes (a gynecologic oncology group study). Gynecol Oncol 1984; 19:8.

Berman ML, Lagasse LD, Watring WG, et al. The operative evaluation of patients with cervical carcinoma by an extraperitoneal approach. Obstet Gynecol 1977;50:658.

Bloss JD, Berman ML, Mukherjee J, Manetta, Rettenmaier ED, DiSaia PJ. Bulky stage IB cervical carcinoma managed by primary radical hysterectomy followed by tailored radiotherapy (abstract). 23rd Annual Meeting of the Society of Gynecologic Oncologists, San Antonio, Texas, March 15–18, 1992.

Bolli JN, Bosscher JR, Doering DL, Day TG, Florman S, Owens KJ, Kelly BA. Squamous cell carcinoma antigen; clinical utility in squamous cell carcinoma of the uterine cervix. Presented at the 25th annual meeting of the Society of Gynecologic Oncologists, Orlando, Florida, February 6–9, 1994. Abstract.

Bonanno JP, Boyce J, Fruchter R, Khulpateea N, Macasaet M, Remy JC. Involvement of para-aortic lymph nodes in carcinoma of the cervix. J Am Osteopath Assoc 1980;79:567.

Boronow RC. Stage I cervix cancer and pelvic metastasis. Special reference to the implications of the new and recently replaced FIGO classifications of stage Ia. Am J Obstet Gynecol 1977;127:135.

Borras G, Molina R, Xercavins J, Ballesta A, Iglasias X. Squamous cell carcinoma antigen in cervical cancer. Eur J Gynaecol Oncol 1992;13:414.

Bortolozzi G, Rossi F, Mangioni C, Candiani GB. A contribution to the therapy of cervicocarcinoma: remarks on 40 patients presenting paraaortic metastases (1970–1979). Europ J Gynaecol Oncol 1983;4:9.

Brandt B, Lifshitz S. Scalene node biopsy in advanced carcinoma of the cervix uteri. Cancer 1981;47:1920.

Brenner DE, Whitley NO, Prempree T, Villasanta U. An evaluation of the computed tomographic scanner for the staging of carcinoma of the cervix. Cancer 1982; 50:2323.

Brioschi PA, Bischof P, Delafosse C, Krauer F. Squamous-cell carcinoma antigen (SCC-A) vaules related to clinical outcome of pre-invasive and invasive carvical carcinoma. Int J Cancer 1991;47:376.

Brodman M, Friedman F Jr, Dottino P, et al. A comparative study of computerized tomography, magnetic resonance imaging, and clinical staging for the detection of early cervix cancer. Gynecol Oncol 1990;36:409.

Brown RC, Buchsbaum HJ, Platz CE. Accuracy of lymphangiography in the diagnosis of paraaortic lymph node metastases from carcinoma of the cervix. Obstet Gynecol 1979;54:571.

Buchsbaum HJ. Extrapelvic lymph node metastases in cervical carcinoma. Am J Obstet Gynecol 1979;133:814.

Burghardt E, Hofmann HMH, Ebner F, Haas J, Tamussino

K, Justich E. Magnetic resonance imaging in cervical cancer: a basis for objective classification. Gynecol Oncol 1989;33:61.

Burghardt E, Pickel H. Local spread and lymph node involvement in cervical cancer. Obstet Gynecol 1978; 52:138.

Burghardt E, Pickel H, Haas J, Lahousen M. Prognostic factors and operative treatment of stages IB and IIB cervical cancer. Am J Obstet Gynecol 1987;156:988.

Camilien L, Gordon D, Fruchter RG, Maiman M, Boyce JG. Predictive value of computerized tomography in the presurgical evaluation of primary carcinoma of the cervix. Gynecol Oncol 1988;30:209.

Cheng MCE. Role of surgery in the treatment of cancer of the cervix. Singapore Med J 1990;31:253.

Childers J, Surwit E, Hatch K. The role of laparoscopic lymphadenectomy in the management of cervical carcinoma (abstract). 23rd Annual Meeting of the Society of Gynecologic Oncologists, San Antonio, Texas, March 15–18, 1992.

Christopherson WA. The spread and staging of cervical carcinoma 1992. In Lurain JR, Sciarra JJ (eds). Gynecology and Obstetrics. Philadelphia: JB Lippincott 1992.

Christopherson WA, Buchsbaum HJ. The influence of pretreatment celiotomy and para-aortic lymphadenectomy on the management of advanced stage squamous cell carcinoma of the cervix. Eur J Gynaecol Oncol 1987; 8:90.

Chung CK, Nahhas WA, Zaino R, Stryker JA, Mortel R. Histologic grade and lymph node metastasis in squamous cell carcinoma of the cervix. Gynecol Oncol 1981; 12:348.

Cochand-Proillet B, Roger, Boccon-Gibod I, Ferrand J, Faure B, Blery M. Retroperitoneal lymph node aspiration biopsy in staging of pelvic cancer: a cytological study of 228 consecutive cases. Diagn Cytopathol 1987;3:102.

Cohen C, Schulman G, Budgeon LR. Endocervical and endometrial adenocarcinoma: an immunoperoxidase and histochemical study. Am J Surg Pathol 1982;6:151.

Copeland LJ. Staging laparotomy. In Greer BE, Berek JS, eds. Gynecologic oncology: treatment rationale and techniques. New York: Elsevier, 1991:3.

Creasman WT, Soper JT, Clarke-Pearson D. Radical hysterectomy as therapy for early carcinoma of the cervix. Am J Obstet Gynecol 1986;155:964.

Crombach G, Scharl A, Vierbuchen M, Wurz H, Bolte A. Detection of squamous cell carcinoma antigen in normal squamous epithelia and in squamous cell carcinomas of the uterine cervix. Cancer 1989;63:1337.

Cullhead S. Carcinoma cervicis uteri stages I and IA. Acta Obstet Gynecol Scand (Suppl) 1978;75:1.

Dargent D, Arnould P, Roy M. The value and the limits of panoramic retroperitoneal pelviscopy (PRPP) in gynecological cancer (abstract). 23rd Annual Meeting of the Society of Gynecologic Oncologists, San Antonio, Texas, March 15–18, 1992.

Delgado G. Stage IB squamous cancer of the cervix: the choice of treatment. Obstet Gynecol Surv 1978;33:174.

de Muylder X, Belanger R, Vauclair R, Audet-Lapointe P, Cormier A, Methot Y. Value of lymphography in stage

IB cancer of the uterine cervix. Am J Obstet Gynecol 1984;148:610.

Dolan TE, McIntosh PK. Percutaneous retroperitoneal lymph node biopsy: an appraisal for a substitute to laparotomy in far advanced metastatic carcinoma. Gynecol Oncol 1981;11:364.

Downey GO, Potish RA, Adcock LL, Prem KA, Twiggs LB. Pretreatment surgical staging in cervical carcinoma: therapeutic efficacy of pelvic lymph node resection. Am J Obstet Gynecol 1989;160:1055.

Duk JM, de Bruun HWA, Groenier KH, et al. Cancer of the uterine cervix: sensitivity and specificity of serum squamous cell carcinoma antigen determinations. Gynecol Oncol 1990;39:186.

du Toit JP, Med M, Grove DV. Radioisotope bone scanning for the detection of occult bony metastases in invasive cervical carcinoma. Gynecol Oncol 1987;28:215.

Eifel PJ, Burke TW, Delclos L, Wharton JT, Oswald MJ. Early stage I adenocarcinoma of the uterine cervix: treatment results in patients with tumors 4cm in diameter. Gynecol Oncol 1991;41:199.

Engelshoven JMA, Versteege CWM, Ruys JHJ, et al. Computed tomography staging untreated patients with cervical cancer. Gynecol Obstet Invest 1984;18:289.

Ewing TL, Buchler DA, Hoogerland DL, Sonek MG, Wirtanen GW. Percutaneous lymph node aspiration in patient with gynecologic tumors. Am J Obstet Gynecol 1982;143:824.

Feigan M, Crocker EF, Read J, Crandon AJ. The value of lymphoscintigraphy, lymphangiography and computed tomography scanning in the preoperative assessment of lymph nodes involved by pelvic malignant conditions. Surg Gynecol Obstet 1987;165:107.

Fenton D, Beck S, Slater D, Peel J. Occult cervical carcinoma revealed by large loop diathermy. Lancet 1989; 8666:807.

Fortier KJ, Clarke-Pearson DL, Creasman WT, Johnston WW. Fine-needle aspiration in gynecology: evaluation of extrapelvic lesions in patients with gynecologic malignancy. Obstet Gynecol 1985;65:67.

Friedberg V. Operative therapy for stage IIB cervical cancer. Baillieres Clin Obstet Gynaecol 1988;2:973.

Fuller AF Jr, Elliott N, Kosloff C, Hoskins W, Lewis JL Jr. Determinants of increased risk for recurrence in patients undergoing radical hysterectomy for stage IB and IIA carcinoma of the cervix. Gynecol Oncol 1989;33:34.

Gal D, Buchsbaum HJ. The staging of cervical carcinoma. In Lurain JR, Sciarra JJ, eds. Gynecology and obstetrics, vol 4. Philadelphia: JB Lippincott, 1990.

Gallion HH, van Nagell JR, Donaldson ES, et al. Combined radiation therapy and extrafascial hysterectomy in the treatment of stage IB barrel-shaped cervical cancer. Cancer 1985;56:262.

Gallup DG, King LA, Messing MJ, Talledo OE. Paraaortic lymph node sampling by means of an extraperitoneal approach with a supraumbilical transverse "sunrise" incision. Am J Obstet Gynecol 1993;169:307.

Giuntoli RL, Atkinson BF, Ernst CS, Rubin MM, Egan VS, eds. Atkinson's correlative atlas of colposcopy, cytology, and histopathology. Philadelphia: JB Lippincott, 1987: 175.

Goldberg GL, Sklar A, O'Hanlan KA, Levine PA, Runowicz CD. CA-125: a potential prognostic indicator in patients with cervical cancer. Gynecol Oncol 1991; 40:222.

Gonzalez DG, Ketting BW, van Bunningen B, van Dijk JDP. Carcinoma of the uterine cervix stage IB and IIA: results of postoperative irradiation in patients with microscopic infiltration in the parametrium and/or lymph node metastasis. Int J Radiat Oncol Biol Phys 1989;16:389.

Goodman HM, Buttlar CA, Niloff JM, Welch WR, Marck A, et al. Adenocarcinoma of the uterine cervix: prognostic factors and patterns of recurrence. Gynecol Oncol 1989;33:241.

Gordon RE, Mettler FA Jr, Wicks JD, Bartow SA. Chest x-rays and full lung tomograms in gynecologic malignancy. Cancer 1983;52:559.

Greco A, Mason P, Leung AWL, et al. Staging of carcinoma of the uterine cervix: MRI-surgical correlation. Clin Radiol 1989;40:401.

Grumbine FC, Rosenshein NB, Zeerhoyni EA, Siegelman SS. Abdomino-pelvic computed tomography in the preoperative evaluation of early cervical cancer. Gynecol Oncol 1981;12:286.

Gynning I, Johnsson JE, Alm P, Trope C. Age and prognosis in stage IB squamous cell carcinoma of the uterine cervix. Gynecol Oncol 1983;15:18.

Hall SW, Monaghan JM. Invasive carcinoma of the cervix in younger women (letter). Lancet 1983;II:731.

Hanks GE, Herring DF, Kramer S. Patterns of care outcome studies: results of the national practice in cancer of the cervix. Cancer 1983;51:959.

Heaps JM, Berek JS. Surgical staging of cervical cancer. Clin Obstet Gynecol 1990;33:852.

Heller PB, Malfetano JH, Bundy BN, Barnhill DR, Okagaki T. A clinical-pathologic study of stages IIB, III and IVA carcinoma of the cervix: extended diagnostic evaluation for paraaortic node metastasis—a gynecologic oncology group study. Gynecol Oncol 1990;38:425.

Helm CW, Gore H, Soong S-J, Partridge EE, Shingleton HM. Adenosquamous carcinoma of the cervix stage IB—low risk and high risk criteria can guide selection for adjuvant therapy (abstract). 24th Annual Meeting, Society of Gynecologic Oncologists, Palm Desert, CA, February 1993.

Hillman BJ, Clark RL, Babbitt G. Efficacy of the excretory urogram in the staging of gynecologic malignancies. Am J Roentgenol 1984;143:997.

Hofmann HMH, Ebner F, Haas J, et al. Magnetic resonance imaging in clinical cervical cancer: pretherapeutic tumor volumetry. Baillieres Clin Obstet Gynaecol 1988; 2:789.

Hopkins MP, Morley GW. A comparison of adenocarcinoma and squamous cell carcinoma of the cervix. Obstet Gynecol 1991;77:912.

Hricak H. Carcinoma of the female reproductive organs. Value of cross-sectional imaging. Cancer 1991;67:1209.

Hricak H, Lacey GC, Sanles GL, Chang YC, et al. Invasive cervical carcinoma: comparison of MR imaging and surgical findings. Radiology 1988;166:623.

Hsieh CY, Chang DY, Huang SC, Yen ML, Juang GT,

Ouyang PC. Serum squamous cell carcinoma antigen in gynecologic malignancies with special reference to cervical cancer. J Formos Med Assoc 1989;88:797.

Hsu C-T, Cheng Y-S, Su S-C. Prognosis of uterine cervical cancer with extensive lymph node metastases. Am J Obstet Gynecol 1972;114:954.

Hughes RR, Brewington KC, Hanjani P, et al. Extended field irradiation for cervical cancer based on surgical staging. Gynecol Oncol 1980;9:153.

Hurlimann J, Gloor E. Adenocarcinoma in situ and invasive adenocarcinoma of the uterine cervix. An immunohistologic study with antibodies specific for several epithelial markers. Cancer 1984;54:63.

Inoue T, Morita K. The prognostic significance of number of positive nodes in cervical carcinoma stages IB, IIA, and IIB. Cancer 1990;65:1923.

Ireland D, Hardiman P, Monaghan JM. Adenocarcinoma of the uterine cervix: a study of 73 cases. Obstet Gynecol 1985;65:82.

Jiminez J, Alert J, Beldarrain L, Montalvo J, Roca C. Carcinoma of the uterine cervix. Acta Radiol Oncol Rad Phys Biol 1979;18:465.

Jones HW III. The value of operative staging in the treatment of invasive carcinoma of the cervix. In Ballon SC, ed. Gynecologic oncology; controversies in cancer treatment. Boston, GK Hall, 1981:167.

Kamath CR, Maruyama Y, DeLand FH, van Nagell JR. Role of bone scanning for evaluation of carcinoma of the cervix. Gynecol Oncol 1983;15:171.

Kennedy AW, Flagg JS, Webster KD. Gynecologic cancer in the very elderly. Gynecol Oncol 1989;32:49.

Kerr-Wilson RH, Shingleton HM, Orr JM Jr, Hatch KD. The use of ultrasound and computed tomography scanning in the management of gynecologic cancer patients. Gynecol Oncol 1984;18:54.

Kilgore LC, Soong S-J, Gore H, Shingleton HM, Hatch KD, Partridge EE. Analysis of prognostic features in adenocarcinoma of the cervix. Gynecol Oncol 1988;31:137.

King LA, Talledo E, Gallup DG, Gammal FL. Computed tomography in evaluation of gynecologic malignancies: a retrospective analysis. Am J Obstet Gynecol 1986; 155:960.

Kjorstad JE. Carcinoma of the cervix in the young patient. Obstet Gynecol 1977;50:28.

Kjorstad JE, Orjasaester H. The prognostic significance of carcinoembryonic antigen determinations in patients with adenocarcinoma of the cervix. Gynecol Oncol 1984;19:284.

Kjorstad KE. The management of the high risk patient with early invasive carcinoma of the cervix. In Surwit EA, Alberts DS, eds. Cervix cancer. Boston, Martinus Nijhoff, 1987.

Kjorstad KE, Osjasaester H. The prognostic vaule of CEA determinations in the plasma of patients with squamous cell cancer of the cervix. Cancer 1982;50:283.

Kleine W, Rau K, Schwoeorer D, Pfleiderer A. Prognosis of the adenocarcinoma of the cervix uteri: a comparative study. Gynecol Oncol 1989;35:145.

Korhonen M, Stenback F. Adenocarcinoma metastatic to the uterine cervix. Gynecol Obstet Invest 1984;17:57.

Krebs H-B, Wilstrup MA, Wheelock JB. Partial trachelectomy in the elderly patient with abnormal cytology. Obstet Gynecol 1985;65:579.

Lagasse LD, Ballon SC, Berman ML, Watring WG. Pretreatment lymphangiography and operative evaluation in carcinoma of the cervix. Am J Obstet Gynecol 1979; 134:219.

Lagasse LD, Creasman WT, Shingleton HM, Ford JH, Blessing JA. Results and complications of operative staging in cervical cancer: experience of the gynecologic oncology group. Gynecol Oncol 1980;9:90.

Lam CP, Yuan CC, Jeng FS, Tsai LC, Yeh SH, Ng HT. Evaluation of carcinoembyronic antigen, tissue polypeptide antigen, and squamous cell carcinoma antigen in the detection of cervical cancers. Chin Med J (Engl) 1992; 50:7.

Langley II, Moore DW, Tarnasky JW, Roberts PHR. Radical hysterectomy and pelvic Iymph node dissection. Gynecol Oncol 1980;9:37.

LaPolla JP, Schlaerth JB, Gaddis O, Morrow SP. The influence of surgical staging on the evaluation and treatment of patients with cervical carcinoma. Gynecol Oncol 1986;24:194.

Lee RB, Weisbaum GS, Heller PB, Park RC. Scalene node biopsy in primary and recurrent invasive carcinoma of the cervix. Gynecol Oncol 1981;11:200.

Lee Y-N, Wang KL, Lin M-H, et al. Radical hysterectomy with pelvic lymph node dissection for treatment of cervical cancer: a clinical review of 954 cases. Gynecol Oncol 1989;32:135.

Lehtovirta P, Viinikka L, Ylikorkala O. Comparison between squamous cell carcinoma-associated antigen and CA-125 in patients with carcinoma of the cervix. Gynecol Oncol 1990;37:276.

Leminen A. Tumor markers CA 125, carcinoembryonic antigen and tumor-associated trypsin inhibitor in patients with cervical adenocarcinoma. Gynecol Oncol 1990;39: 358.

Levrant SG, Fruchter RG, Maiman M. Radical hysterectomy for cervical cancer: morbidity and survival in relation to weight and age. Gynecol Oncol 1992;45:317.

Lichtenegger W. Tumor volumetric measurement on MRI in cervical cancer. Presented at the 43rd annual meeting of the Society of Pelvic Surgeons, Birmingham AL, November 3–7, 1993. Abstract.

LiVolsi VA, Merino MJ, Schwartz PE. Coexistent endocervical adenocarcinoma and mucinous adenocarcinoma of ovary: a clinico-pathologic study of four cases. Int J Gynecol Pathol 1983;1:391.

Maiman M, Geuer G, Fruchter RG, Shaw N, Boyce J. Value of squamous cell antigen levels in invasive cervical carcinoma. Gynecol Oncol 1989;34:312.

Mann WJ, Hatch KD, Levy DS, Shingleton HM, Soong S-J. Prognostic significance of age in stage I carcinoma of the cervix. South Med J 1980;73:1186.

Martimbeau PW, Kjorstad KE, Iversen T. Stage IB carcinoma of the cervix, the Norwegian Radium Hospital. Results of treatment and major complications. II. Results when pelvic nodes are involved. Obstet Gynecol 1982;60:215.

Matsukuma K, Tsukamoto N, Matsuyuma T, Ono M, Nakano H. Preoperative CT study of lymph nodes in cervical cancer—its correlation with histological findings. Gynecol Oncol 1989;33:168.

Matsuyama T, Inoue I, Tsukamoto N, et al. Stage IB, IIA, and IIB cervix cancer, postsurgical staging, and prognosis. Cancer 1984;54:3072.

McDonald TW, Morley GW, Choo YL, et al. Fine needle aspiration of para-aortic and pelvic lymph nodes showing lymphangiographic abnormalities. Obstet Gynecol 1983; 61:383.

Meier W, Eiermann W, Stieber P, Fateh-Moghadam A, Schneider A, Hepp H. Squamous cell carcinoma antigen and carcinoembryonic antigen levels as prognostic factors for the response of cervical carcinoma to chemotherapy. Gynecol Oncol 1990;38:6.

Milsom I, Friberg LG. Primary adenocarcinoma of the uterine cervix. A clinical study. Cancer 1983;52:942.

Nelson JH Jr, Boyce J, Macasaet M, et al. Incidence, significance and follow-up of para-aortic lymph node metastases in late invasive carcinoma of the cervix. Am J Obstet Gynecol 1977;128:336.

Newton WA, Roberts WS, Marsden DE, Cavanagh D. Value of computerized axial tomography in cervical cancer. Oncology 1987;44:124.

Noguchi H, Shiozawa I, Sakai Y, Yamazaki T, Fukuta T. Pelvic lymph node metastasis in uterine cervical cancer. Gynecol Oncol 1987;27:150.

Nordqvist SRB, Sevin B-L, Nadji M, Greening SE, Ng ABP. Fine-needle aspiration cytology in gynecologic oncology. I. Diagnostic accuracy. Obstet Gynecol 1979; 54:719.

O'Brien DM, Carmichael JA. Presurgical prognostic factors in carcinoma of the cervix, stages IB and IIA. Am J Obstet Gynecol 1988;158:2508.

O'Leary JA, Symmonds RE. Radical pelvic operations in the geriatric patient: a 15-vear review of 133 cases. Obstet Gynecol 1966;28:745.

Orr JW Jr, Kerr-Wilson RH, Bodiford C, et al. Nutritional status of patients with untreated cervical cancer. Am J Obstet Gynecol 1985;151:625.

Parker LA, McPhail AH, Yankankas BC, Mauro MA. Computed tomography in the evaluation of clinical stage IB carcinoma of the cervix. Gynecol Oncol 1990;37:332.

Parkin DE. Lower urinary tract complications of the treatment of cervical carcinoma. Obstet Gynecol Surv 1989;44:523.

Patricio MB, Baptista AM. Renographic analyses in radiation therapy for carcinoma of the uterus. Acta Radiol Ther Phys Biol 1968;7:97.

Patsner B, Orr JW Jr, Allmen T. Does preoperative serum squamous cell carcinoma antigen level predict occult extracervical disease in patients with stage IB invasive squamous cell carcinoma of the cervix? Obstet Gynecol 1989;74:786.

Pellegrino A, Vanzulli A, Parma G, et al. Magnetic resonance imaging (MRI) in early carcinoma of uterine cervix: evaluation of residual uninvolved myometrium and pericervical tissues (abstract). Int J Gynecol Cancer 1993;3:13.

Perez CA, Zivnuska F, Askin F, Camel HM, Ragan D, Powers WE. Mechanisms of failure in patients with carcinoma of the uterine cervix extending into the endometrium. Int J Radiat Oncol Biol Phys 1977;2:651.

Phipps JH, Gunasekara PC, Lewis BV. Occult cervical carcinoma revealed by large loop diathermy. Lancet 1989; 8660:453.

Photopulos G, McCartney WH, Walton LA, Staab EV. Computerized tomography applied to gynecologic oncology. Am J Obstet Gynecol 1979;135:381.

Piver MS, Barlow JJ. Para-aortic lymphadenectomy, aortic node biopsy, and aortic lymphangiography in staging patients with advanced cervical cancer. Cancer 1973; 32:367.

Piver MS, Wallace S, Castro JR. The accuracy of lymphangiography in carcinoma of the uterine cervix. Am J Roentgenol Rad Ther Nuclear Med 1971;CXI:278.

Podczaski ES, Palombo C, Manetta A, Andrews C. Assessment of pretreatment laparotomy in patients with cervical carcinoma prior to radiotherapy. Gynecol Oncol 1989;33:71.

Prempree T, Amornmarn R, Wizenberg MJ. A therapeutic approach to primary adenocarcinoma of the cervix. Cancer 1985;56:1264.

Prempree T, Patanaphan V, Sewchand W, Scott RM. The influence of patients' age and tumor grade on the prognosis of carcinoma of the cervix. Cancer 1983;51:1764.

Pretorius R, Semrad N, Watring W, Fotherongham N. Presentation of cervical cancer. Gynecol Oncol 1991; 42:48.

Querleu D, Leblanc E, Castelain B. Laparoscopic pelvic lymphadenectomy in the staging of early carcinoma of the cervix. Am J Obstet Gynecol 1991;164:579.

Rabin S, Browde S, Nissenbaum M, Koller AB, DeMoor NG. Radiotherapy and surgery in the management of stage IB and IIA carcinoma of the cervix. S Afr Med J 1984;65:374.

Reisenger SA, Palazzo JP, Talerman A, Carlson J, Jahshan A. Stage IB glassy cell carcinoma of the cervix diagnosed during pregnancy and recurring in a transposed ovary. Gynecol Oncol 1991;42:86.

Rubens D, Thornbury JR, Angel C, et al. Stage IB cervical carcinoma: comparison of clinical, MR, and pathologic staging. Am J Roentgenol 1988;150:135.

Rutledge FN, Galakatos AE, Wharton JT, Smith JP. Adenocarcinoma of the uterine cervix. Am J Obstet Gynecol 1975;122:236.

Rutledge FN, Seski J. More or less radical surgery. Int J Radiat Oncol Biol Phys 1979;5:1881.

Schellhas HF. Extraperitoneal para-aortic node dissection through an upper abdominal incision. Obstet Gynecol 1975;46:444.

Schwartz PE, Chambers JT, Gutman J, Katopodis N, Foemmel R. Circulating tumor markers in the monitoring of gynecologic malignancies. Cancer 1987;60:353.

Senekjian EK, Young JM, Weiser PA, Spencer CE, Magic Se, Herbst AL. An evaluation of squamous cell carcinoma antigen in patients with cervical squamous cell carcinoma. Am J Obstet Gynecol 1987;157:433.

Sevin BU, Greening SE, Nadji M, Ng AB, Averette HE, Nordqvist SR. Fine needle aspiration cytology in gynecologic oncology. I: Clinical aspects. Acta Cytol 1979; 23:277.

Shepherd JH, Cavanagh D, Ruffolo E, Praphat H. The value of needle biopsy in the diagnosis of gynecologic cancer. Gynecol Oncol 1981;11:309.

Shingleton HM. American College of Surgeons patterns of care study—invasive cervical cancer. 1995. In preparation.

Shingleton HM, Fowler WC, Koch GG. Pretreatment evaluation in cervical cancer. Am J Obstet Gynecol 1971; 110:385.

Shingleton HM, Gore H, Soong S-J, Bradley D. Adenocarcinoma of the cervix: 1. Clinical evaluation and pathological features. Am J Obstet Gynecol 1981;138:799.

Sironi S, Belloni C, Taccagni GL, DelMaschio A. Carcinoma of the cervix: value of MR imaging in detecting parametrial involvement. Am J Roentgenol 1991;156:753.

Spanos WJ Jr, King A, Keeney E, Wagner R, Slater JM. Age as a prognostic factor in carcinoma of the cervix. Gynecol Oncol 1989;35:66.

Stanhope CR, Smith JP, Wharton JT, Rutledge FN, Fletcher GH, Gallagher HS. Carcinoma of the cervix: the effect of age on survival. Gynecol Oncol 1980;10:188.

Stehman FB, Bundy BN, DiSaia PJ, Keys HM, Larson JE, Fowler WC. Carcinoma of the cervix treated with irradiation therapy. I. A multivariate analysis of prognostic variables in the Gynecologic Oncology Group. Cancer 1991;67:2776.

Sudarsanam A, Charyulu K, Belinson J, et al. Influence of exploratory celiotomy on the management of carcinoma of the cervix. Cancer 1978;41:1049.

Sugimori H, Kawarabayashi T, Iwasaka T, Fukuda K, Hachisuga T, Hayashi Y. Colposcopic assessment of stage I cervical cancer. Int J Gynecol Cancer 1991;1:179.

Tamimi HK, Gown AM, Kim-Deobold J, Figge DC, Greer BE, Cain JM. The utility of immunohistochemistry in invasive adenocarcinoma of the cervix. Am J Obstet Gynecol 1992;166:1655.

te Velde ER, Persijn JP, Ballieux RE, Faber J. Carcinoembryonic antigen serum levels in patients with squamous cell carcinoma of the uterine cervix: clinical significance. Cancer 1982;49:1866.

Tinga DJ, Bouma J, Aalders JG. Patients with squamous cell versus adeno(squamous) carcinoma of the cervix, what factors determine the prognosis? Int J Gynecol Cancer 1992;2:83.

Togashi K, Nishimura K, Itoh K, et al. Uterine cervical cancer: assessment with high-field MR imaging. Radiololgy 1986;160:431.

Tulusan AH, Egger H, Lang N, Ober KG. Surgery for cervical cancer. Baillieres Clin Obstet Gynaecol 1988;2:981.

Ueda S, Tsubura A, Izumi H, Sasaki M, Morii S. Immunohistochemical studies on carcinoembryonic antigen in adenocarcinoma of the uterus. Acta Pathol Jpn 1983;33:59.

van Nagell JR Jr, Roddick JW Jr, Lowin DM. The staging of cervical cancer: inevitable discrepancies between clinical staging and pathological findings. Am J Obstet Gynecol 1971;110:973.

van Nagell JR Jr, Sprague AD, Roddick JW Jr. The effect of intravenous pyelography and cystoscopy on the staging of cervical cancer. Gynecol Oncol 1975;3:87.

Vas W, Wolverson M, Freel J, Salimi Z, Sundaram M. Computed tomography in the pretreatment assessment of carcinoma of the cervix. J Comput Tomogr 1985; 9:359.

Vercamer R, Janssens J, Usewills R, et al. Computed tomography and lymphography in the presurgical staging of early carcinoma of the uterine cervix. Cancer 1987; 60:1745.

Verlooy H, Devos P, Janssens J, et al. Clinical significance of squamous cell carcinoma antigen in cancer of the human uterine cervix. Comparison with CEA and CA–125. Gynecol Obstet Invest 1991;32:55.

Vick CW, Walsh JW, Wheelock JB, Brewster WH. CT of the normal and abnormal parametria in cervical cancer. Am J Roentgenol 1984;143:597.

Villasanta U, Prempree T, Kwon T. Late recurrent squamous cell carcinoma of the cervix uteri or vagina after successful initial treatment. Md State Med J 1983;32:111.

Volterrani F, Sigurta D, Gardani G, Milani A, Musumeci R. Role of lymphography in cancer of the uterine cervix. Radiol Med (Torino) 1980;66:611. Abstract.

Waggonspeck GA, Amparo EG, Hannigan EV, O'Neal MF. MRI of cervical carcinoma. Semin Ultrasound CT MR 1988;9:158.

Wallace S, Jing B-S, Zornoza J. Lymphangiography in the determination of the extent of metastatic carcinoma: the potential value of percutaneous lymph node biopsy. Cancer 1977;39:706.

Walsh JW, Goplerud DR. Prospective comparison between clinical and CT staging in primary cervical carcinoma. Am J Radiol 1981;137:977.

Welander CE, Pierce VK, Nori D, et al. Pretreatment laparotomy in carcinoma of the cervix. Gynecol Oncol 1981;12:336.

Wharton JT, Jones HW III, Day TG Jr, Rutledge FN, Fletcher GH. Preirradiation celiotomy and extended field irradiation for invasive carcinoma of the cervix. Obstet Gynecol 1977;49:333.

Whitley NO, Brenner DE, Francis A, et al. Computed tomographic evaluation of carcinoma of the cervix. Radiology 1982;142:439.

Winter R, Petru E, Haas J. Pelvic and para-aortic lymphadenectomy in cervical cancer. Baillieres Clin Obstet Gynaecol 1988;2(4):857.

Worthington LJ, Balfe MD, Lee TKJ, et al. Uterine neoplasms: MR imaging. Radiology 1986;159:725.

Yazigi R, Munoz AK, Richardson B, Risser R. Correlation of squamous cell carcinoma antigen levels and treatment response in cervical cancer. Gynecol Oncol 1991; 41:135.

Zander J, Baltzer J, Lohe KJ, Ober KG, Kaufmann C. Carcinoma of the cervix: an attempt to individualize treatment; results of a 20-year cooperative study. Am J Obstet Gynecol 1981;139:752.

Zornoza JJ, Jonsson K, Wallace S, Lukeman JM. Fine needle aspiration biopsy of retroperitoneal lymph nodes and abdominal masses: an update report. Radiology 1977; 125:87.

Cancer of the Cervix by Hugh M. Shingleton and James W. Orr, Jr.
J. B. Lippincott Company, Philadelphia, © 1995.

7

Primary Surgical Treatment
of Invasive Cancer

Various surgical procedures to excise the cervical tumor mass have been used for centuries. In the latter part of the nineteenth century, it became apparent that excision of the malignant mass on the cervix was not curative. An extended operation to resect the tumor and a margin of surrounding normal tissue was developed and is the basis for modern surgical therapy of early-stage invasive disease in otherwise healthy women. Gynecologists and some family physicians and surgeons must initially evaluate abnormal Papanicolaou (Pap) smears to determine the presence and extent of cervical disease. Usually, the therapeutic decision involves the use of simple excision or destruction, as is the case with precursor lesions, or an extended operation or radiation therapy when invasive disease is present. The surgical treatment for invasive cancer spans a spectrum of tumor-volume configurations and histologies and requires a knowledge of the surgical options that are available to offer the best chance for cure. Preoperative patient preparation is important, as is knowledge of intraoperative and postoperative factors. Many different physicians provide some of the care and follow-up. These considerations form the basis for this chapter.

SELECTION OF OPERATION FOR INVASIVE LESIONS

Squamous Microcarcinoma

Microcarcinoma was defined by Lohe (1978) as a lesion of measurable width and depth, the stromal invasion not exceeding 5 mm and the width not exceeding 10 mm. We recommend treating patients who have le-

sions invading the stroma between 3 and 5 mm in depth by extended abdominal (class II) hysterectomy (Fig. 7-1). A diagnostic and (perhaps therapeutic) lymphadenectomy is performed because of the 8% incidence of nodal metastases in these patients (Table 7-1). We do not believe that the pelvic node dissection adds appreciably to operative morbidity. The excision of the medial third or half of the cardinal ligament and a 2- to 3-cm vaginal cuff provides adequate local resection for these small (microscopic) tumors, yet decreases the risk of bladder denervation associated with more radical resection of the cardinal ligaments and paracolpos at the pelvic side wall. This conservative approach is supported by the parametrial tissues only rarely containing metastatic tumor in those microinvasive lesions invading 5 mm or less in depth. This treatment approach is endorsed by Copeland and associates (1992), for lesions invading 3 to 5 mm in depth, and by Photopulos and Zwaag (1991), who favor it for early cancers when there is a question regarding depth of invasion because of involved margins or artifact after a cone biopsy. We also advocate this treatment with tumor involvement of lymphvascular spaces in the conization specimen because these patients are at a presumed greater risk of parametrial or pelvic node involvement.

Kudo and coworkers (1984) advocated a radical vaginal approach for microcarcinoma. Important features of their surgical procedure include removal of at least 1 cm of vaginal cuff, partial resection of the vesicouterine ligament, and resection of 2 cm or more of the parametrial tissues. They indicated that operative time and blood loss for this operation were similar to those of total vaginal hysterectomy and reported no serious postoperative complications in the 25 patients

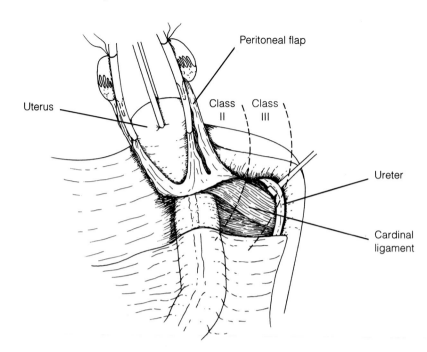

FIGURE 7-1. Class II and class III hysterectomies. (Shingleton HM, Gusberg SB. Radical hysterectomy. In Gusberg SB, Shingleton HM, Deppe G (eds). Female genital cancer. New York, Churchill Livingstone, 1988:536.)

undergoing this procedure. Perhaps in the near future, laparoscopic pelvic lymph node sampling, as advocated by Querleu and colleagues (1991), will assume a role in the treatment of microscopically invasive lesions; radical tumor resection may be performed vaginally, and lymph node sampling may be completed laparoscopically, with a resultant shorter hospital stay and potentially less postoperative morbidity.

Modified Radical Hysterectomy for Small Volume Lesions

It may be possible to reduce the radicality of the surgery in women with small invasive lesions of the cervix. In the United States, before the definition of microinvasion by the Society of Gynecologic Oncologists (1974), surgery for *any* degree of stromal inva-

TABLE 7-1
Squamous Cell Carcinoma Node Metastases According to Depth of Invasion

STUDY	YEAR	PATIENTS (N) (0–3 MM)	NODE METASTASES (N)	PATIENTS (N) (3.1–5 MM)	NODE METASTASES (N)
Leman, et al	1976	44	0	7	0
Seski, et al	1977	37	0	—	—
Taki, et al	1979	125	0	—	—
Yajima, et al	1979	90	0	—	—
Boyce, et al	1981	28	1	19	1
Hasumi, et al	1981	106	1	29	4
van Nagell, et al	1983	52	0	32	3
Simon, et al	1986	43	0	26	1
Maiman, et al	1988	65	1	30	4
Copeland, et al	1992	43	0	28	1
TOTALS		633	3 (0.5%)	171	14 (8.2%)

Adapted from Cavanagh D, Ruffalo EH, Marsden DE. Gynecologic cancer: a clinico-pathologic approach. East Norwalk, CT, Appleton-Lange, 1985:79.

sion often consisted of the class III or Meigs radical operation (see Fig. 7-1). Most American gynecologic oncologists perform the radical Meigs operation for lesions invading more than 3 mm (and those less invasive lesions with lymphvascular space involvement), although some persist in the more radical approach, even for early stromal invasion (0 to 3 mm; Jones 1993). Newer literature suggests that even larger-volume lesions may be treatable by a modified radical hysterectomy. Inoue (1984), using the class III operation, reported a 94% 5-year survival for women with stromal invasion to 1 cm, and Burghardt and associates (1988), using the same operation, reported a 92.5% 5-year survival for women with lesions involving less than 20% of the volume of the cervix. Importantly, the parametrium was found to contain tumor in only 2% and 5.2% of their patients, respectively, suggesting that a less radical parametrial dissection offers effective treatment. Other studies that support the concept of a less radical operation for small lesions are those of Fuller and coworkers (1989) and Alvarez and colleagues (1991), each reporting 97% 5-year survival for surgically treated patients with lesions up to 1 cm in greatest diameter. Tulusan and associates (1991) reported a 95% 5-year survival for women with lesions with a 1.49 cm^3 volume (Table 7-2). Tulusan and Burghardt noted that the medial parametrium is more likely to contain metastatic tumor than is the lateral parametrium, supporting the use of the modified (class II) operation for small cervical tumors (Fig. 7-2; see Fig. 7-1). It is logical to assume that the risk of tumor involvement of parametrial tissues is primarily related to the cervical tumor volume and that parametrial involvement is unlikely in small (one quadrant or lesions of 1 cm or less). Kinney and associates (1993) proposed that volumes less than or equal to that of a 2-cm sphere (4.19 cm^3) are suited to less radical surgery, based on Mayo Clinic data. Clearly, prospective studies are needed to define the size or volume above which a radical or conservative parametrial resection is indicated.

Surgery for Clinical Stage IB and IIA Tumors

Many American gynecologic oncologists confine the use of the class III radical hysterectomy to small IB and IIA lesions because of their concern for the risks and difficulties associated with parametrial extension, the risk of inadequate surgical margins, and increased nodal metastasis encountered with more bulky tumors, especially those lesions involving the entire cervical circumference or those thought to extend into the parametrial tissues (International Federation of Gynecology and Obstetrics [FIGO] stage IIB).

Creasman and coworkers (1986) questioned the need to confine the use of radical hysterectomy for treatment of small lesions. Operating on 27 women having stage IB tumors 4 cm or larger in size, they reported pelvic node metastasis in only 4 (15%) and a 5-year survival rate of 82% for women having lesions 4 to 6 cm in size and 66% for women having lesions larger than 6 cm. Alvarez and colleagues (1993) reported 48 surgically treated patients having bulky (larger than 4 cm diameter) stage IB tumors who were treated at the University of Alabama at Birmingham. Although he observed a high pelvic node metastasis rate (29.2%), he reported excellent 5- and 10-year survival rates (73.6% and 60.6%, respectively). In both series, some adjunctive postoperative irradiation was used, however. Bloss (1993) reported 84 women treated by radical hysterectomy for lesions 4 cm or larger in size, as measured on the formalin-fixed pathology specimen. Half of the women received postoperative radiation therapy based on findings of positive lymph nodes, parametrial spread, or compromised margins. Despite the bulky nature of the tumors, major operative complications were low (6%). Five-year survival was 70.4% (75.6% in the surgery only group and 65.0% in the combined treatment group). Most recurrences or deaths occurred in women who had lesions measuring in excess of 6 cm (Table 7-3).

Although it is true that in retrospective series

TABLE 7-2
Support for Modified (Class II) RHPND for Small Cervical Lesions

STUDY	YEAR		PARAMETRIAL EXTENSION	5-YEAR SURVIVAL (%)
Inoue	1984	Depth to 1 cm	2.0	93.0
Burghardt, et al	1987, 88	≤ 20% volume of cervix	5.2	97.5
Fuller, et al	1989	≤ 1 cm	—	97.0
Alvarez, et al	1991	≤ 1 cm	—	97.0
Tulusan, et al	1991	0–1.49 cm^3	—	95.0

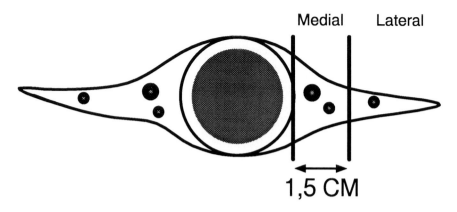

Author	Year	# Pts.	Stage II %	Pos. Nodes # Pts.	Pos. Nodes %	Medial %	Lateral %
Burghardt	1987	325	62	58 (17.8%)		54	46
Tulusan	1991	326	28	28 (8.6%)		75	25

FIGURE 7-2. Schematic of the areas of the parametrium in which the parametrial lymph nodes are found. (Modified from Tulusan AH, Wilczek-Engelmann T, Kaufmann W, et al. Operative Therapie des Zervixkarzinoms in der Univ.-Fauenklinik Erlangen. In Köchli, Sevin, Benz, Petru, Haller (eds). Gynäkologishe Onkologie. Berlin: Springer 1991;172, with permission.)

these surgically treated patients were selected, radiotherapists who treat bulky stage IB and IIA cervical lesions experience considerable difficulty achieving equal pelvic control and cure rates.

Surgery for Clinical Stage IIB Disease

In Europe and in the Orient, radical surgery is frequently performed for the treatment of clinical stage IIB disease. Numerous authors (Matsuyama et al 1984, Burghardt et al 1987, Friedberg et al 1988, Tulusan et al 1988, Lee et al 1989, Cheng 1990, Inoue 1990) make compelling arguments for offering radical

surgery to women who have clinical stage IIB disease. Lee and coworkers reported a 60.1% 5-year survival rate in 109 women undergoing radical hysterectomy for stage IIB disease. Others (Matsuyama et al, Burghardt et al, Cheng, and Inoue et al) reported negative parametria in 58%, 70%, 80%, and 66% of clinical stage IIB lesions, respectively, emphasizing that most of these lesions are actually confined to the cervix. Burghardt and associates reported an insignificant difference in 5-year survival rates of 82.2% and 76.9% in surgically treated patients having stage IB and IIB, respectively. Tulusan and colleagues indicated a 66% 5-year survival rate in 101 surgically treated patients (mostly clinical stage IIB) having tumor vol-

TABLE 7-3
RHPND for Large-Volume Tumors: Stage IB

STUDY	YEAR	PATIENTS (N)	SIZE (CM)	POSITIVE NODES (%)	SURVIVAL (%) 5-Year	SURVIVAL (%) 10-Year
Creasman, et al	1986	27	4–6	15	82	—
			> 6		66	—
Alvarez, et al	1993	48	≥ 4	29	74	61
Bloss	1993	84	≥ 4		70	—

umes exceeding 6.5 cm^3, despite a 57% frequency of pelvic lymph node involvement. Friedberg and associates reported a 5-year survival rate of 77% in surgically treated women who had stage IIB tumors. They concluded that radical surgery for women with stage IIB disease may offer better cure rates than radiation therapy because radiotherapists must rely on and base treatment on palpation or imaging studies only, without exact knowledge of tumor volume or the status of regional lymph nodes.

For Cervical Stump Cancer

Cancers of the cervical stump may be treated by surgery or radiation therapy. The rarity of this presentation is exemplified by little mention of it in the newer literature. Selection of therapy involves the same considerations as for carcinoma in the intact uterus (i.e, estimation of tumor volume and of the likelihood of adequate margins). The radical surgical technique is little different from radical hysterectomy, except that bowel adhesions are often present and the bladder may extend over the cervcial stump as part of the previous peritonealization. After identifying and mobilizing the bladder, the stump can be grasped for traction and the radical parametrial resection can proceed routinely. If the lesion is only focally microinvasive (invasion to less than 3 mm, with no evidence of lymphvascular space involvement), a total vaginal trachelectomy may be adequate treatment.

For Tumor Discovered After a Total Hysterectomy

Patients in whom invasive carcinoma has been found in a conventional vaginal or abdominal hysterectomy specimen may be successfully treated by radical reoperation to complete their therapy. Radical parametrectomy should be considered as treatment for younger women in whom ovarian conservation and vaginal preservation are important or in older women with relative contraindications to irradiation. The distorted post-hysterectomy mid-pelvic anatomic relations require attention; after bladder and rectal dissection, the vaginal cuff can be grasped for traction and the paravaginal tissues and upper vagina excised without undue difficulty. Care in dissecting the ureter and the ureterovesical junctions free from the vaginal cuff angles is critical because adhesions are to be expected secondary to the previous surgery. It appears that this procedure can be completed successfully, with operative time, infectious morbidity, or blood loss no greater than that of radical hysterectomy (Orr et al 1985). If no residual cancer is present in the radical parametrectomy specimen, survival rates approach 100% (Orr et al 1985, Ayhan et al 1991, Kinney et al 1992) and the patient is spared the effects of pelvic irradiation, with its possible long-term sequelae.

For Stage IVA Tumors

The argument has been raised that patients with stage IVA disease are at risk for bladder or rectal fistula if treated with pelvic irradiation. For this reason, some advocate primary pelvic exenteration for patients having advanced disease in which tumor has not reached the pelvic side walls (Cheng 1990). Actually, most such patients do not develop bladder fistulas with or after radiation treatment (see Chap. 8). These factors make us hesitant to recommend initial exenterative surgery but we do not hesitate to intervene if the central pelvic tumor mass fails to rapidly respond during radiation treatment or if viable tumor remains in the central pelvis at the time of completion of the radiation therapy.

TECHNIQUE OF RADICAL ABDOMINAL HYSTERECTOMY AND PELVIC LYMPHADENECTOMY

Preoperative Considerations

Cruse and Foord (1980) suggested several important methods to decrease the incidence of surgical wound infections after abdominal operations. Significant factors include shortening the preoperative hospital stay; using preoperative hexachlorophene showers; minimizing the amount of abdominal hair removal (using a clipper, if necessary); avoiding the use of pelvic drains; using good surgical technique; and minimizing operative time. Other authors indicate that using polyglycolic acid sutures and minimizing the use of electrocautery may also decrease the risk of infection (Orr et al 1987).

Prophylactic antibiotics significantly decrease infectious morbidity in premenopausal women undergoing total vaginal hysterectomy; effective prophylaxis for these procedures is a single dose of preoperative antibiotic. It is less clear, however, that perioperative antibiotics are effective in reducing febrile morbidity in patients undergoing radical hysterectomy. Fewer than ten studies address this subject (Table 7-4). Perioperative (nine-dose) cefoxitin has been reported to decrease the risk of postoperative infection (Sevin et al 1984). Orr and coworkers (1990) evaluated the comparative use of a single dose of antibiotics suggesting equal efficacy; surgical-site infections occurred in only 4% of treated patients. Although the risk of infectious morbidity is related to many factors, we believe that

TABLE 7-4
Extended Hysterectomy and Infectious Morbidity

STUDY	PATIENTS (N)	ANTIBIOTIC	FEBRILE MORBIDITY (%)	MAJOR MORBIDITY (%)	HOSPITAL STAY (DAYS)	OPERATIVE TIME (H)	BLOOD LOSS (ML)
Orr, et al (1982)	270	Cephalosporin (5–7 days)	32.4	18.9	9.8	3.7	1800
	41	None	41.5	26.8	12.0		
Rosenshein, et al (1983)	34	Doxycycline (1 dose)*	64.5†	11.8	16.1	3.9	2400
	30	None	84.5	26.7	15.6	3.7	1600
Sevin, et al (1984)	26	Cefoxitin (12 dose)	41.7	15.3	15.6	6.1	
	27	None	88.9	52.8	18.0	5.5	
Marsden (1985)	31	Cefoxitin (12 dose)		3.0	12.0	3.1	765
	43	None		16.0	12.0	3.6	832
Micha (1987)	15	Mezlocillin (3 dose)	26.6	6.6	10.1	3.7	840
	15	None	80.0	67.7	10.4	4.0	1013
Miyazawa (1987)	8	None	109†	87.5		5.4	2196
	11	Cefamandole/doxycycline (< 48 hr)	71	63.6		4.6	1851
	26	Cefamandole/doxycycline (< 48 hr) + cefamandole irrigation	30	3.8		4.4	1544
Bendvold & Kjorstad (1987)	35	None	17	0	10.1	2.6	525
Creasman (1982)	24	Mandol (5 dose)	12.5	4.2	8.2	3.2	
	25	None	45.8	36.0	9.0	3.2	
Orr, et al (1990)	24	Single dose Cefotan	41.7	4.2	6.9	2.25	1104
	22	Multiple dose Cefotan	45.4	4.5	7.1	2.45	1126

*Bowel preparation.
†Fever index.

From Orr JW Jr, Sisson PF, Patsner B, et al. Single-dose antibiotic prophylaxis for patients undergoing extended pelvic surgery for gynecologic malignancy. Am J Obstet Gynecol 1990;162:718.

the use of prophylactic antibiotics is justified; whereas the optimal drug is not yet determined, long-term use (3 or more doses) has little theoretic or scientific justification and only increases drug exposure and costs.

The risk of clinical deep vein thrombosis or thromboembolism is 1% to 3% (Shingleton 1994) and risk factors associated with thromboembolism are weight in excess of 188 lbs (85.5 kg), advanced clinical stage of malignancy, and radiation therapy within 6 weeks of the operative procedure. We do not use or recommend minidose heparin because its efficacy is unproved and it is associated with a significant increase in blood loss during pelvic surgery (Orr et al 1982, Clarke-Pearson et al 1984).

Pneumatic calf compression by an externally applied device appears to be effective as prophylaxis against venous thrombosis in patients with gynecologic cancer (Clarke-Pearson et al 1984, Farquharson et al 1984). We use this technique routinely for patients undergoing abdominal surgery. The prophylactic use of intravenous dextran against thromboses is unproved in radical gynecologic surgery patients, although it is thought to be effective in general surgical patients (Farquharson et al 1984).

Selection of Incision

The proper interval between cervical conization and radical abdominal hysterectomy is worthy of mention. Orr and colleagues (1982), reviewing the material at the University of Alabama, and Webb and Symmonds (1979), reviewing the material from the Mayo Clinic, indicated that the conization–hysterectomy interval was not an important factor in relation to perioperative morbidity and surgical difficulty. With this information, we believe that it is safe to proceed with a radical hysterectomy at any interval after conization.

In most cases, a midline incision is appropriate and adequate for abdominal operations for invasive cervical cancer. Because many of the patients are either obese or malnourished, we prefer a Smead-Jones–type closure, using prolene or some other nonreactive long-acting or nonabsorbable suture. Gallup (1984) believes that such a closure technique, including use of hemovacs subfascially and omission of subcutaneous sutures, decreases morbidity. Orr and associates (1990) reported a prospective randomized study comparing continuous with interrupted closures. Their conclusions from more than 400 patients indicated no difference in acute wound complications (infection, seroma, dehiscence, evisceration) or late wound problems (hernia). A continuous closure was associated with significant time-savings. There appears to be no benefit of subcutaneous drainage in clean uncontaminated operations (Orr et al 1986). Generally, subcutaneous sutures are to be discouraged because they potentially

increase the risk of infection (Orr et al 1986). Newer data, however, suggest that widely placed subcutaneous retention sutures may decrease the risk of poor wound outcome in the morbidly obese woman (Soisson et al 1993). Transverse lower abdominal incisions offer exceptional exposure for the pelvic lymphadenectomy and uterine resection but may restrict upper abdominal exposure. If a transverse incision is selected, a Pfannenstiel or Maylard muscle-cutting incision can be used. In the Maylard incision, all layers are opened transversely, with sacrifice of the inferior epigastric vessels. Initial data suggest that Pfannenstiel's incision can be used without compromise.

Peritoneal Washings

Several investigators have routinely submitted multiple intraoperative washings for peritoneal cytology. Hughes and coworkers (1980), Welander and associates (1981), and Abu-Ghazelah and colleagues (1984) reported malignant peritoneal cytology in washings in 9.3%, 12.6%, and 8.1% of surgical patients, respectively. Kilgore and associates (1984), reviewing the Alabama material, failed to demonstrate any abnormal cytology in 77 consecutive radical hysterectomy operations for stage IB but found a 2.5% incidence of positive washings in a group of patients with advanced stage disease who were undergoing surgical staging procedures. Delgado and coworkers (1989) reported only two positive washings in 627 patients with stage I disease, whereas Imachi (1987) reported three positive washings in 57 stage IB (5.3%) disease cases and overall positivity rate of 11.2% in a total of 125 women, many having clinical stage II and stage III disease. Podczaski and colleagues (1989) observed that peritoneal metastases were present in 23% of women with documented paraaortic node metastases. Most of these investigators conclude that positive cytology is associated with other poor-risk factors and is of little value as an independent prognostic or treatment variable. If a rapid cytologic evaluation technique were available and microscopic peritoneal involvement could be proved intraoperatively, it constitutes an indication for abandoning a radical surgical procedure. At this time, however, no such cytologic technique is available to the pelvic surgeon. If visible metastases to peritoneal surfaces are encountered, we believe that a radical procedure should be terminated.

Intraoperative Assessment

After entering the peritoneal cavity, an evaluation including palpation and visualization of all peritoneal surfaces, omentum, subdiaphragmatic, and retroperitoneal areas is undertaken. Particular attention is paid to the pelvic, common iliac, and aortic nodes. Unfortunately, clinical assessment of nodal status is subject to error: Welander and colleagues (1981) reported that if the nodes were negative to palpation, the surgeon was correct 94% of the time; if the nodes were clinically suspicious, the accuracy of the assessment was only 59%. Bjornsson and coworkers (1993) reported that the clinical evaluation of node status had a sensitivity and specificity of 68% and 100%, respectively. Sensitivity increased to 87% if micrometastases (less than 2 mm) were excluded from the evaluation.

If the secondary or high nodes (common iliac, precaval, aortic) contain macroscopic metastatic tumor, we ordinarily abandon the radical hysterectomy because of our belief that the significantly reduced survival in this situation does not justify the morbidity of a radical pelvic operation (Table 7-5). Martimbeau and associates (1982), reporting the surgical experience with stage IB tumors at the Norwegian Radium Hospital, state that metastases to common iliac or aortic nodes are an ominous finding, associated with only a 23% 5-year survival, whereas metastasis to nodes below the level of the common iliac arteries were associated with a 60% 5-year cure rate. Curtin and Morrow (1990), however, expressed the opinion that one might proceed with the radical hysterectomy if only micrometastases to aortic nodes are present. Resection of the primary tumor by the class II or class III hysterectomy and dissection of the pelvic and paraaortic nodes may well be therapeutic in this circumstance. Robertson and coworkers (1993), however, were not able to demonstrate a survival advantage of routine dissection of paraaortic nodes in patients with or without metastatic spread to pelvic or paraaortic nodes, raising a question regarding the use of paraaortic dissections other than to determine prognosis.

A decision to abandon the radical hysterectomy because of isolated metastases to the primary nodes (external iliac, obturator, or hypogastric) is even more difficult. Occasionally, we have stopped the radical operation if multiple (three or more) macroscopically positive pelvic nodes are present, especially if more than one group of nodes is involved or if a cancerous node is unresectable or densely adherent to a major pelvic vessel or nerve. These are not common findings. Heller and Park (1981) favored continuation of the surgical procedure, reporting a 71% 5-year survival in surgical patients having resected pelvic node metastases treated adjunctively by 50-Gy pelvic irradiation, compared with only a 34% 5-year survival in women who had only node sampling followed by irradiation or chemotherapy. Bortolozzi and colleagues (1983) also reported a 15-month mean increase in survival when the radical hysterectomy was completed before radiation therapy. Potter and associates (1990), reporting the experience at the University of Alabama, noted a trend toward better survival if the hysterectomy was completed and followed by pelvic irradiation, compared with abandonment of the hysterectomy and treatment by irradiation alone. Perhaps because of the small numbers (15 patients in each group and maldistribution by lesion size and number of positive nodes in the two study groups), the 5-year survival rates were not significantly different (46% with hysterectomy, 35% without hysterectomy). Kinney and coworkers (1993) reported a 45.8% 5-year survival rate in 51 women who had palpably positive pelvic nodes at the time of surgery; these women were treated by radical hysterectomy, although 29 also received adjunctive postoperative pelvic radiation therapy.

Lacking clear evidence that primary irradiation is superior in these patients, we ordinarily favor completion of the radical hysterectomy if clinically apparent node metastases have not extended to the level of the secondary nodes (common iliac, precaval, aortic) and if the primary tumor and pelvic nodes are otherwise easily resected. Citing almost identical criteria, Delgado and colleagues (1989) reported that only 12% of 732 patients explored in a Gynecologic Oncology Group (GOG) protocol had findings that led to abandonment of the radical hysterectomy (GOG study: 732 patients).

TABLE 7-5
Intraoperative Findings That May Alter
the Planned Procedure

1. Intraoperative metastases (bladder or cul-de-sac, peritoneum, other surfaces)
2. Direct parametrial extension
3. Multiple (three or more) or bilateral pelvic node metastases
4. Unresectable pelvic node disease
5. Macroscopic metastases to secondary nodes (common iliac, pre-caval, paraaortic)

Protecting the Small Bowel in Those Receiving Postoperative Radiation

In the clinical situation suggesting the need for postoperative radiation therapy, a biodegradable mesh to maintain superior placement of the intestinal tract should be considered. Some suggest a potential benefit in decreasing small bowel injury; however, this opinion is not shared by all (Patsner et al 1990). Dasmahapatra and Swaminathan (1991) reported the use of polyglycolic and polyglactin 910 mesh in 45 patients undergoing radical pelvic cancer operations, with minimal acute or long-term sequelae. Postradiation roent-genography in this situation demonstrated the small bowel to be consistently above the pelvic inlet at 12 weeks. Mesh absorption and small bowel descent occurred after 4 months (Dasmahapatra et al 1991). In patients undergoing exploration for other indications, minimal adhesions were related to the mesh.

Rodier and associates (1991), reporting a 60-patient multicenter study, indicated the safety and probable decrease in intestinal complications using an absorbable polyglycolic acid suture mesh. It was completely absorbed by the third to fifth month. They believed it to be necessary to interpose omentum and use prolonged submesh drainage.

The omentum (J flap) may be successfully used to create a hammock to support the small intestine above the pelvic floor (Granai et al 1990). Its use may decrease adhesions or allow an increase in the deliverable tumoricidal dose (inverse square law). Dockendorf and coworkers (1993), studying the effect of an omental graft on intestinal anastomosis in an animal model, reported that the omentum acted as a "sealant" and provided an ingrowth of blood supply (even to the mucosa) by 10 days but not at 3 days. Hindley and Cole (1993) reported the successful use of peritoneal insufflation as an alternative to displace the intestinal tract during treatment.

Comprehensiveness of Lymphadenectomy

The comprehensiveness of the pelvic lymphadenectomy may affect survival. In surgical series from around the world, the reported mean number of nodes dissected ranges between 16 and 38 (Table 7-6). The number of nodes retrieved and the percentage of node metastases are directly related (Fig. 7-3). Kjorstad and colleagues (1984), who performed pelvic node dissections under lymphangiographic control, also demonstrated that node metastases rate (in this case, by 8%) can be increased by extending the surgery. The concept of a need for a complete meticulous node dissection persists, particularly in the German-speaking countries. Although from a theoretic standpoint the most complete lymphadenectomy (i.e., involving mobilization of all major vessels and circumferential meticulous removal of nodes) seems to offer the most therapeutic benefit, this does not actually seem to be the case. Neither Kjorstad and associates (1984), Pilleron and coworkers (1974), Burghardt and colleagues (1992), nor Winter and associates (1988) have demonstrated a difference in 5-year survival related solely to the comprehensiveness of the dissection. Gitsch and associates (1984,1987) reported a trend toward improved survival of those women subjected to dissections under ^{99m}Tc labeling but their data are not controlled for other important prognostic

TABLE 7-6
Cancer of the Cervix Pelvic Nodes Dissected

STUDY	YEAR	PATIENTS	MEAN NODES (N)	RANGE OR MAXIMUM NODES (N)
Pilleron, et al	1974	140	26	10–47
Baltzer, et al	1979	684	17	Max, 57
Zander, et al	1981	1092	18	NS
Inoue, et al	1984	628	20	9–49
Creasman, et al	1986	268	29	Max, 83
Kjorstad	1987	304	30	—
Ng, et al	1987	908	18	11–64
Ferraris, et al	1988	402	22	15–60
Winter, et al	1988	359	35	25–46
Inoue, et al	1990	875	32	9–73
Hale, et al	1991a	49	16	6–38
Panici, et al	1991	208	38	NS
Querleu, et al*	1991	39	8.7	3–22
Dargent, et al*	1992	176	10.4	NS
Fowler, et al*	1994	12	23.5	7–33

*Laparoscopic sampling
NS, no sample

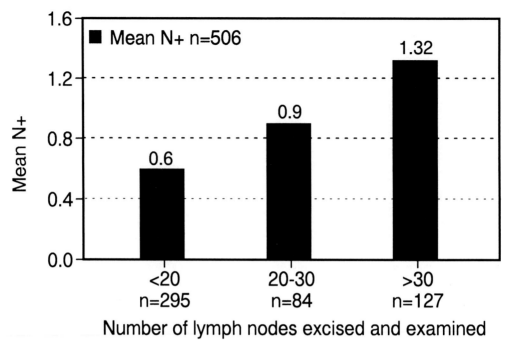

Number of lymph nodes excised and examined

FIGURE 7-3. Mean number of positive lymph nodes versus number excised and examined. (Modified from Friedberg V. Operative therapy for stage IIB cervical cancer. Baillieres Clin Obstet Gynaecol 1988;2:973, with permission.)

variables, such as histologic type, tumor stage, or tumor volume and did not show a significant difference.

COMPLICATIONS RELATED TO NODE DISSECTION

The risks of pelvic lymphocyst and lower extremity edema are associated with more extensive lymph node dissections. Martimbeau and coworkers (1982) reported lower-extremity edema in 23% of postoperative patients (5% with severe edema) as a consequence of the comprehensive dissection technique practiced in Oslo. This complication rate is higher than reported with more routine dissections (Author's data; Kenter et al 1989, 8.6%; Clarke-Pearson et al 1992, 8%). We believe that nodal tissue should be removed superficial and lateral to the major vessels; however, little is gained by a more extensive lymphadenectomy, and increased complications are likely to occur with extended procedures. We advocate dissection of all nodes lateral and medial to the common iliac, the external iliac, and hypogastric vessels and those in the obturator fossa superior to the obturator nerve. We do not routinely mobilize or dissect behind the vessels (with the exception of the external iliac artery) nor do we use or advocate use of lymphangiography or radionuclide labeling to increase the completeness of the dissection. With this approach, 5-year survival of our stage IB patients is equal to that reported by Gitsch and colleagues (1984, 1987) and Martimbeau and as-

sociates (1982) for the more extensive dissection. In contrast to Martimbeau and coworkers' reporting more than 1 in 5 women with chronic leg edema, we have seen chronic leg edema rarely (0.1%) and mostly in women who had postoperative whole-pelvis irradiation (Fig. 7-4).

Excision of the Uterus

More extensive dissection of the ureter and the bladder base distinguishes the class II and III operations (Piver et al 1974; see Fig. 7-1). During the class II operation, the broad ligament is opened and the ureter is

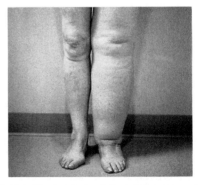

FIGURE 7-4. Elephantiasis of the left leg after radical hysterectomy with pelvic node dissection.

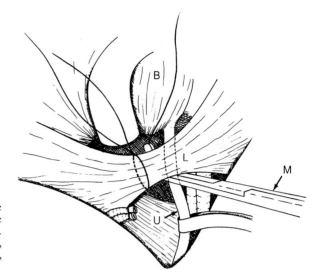

FIGURE 7-5. Dissection of the anterior vesicouterine ligament to free the ureter from its tunnel. Ligatures are placed around the tissue. (Shingleton HM, Gusberg SB. Radical hysterectomy. In Gusberg SB, Shingleton HM, Deppe G (eds). Female genital cancer. New York, Churchill Livingstone, 1988:542.)

identified on the medial peritoneal flap. After identifying the ureteral tunnel through the cardinal ligament and after partial mobilization of the bladder from the cervix, the vesicouterine ligament anterior to the ureter is incised, "unroofing" the ureter (Fig. 7-5). For this less radical operation, the posterior attachments of the ureter can be left in place and the ureterovesical junction can be pushed aside to allow resection of the medial half of the parametrium. For the more radical (class III) operation, further dissection to mobilize the ureter, the ureterovesical junction, and bladder base from attachments to the cardinal ligament and vagina is necessary; only in this way is one able to isolate the entirety of the cardinal ligaments (Fig. 7-6).

Ovarian Resection or Transposition

The surgeon may elect to remove the ovaries when diseased or in women who are 40 or older. Based on the negligible chance of ovarian metastasis in squamous lesions (less than 1%) and only a slightly higher rate (1.4%) in adenocarcinoma of the cervix (Table 7-7), it seems justifiable to conserve normal-appearing ovaries in young women undergoing radical surgery. Evaluating the concern of some about adenocarcinoma of the cervix, Brown and colleagues (1990) noted that all women with ovarian metastases also had at least one of the following: they were postmenopausal and had positive pelvic nodes or obvious adnexal pathology. Clinically, each of these situations suggests the need for ovarian removal in any radical hysterectomy.

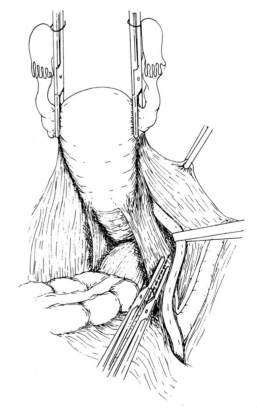

FIGURE 7-6. Resection of the cardinal ligaments at the pelvic sidewall, in the class III or Meigs radical hysterectomy. (Shingleton HM, Gusberg SB. Radical hysterectomy. In Gusberg SB, Shingleton HM, Deppe G (eds). Female genital cancer. New York, Churchill Livingstone, 1988:543.)

TABLE 7-7
Incidence of Ovarian Metastases in Stage IB Carcinoma of the Cervix

STUDY	YEAR	SQUAMOUS CELL CARCINOMA		ADENOCARCINOMA	
		(n)	(%)	(n)	(%)
Parente, et al	1964	105	0	—	—
Baltzer, et al	1982	749	0.5	—	—
Kaminski, et al	1984	161	—	161	0.6
Kjorstad, et al	1984	—	—	150	1.3
Shingleton*	1987	258	0.4	—	—
Tabata, et al	1987	122	0	26	7.7
Hopkins	1988	—	—	32	0
Kilgore, et al*	1988	—	—	78	0
Owens, et al	1989	77	0	22	0
Brown, et al	1990	—	—	25	4.0
Toki, et al	1991	355	0	36	5.5
Angel, et al	1992	—	—	41	0
TOTALS		1666	< 0.5	571	1.4

Modified from Reisenger SA, Palazzo JP, Talerman A, et al. Stage IB glassy cell carcinoma of the cervix diagnosed during pregnancy and recurring in a transposed ovary. Gynecol Oncol 1991;42:86; with permission.

Many authors advocate ovarian transposition to displace the ovaries from the pelvic irradiation field, should postoperative pelvic irradiation be given. We have made a practice of relocating at least one ovary in the paracolic gutter in patients 35 years or younger having bulky cervical lesions or known pelvic node metastases. Most patients who undergo radical hysterectomy do not receive adjunctive irradiation; thus, routine transposition may be unnecessary. It may be important, however, to stabilize the conserved ovarian pedicle on the lateral pelvic side wall.

Operative Time and Blood Loss

The operative time for radical hysterectomy and pelvic lymphadenectomy varies between 2 and 5 hours, and the usual blood loss is 1000 to 1900 mL (Hoskins et al 1976, Orr et al 1982). The portion of the procedure usually associated with the greatest blood loss is the dissection and mobilization of the bladder base and ureterovesical junction, where bleeding occurs from large veins in the vicinity of the vesicouterine ligament. We believe that patients should have an adequate volume (4 units) of blood cross-matched before the surgical procedure. We prefer to maintain a conservative approach to perioperative transfusion because theoretic and clinical data (Eisenkop et al 1990) support the contention that perioperative transfusion may adversely affect prognosis.

Pelvic Drainage

After a hemostatic suture is placed along the cut vaginal edges (or after vaginal closure), the peritoneum of the pelvis is left open and inspected for hemostasis. There appears to be little benefit in reperitonealizing or covering the vaginal cuff and denuded pelvic vessels. If the ovaries have been retained, they should be stabilized to the pelvic side wall with a suture to minimize later torsion on their vascular pedicles. For many years, we placed extraperitoneal Penrose drains in the obturator fossae, which were externalized through an open vaginal cuff. For the past 10 to 15 years, we have frequently used closed suction pelvic drainage because we (and many authors) sought to reduce ureteral fistula and lymphocyst risk. Two papers provide additional information about the use of suction drainage. Barton and associates (1992) studied two closed-suction drainage methods in 96 patients after radical hysterectomy. In the first group, they used two pelvic side wall drains and a vaginal drain; in the second group, only the vaginal drain was used. They found that the single vaginal drain was more acceptable, more cost-effective, and equally effective as the three-drain method. Clarke-Pearson and coworkers (1992) evaluated retroperitoneal suction drains in relation to their ability to reduce the occurrence of lymphocysts and pelvic infections in 493 gynecologic patients undergoing selective pelvic lymphadenectomy for a variety of indications. They concluded that suction drainage does not benefit patients and may actually be associated with an increase in febrile morbidity, pulmonary embolism, and urinary fistula. Jensen and colleagues (1993) reported a similar study, with almost identical conclusions. The incidence of postoperative pelvic infection is low (Orr 1991) and we do not advocate routine pelvic suction drainage but consider using it if a bladder or ureteral injury has occurred.

Bladder Drainage

For 20 or more years, we have employed suprapubic Foley catheters (16 French), placed directly in the dome of the bladder at the time of the abdominal closure, as the method of postoperative urinary drainage. Alternate suprapubic urinary drainage systems are available, all (in our opinion) preferable to transurethral indwelling catheters. Although some authors advocate early removal, we believe that longer (about 2 to 3 weeks) drainage carries little morbidity and assures adequate drainage to decrease the risk of bladder distention.

The Surgical Specimen

At the end of the procedure, the surgical specimen (Fig. 7-7) is carefully inspected and in most cases, the surgical pathologist is directly consulted to discuss areas of special concern, such as the margins of excision. This may provide information that allows the pathologist to better evaluate the excised tissues and consequently better serve the patient.

Early Postoperative Care

The usual postoperative stay of our patients undergoing radical hysterectomy is 5 days. About a third of the patients experience febrile morbidity, which prolongs

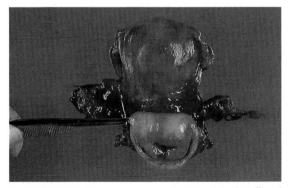

FIGURE 7-7. Excised uterus with wide vaginal cuff and parauterine tissues. The ovaries were not removed in this patient. See Color Figure 7-7.

the hospital stay. Early ambulation is practiced. The patient is encouraged to be out of bed on the first postoperative day and barring complications is placed on a regular diet and is freely ambulatory within the week. The suprapubic catheter is connected to straight drainage during the hospitalization and no trial of voiding is attempted; the patient is discharged with the suprapubic catheter in place. If at 10 to 14 days the patient has bladder sensation, she is asked to void. If this can be accomplished with a low residual urine (less than 50 mL), the suprapubic catheter is removed. Instruction regarding bladder care should emphasize prevention of overdistention because this can further damage the bladder. Suprapubic drainage has an advantage over transurethral catheters because the patient can open and close the catheter herself and thus can attempt voiding without the necessity of removal and replacement of the catheter. Using this regimen, we have experienced few long-term bladder complications. We rarely prescribe intermittent self-catheterization for patients, although it is an acceptable technique and is preferable to long-term indwelling catheter use.

COMPLICATIONS OF RADICAL ABDOMINAL HYSTERECTOMY

Urologic

BLADDER DENERVATION

The exact etiology and nature of the bladder damage associated with the radical hysterectomy has been the subject of many studies and is still under investigation. Petri (1984) identified three types of surgical injury to the lower urinary tract: type I, parasympathetic damage, leading to a contractile detrusor; type II, partial lesion of the pelvic ganglia, resulting in a hypertonic low-compliance bladder, which also collects residual urine because of functional bladder outlet obstruction; and type III, complete destruction of the pelvic ganglia, resulting in a contractile bladder, with sensory loss and sphincter incompetence due to an atonic urethra. Any operation involving excision of the paracervical and paravaginal web invariably interrupts some portion of bladder innervation.

The three major urinary symptom complexes after radical hysterectomy are diminished bladder sensation, bladder dysfunction, and stress incontinence. Most women complain of some loss of bladder sensation; however, in most patients this problem seems to improve with time. Post–radical hysterectomy bladder dysfunction is manifest by early postoperative bladder hypertonicity due to muscle trauma. The hypertonic phase is often replaced by a flaccid bladder phase, as a consequence of damage to the vesical plexus. Farquharson and Orr (1987), at Alabama, observed a significant reduction in functional urethral length and urethral closure pressure after surgery; however, pressure transmission ratios were maintained, indicating no evidence of loss of bladder neck support with stress. Their findings regarding reduction in urethral closure pressures were similar to those of Scotti and colleagues (1986) in their review of the subject.

Kindermann and Debus-Thiede (1988) indicated that the pathology of voiding dysfunction after radical hysterectomy is still not clearly understood. They note that normal micturition requires a detrusor muscle contraction and simultaneous relaxation of the periurethral striated muscle and believe that this synchrony is disturbed in the early postoperative period. They also believe that after the surgery, a temporary functional obstruction occurs that disappears by the sixth to eighth postoperative week.

DISTURBANCES IN BLADDER FUNCTION RELATED TO RADICALITY OF SURGERY

Christ (1979) examined two groups of women—one group had the class III radical operation and one had the class II modified radical operation—and found no difference in subjective complaints or objective urodynamic results. Forney (1980) and Sasaki and coworkers (1982) also addressed the disturbances of bladder innervation related to the radicality of the parametrial–paravaginal excision. Kindermann and Debus-Thiede (1988) concluded that the extent of cardinal ligament resection may be less important for bladder disturbances than the radicality of resection of the deep paravaginal tissues. They make an analogy to individuals who have voiding difficulties after abdominoperineal resection. Vervest and associates (1989) reported urodynamic evaluation of patients undergoing pre- and postoperative testing of modified radical hysterectomy. The most prominent finding in postoperative patients was a significant reduction in detrusor contractility and the development of the need for abdominal straining to empty the bladder successfully. Not all investigators have reported changes related to radicality of the surgery; for example, Scotti and colleagues (1986) were unable to demonstrate any difference in testing after the different operations. Given the results of studies, it is unclear whether less radical resection of the parametrium–paracolpos preserves bladder function; the difficulty in establishing comparable study groups suggests that this question is unlikely to be resolved in the foreseeable future. Regardless, bladder dysfunction occurs in most patients undergoing radical hysterectomy, and these potential problems and their management should be discussed preoperatively.

STRESS URINARY INCONTINENCE

The incidence of stress urinary incontinence after radical hysterectomy varies between 10% and 74% (Petri 1984, Ralph et al 1990, Carenza et al 1988, Kenter et al 1989). Kindermann and Debus-Thiede (1988) noted that 10% of women studied have preoperative stress incontinence, whereas 22% of his patients developed it after the surgery. Christ and associates (1983) and Farquharson and coworkers (1987) also noted that numerous patients have preexisting bladder dysfunction. Farquharson and colleagues' report suggests that the patients with objective preoperative evidence of an incompetent bladder neck may be predisposed to the development of incontinence after radical hysterectomy, perhaps due to a postsurgical reduction in urethral closure pressure.

Unfortunately, surgical treatment of stress urinary incontinence after radical hysterectomy has proved disappointing. Various suprapubic and vaginal approaches have been advocated but generally with poor results. Although seldom encountered, severe incontinence may be approached surgically but such procedures should be delayed a few months until the early postoperative bladder disturbances have passed.

URINARY TRACT INFECTIONS

Even if perioperative antibiotics are used, urinary tract infections after radical hysterectomy occur in 5% to 10% of patients and may be associated with or secondary to prolonged urethral or suprapubic bladder drainage. Early infection may worsen urinary symptoms and interfere with postoperative recovery. The continued use of urinary prophylaxis during suprapubic catheterization does not prevent the development of serious urinary tract infection and may select out specific urinary pathogens.

UROLOGIC FISTULAS

Ureteral and bladder fistulas, once one of the most dreaded urinary complications after radical pelvic operations, are relatively uncommon (Table 7-8). The incidence of urologic fistulas has decreased markedly from the rates encountered in those series reported in the 1960s or earlier; although there is no immediate explanation for the dramatic decrease in the incidence of urologic fistulas, altered surgical technique, discontinued use of intraoperative indwelling ureteral catheters, use of perioperative antibiotics, improved methods of bladder drainage, and other differences in postoperative care may be responsible. Ureteral fistulas and strictures are managed successfully in most cases by ureteral stenting, using percutaneous techniques, even in patients in whom transvesical retrograde catheter placement is unsuccessful. This advance in

TABLE 7-8
Urinary Fistulas in Nonirradiated Patients Treated by Radical Abdominal Hysterectomy

STUDY	YEAR	PATIENTS (N)	URETERAL FISTULA (%)	VESICAL FISTULA (%)
Kaser, et al	1973	717	3.3	0.6
Park, et al	1973	156	0	0
Hoskins, et al	1976	224	1.3	0.45
Morley, et al	1976	208	4.8	0.5
Sall, et al	1979	349	2.0	0.8
Webb, et al	1979	423	1.4	0.7
Benedet, et al	1980	241	1.2	0.4
Langley, et al	1980	284	5.6	1.4
Lerner, et al	1980	108	0.9	0
Bostofte, et al	1981	479	3.8	1.4
Powell, et al	1981	135	1.5	0
Zander, et al	1981	1092	1.4	0.3
Gitsch, et al	1984	187	0.5	NS
Shingleton	1985	444	1.4	0.23
Artman, et al	1987	153	1.3	1.3
Larson, et al	1987	233	0.8	NS
Ralph, et al	1988	320	1.9	2.5
Lee, et al	1989	954	1.2	1.2
Kenter, et al	1989	213	3.3	3.3
Burghardt, et al	1989	325	2.5	2.8
Massi, et al	1993	228	0.9	0.4
TOTAL		7473	2.0	0.9

NS,. no sample.

Modified from Shingleton HM, Orr JW Jr. Cancer of the cervix: diagnosis and treatment. New York, Churchill Livingstone, 1987:133.

management reduces the necessity for repeat operations in most cases.

FEBRILE MORBIDITY

Febrile morbidity is common and is reported to occur in 25% to 30% of patients after radical hysterectomy, depending on the definitions used by the authors. Orr and associates (1982), reporting 311 patients followed-up at the University of Alabama, observed postoperative febrile morbidity in 33%. The major causes include pulmonary atelectasis, urinary tract infections, wound infections or hematoma, pelvic cellulitis, pelvic or deep vein thrombosis, and pelvic abscess.

Deep Vein Thrombosis

Crandon and Koutts (1983), using ^{125}I fibrinogen scanning, reported a 38% incidence of postoperative deep vein thrombosis in patients with gynecologic malignancies, substantially higher than the 10% to 15% expected in a general gynecology population. Twenty percent of the total group had bilateral venous thromboses. This indicates the inaccuracy of clinical diagnosis and the need to investigate both lower limbs if thrombosis is suspected. Surprisingly, the incidence of postoperative venous thrombosis was found to be significantly lower in smokers than in nonsmokers. The high risk of postoperative venous thrombosis clearly indicates the need for perioperative prophylaxis. Newer recommendations include the use of pneumatic calf compression, which not only improves venous flow but decreases plasminogen activation.

Pulmonary Morbidity

Pulmonary febrile morbidity is usually secondary to atelectasis; this is usually minor and responds well to conservative measures. Given the alterations in postoperative pulmonary function, we believe aggressive pulmonary intervention in the form of postoperative incentive spirometry is in order (Orr et al 1994a).

Pneumonia after this procedure is rare, occurring in 1% to 3% of patients.

Pelvic Cellulitis

Morbidity of pelvic etiology due to pelvic cellulitis or abscess may occur in as many as 10% of patients. These infections are potentially serious because they may predispose patients to the development of a urinary fistula and increase the risk of pulmonary emboli and increase patient treatment costs. Some authors indicate that vaginal cuff closure may decrease these risks because an open vaginal cuff may allow ascending infection. It has become clear that the use of perioperative antibiotics decreases this risk. Although the optimal drug selection remains unknown, there is little benefit in the use of prolonged perioperative coverage. Using a single-dose prophylactic regimen results in a 4.1% risk of surgical-site infectious morbidity and is no different than three doses (Orr 1991). Closed-suction drainage contributes to increased nursing costs and loss of important proteins, without decreasing infectious risks.

Pelvic Lymphocysts

While commonly reported (Table 7-9), the cause of pelvic lymphocysts after radical hysterectomy is not readily apparent; however, they are usually asymptomatic and seldom present a clinical problem requiring intervention. Pilleron and colleagues (1974) indicated that they were more common in patients undergoing extensive lymph node dissection. Others have observed that incomplete dissections cause collection of

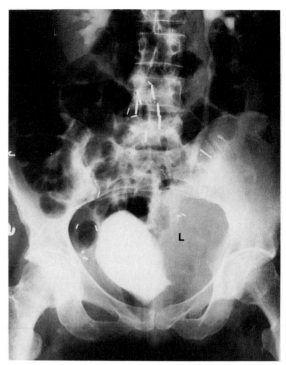

FIGURE 7-8. Postoperative symptomatic lymphocyst after radical hysterectomy. The lymphocyst (*L*) displaces the bladder and the left ureter medially. (Shingleton HM, Orr JW Jr. Cancer of the cervix: diagnosis and treatment. New York, Churchill Livingstone, 1987:147.)

TABLE 7-9
Incidence of Pelvic Lymphocysts
after Radical Abdominal Hysterectomy
and Pelvic Lymphadenectomy

STUDY	YEAR	PATIENTS (N)	LYMPHOCYSTS (%)
Benedet, et al	1980	241	2
Allen, et al	1982	191	1.6
Shingleton	1985	444	1
Artman, et al	1987	153	1
Ilancheran, et al	1988	221	25
Fuller, et al	1989	418	1.4
Kenter, et al	1989	213	6.7
Mann, et al	1989	124	2
Moore, et al	1989	111	2.7
Petru, et al	1989	173	20*
Massi, et al	1993	228	0.4

*Diagnosed by computed tomography scan.

lymph in the retroperitoneal space that results in lymphocysts. Some surgeons have advocated ligating the afferent lymphatics to decrease risks. Although some believe that proper drainage of the retroperitoneal area may prevent lymphocyst formation, others (Lopes et al 1993), in a randomized study of 60 patients, could not show a reduction in lymphocyst formation by use of pelvic drainage. Although we have only occasionally practiced ligation of the lymphatics and have provided only short-term retroperitoneal drainage, we have rarely seen the condition. Elimination of pelvic peritoneal closure, which was used in former years, may prevent lymphocyst formation (Monaghan et al 1990).

The occasional symptomatic lymphocyst (Fig. 7-8) requires treatment. Simple needle aspiration is not usually curative; however, percutaneous catheters may be placed to drain and allow collapse and healing (Mann et al 1989). Others advocate operative management, with transperitoneal marsupialization of the lymphocyst for drainage (Aronowitz et al 1983). These patients require evaluation to exclude the presence of recurrent cancer. Cytologic samples should be submitted, if aspirated. A portion of the wall of the lymphocyst should be submitted during an open procedure.

Neurologic Injury

Nerve injury may occur during the course of the radical hysterectomy operation. Obturator nerve damage is the most likely; however, the femoral or peroneal nerves can also be injured. The obturator nerve can be severed, compressed by a hemoclip, or cauterized during the obturator fossa lymph node dissection. If transected, it can be resutured and may regenerate but weakness in adduction of the thigh of varying degrees may result. In most situations, this weakness can be compensated with physical therapy. Femoral neuropathies may result from pressure by the blades of self-retaining retractors, and care should be exercised during placement, so that they do not rest on the psoas muscle. Peroneal nerve damage may occur as a result of pressure on the popliteal fossa when the patient is placed in knee stirrups. Careful attention to leg placement and stirrup padding decreases the risk of this type of nerve injury, which may result in "foot drop" that lasts for weeks or months. The use of specific stirrups (Allen universal) significantly decreases the risks.

Vascular Injuries

Vena cava lacerations or lacerations of the external iliac, the hypogastric, or obturator veins may occur in the course of the node dissections. Hemorrhage from such large-vein injuries may be difficult to control and may result in major blood losses. Intraoperative control may require clips, sutures, vascular patches, or ligation. Obturator fossa venous bleeding may respond best to initial packing of the fossa, whereas vena cava and iliac vein injuries require suturing of the vessels.

OPERATIVE DEATHS

Operative deaths (which plagued the pelvic surgeons in the early part of the century before Meigs' 1951 report of only 1.7% deaths) are rare occurrences, resulting in about six deaths per 1000 operations (Table 7-10).

POSSIBLE EFFECT OF TRANSFUSIONS

Eisenkop and associates (1990) reported 126 women treated by radical hysterectomy for clinical stage IB tumors. His patients had clear surgical margins, negative nodes, no other high-risk factors in the specimen, and no postoperative irradiation therapy. They also had no history of immunosuppression with medication and had at least 18 months of follow-up. The operative

TABLE 7-10
Operative Deaths in Patients Treated by Primary Radical Abdominal Hysterectomy

STUDY	YEAR	PATIENTS (N)	OPERATIVE DEATHS (%)
Park, et al	1973	156	0.64
Hoskins, et al	1976	224	0.89
Morley, et al	1976	208	1.4
Sall, et al	1979	349	0
Webb, et al	1979	423	0.3
Benedet, et al	1980	241	0.4
Langley, et al	1980	284	0
Lerner, et al	1980	108	0
Bostofte, et al	1981	479	0.2
Powell, et al	1981	135	0.74
Zander, et al	1981	1092	1.0
Shingleton	1985	444	0.23
Artman, et al	1987	153	0.7
Burghardt, et al	1988	359	1.4
Lee, et al	1989	954	0.4
Kenter, et al	1989	213	0
Monaghan, et al	1990	498	0.6
TOTAL		6320	0.6

Modified from Shingleton HM, Orr JW Jr. Cancer of the cervix: diagnosis and treatment. New York, Churchill Livingstone, 1987:133.

time, node yields, mean tumor diameters, median depths of invasion, and histologic subtypes were not statistically different between transfused and nontransfused groups. Among the 68 women who received blood perioperatively, the recurrence rate (14.7%) was statistically different from the 3.4% rate of 58 patients who did not receive blood ($p = .035$) after a short follow-up (18 months); perhaps with longer follow-up, this difference would disappear. Dalrymple and Monaghan (1988), in a similar study with longer observation, reported 83% versus 78% 5-year survival in 151 women treated for cervical cancer (non-transfused versus transfused, respectively). Soper (1991), using multivariate analysis techniques, reported no support for concern regarding adverse survival in patients who received transfusions in a series of 236 women with negative nodes and margins. Many women undergoing radical hysterectomy have significant blood loss and may be considered to be candidates for transfusion. Blood is administered based on the overall clinical situation; tolerance of physicians to lower hemoglobin levels in their operative patients has increased relative to potential infectious risks, especially that of human immunodeficiency virus infection. Surgeons tolerate a lower postoperative serum hemoglobin in those women having no evidence of coronary artery disease.

OVARIAN FUNCTION AFTER RADICAL HYSTERECTOMY

Ellsworth and coworkers (1983) studied ovarian function in 16 patients after radical hysterectomy and pelvic node dissection. The fact that 20% of patients had diminished ovarian function after surgery was thought to be related to blood supply problems of the retained ovaries. Reoperation for a pathologic condition of the retained adnexa was necessary in 5% of the patients, a complication rate that is similar to our experience. Owens and colleagues (1989) reported a follow-up of 14 patients with transposed ovaries; only 1 of these patients developed symptoms of ovarian failure and none developed metastatic disease or required reoperation due to ovarian cysts or other pathology. Chambers and associates (1990) studied 25 patients with transposed ovaries and compared them with 59 other patients treated during the same period. They reported a 24% incidence of symptomatic ovarian cysts, most of which required reoperation, compared with 7.4% cysts in women who had retained ovaries but who did not have transposition. Incidence of ovarian failure in the transposed ovary patients was the same as in those without transposition (4.3% versus 4.1%). Anderson and coworkers (1993) reported 82 women younger than 42 who underwent transposition of ovaries to the paracolic gutter. Of the 24 in the transposed group who had postoperative radiation therapy, only 4 (17%) had continued ovarian function, in contrast to 40 of 44 (91%) with transposition who received no postoperative radiation therapy. After transposition, 17.6% required surgical treatment for ovary-associated pain or cysts. Anderson and colleagues concluded that 71% of individuals who had ovaries left in place without transposition retained ovary function without problems, more than the group who had transposition of the ovaries (only 53% retention of function). This raises the question whether lumbar gutter transposition actually achieves its goal of protecting the ovaries.

FACTORS AFFECTING SURVIVAL AFTER RADICAL ABDOMINAL HYSTERECTOMY

Lesion Size and Pelvic Node Metastases

Many investigators have related survival to lesion size and pelvic node metastases. Five and ten-year survival is excellent for lesions up to 2 cm in diameter (Fig. 7-9),

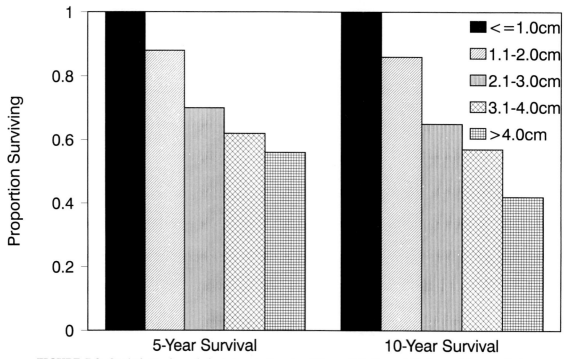

FIGURE 7-9. Survival rates by pathologic tumor diameter. (Alvarez RD, Potter ME, Soong S-J, et al. Rationale for using pathologic tumor dimensions and nodal status to subclassify surgically treated stage IB cervical cancer patients. Gynecol Oncol 1991;43:108, with permission.)

whereas larger lesions result in survival similar to that of patients with stage II disease. As tumors increase in size, the node metastasis rates also increase (Fig. 7-10). The size of metastatic foci in nodes and their location within nodes vary widely (Fig. 7-11*A* and *B*). Metastatic disease to pelvic nodes has a significant impact on the chances of 5- and 10-year survival (Table 7-11). Patients with an adequately resected primary lesion and one to three positive pelvic nodes have a better prognosis than do those with more than three nodes (Table 7-12).

Inoue and coworkers (1984) studied the size of the largest metastatic node as a prognostic factor in 152 patients having stage IB and IIA cervical cancer treated by radical hysterectomy and postoperative irradiation. They found that 60% of the patients had nodes less than 1 cm in size, 39% had largest nodes between 1 and 2 cm, and an additional 24% had nodes larger than 2 cm. Eleven percent of the nodes were unresectable. They noted an inverse relation between increasing size of the tumor-containing node and the length of disease-free interval.

Many investigators through the years have reported decreased survival when comparing unilateral pelvic node metastasis with bilateral primary pelvic nodes (Hsu et al 1972, Pilleron et al 1974, Delgado et al 1978, Shingleton et al 1983), whereas some (Webb et al 1979, Martimbeau et al 1982) ascribe no significance to bilaterality of node metastases. When considering the number of involved nodes, however, this seems to make the effect of bilaterally involved nodes less important.

Surgical Margins

The survival of patients after radical hysterectomy largely depends on adequate tumor resection (i.e., wide margins around the tumor). Extension to the anterior margin of resection (i.e., deep invasion to or into the bladder muscularis) is a finding on some surgical specimens after radical hysterectomy. This may not be anticipated on pelvic examination alone; it is usually associated with larger-volume stage IB and stage IIA tumors. If the anterior margins are considered suspicious intraoperatively, one may make the case that the operation should be abandoned; however, at that point in the dissection, the blood supply to the uterus may have been sacrificed.

Tumor extending near or to the surgical margins predicts central pelvic recurrence (Creasman et al 1986). Extension of tumor into the parametrial tissues or parametrial nodes increases the risk of more distal node metastases or lateral pelvic recurrence. Extension of tumor through the thickness of the cervix to involve the cul-de-sac peritoneum may be associated with free tumor cells in pelvic fluid or washings and is associated with a worse prognosis.

Parametrial Involvement

The risk of parametrial involvement varies by stage (Table 7-13) and to some degree reflects the method and completeness of the study of the operative specimen (Fig. 7-12).

Giant sections of radical hysterectomy specimens,

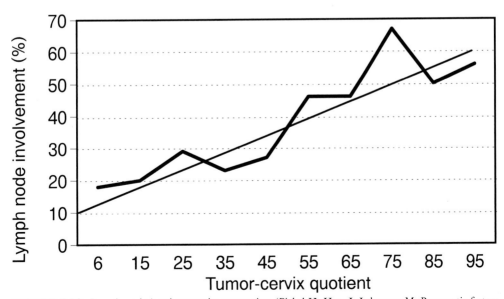

FIGURE 7-10. Lymph node involvement by tumor size. (Pickel H, Haas J, Lahousen M. Prognostic factors in cervical cancer on the basis of morphometric evaluation. Baillieres Clin Obstet Gynaecol 1988;2:805, with permission.)

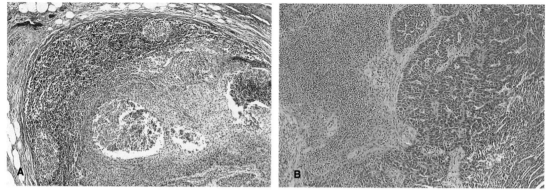

FIGURE 7-11. (**A**) Squamous cell carcinoma with focal necrosis metastatic to lymph node. (**B**) Adenocarcinoma, moderately well- to well-differentiated, metastatic to lymph node. See Color Figure 7-11.

such as those performed (or that have been performed) in some centers in Germany, Austria, and Japan, allow study of the nature of the spread of tumor and in particular, spread to the parametrial tissues and vaginal margins. Extracervical extension of tumor may occur (1) in a direct (continuous) manner, (2) in a dissociated manner, or (3) in parametrial nodes. Burghardt and colleagues (1988) believe strongly that continuous cancer spread into the parametrial tissues is rare, stating, "the idea of cervical cancer spreading continuously via the parametria to the pelvic wall has a shaky foundation. Stage IIIB disease . . . arises by expansion of the primary tumor and by confluence of multiple isolated foci in the parametria." The dearth of actual data supporting this concept relates to the difficulty and expense associated with such studies.

Parametrial Nodes

It has long been appreciated that the parametrium contains lymph nodes (Henriksen 1954), yet only by special assessment of the specimen is one able to appreciate the number, the size, and the location of such nodes (Baltzer et al 1979, Burghardt et al 1988, Tulusan et al 1991). These nodes, often small, may be detected throughout the parametrium and at least one group (Tulusan et al 1991) believes that most nodes

TABLE 7-11
Surgically Treated Stage IB Carcinoma*: Overall 5-Year Survival
and Survival by Pelvic Node Status

STUDY	YEAR	PATIENTS (N)	NEGATIVE NODES (%)	POSITIVE NODES (%)	OVERALL (%)
Morley, et al	1976	149	96.0	55.0	91.3
Zander, et al	1981	747	90.1	68.8	84.5
Noguchi, et al	1987	191	90.6	59.4	85.3
Barber	1988	273	83.4	50.0	78.8
Carenza, et al	1988	105	91.0	56.2	85.7
Fuller, et al	1989	285	94.0	54.0	86.0
Kenter, et al	1989	178	94.0	65.0	87.0
Lee, et al	1989	237	87.7	73.1	86.1
Monaghan, et al	1990	494	91.4	50.5	83.0
Hopkins, et al	1991b	213	93.0	61.0	89.0
Alvarez, et al	1991	401	88.0	53.0	85.0
Burghardt, et al	1992	443	—	—	83.4
Massi, et al	1993	211	85.0	45.0	75.8
Hepp[†]	1993	183	92.5	63.9	86.9

*Predominantly squamous cell.
[†]Hepp H. Written communication, January 1993.

TABLE 7-12
Five-Year Survival by Number of Positive Pelvic Nodes*: Stage IB

STUDY	YEAR	PATIENTS (N)	NUMBER OF POSITIVE NODES					
			1	1–2	1–3	2–3	≥3	≥4
Pilleron, et al	1974	49	71	—	—	—	—	—
Piver, et al	1975	71	—	—	51	—	—	29
Morrow	1980	174	—	—	70	—	—	35
Kjorstad	1987	300	—	75	—	—	12	—
Shingleton	1985	48	—	—	62	—	—	38
Noguchi, et al	1987	177	—	—	54	—	—	43
Fuller, et al	1989	71	—	60	—	—	12	—
Lee, et al	1989	956	62	44	—	—	43	44
Inoue, et al	1990	484	91	—	—	71	—	50
Hopkins, et al	1991	44	—	—	79	—	—	33

*Predominantly squamous cell carcinoma.

and nodes containing metastatic tumor will be found in the medial parametrium (see Fig. 7-2). With negative parametrium and negative pelvic lymph nodes, the survival rate (regardless of lesion size) is excellent (90% to 98%), whereas with positive parametrium and pelvic node metastases, the survival rate falls by about half (Fig. 7-13). When the parametrium is invaded, the incidence of pelvic node involvement rises three to five times (Burghardt et al 1978, Inoue et al 1984, Delgado et al 1989); the risk of multiple (four or more) positive pelvic nodes rises sixfold (Inoue et al 1984); and vascular invasion in the vessel-rich parametrium probably increases, with its attendant effect on survival (Fig. 7-14).

Uterine Extension

Noguchi and associates (1983) and Gonzalez and colleagues (1989) commented on the significance of uterine body extension of tumor, reporting an 82%

and 65% 5-year survival rate in patients with a negative endometrial cavity and 45% and 39% 5-year survival rate with tumor extension into the lower uterine segment, respectively. Some share their view; however, studies using multivariate analysis techniques have not established uterine extension to be an independent variable (Tables 7-14 and 7-15).

Lymphvascular Space Invasion

Tumor in lymphvascular spaces (lymphvascular invasion; Fig. 7-15) has long been considered an ominous finding, even in the absence of demonstrated pelvic node metastases (Noguchi et al 1983, Boyce et al 1984, Matsuyama et al 1984, Delgado et al 1989). For this reason, many have advocated postoperative pelvic irradiation or adjunctive chemotherapy for such patients. Our data (Gauthier et al 1985, Simon et al 1986) and that of others (Nahhas et al 1983, White et

TABLE 7-13
Parametrial Involvement by FIGO Stage*

STUDY	YEAR	PATIENTS (N)	IB	IIA	IIB
Matsuyama, et al	1984	255	15.5	25.9	42.0
Burghardt, et al	1988	359	12.9	25.0	30.6
Tulusan, et al	1988	487	6.3	—	69.0
Delgado, et al	1989	645	6.8	—	—
Cheng	1990	100	—	—	20.0
Inoue, et al	1990	484	6.9	23.3	34.1

FIGO, International Federation of Gynecology and Obstetrics.
*Predominantly squamous cell carcinoma.

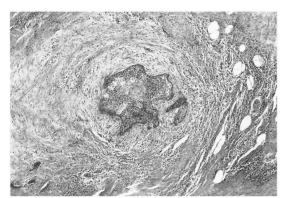

FIGURE 7-12. Venous extension of squamous cell carcinoma, now enveloped by organized thrombus within parametrial tissue. At the right is a small focus of tumor within a lymphvascular space. See Color Figure 7-12.

of tumor volume and pelvic node metastases (Fig. 7-16).

ADENOCARCINOMA OF THE CERVIX—LESS CURABLE?

In comparing women who have surgically treated stage IB squamous cell carcinoma and adenocarcinoma, overall 5-year survival rates are lower for the adenocarcinoma patients (see Table 7-16); the reasons for this are unclear. Several investigators (see Table 7-16) have observed that patients with adenocarcinoma of the cervix and pelvic lymph node metastases have a significantly higher recurrence rate than patients with squamous cell carcinoma. We previously noted (Shingleton et al 1982) a shorter interval to recurrence for adenocarcinoma and adenosquamous tumors than for squamous cell lesions; however, when the data are corrected for tumor diameter, we have never shown worse survival for surgically treated patients with adenocarcinoma.

Some advocate combined irradiation and surgery in adenocarcinomas. Surgery, however, may offer a survival advantage, compared with radiation therapy as sole treatment for stage I and II lesions. For example, Kleine and associates (1989) reported that patients who had stage IB and II adenocarcinoma had 5-year

al 1984) suggest that when data on patients with lymphvascular space invasion is corrected for depth of stromal invasion and for tumor size or volume (i.e., submitted to multivariate analysis), lymphvascular invasion may lose its significance as an independent variable. Combined series analysis leaves the issue unresolved (see Tables 7-14 and 7-15). Baltzer and Koepcke (1979) believe that tumor cell emboli (lymphvascular invasion) are a random event, independent

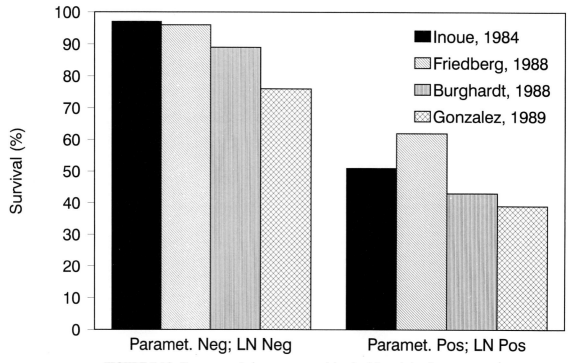

FIGURE 7-13. Five-year survival versus parametrial and pelvic node involvement.

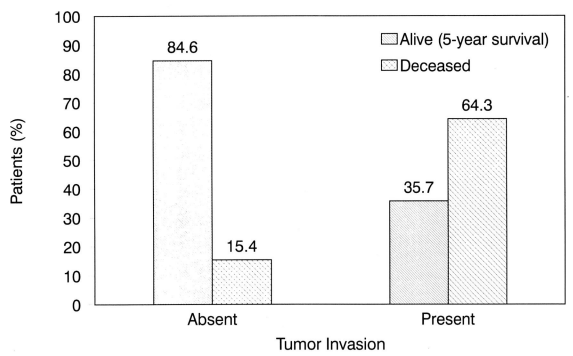

FIGURE 7-14. Prognostic significance of tumor invasion into blood vessels. (Burghardt E, Baltzer J, Tulusan AH, Haas J. Results of surgical treatment of 1028 cervical cancers studied with volumetry. Cancer 1992;70:648, with permission.)

survival rates equal to those who had squamous cell cancer, whereas those in stages I and II who were treated by radiation therapy did worse (85.0% versus 58.6% stage I; 62.3% versus 37.5% stage II; squamous cell carcinoma versus adenocarcinoma, respectively). Eifel and coworkers (1991) expressed concern about a 45% pelvic recurrence rate in patients having stage IB

adenocarcinomas (3 to 4 cm or more in diameter) treated by surgery alone, compared with a 11% recurrence in large lesions treated by radiation therapy or combination therapy. We (Shingleton et al 1981) had also noted a high (57%) recurrence rate in surgically treated adenocarcinomas 3 cm or more in size. Prempree and colleagues (1985) reported improved survival

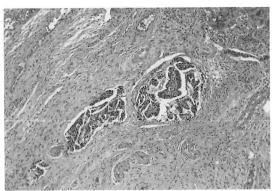

FIGURE 7-15. Adenocarcinoma of cervix, extending within a lymphvascular space. See Color Figure 7-15.

TABLE 7-14
Multivariate Analysis of Most Commonly Analyzed Risk Factors: Squamous Cell Cancer*

Significant
   Size (volume) of tumor
   Metastasis to lymph nodes
   Parametrial invasion
   Lymphvascular invasion
Probably significant
   Depth of stromal invasion
Not significant
   Age of patient
   Grade of tumor

*Some series contain adenocarcinoma patients.
n = 3761

Haas et al 1988, Alvarez et al 1989, Delgado et al 1990, Alvarez et al 1991, Hale et al 1991, Hopkins et al 1991, Kamura et al 1992, Tinga et al 1992, Burghardt et al 1992.

TABLE 7-15
Significant Prognostic Factors in Stage IB
and IIA Cancer

1. Node metastases
    a. Multiple nodes or node groups
    b. Bilateral nodes or node groups
2. Size of tumor equal to or greater than 4 cm
3. Depth of invasion into the cervix equal to or greater than
    10 mm or invasion into the outer third of the cervix
4. Histologic cell type*
5. Histologic grade*
6. Lymphvascular invasion*
7. Extension to the corpus uteri*
8. Age of the patient at diagnosis*
9. Stage IIA*

*Risk factors that may be important but are not clearly established as being independent of the other factors.

Modified from Hoskins WJ. Prognostic factors for risk of recurrence in stages IB and IIA cancer. Baillieres Clin Obstet Gynaecol 1988;2:817; with permission.

using combined treatment for large stage IB and stage II adenocarcinomas of the cervix. There seems to be more risk in choosing surgery as the sole modality for the treatment of large cervical adenocarcinomas when compared with large stage IB squamous lesions, which are highly curable by surgery alone (Alvarez 1993).

In a surgical series totaling 978 women, Averette and associates (1993), comparing 74 surgically treated patients having stage IB or IIA adenosquamous tumors with 108 patients having adenocarcinoma, found no difference in survival between patients with squamous cell or pure adenocarcinoma but a significantly reduced survival rate (63.5%) in those having adenosquamous tumors. This has not been our experience; in a matched control study of surgically treated stage IB adenocarcinomas (A) and adenosquamous tumors (AS; Helm et al 1992), all pathology was reviewed by a panel of three gynecologic pathologists for uniformity. Thirty-two (37.6%) of the 85 cases originally called adenosquamous type were excluded because no squamous component was found on review. Five-year survival for the matched groups (A versus AS) was not significantly different (A = 91%, AS = 80%; $p = .146$); however, a significantly shorter time to recurrence in the AS group was noted. It is also noteworthy that in several series in which multivariate analysis techniques were applied to the data, adenosquamous tissue type did not prove to be a significant variable (Table 7-18). The lack of an accepted pathologic classification of adenocarcinomas of the cervix and lack of uniformity in diagnosis of subpatterns of adenocarcinoma by individual pathologists may explain the different results that are reported on the subject.

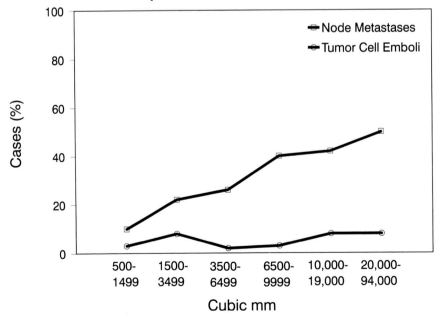

FIGURE 7-16. Tumor cell emboli and lymph node metastases versus tumor volume. (Modified from Baltzer J, Koepcke W. Tumor size and lymph node metastases in squamous cell carcinoma of the uterine cervix. Arch Gynecol 1979;227:271, with permission.)

TABLE 7-16
Surgically Treated Stage IB Adenocarcinoma of the Cervix 5-Year Survival:
Positive Versus Negative Nodes

STUDY	YEAR	PATIENTS (N)	NEGATIVE NODES (%)	POSITIVE NODES (%)	OVERALL (%)
Tamimi, et al	1982	32	92.0	25.0	81.1
Inoue, et al	1984	53	92.9	36.4	81.1
Berek, et al	1985	51	91.7	10.0	82.9
Ireland, et al	1985	50	91.1	50.0	79.2
Hopkins	1988	63	82.0	28.0	76.0
Kilgore, et al	1988	78	81.3	42.7	77.7
Angel, et al	1992	53	93.0	15.0	80.0
Averette, et al*	1993	108	NS	NS	80.5
McLellan, et al	1994	55	97.8	22.2	85.5

*Some IIa

Surgical Studies Using Multivariate Analysis of Risk Factors

The literature on cervical cancer is difficult to interpret. Most authors fail to separate the results in patients with squamous cell carcinoma or adenocarcinoma. Each set of authors uses different clinical and pathologic study variable—to some degree related to whether a coauthor pathologist was involved—in review of the radical specimens. In nine publications reporting 3761 patients with predominantly squamous cell carcinoma (see Table 7-16), 28 different risk factors were analyzed. Regarding the risk factors most commonly considered, the two most significant were size (or volume) of tumor and metastasis of tumor to lymph nodes. Other variables that may be important

include depth of stromal invasion, lymphvascular invasion, and parametrial invasion. Two variables found to have no significance were age of the patient and grade of the tumor. Although the variable of parametrial invasion was not considered in the reports he reviewed (see Table 7-17), Hoskins (1988), evaluated more than 1400 patients from nine series reported between 1975 and 1987 and reached essentially the same conclusions.

Adenocarcinoma of the cervix presents special problems when attempting to interpret the literature. The lack of an accepted classification of adenocarcinoma presents the most serious problem and every investigator seems to use a different classification. In eight studies using multivariate analysis, 577 patients are reviewed. The strongest independent variables (as

TABLE 7-17
Recurrences in Surgically Treated Stage IB Cervical Squamous Cell and Adenocarcinomas by Node Status

STUDY	YEAR	SCC (N)	ADENOCA (N)	RECURRENCE (%)			
				SCC (−Nodes)	Adenoca (−Nodes)	SCC (+Nodes)	Adenoca (+Nodes)
Burke, et al	1987	206	69	6.2	12	29	50
Larson, et al	1988	200	49	5.7	16	25	67
Greer, et al	1989	—	55	—	11.0	—	78
Angel, et al	1992	—	53	—	8.5	—	66.7
Hopkins, et al*	1992	213	63	6.8	20.8	27	58
Shingleton	1992	378	94	10.4	15.9	30	33.3
Tinga, et al	1992	130	38	2.8	13.8	18.2	75

*Personal communication.
Adenoca, adenocarcinoma; *SCC,* squamous cell carcinoma.

TABLE 7-18
Multivariate Analysis of Most Commonly Analyzed
Risk Factors: Adenocarcinoma of the Cervix

Highly significant
    Lesion size (volume)
    Metastasis to lymph nodes
Probably significant
    Grade of tumor
    Depth of stromal invasion
Not significant
    Age of patient
    Type of treatment
    Adenosquamous tissue type

n = 577

Saigo 1986, Kilgore et al 1988, Goodman et al 1989, Hopkins et al 1991, Angel et al 1992, Tinga et al 1992, Favalli et al 1993, Eisner et al 1993, McLellan et al 1994.

with squamous cell lesions) are lesion size and node metastasis. Grade of tumor seems to be more important in cervical adenocarcinoma than it is in squamous cell carcinoma; another factor that may be of importance is depth of stromal invasion. Variables that were found not to be significant are age of patient, type of treatment, or adenosquamous tissue type (see Table 7-18).

SHOULD RADICAL VAGINAL HYSTERECTOMY BE REVISITED?

Massi and coworkers (1993) raised the issue of whether there is a place for radical vaginal hysterectomy in the modern treatment of cervical cancer. Comparing 283 patients subjected to radical vaginal hysterectomy (no lymphadenectomy) and postoperative pelvic irradiation (some patients) with 175 patients undergoing Wertheim-Meigs abdominal operations (with lymphadenectomy), Massi's group reported no significant difference in the 5-year survival for the two groups. In commenting on the series, Massi and associates postulate that radical vaginal hysterectomy without lymphadenectomy is as effective as the Wertheim-Meigs operation with lymphadenectomy in the surgical management of cervical cancer, and they raise the question regarding the value of pelvic lymphadenectomy in this disease. They also pose questions regarding whether it is useful or harmful to remove uninvolved pelvic or abdominal lymph nodes in these patients and whether the excision of metastatic nodes results in improved survival. Massi and colleagues referred to work by Rauscher and Spurney (1959), who compared two groups of patients

who were submitted to radical hysterectomy, with or without lymphadenectomy. The 5-year survival rate for the lymphadenectomy group was 75%, whereas the survival rate for those without lymphadenectomy was 74% (315 patients total).

LAPAROSCOPIC LYMPHADENECTOMY

Techniques have been reported for laparoscopic evaluation of the pelvic and paraaortic lymph nodes, both in animals (Herd et al 1992) and in humans (Schuessler et al 1991, Querleu et al 1991, Childers 1992, Fowler et al 1994). Such techniques could replace all laparotomies that are solely performed for surgical staging in cervical cancer patients. An extensive pelvic lymph node sampling procedure is possible and with experience and expertise, can be performed safely. Because the most important feature of curative surgery for invasive cervical cancer appear to be wide excision of the primary tumor, this may be accomplished vaginally and when combined with laparoscopic lymphadenectomy may offer results equal or superior to the abdominal Wertheim-Meigs operation—possibly with less morbidity and a shorter hospital stay.

The emerging literature on this subject suggests a need for reevaluation of the role of radical vaginal hysterectomy, particularly when combined with laparoscopic staging of the aortic and pelvic nodes. Such a shift in approach to surgical treatment requires changes in training of gynecologic pelvic surgeons in this country because few possess the skills and experience to accomplish the radical surgical excision of the cervical tumor from the vaginal approach.

References

Abu-Ghazaleh S, Johnston W, Creasman WT. The significance of peritoneal cytology in patients with carcinoma of the cervix. Gynecol Oncol 1984;17:139.

Allen HH, Nisker JA, Anderson RJ. Primary surgical treatment in one hundred ninety-five cases of stage IB carcinoma of the cervix. Am J Obstet Gynecol 1982; 143:581.

Alvarez RD, Gelder MS, Gore H, Soong S-J, Partridge EE. Radical hysterectomy in the treatment of patients with bulky early stage carcinoma of the cervix uteri. Surg Gynecol Obstet 1993;176:539.

Alvarez RD, Potter ME, Soong S-J, et al. Rationale for using pathologic tumor dimensions and nodal status to subclassify surgically treated stage IB cervical cancer patients. Gynecol Oncol 1991;43:108.

Alvarez RD, Soong S-J, Kinney WK, et al. Identification of prognostic factors and risk groups in patients found to have nodal metastasis at the time of radical hysterectomy for early-stage squamous carcinoma of the cervix. Gynecol Oncol 1989;35:130.

Anderson B, LaPolla J, Turner D, Chapman G, Buller R. Ovarian transposition in cervical cancer. Gynecol Oncol 1993;40:206.

Angel C, DuBeshter B, Lin J. Clinical presentation and management of stage I cervical adenocarcinoma: a 25 year experience. Gynecol Oncol 1992;44:71.

Aronowitz J, Kaplan AL. The management of a pelvic lymphocele by the use of a percutaneous indwelling catheter inserted with ultrasonic guidance. Gynecol Oncol 1983;16:292.

Artman LE, Hoskins WJ, Bibro MC, et al. Radical hysterectomy and pelvic lymphadenectomy for stage IB carcinoma of the cervix: 21 years experience. Gynecol Oncol 1987;28:8.

Averette HE, Nguyen HN, Donato DM, et al. Radical hysterectomy for invasive cervical cancer: a 25-year prospective experience with the Miami technique. Cancer 1993;71:1422.

Ayhan A, Tuncer ZS. Radical hysterectomy with lymphadenectomy for treatment of early stage cervical cancer: clinical experience of 278 cases. J Surg Oncol 1991;47:175.

Baltzer J, Koepcke W. Tumor size and lymph node metastases in squamous cell carcinoma of the uterine cervix. Arch Gynecol 1979;227:271.

Baltzer J, Lohe KJ, Kopcke W, Zander J. Histological criteria for the prognosis in patients with operated squamous cell carcinoma of the cervix. Gynecol Oncol 1982; 13:184.

Barber HRK. Cervical cancer: pelvic and para-aortic lymph nodes sampling and its consequences. Baillieres Clin Obstet Gynaecol 1988;2:768.

Barton DPJ, Cavanagh D, Roberts WS, Hoffman MS, Fiorica JV, Finan MA. Radical hysterectomy for treatment of cervical cancer: a prospective study of two methods of closed-suction drainage. Am J Obstet Gynecol 1992; 166:533.

Bendvold E, Kjorstad KF. Antibiotic prophylaxis for radical abdominal hysterectomy. Gynecol Oncol 1987;28:201.

Benedet JL, Turko M, Boyes DA, Nickerson KG, Bienkowska BT. Radical hysterectomy in the treatment of cervical cancer. Am J Obstet Gynecol 1980;137:254.

Berek JS, Hacker NF, Fu Y-S. Sokale JR, Leuchter RC, Lagasse LD. Adenocarcinoma of the uterine cervix: histologic variables associated with lymph node metastasis and survival. Obstet Gynecol 1985;65:46.

Bjornsson, Nelson, Reale, Rose. Accuracy of frozen section (FS) for lymph node metastasis in patients undergoing radical hysterectomy (RH) for carcinoma of the cervix (abstract). 24th Annual Meeting, Society of Gynecologic Oncologists, Palm Desert, California, 1993.

Bloss JD, Berman NL, Mukhererjee J, et al. Bulky stage IB cervical carcinoma managed by primary radical hysterectomy followed by tailored radiotherapy. Gynecol Oncol 1992;47:21.

Bortolozzi G, Rossi F, Mangioni C, Candiani GB. A contribution to the therapy of cervicocarcinoma: remarks on 40 patients presenting paraaortic metastases (1970–1979). Eur J Gynaecol Oncol 1983;4:9.

Bostofte E, Serup J. Urological complications of Okabayashi's operation for cervical cancer. Acta Obstet Gynecol Scand 1981;60:39.

Boyce J, Fruchter RG, Nicastri AD, Ambinvagar PC, Reinis MS, Nelson JH Jr. Prognostic factors in stage I carcinoma of the cervix. Gynecol Oncol 1981;12:154.

Boyce J, Fruchter RG, Nicastri AD, Ambinvagar PC, Reinis MS, Nelson JH Jr. Vascular invasion in stage I carcinoma of the cervix. Cancer 1984;53:1175.

Brown JV, Fu Y-S, Berek JS. Ovarian metastases are rare in stage I adenocarcinoma of the cervix. Obstet Gynecol 1990;76:623.

Burghardt E, Baltzer J, Tulusan AH, Haas J. Results of surgical treatment of 1028 cervical cancers studied with volumetry. Cancer 1992;70:648.

Burghardt E, Hofmann HMH, Ebner F, Haas J, Tamussino K, Justick E. Magnetic resonance imaging in cervical cancer: a basis for objective classification. Gynecol Oncol 1989;33:61.

Burghardt E, Pickel H. Local spread and lymph node involvement in cervical cancer. Obstet Gynecol 1978; 52:138.

Burghardt E, Pickel H, Haas J, Lahousen M. Objective results of the operative treatment of cervical cancer. Baillieres Clin Obstet Gynaecol 1988;2:987.

Burghardt E, Pickel H, Haas J, Lahousen M. Prognostic factors and operative treatment of stages IB to IIB cervical cancer. Am J Obstet Gynecol 1987;156:988.

Burke TW, Hoskins WJ, Heller PB, Bibro MC, Weiser EB, Park RC. Prognostic factors associated with radical hysterectomy failure. Gynecol Oncol 1987;26:153.

Carenza L, Villani C. Parametrial involvement and therapeutic programming in stage IB cervical cancer. Baillieres Clin Obstet Gynaecol 1988;2:889.

Chambers TK, Chambers JT, Holm C, Peschel RE, Schwartz PE. Sequelae of lateral ovarian transposition in unirradiated cervical cancer patients. Gynecol Oncol 1990; 39:155.

Cheng MCE. Role of surgery in the treatment of cancer of the cervix. Singapore Med J 1990;31:253.

Childers J. The role of laparoscopic lymphadenectomy in the management of cervical carcinoma (abstract). 23rd Annual Meeting, Society of Gynecologic Oncologists, San Antonio, Texas, March 15–18, 1992.

Christ F. Prospektive und retrospektive Untersuchungen zur Urodynamik von Harnblase und Harnröhre nach Zervixkrebs-operationen Habilitationsschrist Erlangen, 1979.

Christ F, Wagner U, Debus G. Early bladder function disorders following Wertheim surgery. Causes and therapeutic consequences. Geburtshilfe Frauenheilkd 1983; 43:380.

Clarke-Pearson DL, DeLong ER, Synan IS, Creasman WT. Complications of low-dose heparin prophylaxis in gynecologic oncology surgery. Obstet Gynecol 1984;64: 689.

Clarke-Pearson DL, Jelovsek FR, Creasman WT. Thromboembolism complicating surgery for cervical and uterine malignancy: incidence, risk factors and prophylaxis. Obstet Gynecol 1983;61:87.

Clarke-Pearson DL, Soper J, Berchuck A, et al. Closed

retroperitoneal suction drainage following selective lymphadenectomy: risks and benefits (abstract). 23rd Annual Meeting, Society of Gynecologic Oncologists, San Antonio, Texas, March 15–18, 1992.

Copeland LJ, Silva EG, Gershenson DM, et al. Superficially invasive squamous cell carcinoma of the cervix. Gynecol Oncol 1992;45:307.

Crandon AJ, Koutts J. Incidence of post-operative deep vein thrombosis in gynaecological oncology. Aust NZ J Obstet Gynaecol 1983;23:216.

Creasman WT, Hill GB, Weed JC, et al. A trial of prophylactic cefamandole in extended gynecologic surgery. Obstet Gynecol 1982;59:309.

Creasman WT, Soper JT, Clarke-Pearson D. Radical hysterectomy as therapy for early carcinoma of the cervix. Am J Obstet Gynecol 1986;155:964.

Cruse PJ, Foord R. The epidemiology of wound infection. A 10-year prospective study of 62,939 wounds. Surg Clin North Am 1980;60:27.

Curtin JP, Morrow CP. Therapy of patients with positive nodes. Clin Obstet Gynecol 1990;33:883.

Dalrymple JC, Monaghan JM. Blood transfusion and disease free survival in cervical cancer. J Obstet Gynaecol 1988;8:356.

Dargent D. The value and the limits of panoramic retroperitoneal pelviscopy (PRPP) in gynecologic cancer (abstract). 23rd Annual Meeting, Society of Gynecologic Oncologists, San Antonio, Texas, March 15–18, 1992.

Dasmahapatra KS, Swaminathan AP. The use of a biodegradable mesh to prevent radiation-associated small bowel injury. Arch Surg 1991;126:366.

Delgado G, Bundy BN, Fowler WC Jr, et al. A prospective surgical pathological study of stage I squamous carcinoma of the cervix: a gynecologic oncology group study. Gynecol Oncol 1989;35:314.

Delgado G, Bundy B, Zaino R, Sevin B-U, Creasman WT, Major F. Prospective surgical-pathological study of disease-free interval in patients with stage IB squamous cell carcinoma of the cervix: a gynecologic oncology group study. Gynecol Oncol 1990;38:352.

Dockendorf BL, Frazee RC, Matheny RG. Omental pedicle graft to improve ischemic anastomoses. South Med J 1993;86:628.

Eifel PJ, Burke TW, Delclos L, et al. Early stage I adenocarcinoma of the uterine cervix: treatment results in patients with tumors 4 cm in diameter. Gynecol Oncol 1991;41:199.

Eisenkop SM, Spirtos NM, Montag TW, Moossazadeh J, Warren P, Hendrickson M. The clinical significance of blood transfusion at the time of radical hysterectomy. Obstet Gynecol 1990;76:110.

Eisner RF, Cirisano F, Berek JS. The influence of histology on outcome in stage IB cervical cancer treated with radical hysterectomy followed by pelvic irradiation (abstract). Int J Gynecol Cancer 1993;3:19.

Ellsworth LR, Allen HH, Nisker JA. Ovarian function after radical hysterectomy for stage IB carcinoma of cervix. Am J Obstet Gynecol 1983;145:185.

Farquharson DIM, Orr JW Jr. Prophylaxis against thromboembolism in gynecologic patients. J Reprod Med 1984;29:845.

Farquharson DIM, Shingleton HM, Soong S-J, Sanford SP, Levy DS, Hatch KD. The adverse effects of cervical cancer treatment on bladder function. Gynecol Oncol 1987;27:15.

Favalli G, Garbelli R, Ravelli V, Santin A, Pecorelli S, Bianchi UA. Adenocarcinoma of the uterine cervix: still a controversial issue (abstract). Int J Gynecol Cancer 1993;3:15.

Ferraris G, Lanza A, Daddato F, et al. Technique of pelvic and paraaortic lymphadenectomy in the surgical treatment of cervix carcinoma. Eur J Gynaecol Oncol 1988;9:83.

Forney JP. The effect of radical hysterectomy on bladder physiology. Am J Obstet Gynecol 1980;138:374.

Fowler JM, Carter JR, Carlson JW, et al. Lymph node yield from laparoscopic lymphadenectomy in cervical cancer: a comparative study. Gynecol Oncol 1993;51:187.

Friedberg V. Operative therapy for stage IIB cervical cancer. Baillieres Clin Obstet Gynaecol 1988;2:973.

Fuller AF Jr, Elliott N, Kosloff C, Hoskins W, Lewis JL Jr. Determinants of increased risk for recurrence in patients undergoing radical hysterectomy for stage IB and IIA carcinoma of the cervix. Gynecol Oncol 1989;33:34.

Gallup DG. Modifications of celiotomy techniques to decrease morbidity in obese gynecologic patients. Am J Obstet Gynecol 1984;150:171.

Gauthier P, Gore I, Shingleton HM, Soong S-J, Orr JW, Hatch KD. Identification of histopathologic risk groups in early stage cervical cancer. Obstet Gynecol 1985; 66:569.

Gitsch E, Patelsky N, Philipp K. Radical isotope surgery: an enrichment for the surgical therapy of gynecological malignancies. Eur J Gynaecol Oncol 1987;8:71.

Gitsch E, Philipp K, Patelsky N. Intraoperative lymph scintigraphy during radical surgery for cervical cancer. J Nucl Med 1984;25:486.

Gonzalez DG, Ketting BW, van Bunningen, van Dijk JDP. Carcinoma of the uterine cervix stage IB and IIA: results of postoperative irradiation in the parametrium and/or lymph node metastasis. Int J Radiat Oncol Biol Phys 1989;16:389.

Goodman HM, Buttlar CA, Niloff JM, et al. Adenocarcinoma of the uterine cervix: prognostic factors and patterns of recurrence. Gynecol Oncol 1989;33:241.

Granai CO, Gajewski W, Madoc-Jones H, Moukhtar M. Use of the omental J flap for better delivery of radiotherapy to the pelvis. Surg Gynecol Obstet 1990;171:71.

Greer BE, Figge DC, Tamimi HK, Cain JM. Stage IB adenocarcinoma of the cervix treated by radical hysterectomy and pelvic lymph node dissection. Am J Obstet Gynecol 1989;160:1509.

Haas J, Friedl H. Prognostic factors in cervical carcinoma: a multivariate approach. Baillieres Clin Obstet Gynaecol 1988;2:829.

Hale RJ, Buckley CH, Fox H, Wilcox FL, Tindall VR, Logue JP. The morphology and distribution of lymph node metastases in stage IB/IIA cervical carcinoma; a relationship to prognosis. Int J Gynecol Cancer 1991a: 1:233.

Hale RJ, Wilcox FL, Buckley CH, Gindall VR, Ryder WDJ, Logue JP. Prognostic factors in uterine cervical carcinoma: a clinicopathological analysis. Int J Gynecol Cancer 1991b;1:19.

Hasumi K, Sakamoto A, Sugano H. Microinvasive carcinoma of the uterine cervix. Cancer 1980;45:928.

Heller PB, Park RC. Lymph node positivity in cervical cancer. Gynecol Oncol 1981;12:328.

Helm CW, Soong S-J, Partridge EE, Shingleton HM. A matched study of surgically treated IB adenosquamous carcinoma and adenocarcinoma of the cervix (abstract). 23rd Annual Meeting, Society of Gynecologic Oncologists, San Antonio, Texas, March 15–18, 1992.

Henriksen E. Surgical Treatment of Cancer of the Cervix. In Meigs JV, ed. New York, Grune & Stratton, 1954:65.

Herd J, Fowler JM, Shenson D, Lacy S, Montz FJ. Laparoscopic para-aortic lymph node sampling: development of a technique. Gynecol Oncol 1992;44:271.

Hindley A, Cole H. Use of peritoneal insufflation to displace the small bowel during pelvic and abdominal radiotherapy in carcinoma of the cervix. Br J Radiol 1993;66:67.

Hopkins MP, Schmidt RW, Roberts JA, Morley GW. The prognosis and treatment of stage 1 adenocarcinoma of the cervix. Obstet Gynecol 1988;72:915.

Hopkins MP, Morley GW. A comparison of adenocarcinoma and squamous cell carcinoma of the cervix. Obstet Gyecol 1991a;77:912.

Hopkins MP, Morley GW. Squamous cell cancer of the cervix: prognostic factors related to survival. Int J Gynecol Cancer 1991b;1:173.

Hoskins WJ. Prognostic factors for risk of recurrence in stages IB and IIA cervical cancer. Baillieres Clin Obstet Gynaecol 1988;2:817.

Hoskins WJ, Ford JH Jr, Lutz MH, Averette HE. Radical hysterectomy and pelvic lymphadenectomy for the management of early invasive cancer of the cervix. Gynecol Oncol 1976;4:278.

Hsu C-T, Cheng Y-S, Su S-C. Prognosis of uterine cervical cancer with extensive lymph node metastases. Am J Obstet Gynecol 1972;114:954.

Hughes RR, Brewington KC, Hanjani P, et al. Extended field irradiation for cervical cancer based on surgical staging. Gynecol Oncol 1980;9:153.

Ilancheran A, Monaghan JM. Pelvic lymphocyst—a 10 year experience. Gynecol Oncol 1988;29:333.

Inoue T, Okumura M. Prognostic significance of parametrial extension in patients with cervical carcinoma stages 1B, IIA and IIB. Cancer 1984;54:1914.

Inoue T. Prognostic significance of the depth of invasion relating to nodal metastases, parametrial extension and cell types. Cancer 1984;54:3035.

Inoue T, Chihara T, Morita K. The prognostic significance of the size of the largest nodes in metastatic carcinoma from the uterine cervix. Gynecol Oncol 1984;19:187.

Inoue T, Morita K. The prognostic significance of number of positive nodes in cervical carcinoma stages IB, IIA, and IIB. Cancer 1990;65:1923.

Ireland D, Hardiman P, Monaghan JM. Adenocarcinoma of the uterine cervix: a study of 73 cases. Obstet Gynecol 1985;65:82.

Jensen JK, DiSaia PJ, Lucci JA III, Manetta A, Berman ML. To drain or not to drain: a retrospective study of closed-suction drainage following radical hysterectomy with pelvic lymphadenectomy (abstract). 24th Annual Meeting, Society of Gynecologic Oncologists, Palm Desert, California, February 7–10, 1993.

Kaminski PF, Norris HJ. Coexistence of ovarian neoplasms and endocervical adenocarcinoma. Obstet Gynecol 1984;64:553.

Kamura T, Tsukamoto N, Tsuruchi N, et al. Multivariate analysis of the histopathologic prognostic factors of cervical cancer in patients undergoing radical hysterectomy. Cancer 1992;69:181.

Kaser G, Ike FA, Hirsch HA. Atlas der gytnakologischen operationen unter berucksichtigung. Gynakologischen Urologischer Eingriffe 3, Stuttgart, Aufluger Thieme, 1973.

Kenter GG, Ansink AC, Heintz APM, Aartsen EJ, Delemarre JFM, Hart AAM. Carcinoma of the uterine cervix stage I and IIA: results of surgical treatment: complications, recurrence and survival. Eur J Surg Oncol 1989;15:55.

Kilgore LC, Orr JW Jr, Hatch KD, Shingleton HM, Roberson J. Peritoneal cytology in patients with squamous cell carcinoma of the cervix. Gynecol Oncol 1984;19:24.

Kilgore LC, Soong S-J, Gore H, Shingleton HM, Hatch KD, Partridge EE. Analysis of prognostic features in adenocarcinoma of the cervix. Gynecol Oncol 1988;31:137.

Kindermann G, Debus-Thiede G. Postoperative urological complications after radical surgery for cervical cancer. Baillieres Clin Obstet Gynecol 1988;2:933.

Kinney WK, Egorshin EV, Ballard DJ, Podratz KC. Long–term survival and sequelae after surgical management of invasive cervical carcinoma diagnosed at the time of simple hysterectomy. Gynecol Oncol 1992;44:24.

Kinney W, Hodge D, Egorshin E, Ballard D, Podratz K. Identification of a low risk subset of patients with stage IB invasive squamous carcinoma of the cervix possibly suited to less radical surgical treatment (abstract). 24th Annual Meeting, Society of Gynecologic Oncologists, Palm Desert, California, February 7–10, 1993.

Kjorstad KE. The management of the high risk patient with early invasive carcinoma of the cervix. In Surwit EA, Alberts DS, eds. Cervix cancer. Boston, Martinus Nijhoff Publishers, 1987.

Kjorstad KE, Kolbenstvedt A, Strickert T. The value of complete lymphadenectomy in radical treatment of cancer of the cervix, stage IB. Cancer 1984;54:2215.

Kleine W, Rau K, Schwoeorer D, Pfleiderer A. Prognosis of the adenocarcinoma of the cervix uteri: a comparative study. Gynecol Oncol 1989;35:145.

Kudo R, Kusanagi T, Hashimoto M. Vaginal semiradical hysterectomy: a new operative procedure for microinvasive carcinoma of the cervix. Obstet Gynecol 1984;64:810.

Langley II, Moore DW, Tarnasky JW, Roberts PHR. Radical hysterectomy and pelvic lymph node dissection. Gynecol Oncol 1980;9:37.

Larson DM, Copeland LJ, Stringer CA, Gershenson DM, Malone JM Jr, Edwards CL. Recurrent cervical carcinoma after radical hysterectomy. Gynecol Oncol 1988;30:381.

Larson DM, Stringer CA, Copeland LJ, Gershenson DV, Malone JM Jr, Rutledge FN. Stage IB cervical carcinoma treated with radical hysterectomy and pelvic lymphadenectomy: role of adjuvant radiotherapy. Obstet Gynecol 1987;69:378.

Lee Y-N, Wang K⊤, Lin M-H, et al. Radical hysterectomy with pelvic lymph node dissection for treatment of cervical cancer: a clinical review of 954 cases. Gynecol Oncol 1989;32:135.

Leman MH, Benson WL, Kurman RJ, Park RC. Microinvasive carcinona of the cervix. Obstet Gynecol 1976; 48:571.

Lerner HM, Jones HW III, Hill EC. Radical surgery for the treatment of early invasive cervical carcinoma (stage IB): review of 15 years experience. Obstet Gynecol 1980; 56:413.

Lohe KJ. Early squamous cell carcinoma of the uterine cervix. I. Definition and histology. Gynecol Oncol 1978;6:10.

Lopes A, Hall J, Monaghan JM. Drainage following radical hysterectomy and pelvic node dissection—dogma or need (abstract). Int J Gynecol Cancer 1993;3:23.

Maiman MA, Fruchter RG, DiMaio TM, Boyce JG. Superficially invasive squamous cell carcinoma of the cervix. Obstet Gynecol 1988;72:399.

Mann WJ, Vogel F, Pastner B, Chalas E. Management of lymphocysts after radical gynecologic surgery. Gynecol Oncol 1989;33:248.

Marsden DE, Cavanagh D, Wisniewski BJ, Roberts WS, Lyman GH. Factors affecting the incidence of infectious morbidity after radical hysterectomy. Am J Obstet Gynecol 1985;152:817.

Martimbeau PW, Kjorstad KE, Iversen T. Stage IB carcinoma of the cervix, the Norwegian Radium Hospital. II. Results when pelvic nodes are involved. Obstet Gynecol 1982;60:215.

Massi G, Savino L, Susini T. Schauta-Amreich's vaginal hysterectomy and Wertheim-Meigs abdominal hysterectomy in the treatment of cervical cancer: a retrospective analysis. Am J Obstet Gynecol 1993;168:928.

Matsuyama T, Inoue I, Tsukamoto N, et al. Stage IB, IIA, and IIB cervix cancer, postsurgical staging, and prognosis. Cancer 1984;54:3072.

McLellan R, Dillon MB, Woodruff JD, Heatley GJ, Fields AL, Rosenshein NB. Long-term follow-up of stage I cervical adenocarcinoma treated by radical surgery. Gynecol Oncol 1994;52:253.

Micha JP, Kucera PR, Burkett JP, et al. Prophylactic mezlocillin in radical hysterectomy. Obstet Gynecol 1987;69:251.

Miywzawa K, Hernandez E, Dillon MD. Prophylactic topical Mandol in radical hysterectomy. Int J Gynecol Obstet 1987;25:133.

Monaghan JM, Ireland D, Mor-Yosef S, Pearson SE, Lopez A, Sinha DP. Role of centralization of surgery in stage IB carcinoma of the cervix: a review of 498 cases. Gynecol Oncol 1990;37:206.

Moore DH, Fowler WC Jr, Walton LA, Droegemueller W. Morbidity of lymph node sampling in cancers of the uterine corpus and cervix. Obstet Gynecol 1989; 74:180.

Morley GW, Seski JC. Radical pelvic surgery versus radiation therapy for stage I carcinoma of the cervix (exclusive of microinvasion). Am J Obstet Gynecol 1976;126:785.

Morrow CP. Is pelvic radiation beneficial on the postopera-

tive management of stage IB squamous cell carcinoma of the cervix with pelvic node metastasis treated by radical hysterectomy and pelvic lymphadenectomy? Gynecol Oncol 1980;10:105.

Nahhas WA, Sharkey FE, Whitney CW, Husseinzadeh N, Chung CK, Mortel R. The prognostic significance of vascular channel involvement and deep stromal penetration in early cervical carcinoma. Am J Clin Oncol 1983;6:259.

Ng H-T, Kan Y-Y, Chao K-C, Huan C-C, Shyu S-K. The outcome of the patients with recurrent cervical carcinoma in terms of lymph node metastasis and treatment. Gynecol Oncol 1987;26:355.

Noguchi H, Shiozawa I, Sakai Y, Yamazaki T, Fukuta T. Pelvic lymph node metastasis of uterine cervical cancer. Gynecol Oncol 1987;27:150.

Noguchi H, Shiozawa K, Tsukamoto T, Tsukahara Y, Iwai S, Fukuta T. The postoperative classification for uterine cervical cancer and its clinical evaluation. Gynecol Oncol 1983;126:219.

Orr JW Jr, Ball GC, Soong S-J, Shingleton HM, et al. Surgical treatment of women found to have invasive cervical cancer at the time of total hysterectomy. Obstet Gynecol 1985;68:353.

Orr JW Jr, Barter JF, Kilgore LC, Soong SJ, Shingleton HM, Hatch, KD. Closed suction pelvic drainage after radical pelvic surgical procedures. Am J Obstet Gynecol 1986;155:867.

Orr JW Jr, Holloway RW. Surgical aspects of cervical cancer. Surg Clin North Am 1991;71:1067.

Orr JW Jr, Holloway RW, Orr PJ. Pulmonary complications. In Orr JW Jr, Shingleton HM, eds. Complications in gynecologic oncology: prevention, recognition and management. Philadelphia, JB Lippincott, 1994.

Orr JW Jr, Orr PF, Barrett JM, et al. Continuous or interrupted fascial closure: a prospective evaluation of No. 1 Maxon suture in 402 gynecologic procedures. Am J Obstet Gynecol 1990;163:1485.

Orr JW Jr, Shingleton HM, Hatch KD, Mann WJ, Austin JM Jr, Soong SJ. Correlation of perioperative morbidity and conization-radical hysterectomy interval. Obstet Gynecol 1982;59:726.

Orr JW Jr, Sisson PF, Patsner B, et al. Single-dose antibiotic prophylaxis for patients undergoing extended pelvic surgery for gynecologic malignancy. Am J Obstet Gynecol 1990;162:718.

Orr JW Jr, Taylor PT. Avoiding postoperative infection in the patient with gynecologic cancer. Infect Surg 1987;12:361.

Orr JW Jr, Taylor PT Jr. Wound healing. In Orr JW Jr, Shingleton HM, eds. Complications in gynecologic surgery: prevention, recognition and management. Philadelphia, JB Lippincott, 1994:175.

Owens S, Roberts WS, Fiorica JV, Hoffman MS, LaPolla JP, Cavanagh D. Ovarian management at the time of radical hysterectomy for cancer of the cervix. Gynecol Oncol 1989;35:349.

Panici PB, Scambia G, Baiocchi G, Greggi S, Mancuso S. Technique and feasibility of radical para-aortic and pelvic lymph adenectomy for gynecologic malignancies: a prospective study. Int J Gynecol Cancer 1991;1:133.

Parente JT, Silberblatt W, Stone M. Infrequency of metastasis to ovaries in stage I carcinoma of the cervix. Am J Obstet Gynecol 1964;90:1362.

Park RC, Partow WE, Rogers RE, Zimmerman EA. Treatment of stage I carcinoma of the cervix. Obstet Gynecol 1973;41:117.

Patsner B, Mann WJ Jr, Chalas E, Orr JW Jr. Intestinal complications associated with use of the Dexon mesh sling in gynecologic oncology patients. Gynecol Oncol 1990; 38:146.

Petri E. Bladder after radical pelvic surgery. In Stanton SL, ed. Clinical gynecologic urology. St. Louis, CV Mosby, 1984:220.

Petru E, Tamussino K, Lahousen M, Winter R, Rickel H, Haas J. Pelvic and para-aortic lymphocysts after radical surgery because of cervical and ovarian cancer. Am J Obstet Gynecol 1989;161:937.

Photopulos GJ, Zwaag RV. Class II radical hysterectomy shows less morbidity and good treatment efficacy compared to class III. Gynecol Oncol 1991;40:21.

Pilleron JP, Durand JC, Hamelin JP. Prognostic value of node metastasis in cancer of the uterine cervix. Am J Obstet Gynecol 1974;119:458.

Piver MS, Chung WS. Prognostic significance of cervical lesion size and pelvic node metastases in cervical carcinoma. Obstet Gynecol 1975;46:507.

Piver MS, Rutledge F, Smith JP. Five classes of extended hysterectomy for women with cervical cancer. Obstet Gynecol 1974;44:265.

Podczaski ES, Palombo C, Manetta A, et al. Assessment of pretreatment laparotomy in patients with cervical carcinoma prior to radiotherapy. Gynecol Oncol 1989; 33:71.

Potter ME, Alvarez RD, Shingleton HM, et al. Early invasive cervical cancer with pelvic lymph node involvement: to complete or not to complete radical hysterectomy? Gynecol Oncol 1990;37:78.

Powell JL, Burrell MO, Franklin EW III. Radical hysterectomy and pelvic lymphadenectomy. Gynecol Oncol 1981;12:23.

Prempree T, Amornmarn R, Wizenberg MJ. A therapeutic approach to primary adenocarcinoma of the cervix. Cancer 1985;56:1264.

Querleu D, Leblanc E, Castelain B. Laparoscopic pelvic lymphadenectomy in the staging of early carcinoma of the cervix. Am J Obstet Gynecol 1991;164:579.

Ralph G, Tamussino K, Lichtenegger W. Urological complications after radical abdominal hysterectomy for cervical cancer. Ballieres Clin Obstet Gynaecol 1988;2:943.

Ralph G, Tamussino K, Lichtenegger W. Urological complications after radical hysterectomy with or without radiotherapy for cervical cancer. Arch Gynecol Obstet 1990;248:61.

Rauscher VH, Spurney J. Ergebnisse der Wertheimschen radikaloperation ohne und mit obligatischer lymphadenectomie. Geburtshilf Frauenheilkd 1959;19(8):651.

Reisenger SA, Palazzo JP, Talerman A, Carlson J, Jahshan A. Stage IB glassy cell carcinoma of the cervix diagnosed during pregnancy and recurring in a transposed ovary. Gynecol Oncol 1991;42:86.

Robertson G, Lopes A, Monaghan JM. Stage IB carcinoma of the cervix: is there a place for para-aortic lymph node dissection? (abstract). Int J Gynecol Cancer 1993;3:2.

Rodier JF, Janser JD, Rodier D, et al. Prevention of radiation enteritis by an absorbable polyglycolic acid mesh sling. Cancer 1991;68:2545.

Rosenshein NB, Ruth JC, Villar J, Grumbine FB, Dillon MB, Spence MR. A prospective randomized study of doxycycline as a prophylactic antibiotic in patients undergoing radical hysterectomy. Gynecol Oncol 1983;15:210.

Sall S, Pineda AA, Calanog A, Heller P, Greenberg H. Surgical treatment of stages IB and IIA invasive carcinoma of the cervix by radical abdominal hysterectomy. Am J Obstet Gynecol 1979;135:442.

Sasaki H, Yoshida T, Noda K, Yochiku S, Minami K, Kaneko S. Urethral pressure profiles following radical hysterectomy. Obstet Gynecol 1982;59:101.

Schuessler WW, Vancaillie TG, Reich H, Griffith DP. Transperitoneal endosurgical lymphadenectomy in patients with localized prostate cancer. J Urol 1991; 145:988.

Scotti RJ, Bergman A, Bhatia NN, Ostergard DR. Urodynamic changes in uretrovesical function after radical hysterectomy. Obstet Gynecol 1986;68:111.

Seski JC, Abell MR, Morley GW. Microinvasive squamous carcinoma of the cervix. Definition, histologic analysis, late results of treatment. Obstet Gynecol 1977;50:410.

Sevin B-U, Ramos R, Lichtinger M, Girtanner RE, Averette H. Antibiotic prevention of infections complicating radical abdominal hysterectomy. Obstet Gynecol 1984; 64:539.

Shingleton HM. American College of Surgeons invasive cervical cancer patterns of care study. 1995. In preparation.

Shingleton HM. Surgical treatment of cancer of the cervix. Eur J Gynaecol Oncol 1992;XIII:45.

Shingleton HM, Gore H, Soong S-J, Bradley DH. Adenocarcinoma of the cervix: 1. Clinical evaluation and pathologic features. Am J Obstet Gynecol 1981;138:799.

Shingleton HM, Gore H, Soong S-J, et al. Tumor recurrence and survival in stage IB cancer of the cervix. Am J Clin Oncol 1983;6:265.

Shingleton HM, Gore H, Wilters JH. Adenocarcinoma of the cervix: histopathologic and clinical features. In Hafez ESE, Smith JP, eds. Carcinoma of the cervix: biology and diagnosis. The Hague, Martinus Nijhoff, 1982: 200.

Shingleton HM, Gusberg SB. Radical hysterectomy. In Gusberg SB, Shingleton HM, Deppe G, eds. Female genital cancer. New York, Churchill Livingstone, 1988:536.

Simon NL, Gore H, Shingleton HM, Soong S-J, Orr JW Jr, Hatch KD. A study of superficially invasive carcinoma of the cervix. Obstet Gynecol 1986;68:19.

Soisson AP, Olt G, Soper JT, Berchuck A, Rodriguez G, Clarke-Pearson DL. Prevention of superficial wound separation with subcutaneous retention sutures. Gynecol Oncol 1993;51:330.

Soper JT. The clinical significance of blood transfusion at the time of radical hysterectomy. Obstet Gynecol 1991; 77:165.

Tabata M, Ichinoe K, Saburagi N, Shima Y, Yamaguchi T, Mabuchi Y. Incidence of ovarian metastasis in patients with cancer of the uterine cervix. Gynecol Oncol 1987;28:255.

Taki I, Sugimuri H, Matsuyama T, et al. Treatment of microinvasive carcinoma. Obstet Gynecol Surv 1979;34:839.

Tamimi HK, Figge DC. Adenocarcinoma of the uterine cervix. Gynecol Oncol 1982;13:335.

Tinga DJ, Bouma J, Aalders JG. Patients with squamous cell versus adeno(squamous) carcinoma of the cervix: what factors determine the prognosis? Int J Gynecol Cancer 1992;2:83.

Toki N, Tsukamoto N, Kaku T, et al. Microscopic ovarian metastasis of the uterine cervical cancer. Gynecol Oncol 1991;41:46.

Tulusan AH, Egger H, Lang N, Ober KG. Surgery for cervical cancer. Baillieres Clin Obstet Gynaecol 1988;2:981.

Tulusan AH, Wilczek-Engelmann T, Kaufmann W, et al. Operative therapie des Zervixkarzinoms in der Univ. Frauenklinik Erlangen. In Köchli, Sevin, Benz, Petree, Heller, eds. Gynäkologisch Onkologie—Manual für Klinik und Praxia. Berlin: Springer 1991;172.

van Nagell JR, Greenwell N, Powell DF, Donaldson ES, Hanson MG, Gay EC. Microinvasive carcinoma of the cervix. Am J Obstet Gynecol 1983;145:981.

Vervest HAM, Barents JW, Haspels AA, Debruyne FM. Radical hysterectomy and the function of the lower urinary tract. Acta Obstet Gynecol Scand 1989;68:331.

Webb MJ, Symmonds RE. Wertheim hysterectomy: a reappraisal. Obstet Gynecol 1979;54:140.

Welander CE, Pierce VK, Nori D, Hilaris BS, Kosloff C, Clark DG. Pretreatment laparotomy in carcinoma of the cervix. Gynecol Oncol 1981;12:336.

White CD, Morley GW, Kumar NB. The prognostic significance of tumor emboli in lymphatic or vascular spaces of the cervical stroma in stage IB squamous cell carcinoma of the cervix. Am J Obstet Gynecol 1984;149:342.

Winter R, Petru E, Haas J. Pelvic and para-aorticlymphadenectomy in cervical cancer. Baillieres Clin Obstet Gynaecol 1988;2:857.

Yajima A, Noda K. The results of treatment of microinvasive carcinoma (stage IA) of the uterine cervix by means of simple and extended hysterectomy. Am J Obstet Gynecol 1979;135:685.

Zander J, Baltzer J, Lohe KJ, Ober KG, Kaufmann C. Carcinoma of the cervix: an attempt to individualize treatment; results of a 20 year cooperative study. Am J Obstet Gynecol 1981;139:752.

Cancer of the Cervix by Hugh M. Shingleton and James W. Orr, Jr.
J. B. Lippincott Company, Philadelphia, © 1995.

8

Radiation Therapy

Radiation therapy represents a potentially curative treatment option for patients who have localized cervical cancer. Additionally, all gynecologic oncologists recognize radiation therapy as an important primary treatment for women with large-volume advanced-stage disease or postsurgical recurrent cervical cancer.

Gynecologists, gynecologic oncologists, and primary-care physicians diagnose, evaluate, and refer patients for radiation treatment. They often assume responsibility for posttreatment surveillance. Unfortunately, the lack of formal education in radiation physics or radiation biology and changes in technology can inhibit communication between the primary-care physician and the radiation therapist. Practicing gynecologists and other women's healthcare providers need a basic understanding of these radiation concepts because they are often the woman's initial source of pretreatment counseling and are frequently responsible for the recognition, management, treatment, or referral for therapy-related complications.

FUNDAMENTALS OF RADIATION PHYSICS

Ionizing radiation results in sufficient energy to eject one or more orbital electrons from an atom or molecule, resulting in the production of abnormal atomic and molecular species in irradiated tissues. Electromagnetic and particulate radiation represent two types of ionizing radiation. X-rays and gamma rays, two forms of electromagnetic radiation, differ only in the manner in which they are produced. X-rays are produced extranuclearly when an electrical device accelerates and directs a high-energy beam of electrons to strike a target, usually tungsten or gold, converting electron kinetic energy to x-rays. Gamma rays, pro-

duced intranuclearly, represent excess energy emitted from the unstable nuclei of certain radioactive isotopes (i.e., cobalt 60). The characteristics of these electromagnetic radiations include an energy wave and a "packet of energy" called a photon. Low-energy photons have a long wavelength and a low oscillatory frequency. Conversely, high-photon energies occur with electromagnetic radiations of short wavelengths and high frequencies. Generally, higher energy photons penetrate tissue to a greater depth before they interact with tissue to cause ionizations (Fig. 8-1). Therefore, higher energy photons (i.e., 10 million V or higher) deliver a higher effective radiation dose to the pelvic structures while sparing superficial (i.e., skin) tissues. When x-rays or gamma rays are absorbed by tissue, energy is unevenly deposited in discrete packets some distance apart in the absorber. Each absorptive event can culminate in a biologic event by breaking chemical bonds and initiating actions at the molecular level. Generally, electromagnetic radiation produces biologic events with tissue ionization if the corresponding wavelength is less than 10^{-6} cm.

Electromagnetic radiations interact primarily with absorbing tissues in three ways. The first, a process called photoelectric absorption, occurs when all of the photon's energy is expended as it interacts with an inner-shell orbital electron, thereby ejecting that electron from its parent nucleus. In the photoelectric process, which dominates at low energies generally in the diagnostic range, x-rays are absorbed preferentially in bone, allowing high resolution of bone on film. The second process, referred to as the Compton effect, dominates with cobalt 60 and low-energy linear accelerator x-rays when an incident photon interacts with an orbital electron, resulting in the ejection of that electron (as in the case of photoelectric effect), with incomplete energy transfer. This process results in a scatter photon, with reduced kinetic energy. This scat-

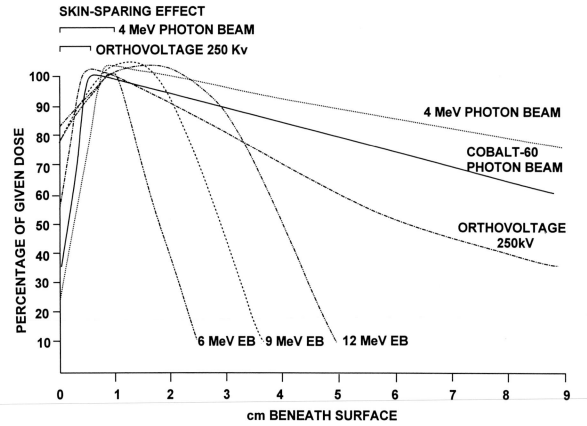

FIGURE 8-1. The depth at which maximum radiation dose occurs is related to the photon. Whereas 100% of the given dose of superficial radiation (not pictured) is at the air–skin interface, less of the given dose occurs at the air–skin interface with higher energy sources such as orthovoltage (about 50%), cobalt (30%), or 4-MeV photons (20%). This explains the skin-sparing effect of higher energy radiation. A greater percentage of a given dose is realized at greater depths of tissue penetration; that is, at 9 cm, only 40% of the given dose of orthovoltage is available to cause ionizing events. This percentage is increased substantially with ^{60}Co photons (60%), 4-MeV photons (75%), and is higher with 18-MeV or 22-MeV photons. This combination (skin-sparing effect of higher energy and increased depth of penetration) allows radiotherapists to treat tumor-bearing tissues with higher doses. *EB,* electron beam. (Shingleton HM, Orr JW Jr. Cancer of the cervix: diagnosis and treatment. New York, Churchill Livingstone, 1987:168.)

ter photon may interact again, and the ejected electron may also interact within the absorber to alter other atoms or vital chemical bonds. The third possible process of tissue interaction is pair production, generally seen at linear accelerator energies greater than 10 mV. During this process, a high-energy photon (more than 1.02 MeV) undergoes a reaction in the vicinity of the nucleus, in which a portion of the photon energy is used to create an electron (e−) positron (e+) pair. The kinetic energy is distributed to the two newly created particles, which ultimately may annihilate each other, creating two 0.51-MeV photons emitted in opposite directions, causing ionization along their paths of travel.

As discussed in the section on radiation biology, electromagnetic radiation interacts with the medium of the cell (i.e., water) to produce free radicals, which diffuse through the cell and interact with critical targets such as the DNA; this is called *indirect* action. High linear energy transfer (LET) radiation directly damages critical targets such as DNA strands and is called *direct* action.

Particulates used for radiation therapy are subatomic particles (electrons, protons, alpha particles, neutrons, negative pi-mesons, and atomic nuclei), which are accelerated to a high energy for tissue penetration. All of these particles, except neutrons, possess two characteristics uniquely different from electromagnetic radiations: mass and charge. Thus, particulate radiation has a greater potential to cause ionization along its path of travel through the absorber. This potential is directly related to particle mass size and charge value. Depth of tissue penetration by particulate radiation depends on both the particle's mass and charge in addition to the initial energy of the particle. For example, an alpha particle with its large mass (2 protons and 2 neutrons) and strong (+2) positive charge must be accelerated to high energy to penetrate a significant tissue depth. The electron is the most commonly used particulate radiation in clinical practice, and linear accelerators can produce electron beams of variable energy. The electron's ionization potential is greater than that of an equivalent energy photon and can be easily regulated regarding depth of tissue penetration (see Fig 8-1). Thus, electron-beam radiation can be used advantageously for the treatment of superficially located tumors (i.e., skin metastases). Neutron or other high LET radiation has been used in the primary treatment of cervical cancer. This form of brachytherapy (californium 252) involves a shorter treatment time (measured in hours, compared with days) and has the ability to eradicate large hypoxic tumors. The radiobiologic effectiveness of neutron radiation may be sixfold greater than conventional photon therapy (Maruyama et al 1982, Cohen et al 1985). Unfortunately, neutrons are difficult to shield, and protection of radiology personnel has limited the clinical usefulness of neutron therapy.

Quantities of radiation are usually expressed in units defined as roentgen, rad, or gray (Gy). The roentgen, a unit of radiation exposure, is not used in therapeutic radiology but is important in the field of radiation health safety to monitor radiation output. A roentgen is that amount of X or gamma radiation that produces an electrostatic unit of charge in 1 cm^3 of dry air. The rad, a unit of absorbed dose commonly used in therapeutic radiology, represents the energy absorbed per gram of absorber material because of electromagnetic or particulate ionizing radiation. By definition, 1 rad represents 100 ergs of energy absorbed per gram of absorber substance, or 0.01 J/kg. The recommended nomenclature for measurement of absorbed radiation dose is the gray (Gy); 1 Gy is equal to one J of energy absorbed per kg of substance (1 Gy = 100 rad; 1 cGy = 1 rad).

FUNDAMENTALS OF RADIATION BIOLOGY

Ionizing radiation can injure mammalian cells by direct interaction of photons or particles with essential cellular molecules, causing their ionization, or by ionization of nonessential cellular components, which in turn transfer and dissipate their radical electrical energies to vital molecular species. Nuclear DNA is accepted as the critical end target for both of these processes of radiation injury (Hall 1978, 1985).

Water, comprising nearly 80% of most mammalian cells, is a likely candidate for photon or particle radiation interaction. Ionization of water produces free radicals, which combine with oxygen and give rise to molecular species with lifespans and chemical characteristics capable of injuring critical targets within the cell. It is commonly accepted that most irradiation-related cell injury (about 70%) results from the indirect actions mediated by ionized water in the presence of oxygen. Without the presence of molecular oxygen (i.e., associated with large hypoxic tumors) this effect is dramatically diminished. The oxygen-enhancement ratio forms the basis of radiation treatment for certain human tumors with hyperbaric oxygen (Dische 1983a). Unfortunately, the use of hyperbaric oxygen is associated with increased normal-tissue radiosensitivity and clinically results in an increased risk of moderate or severe morbidity (Dische 1983b).

Particle radiations produce a dense path of ionization along their path and have a high probability of interacting with critical target molecules (direct action; Richter et al 1984). Particulate radiations with high ionization potential (e.g., neutrons, protons, alpha particles, pi-mesons, and atomic nuclei) are less dependent on tissue oxygenation and cause cell injury primarily through direct interaction with critical target molecules (i.e., DNA).

All proliferating human cells traverse the cell cycle (Fig. 8-2), the components of which include mitosis or cell division phase, synthesis, DNA synthesis, and preparation for cell division. Most mammalian cells are most sensitive to the effects of ionizing radiation during mitosis and least sensitive during the latter portion of DNA synthesis. Noncycling or "nonmetabolizing" cells (G_0), usually present in greater proportion in larger tumors, are considered relatively radioresistant. In contrast, cells undergoing rapid division or with long mitotic futures (stem cells) are relatively more radiosensitive. Unfortunately, the growth fraction—that portion of tumor cells actively cycling (and radiosensitive)—is significantly reduced by the time cervical malignancy becomes clinically apparent. The radiation enhancement effect of oxygen, occurring only when oxygen is present concurrently with the irradiation, is constant across all phases of the cell cycle.

For a given increment of radiation dose, a constant proportion rather than an absolute number of cells is killed (Fig. 8-3). D_0 represents the dose of irradiation required to reduce the surviving fraction of treated cells to 37% of their original number on the exponential curve. Cells with smaller D_0 are more sensitive to irradiation injury. The D_0 for most mammalian cells ranges between 100 and 200 cGy. Experimental studies suggest little difference of in vitro or in vivo radiosensitivity between normal and malignant cells of the same tissue origin. Finally, the survival

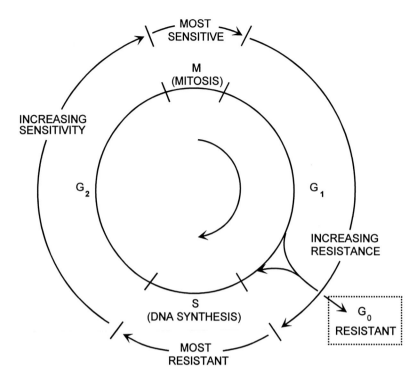

FIGURE 8-2. Radiosensitivity differs during the cell cycle. Increasing radioresistance is present during G_1 and S phases; however, cells proceeding through phase G_2 have increased sensitivity to ionizing radiation, and those in mitosis are the most sensitive. Most tumors have a large number of cells in phase G_0 (non-ionizing); however, these cells may be recalled into the cycle after cell kill during fractional radiotherapy. (Shingleton HM, Orr JW Jr. Cancer of the cervix: diagnosis and treatment. New York, Churchill Livingstone, 1987:171.)

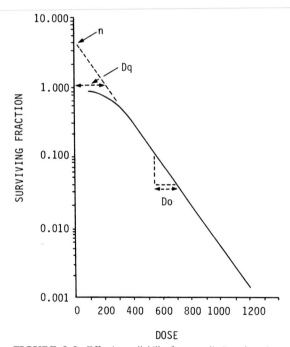

FIGURE 8-3. Effective cell kill after a radiation dose is a constant proportion and not an absolute number. The D_0 dose is that which reduces the surviving fraction to 37% on the exponential curve. The fall-off of the curve at lower doses (Dq) is related to the repair of sublethal damage. (Shingleton HM, Orr JW Jr. Cancer of the cervix: diagnosis and treatment. New York, Churchill Livingstone, 1987:172.)

curves of most mammalian cells have a shoulder (Dq) within the low radiation dose region that allows repair of sublethal damage and results in reduced efficiency of irradiation cell kill.

Clinically, radiation fractionation (dose delivered over multiple exposures) is more effective than a single dose in eradicating tumor cells and lessens the risk of normal tissue damage. Radiation sensitivity is greatly related to the individual cell's position in the cell cycle. Therefore, a single dose of radiation preferentially has a lethal effect on the sensitive (cycling) cells, while producing a partial synchrony of the remaining (non-cycling) cells. Redistribution or reassortment of the remaining malignant cells partially determines the response to additional radiation doses. Hyperfractionation (multiple daily fractions) exploits the ability of late reacting normal tissues to repair sublethal damage. Acute tissue reaction may limit total dose, however.

The advantage of treatment fractionation in tumor treatment is further explained by the process of reoxygenation (Fig. 8-4). Hypoxia can alter cell cycle age, distribution, and tumor proliferation rate and amplify specific oncogenes (Perez 1993a). Regardless of the mechanism, hypoxic cells are more likely to be chemoresistant and radioresistant. The critical diffusion distance for oxygen is 100 to 150 μm from a vascular surface. Thus, all tumors larger than 200 μm have associated zones of hypoxia and necrosis. Between proliferating cells (those less than 100 μm away)

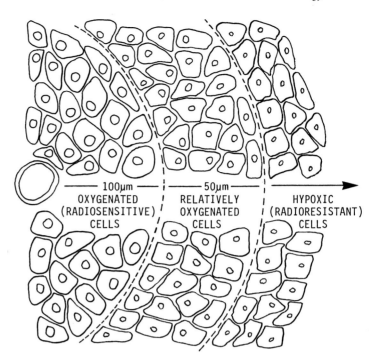

- 100μm -
OXYGENATED
(RADIOSENSITIVE)
CELLS

- 50μm -
RELATIVELY
OXYGENATED
CELLS

HYPOXIC
(RADIORESISTANT)
CELLS

FIGURE 8-4. Well-oxygenated cells, those with less than 100 μm from a vessel, are more radiosensitive than hypoxic cells. During radiation fractionation, the sensitive cells die, allowing reoxygenation of both the relatively hypoxic cells and hypoxic cells. Repeated fractional doses thereby are to affect more oxygenated cells than a single dose. (Shingleton HM, Orr JW Jr. Cancer of the cervix: diagnosis and treatment. New York, Churchill Livingstone, 1987:173.)

and hypoxic cells (those more than 200 μm away) there exists a region of tumor cells in a lowered oxygen tension that allows them to be clonogenic but renders relative protection from the effects of ionizing irradiation. This "relatively" hypoxic cell population would not be killed by a single dose of radiation; however, fractionated doses kill sensitive cells (those less than 100 μm away from oxygen supply) and the interval of fractionation allows those relatively resistant cells (between 100 and 200 μm) to reoxygenate and become sensitive to the radiation delivered with succeeding fractions. These changes clinically correspond to tumor regression during teletherapy. Tissue oxygen tension inversely correlates with interstitial fluid pressure. Roh and coworkers (1991) reported interstitial fluid pressure to be elevated in large cervical cancers, which partly explains the poor penetration and heterogenous distribution of blood-borne therapeutic agents as well as oxygen effects. Interestingly, interstitial fluid pressure decreased with irradiation response.

Heat interacts synergistically with irradiation and hypoxic cells, anoxic cells, and acidotic tumor cells—all of which may be heat sensitive. The role of hyperthermia, which preferentially kills cells during the S phase, is undetermined in the treatment of cervical cancer. Regional hyperthermia and irradiation may offer superior local control but does not contribute to a survival advantage (Hornback 1986).

Small fractionated doses of radiation of normal tissues are better tolerated than a large single dose because they allow time to repair sublethal damage (Bloomer et al 1975), a phenomenon that results when a cell undergoes ionizing events to some but not all of its critical target sites. Most irradiation effects are sublethal (Bedford 1991). Sublethal damage and potentially lethal damage are abstract operationally defined terms relating to alterations in the proportion of surviving cells, depending on the conditions under which treatment is delivered. Because many of these critical cellular target sites are not irreparably damaged, the normal cell may survive if given time for repair. It is postulated that few irradiation-induced chromosomal breaks fail to rejoin or reinstitute, making most irradiation effects sublethal; however, these sublethal events can interact with similar or additional damage from prior or further irradiation to produce lethal cellular damage. If chromosomal or cellular repair occurs before additional therapy, irradiation will be less effective in producing additional cell kill (Bedford 1991). Other specific treatment conditions (including dose rate, position in the cell cycle, tumor ploidy, and other cellular mutations) increase the chance of additional sublethal damage resulting in a lethal cellular effect (Bedford 1991).

A clinical radiobiologic research model that was designed to explain time-dose radiation effects in solid tumors was developed by Whitmore (1969). In this model, four fundamental processes are described as being influencing factors that occur during fractionated radiation treatments of solid tumors: tumor cell repair, reoxygenation, repopulation, and reassortment (redistribution). The fundamental thesis of this model suggests that properly selected radiation time-dose fractionation schemes can take advantage of the physical and physiologic changes that occur within the tumor volume during treatment to maximize the probability of tumor cell kill and minimize normal-tissue injury. Generally, cancer cells are early-reacting tissues, with rapid rates of repopulation. Normal tissues are late-reacting, with little repopulation but possessing a superior ability to repair sublethal damage (Murray 1990).

Tissue Tolerance

Radiation's therapeutic index, defined as the lethal tumor dose–lethal host dose, is narrow in patients with cervical carcinoma because normal-tissue tolerance limits the deliverable dose of radiation. The potential curative dose of radiation increases directly with tumor size in the nonoperated pelvic tumor bed (Fletcher 1973; Table 8-1). These therapeutic doses may increase in the "operated" tumor bed, secondary to the effects of postsurgical fibrosis and scarring. The effect on tumor size and radiosensitivity becomes important when one considers normal-tissue tolerance of surrounding pelvic structures (Table 8-2). The vagina, cervix, uterus, and ureters (with intact blood supply) are relatively radioresistant (Alfert et al 1972); however, the radiation dose that predicts a 50% risk of bladder or rectal injury (Otchy et al 1993) is identical to that necessary to cure large-volume (more than 4 cm) cervical squamous cell cancers. Although tolerance doses frequently allow cure, the associated progressive arteritis and fibrosis in surrounding normal tissue may predispose to complications or interfere with healing if a surgical procedure is performed later.

Histologically, early irradiation-related cellular changes in the intestine include a decreased mitotic rate and a degeneration of crypt cells (Rubin et al 1968, White 1975). Acute mucosal sloughing frequently results in micro-ulceration, submucosal edema, inflammatory infiltrates, and capillary dilation. These changes impair intestinal mucosal absorptive ability, with a resultant excessive secretion of mucous and bleeding. With time, these irradiated tissues demonstrate increased fibrosis and a progressive obliterative arteritis.

Degeneration of radioresponsive cells, suppression of mitotic activity, vascular congestion, edema, and microvascular changes are prominent in the bladder. Suresh and associates (1993) reported the spectrum of irradiation-induced histologic changes, indicating that epithelial changes were most prominent shortly after therapy. Stromal changes predominated later; however, submucosal fibrosis was equally prominent in early or late phases after irradiation.

Reproductive Tract

The kidney and liver, predominantly composed of nonproliferating cells, tolerate irradiation poorly. In fact, fractionated doses in excess of 2000 cGy are associated with nephritis and hepatitis, often unresponsive to medical management. Fortunately, renal and hepatic tissues are rarely incorporated in the treatment field for cervical cancer but need to be considered during paraaortic radiation treatment planning. Although bone has a relatively high irradiation tolerance, prior irradiation can hinder repair if a fracture occurs.

Although acute irradiation-induced changes associated with gastrointestinal or urinary symptoms may be distressing or interrupt therapy, the loss of mitotic activity in cell renewal systems of the vagina only occasionally results in epithelial denudation and acute vaginal symptomatology. Late long-term effects of fibrosis, scarring, and vaginal vault alteration are frequently symptomatic (Abitbol et al 1974b). Structural vaginal alterations may result in pain or dyspareunia but do not hinder systemic absorption of vaginal estrogen administration (Hintz et al 1981). There are no effective prophylactic measures to decrease the incidence or severity of late postirradiation vaginal symptomatology.

Ovarian function is decreased in women receiving pelvic irradiation (Janson et al 1981). Although uncommon, some reports (Gronroos et al 1982) suggest a continued low level of ovarian estradiol production after pelvic irradiation. Generally, women older than 40 may experience ovarian failure after the delivery of 6 Gy; however, doses exceeding 20 Gy are required to eliminate ovarian function in most reproductive-aged women (Orr et al 1993).

Younger women may benefit from pretreatment ovarian transposition to minimize irradiation effect (Nahhas et al 1971, Pitkin et al 1971); however, it appears that the incidence of ovarian metastasis increases

TABLE 8-1
Squamous Cell Carcinoma of the Cervix Dose-Tumor-Volume Relation: Average Dose Radiation Required to Obtain 90% Control in Treated Area

TUMOR VOLUME	DOSE (GY)
<2 cm	50
2 cm	60
2–4 cm	70
4–6 cm	75–89
6 cm	80–100

Shingleton HM, Orr JW. Cancer of the cervix: diagnosis and treatment. New York, Churchill Livingstone, 1987:174.

TABLE 8-2
Radiation Tolerance Levels of Abdominopelvic Organs

	RISK		
ORGAN	T 5/5* (Gy)	TD 50/5[†] (Gy)	TYPE OF INJURY
Bladder	60	80	Ulcer, contracture
Bone	60	150	Necrosis, fracture
Intestine	45	60	Ulcer, stricture, fistula
Muscle	60	80	Fibrosis
Ovary	3	12.5	Sterilization
Rectum	55	80	Ulcer, stricture, fistula
Skin	55	70	Atrophy, ulcer, fibrosis
Spinal cord	50	60	Necrosis, transection
Ureters	75	100	Stricture
Uterus	100	200	Necrosis, perforation
Vagina	90	100	Ulcer, fistula

*Total radiation dose (Gy) that results in a 5% complication rate in patients followed for 5 years.
[†]Total radiation dose (Gy) that results in a 50% complication rate in patients followed for 5 years.

Shingleton HM, Orr JW. Cancer of the cervix: diagnosis and treatment. New York, Churchill Livingstone, 1987:174.

with advanced-stage disease. Sutton (1992), reviewing the Gynecologic Oncology Group (GOG) data, suggested that the risk of ovarian spread in patients with stage IB disease was 0.5% and 1.7% in women with squamous cell carcinoma or adenocarcinoma. Although ovarian metastases are rare in early-stage disease, Toki and associates (1991) reported a 5.5% risk of ovarian metastasis in women having stage IIB disease. This increased risk of surgical morbidity and potential therapy delay argues against routine ovarian transposition before primary radiation therapy.

Post–radical hysterectomy radiation therapy may also result in cessation of ovarian function. Anderson and colleagues' (1993) report indicated that the addition of postoperative radiation therapy resulted in climacteric symptoms in 83% of women who had undergone ovarian transposition. Attention to intraoperative ovarian placement during transposition is paramount to maintaining ovarian function. Anderson and co-workers (1993) reported that 64% of patients had a lower postoperative ovarian position than anticipated at surgery. Although the risk of metastatic disease is low (1%), many women (17%) undergoing transposition may require subsequent oophorectomy for management of painful ovarian cysts, and a significant proportion (14%) require continued medical therapy for ovarian problems (Anderson et al 1993). With these findings, Anderson and associates (1993) suggested that ovarian transposition was not indicated in women at high risk to require postoperative radiation therapy.

In contrast, Chambers and coworkers (1991) sug-

gested maintenance of ovarian function in 71% of patients receiving radiation therapy after ovarian transposition. Menopause occurred more commonly in women receiving scatter doses of more than 300 cGy and in all women whose ovaries were transposed below the iliac crest. Like Anderson and associates' (1993) report, symptomatic ovarian cysts were common, occurring in 18% of patients undergoing transposition. Later ovarian operative intervention was required—three times more common in women undergoing transposition when compared with those with no transposition (Chambers et al 1991).

In a newer report, Parker and colleagues (1993) reported the results of a questionnaire sent to patients after radical hysterectomy and no adjuvant therapy. Although potentially biased by a 32% no-response rate, their report indicated a 20% incidence of early ovarian failure and a 7% risk for subsequent oophorectomy. Although not statistically significant, sexual relations were improved or unchanged in 89% of patients with ovarian conservation and 68% of patients after oophorectomy. Their hypothetical cost comparison favored oophorectomy in premenopausal women.

Given these facts, estrogen-replacement therapy should be considered in all women undergoing or after therapeutic pelvic irradiation. The osteoprotective effects of exogenous estrogen are established and the cardioprotective effects are documented. There is little evidence that estrogen replacement alters cervical cancer prognosis, regardless of histology (Milsom et al 1983).

The irradiated endometrium can respond to hormonal stimulation (Larson et al 1990), and many patients (23%) maintain endometrial sensitivity to exogenous hormones (McKay et al 1990). Unopposed estrogen administration may potentially increase the risk of developing premalignant or malignant corpus lesions. The postradiation cervical stenosis may eliminate the biologic sign of uterine cancer: bleeding. This scenario may explain why endometrial cancers developing after irradiation are more likely to be of higher stage and carry a poor prognosis (Chen et al 1991).

TREATMENT PLANNING

The radiation therapist must consider many factors during treatment planning in an attempt to maximize tumor response and minimize the risk of complications (Table 8-3).

Radiosensitivity cannot be equated to radiocurability. The former relates to the innate sensitivity of a particular cancer cell, whereas the latter implies a favorable tumor–normal tissue relation, such that a potentially curative radiation dose can be delivered with acceptable damage to surrounding normal tissue. Most localized cervical cancers are radiocurable because therapeutic schemas have been developed to protect normal tissue.

Dose

The cumulative radiation dose usually results from a combination of teletherapy and brachytherapy. As one may expect, the total radiation dose necessary to eradicate a 2-cm tumor differs from that which would sterilize a 6-cm tumor. The use of specific reference points or reference treatment volumes aid in the measure-

TABLE 8-3
Factors to be Considered in Treatment Planning

TECHNICAL	CLINICAL
Total radiation dose	Tumor volume
Daily dose	Cell type and grade
Time of delivery	Anatomic factors
Dose rate	Age
Total number of fractions	Nutritional status
Field size	Systemic disease
Sequence of therapy	Previous surgery
Energy source	

Shingleton HM, Orr JW. Cancer of the cervix: diagnosis and treatment. New York, Churchill Livingstone, 1987:175.

ment of the total pelvic and tumor dose to optimize tumor dose and minimize radiation dose to normal pelvic structures (Fig. 8-5).

Alternative calculations to determine the delivered radiation dose and the paracentral and lateral right and left points have been proposed to allow asymmetric treatment. Although advocated by some, this methodology has not gained wide acceptance (Hanks et al 1983). In 1985, the International Commission on Radiation Units and Measurements recommended the use of a reference volume for dose prescription when reporting intracavitary irradiation. Volume reference potentially allows better comparison of specific techniques.

High-energy radiation equipment (cobalt 60, linear accelerators) allows the delivery of a greater-depth dose during teletherapy (Table 8-4). Durrance et al (1969) reported that the risk of central pelvic recurrence in patients with stage I or II cervical carcinoma was decreased by 50% after the introduction of supervoltage units. Kurohara and coworkers (1979), comparing a series of patients treated by orthovoltage and supervoltage, indicated that the use of the latter was associated with increased patient survival across all stages. Johns has demonstrated increased survival in patients with stage III squamous cell carcinoma of the cervix treated with 23-mV photons (Betatron; effective energy greater than 10 mV), compared with those treated with cobalt 60 (Johns 1976). This clinical increase in pelvic control may be associated with a relative increased risk of distant metastases. Actually, autopsy series of cervical cancer deaths indicate less ureteral involvement in patients treated with higher energy equipment (Katz et al 1980).

Higher doses and intracavitary therapy are associated with increased pelvic control in patients with stage II or III disease; however, point A doses above 7000 cGy do not improve pelvic tumor control in patients with stage IB disease (Perez et al 1986). Lanciano, in a Patterns of Care Study (1991a), indicated a dose response for in-field control only for women having stage III disease. The highest rate of pelvic control was noted with a point A dose exceeding 8500 cGy. They were unable to demonstrate a dose-response relation with respect to lateral (PCS point P) dose. These reports indicate the important contribution of intracavitary therapy.

Treatment planning may differ dramatically between institutions. Some use the total dosage to anatomic points in the pelvis or combine external cGy delivery combined with milligram hours or cGy delivery with low dose–rate (LDR) or high dose–rate (HDR) intracavitary application. Reports from those institutions treating numerous cervical cancer patients suggest that the incorporation of appropriate megavoltage and brachytherapy, with specific attention to

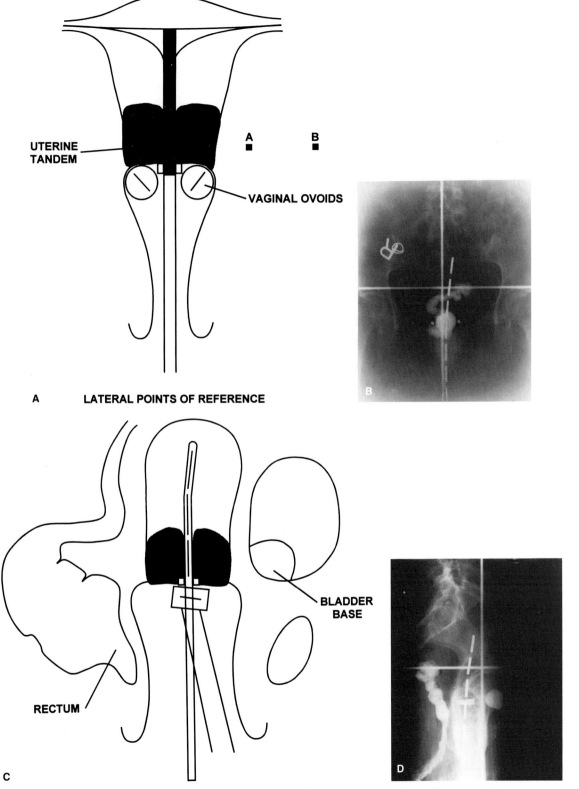

FIGURE 8-5. (**A**) Reference points used during pelvic radiotherapy include point *A* (2 cm lateral from the midline and 2 cm above the lateral vaginal fornix), which corresponds to the paracervical tissues near the ureter, and point *B* (3 cm lateral to point *A*), which represents the pelvic wall. The doses to the base of the bladder and rectum are important reference points in the anterior posterior plane. These reference points may be distorted in women having large cervical tumors. After intracavitary insertion, radio-opaque material (*right*) placed in the rectum and bladder allows tumor localization and dose calculation to the adjacent organs. (Shingleton HM, Orr JW Jr. Cancer of the cervix: diagnosis and treatment. New York, Churchill Livingstone, 1987:177.)

TABLE 8-4
Skin-Sparing and Depth–Dose Comparisons

TELETHERAPY DELIVERY APPARATUS	MAXIMUM-DOSE DELIVERY POINT (CM BELOW SURFACE)	DOSE DELIVERED 10 CM BELOW SURFACE (% OF MAXIMUM)
250 kV(p)	Surface	31
2 MeV	0.4	59
^{60}Co	0.5	59
4 MEV	1.0	65
6 MEV	1.5	69
25 MEV	3.3	81

Shingleton HM, Orr JW. Cancer of the cervix: diagnosis and treatment. New York, Churchill Livingstone, 1987:176.

problem areas, yield excellent results. Combinations vary; however, most centers attempt to deliver 7000 to 8500 cGy to the paracervical tissues (point A) and 6000 cGy to the pelvic side wall (point B; see Fig. 8-5, Figs. 8-6 and 8-7A) while maintaining the bladder and rectal dose at about 6000 cGy. Brady and coworkers (1992) have outlined the treatment policies of primary irradiation and LDR implants by stage (Fig. 8-8B).

Cure rates of 80% to 90% in stage I cancers, 60% to 70% in stage II disease, and 30% to 50% in stage III cancer are usual (Berek et al 1988). Only 5% to 10% of all patients with stage IV disease are cured; however, as many as 30% of selected patients with stage IV disease may be long-term survivors. Although many of the previously acknowledged factors play a significant role in eventual outcome, the radiation therapist must pay close attention to procedural detail and quality control to offer or exceed usual cure rates (Kapp 1983a, Kapp et al 1983b).

Field Size

Effective treatment planning for teletherapy requires close cooperation between gynecologic oncologist and radiation therapist. Decisions regarding field size may be related to computed tomography (CT) scan or lymphangiogram results or the results from fine-needle aspirate or surgical staging. Incorporation of an increased treatment volume increases the risk of complications. Although individualized therapy is vital, the basic pelvic treatment field consists of anterior and posterior opposing portals (15 × 15 cm or 16 × 16 cm), treated daily with a total dose of 180 to 200 cGy. Energies of 10 mV or greater are preferred. Dosimetry may be improved by using lateral pelvic portals, espe-

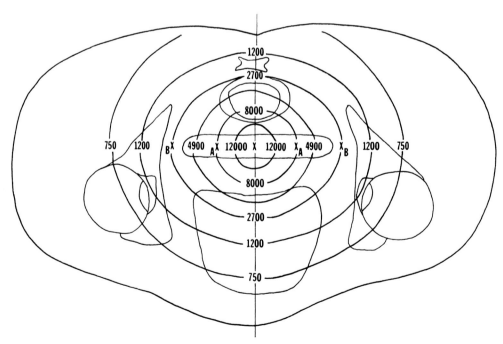

FIGURE 8-6. Typical dosimetry of patients treated with intracavitary therapy alone. This scheme allows a high local dose to the cervix and paracervical area (point *A*); however, the pelvic side wall dose (point *B*) is small. This form of therapy is not to be used in patients with a high risk of node metastases. (Shingleton HM, Orr JW Jr. Cancer of the cervix: diagnosis and treatment. New York, Churchill Livingstone, 1987:180.)

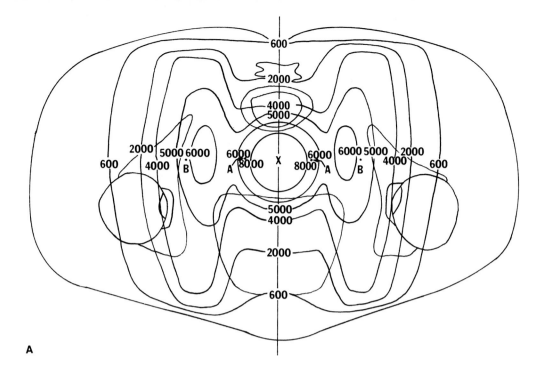

A

B

Tumor Stage	Tumor Extent	External Irradiation (cGy)*		Brachytherapy		
		Whole Pelvis	Additional Parametrial Dose (Midline Shield)	Two Insertions (mg h RaEq) §	Dose to Point A	Total Dose to Point A (cGy)
IA		0	0	6500–8000	7000	6000–7500
IB (small)	Superficial ulceration; less than 2 cm in diameter or involving fewer than two quadrants	0	4500	8000	7000	6500–7000
IB (2–4cm)	Four quadrant involvement; no endocervical component or significant expansion	1000	4000	7000	6500–7500	7500–8500
IIA, IIB	Non-barrel-shaped type	2000	3000	8000	7000	8500
IB-IIA (Bulky)†, IIB, IIIA	Barrel-shaped cervix; parametrial extension	2000	3000	8000	7000	8500–9000
IIIB	Parametrial involvement	2000	4000	8000	7000	8500–9500
IIB, IIIB, IV	Poor pelvic anatomy; patients not readily treated with intracavitary insertions (barrel-shaped cervix not regressing; inability to locate external os)	4000	2000	6500	6000	8500–9500

*180 cGy/day, five weekly fractions, using 15 or higher MV photon beams, two portals treated daily
§ 60–80 cGy/hr at point A. (In patients over 65 years or with history of previous pelvic inflammatory disease or pelvic surgery, reduce doses by 10%)
†In stage IB and IIA, if complete regression is not obtained, perform extrafascial conservative hysterectomy (reduce brachytherapy dose to 6000 mgh).

FIGURE 8-7. (A) Dosimetry of combined teletherapy and brachytherapy. Dose to the paracervical tissues (point *A*) is usually kept at 60 to 80 Gy and the dose to the pelvic side wall (point *B*) is usually 50 to 60 Gy. Bladder and rectal doses are maintained at levels that minimize the risk of complications. (Shingleton HM, Orr JW Jr. Cancer of the cervix: diagnosis and treatment. New York, Churchill Livingstone, 1987:180.) (B) Carcinoma of the uterine cervix: MIR policies of treatment with irradiation. (Brady LW, Perez CA, (eds). Principles and practice of radiation oncology, 2nd ed. Philadelphia, JB Lippincott, 1992:1162.)

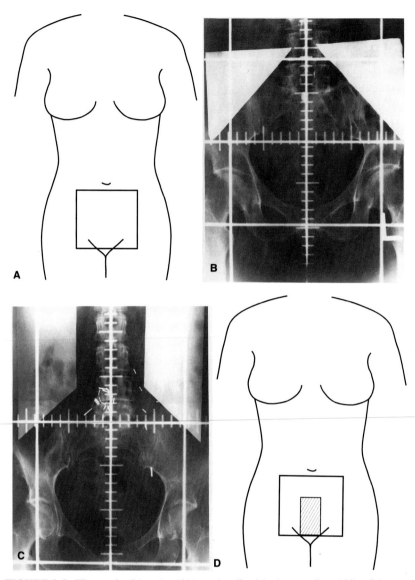

FIGURE 8-8. The usual pelvic point (**A**) includes all pelvic tissue to the middle of the common iliac vessels. The iliac crest is blocked to decrease marrow toxicity. (**B**) An extension of this field to I_{4-5} to include the entire common iliac nodal group and the nodal areas at the bifurcation of the aorta. (**C**) The treatment of metastases in the paraaortic nodes necessitates extending the radiation field to T_{12}. Most treatment schemes necessitate a midline shield (**D**) to decrease the total dose to the rectum and bladder. (Shingleton HM, Orr JW Jr. Cancer of the cervix: diagnosis and treatment. New York, Churchill Livingstone, 1987:179.)

cially in larger patients (those with a anteroposterior pelvic diameter more than 20 to 22 cm) and customized cerrobend (lead alloy) blocks. The usual upper border of the pelvic field is L_5 and should incorporate the common iliac nodes (Fig. 8-8). When treating larger tissue volumes or extended fields (e.g., paraaortic nodes) a decrease in total dose is necessary to lessen the risk of serious gastrointestinal complications. The use of high-energy techniques and daily

four-field treatment may also decrease risks. Smit (1991) suggested the possibility and discussed the rationale for potentially decreasing treatment volume by as much as 60% and increase dose increment by 20%, using proton therapy. Experience with three-dimensional CT simulation (see Fig. 8-9*A–F*) and treatment planning also appears to minimize treatment volume.

Herbert and associates (1991), reporting a population of 115 women treated with pelvic irradiation

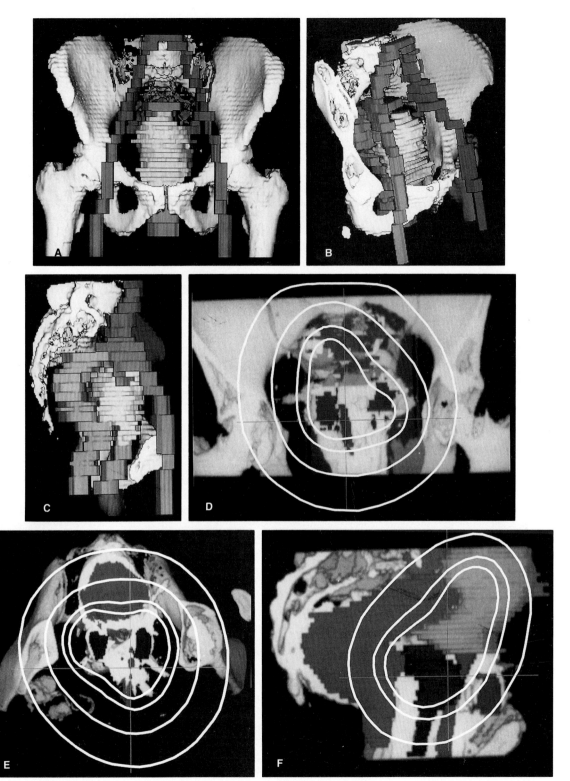

FIGURE 8-9. Computed tomograph dosimetry reconstruction of the vaginal, cervix-uterus, rectum, and nodal tissue in an anterior (**A**), oblique (**B**), and lateral (**C**) view. (**D**) Isodose curves in a coronal three-dimensional reconstruction of the pelvix with a Fletcher applicator in place. Cross-hairs intersect at the cervix with the uterus above, the rectum behind, and the bladder anterior. The 3000-, 2000-, and 1000 cGy isodose curves are depicted after ^{137}Cs loading. (**E**) An axial plane with the cervix at the cross-hairs and the 3000-, 2000-, 1000-, and 500 cGy isodose curves. (**F**) The sagittal plane as visualized through the three-dimensional virtual simulator. (Images generated with a Picker-Varian virtual simulator; courtesy of Dr. A. Wiley and Dr. J. Stephenson, Watson Clinic, Lakeland FL.) See Color Figure 8-9.

after laparotomy, evaluated the possible benefit of small bowel contrast to assist simulation. He surmised that contrast could localize small bowel and allow design of a treatment plan to minimize small bowel exposure. Using these methods, 40% of patients had a treatment modification. Contrast-guided simulation and treatment planning was found to be associated with significantly less diarrhea and fewer long-term irradiation-related complications. Lower (smaller) treatment fields were also associated with fewer complications. Prone treatment with a customized body mold may displace bowel superiorly in some patients (Shanahan et al 1989).

The design of treatment portals has traditionally been determined by palpation of external anatomic landmarks in addition to the radiologic identification of bony architecture. Greer and colleagues (1990) reported that intraoperative measurements dramatically differ from normal external anatomic landmarks. The mean level of the aortic bifurcation when measured intraoperatively was 6.7 cm above the lumbosacral prominence. The common iliac bifurcation was 1.7 cm (left) and 1.4 cm (right) above this reference point. Both common iliac nodes bifurcated cephalad to the lumbosacral prominence in 87% of patients. Their conclusions, based on intraoperative reference points and combined with measured transverse pelvic dimensions at the obturator fossa (12.3 cm) and the outside width of the external iliac vessels (13.0 cm), indicated the need to use the L_4–L_5 interspace as the upper border formation to incorporate the mid–common iliac lymph nodes. Lateral fields should encompass the entire anterior sacral silhouette to consistently cover the entire uterosacral and cardinal ligaments if clinically indicated.

Field size should be determined by actual extent of disease. The continued refinement of CT and other imaging techniques theoretically improves the ability to encompass all macroscopic disease (Fig 8-9). The placement of titanium clips during intraoperative evaluation can be of great assistance to the radiation oncologist, allowing delineation of specific lymph nodes and disease sites.

Dose Size–Fraction

Although numerous combinations of daily dose, total dose, and treatment intervals exist, dose fractions have been conventionally delivered five times per week. Tumor control increases with increasing total dose. An effective or real-dose increment of 10% is the minimum needed to produce a clinically significant (20%) increase in local tumor control (Brown 1985). Minimizing delay and total treatment time is an important axiom of radiation therapy. Generally, treatment delay or long treatment time is not encouraged but is less harmful than therapy interruption. During radiation therapy, many tumors alter their growth-kinetic profiles (accelerated repopulation). After 1 to 3 weeks of treatment, tumor-volume doubling time may be shortened from 100 days to 3 days (Fowler et al 1993) as the spontaneous tumor cell loss (which may average 95% before treatment) falls toward zero. Interruption during this time may be associated with rapid tumor regrowth and failed therapy. Fyles and colleagues (1992) evaluated the effect of treatment duration on pelvic control in 830 patients with cervical cancer. Loss of pelvic tumor control approximated 1% per day of treatment prolongation beyond 30 days, suggesting the clinical importance of accelerated repopulation. In a newer Patterns of Care Study report, Lanciano and coworkers (1993) indicated a highly significant (14%) decrease in survival and pelvic control when treatment time increased from less than 6 weeks to more than 10 weeks. This effect was greatest in women with stage III disease. Prolongation of therapy did not affect the risk of late complications.

Fraction dose size is important, and teletherapy doses in excess of 200 cGy increase the potential for complications, with little effect on tumor cell kill. As previously noted, late-responding tissues (e.g., vaginal, or other tissues that develop fistulas or necrosis) are remarkably efficient in repairing sublethal irradiation damage during delivery of small dose fractions. This ability to repair sublethal damage decreases with increasing dose fraction, however. Early-responding tissues (e.g., intestinal mucosa) and many tumor cells are less efficient in the repair of sublethal damage, and this effect is not affected by fraction size (Fowler et al 1993).

Hypofractionation

Survival results of studies using hypofractionation (large dose fraction delivered less often than five times per week) vary. Two-year survival, acute reactions, and late effects were not different in Marcial and Bosch's (1968) report comparing 150 cGy delivered five times per week and 250 cGy delivered three times per week. The delivery of 150 cGy daily is not a standard treatment schedule. Most of these women also received brachytherapy, however, and treatment regimen differences may have been obscured. Conversely, hypofractionation—when combined with hyperbaric oxygen—has been associated with a decrease in pelvic control (Watson et al 1978). Browde and associates (1984) suggested improved local control using conventional fractionation when compared with a weekly fractionation scheme. Although not statistically significant, serious late complications were increased fourfold in those treated with the weekly regimen. Deore (1992) retrospectively evaluated the effects of hypofractionation on rectal or rectosigmoid complications in 203 patients having stage IIIB cervical disease. Although not predicted by time-dose factors, the incidence of serious (grade II, III) complications increased from 8.2% (daily treatment, 200 cGy) to 33.3% (weekly treatment, 540 cGy). The use of hypofractionation in other tumor systems is also associated with an increased risk of late adverse effects (Cox 1985).

Single-fraction high-dose therapy, a variant of hypofractionation, has been used as a method of pelvic palliation, especially control of bleeding, for some patients with advanced disease. In a nonrandomized study, Chafe and coworkers (1984) reported palliative success of a single 1000 cGy fraction treatment scheme. Hodson and Krepart (1983) reported that single-fraction treatments of 1000 cGy, repeated three times at monthly intervals, were well tolerated, provided effective palliation, and minimized treatment time.

Some clinical results (Marcial et al 1983) suggest that split-course therapy, using higher dose fractions (250 cGy), can accomplish equal cure rates without an associated increase in complications. Using this schema, teletherapy may be completed within a shorter timeframe, with less burden on the patient and the therapy facility. This could be especially useful for selected older and infirm patients. Unfortunately, Marcial and associates' data has not been reproduced.

Hyperfractionation–Accelerated Fractionation

Contemporary radiobiologic knowledge allows delivery of a large total dose while potentially avoiding an increase in late tissue toxicity (complications). Hyperfractionation, using smaller doses per fraction (1.1 to 1.6 Gy), can deliver as much as a 10% increase in total dose and a resultant potential net gain in tumor cell kill (Fowler et al 1993). Using multiple daily fractions (4- to 6-hour minimum interfraction interval) allows tumor cell redistribution with minimal repair of sublethal damage (Stehman et al 1993a). Therefore, in theory, true hyperfractionation (i.e., twice daily treatment with same overall duration) should decrease the risk of late irradiation-induced sequelae by allowing repair of sublethal damage to normal cells. As expected, hyperfractionation increases the incidence of adverse acute normal-tissue reaction (that resolve) but may allow significant dose escalation in patients with cervical cancer (Varghese et al 1992). Komaki and colleagues (1994) reported the results of a phase I–II Radiation Therapy Oncology Group (RTOG) trial evaluating a hyperfractionation scheme. Combined with brachytherapy, total parametrial doses 10% higher

than standard treatment were well tolerated and at least as effective across all stages of disease.

Accelerated fractionation shortens overall treatment time in an attempt to diminish the deleterious effects of tumor cell proliferation during a protracted course of therapy (Fowler et al 1993). Unfortunately, during accelerated fractionation, early-responding healthy tissue is less able to repopulate, and prohibitive acute tissue toxicities occur if the total dose is not decreased (Fowler et al 1993). Most clinical trials use accelerated hyperfractionation (1.2 Gy twice a day) to a slightly higher total dose. Although the effectiveness of altered fractionation appears to be documented for some cancers, the role for accelerated fractionation or hyperfractionation in cervical cancer patients is undetermined (Withers 1985, Fowler et al 1993). In other cancers, hyperfractionation and accelerated fractionation have produced a high incidence of both acute and late toxicity, particularly with high daily doses (Ang et al 1994).

Sequencing Teletherapy and Brachytherapy

Anatomic variations may be extremely important with conventional radiation therapy techniques. Narrow vaginal vaults or asymmetric scarred vaginal fornices may limit the radiotherapeutic contribution of brachytherapy. Increasing the teletherapy component, however, may result in further vaginal stricturing. Therefore, the treatment scheme made before the initiation of therapy should be flexible, to allow necessary changes with tumor response and to allow optimal integration of teletherapy and brachytherapy.

Radiation treatment sequence is often dictated by the tumor volume because brachytherapy alone has a significant ability to sterilize central disease in early-stage cancers (Hamberger 1980). Women who have early invasive cervical disease (focal microinvasion, microinvasion, microcarcinoma) have a low risk of pelvic lymph node involvement and in some situations may be treated with intracavitary sources alone. Using this scheme, Hamberger and coworkers (1978) reported a 100% cure rate in 41 patients having stage IA (less than 3 mm invasion) cervical cancer. None of the 93 patients with stage IB (less than 1 cm in size) disease developed central recurrence. The 5-year survival rate in this latter group was 96% and was associated with a low incidence (1%) of serious complications.

Grigsby and Perez (1991) addressed the use of brachytherapy alone in the management of patients with carcinoma in situ (CIS) or stage IA disease. They reported no pelvic recurrences in 21 patients who were treated for CIS. They also treated 34 patients with stage IA disease (13 with intracavitary therapy alone and 21 with combined therapy). None of the patients treated with brachytherapy alone and only 1 patient treated with combination therapy developed a central failure (3%). When combining their data with those of Kolstad (1989), none of the 149 patients with stage IA1 disease treated with intracavitary therapy alone developed recurrent cancer. We believe that conization alone (with negative margins) is adequate treatment for women with CIS or stage IA1 disease and do not believe that subsequent radiation therapy need be given for these lesions.

Calais and coworkers (1989) reported 70 patients having early-stage IB disease (less than 4 cm) who had only a 13% failure rate when treated with 60-Gy brachytherapy alone. In a retrospective evaluation of 24 patients having clinical stage IB disease, Kim and associates (1988) reported an overall failure rate of 15% (pelvic failure, 9%; distal failure, 6%) when patients were treated with brachytherapy alone. Major complications occurred in 4.1% of their patients. In most situations, the combined delivery of teletherapy and brachytherapy should be considered to be the standard treatment for patients having stage IB disease. After intracavitary treatment, midline shields are placed to protect central pelvic anatomy, and a parametrial boost of teletherapy may be delivered because many women who have stage IB disease have regional spread.

The homogenous characteristic of external therapy favors tumor regression and lessens the anatomic distortion that is often associated with advanced cervical cancer. For this reason, brachytherapy is traditionally used after teletherapy in the treatment of "bulky" disease. Generally, patients with larger-volume tumors usually begin therapy with the delivery of 2000 to 5000 cGy by teletherapy. Hong and colleagues (1992), evaluating 429 patients, suggested that patients who had complete tumor regression at the end of external radiation therapy were more likely to survive (77% versus 31%) and less likely to experience recurrence locally. Arimoto (1993) suggested that CT volumetry provides a prediction of treatment failure. Systematic CT evaluation of 87 patients indicated that post–external irradiation cervical volumes of less than 38 cm^3 were associated with a 90.4% chance of 3-year local control. When CT volumes were more than 38 cm^3, 3-year local control rates fell to 26.1%. Interestingly, pretreatment CT volume did not correlate with local control.

Jacobs and coworkers (1986) evaluated 590 patients having squamous cell cancer treated with a full course of short-term (1 month) radiation therapy. Survival was correlated with complete clinical response (76%), suspicious findings (41.5%), or persistent disease (7.4%). There was no difference in those with sus-

pected or persistent disease at 1 or 3 months, suggesting the need for additional therapy.

The use of surveillance colposcopy (Choo et al 1984) or evaluation of serum levels of copper or ferritin to assess irradiation response are no more predictive than physical examination. Information regarding serum squamous cell antigen suggests a possible role for monitoring treatment. West and associates (1991) reported the local radiation therapy response, or radiosensitivity, as predicted by cell culture of biopsy specimen and calculation of survival fraction after the delivery of 2 Gy (West et al 1991). Survival was significantly different and adversely affected when the survival fraction was elevated (more than 55%).

Type of Intracavitary Treatment

Many different schemes exist—varying in intracavitary exposure, total dosage, type of intracavitary irradiation, or treatment methodology. Attempts to standardize the biologic equivalence of intracavitary and external therapy have been unsuccessful, and the optimal method of conversion remains undetermined. It is understood that the simple addition of cGy delivery by brachytherapy and teletherapy is not correct. Thus, many treatment schemes are based on proved clinical experience when the dosage to specified pelvic reference points is kept within a narrow therapeutic range that results in cure and minimal complications.

Corn and colleagues (1994) evaluated the effects of technical adequacy of brachycavitary therapy from 66 patients in the Patterns of Care Study. When assessing three specific parameters, only 8 of 66 were considered to be ideal implants. Unacceptable implants were noted in 17 of 66 patients and 41 of 66 were considered acceptable. Multivariate analysis indicated that technical adequacy was the most important prognostic discriminate of local control. Although ideal and adequate placements improved local control when compared with unacceptable (68% versus 34%; $p = 0.02$) placement, there was a trend (60% versus 40%) only when evaluating 5-year survival.

The radiobiologic effectiveness of continuous low-dose radiation from intracavitary sources should not be equated to high-dose short-exposure radiation delivered during teletherapy (Allen et al 1980). Low dose–rate brachytherapy has a lower oxygen-enhancement ratio, which reduces the effect of repair of sublethal damage. High dose–rate brachytherapy, delivered with less treatment time, has gained increasing popularity; however, the radiobiologic comparison of HDR and LDR is also extremely complicated (Joslin 1990). Nearly 20% of radiation therapy centers in the United States possess HDR capability (Bastin et al 1993), and some believe that the increased visibility, vigorous marketing, and the call to "high tech" have contributed to the rapid proliferation of these techniques (Eifel 1992).

High Dose–Rate versus Low Dose–Rate Therapy

Decades of experience with thousands of patients have led to the empiric choice of a range of teletherapy–brachytherapy dose combinations that optimize the therapeutic ratio. Review, however, suggests at least 23 different regimens for LDR and teletherapy exist (Brenner et al 1991). Results from the Patterns of Care Study (evaluating 565 patients who were treated with LDR brachytherapy) indicated that 4-year in-field failures were significantly reduced (29% versus 17%) and survival was significantly increased (73% versus 50%) in those patients receiving two or more intracavitary applications (Coia et al 1990). Later studies (Lanciano et al 1992b) indicate the importance of intracavitary therapy but not multiple applications. The use of two LDR intracavitary treatment sessions increases dose to the paracervical point, increases pelvic control, decreases distal recurrences, and improves survival (Marcial et al 1991). Some believe that survival for all stages of disease is increased with multiple intracavitary applications (Marcial et al 1991), whereas others believe that it does not improve survival in all stages of disease (Kraiphibul et al 1992).

Advocates of HDR brachytherapy cite the advantage of outpatient treatment: lessened anesthesia requirement, less potential displacement of the delivery system, and decreased personnel exposure. The use of remote HDR afterloading significantly decreased recorded nurse exposure from 19 mSV to 2.4 mSV (Jones et al 1990). Comparative data evaluating LDR and HDR in terms of therapeutic ratio (tumor control–tissue complications) is difficult to identify. Advocates of LDR therapy indicate the extremely low mortality risk (0.2%), low radiation exposure, and the logistic need for multiple HDR treatments as potential reasons not to use HDR therapy (Eifel 1992). Dusenberry and coworkers (1991), however, described a 6.4% risk of life-threatening complications and a 1.5% 30-day mortality rate associated with anesthesia and perioperative care during LDR brachytherapy. Most complications (76%) were of a cardiac origin. Certainly, the use of general anesthesia, with a 2- to 3-day period of immobilization during therapy, increases the risk of emboli and pneumonia. As expected, these risks are increased in the older patient, those with a history of cardiac disease, or a higher American Society of Anesthesiology (ASA) score (Dusenberry et al 1991). The overall age-related–complication rate in patients

without cardiac disease ranged from 1.9% (age 44) to 5.8% (age 70) and increased from 7.8% (age 40) to 20.8% (age 70) in women with a cardiac history. The Groupe des 9 French collaborative study of more than 1300 patients suggests a 9.8% risk of severe complications and a 27.6% risk of moderate or severe complications using LDR therapy (Orton 1992b). Rotte (1990; in Bastin et al 1993) reported a 7.5% incidence of thromboembolic events with LDR therapy. This information clearly establishes the need for pretreatment medical evaluation for all patients who are undergoing brachytherapy.

High dose–rate brachytherapy (0.5 to 6 Gy/minute) delivers therapy with exposure shorter than the repair half-time of sublethal damage (i.e., shorter than an hour or two), which may increase the risk of complications. The development of small sources (^{192}Ir) allows the use of small catheter size. Additionally, repair of late-responding tissues (bowel, bladder) does not occur as fully with HDR (Stitt et al 1992b). Arguments in favor of using HDR therapy suggest the potential radiobiologic advantage when the rate of sublethal injury repair is greater in tumor cells than in normal cells. Some argue that the relevant end point for evaluating or comparing HDR and LDR therapy should be early complications, not late complications (Brenner et al 1991). A specific number of fractions (about six) are necessary, however, if tumor and tissue doses are equal (Orton 1992a). Advocates of HDR therapy suggest that the physical advantages compensate for the loss of the dose-rate effect; however, many doses and fractionation schemes have been used, with little consensus regarding which is optimal (Eifel 1992). Actually, using different α–β ratios, individual HDR dose equivalents of 13 to 290 Gy have been used. Although the use of as many as 16 HDR insertions have been reported, as few as 4 to 6 fractions can be used if normal tissue dose can be maintained at 80% of the tumor dose (Stitt 1992a). When using HDR, the intracavitary portion of treatment is usually integrated into weekly sessions (Stitt et al 1992b), each treatment incorporating a different (hopefully shrinking tumor) tissue volume. Because of the difference in radiobiologic effect and physical positioning, traditional definitions (i.e., point A, point B) of points of interest may apply poorly to HDR therapy (Thomadsen et al 1992). Preliminary comparisons of HDR with LDR treatment suggests nearly equal 5-year efficacy (Table 8-5) without increased late tissue response (Tables 8-6 and 8-7). Multiple dose fractions can improve this radiobiologic imbalance. Generally, most HDR treatment regimens are based on a compromised radiobiologic theory, patient convenience, and staffing.

Although initial equipment costs are high, in one institution the comparison of LDR therapy (two appli-

TABLE 8-5
High Dose–Rate Versus Low Dose–Rate Intracavitary
Brachytherapy for Carcinoma of the Cervix
(1979–1981)

STAGE	HDR/LDR (N)	5-YEAR SURVIVAL (%)	
		HDR	**LDR**
I	160/422	76.9	71.6
II	358/796	58.1	54.4
III	386/588	38.1	38.4
IV	66/50	15.2	10.0

HDR, high dose rate; *LDR*, low dose rate.

Annual report on the results of treatment in gynecological cancer. In Pettersson F (ed). Twentieth volume statements of results obtained in patients treated in 1979–81, including 5-year survival up to 1986. Stockholm, Sweden, International Federation of gynecology and Obstetrics, 1987;20:52.

cations for 3 days) and HDR therapy (five applications) indicated a 244% higher overall charge for the former (Bastin et al 1993). Moreover, capital expenditure and maintenance expense suggest the need for 770 applications per year to cover costs—a number higher than most academic or private institutions' use (Bastin et al 1993). It would be safe to say that two separate factions of therapists exist: those who believe that established treatment using clinically proved combinations of teletherapy and LDR brachytherapy is superior (Eifel 1992) and those who believe that HDR therapy may be superior (Brenner et al 1991). High dose–rate therapy may be assumed to be a compromise between patient convenience and optimal thera-

peutic advantage (Brenner et al 1991). Efforts and regimen to maximize early tissue effects (tumor control) and minimize late tissue effects (normal tissue damage) continue. Guidelines for comparing teletherapy–LDR with teletherapy–HDR regimens have been postulated. Although the actual optimal number of HDR fractions remains to be determined, it is clear that multiple HDR fractions are important. The benefit of one or two HDR fractions is likely small because of the lack of effect of reoxygenation (Brenner et al 1991). Despite the optimal dose rate and technique being unknown, nonrandomized studies suggest nearly equal cure without associated increase in complications (Fu et al 1990).

Orton and associates (1991) analyzed HDR data from 56 institutions treating 17,000 patients. Comparison across these institutions showed a statistically significant increase in pooled survival. The average number of fractions was five (7.5 Gy each). Although the effect of dose fraction on cure rate was equivocal, dose–fraction rate to point A for more than 7 Gy was associated with an increased risk of severe injury.

Additionally, Arai and colleagues (1992) reported a retrospective comparison of HDR with LDR in 1022 patients having squamous cell carcinoma of the cervix, indicating a comparable stage-related survival and incidence of severe complications.

Finally, in a prospective evaluation of HDR and LDR therapy, Teshima and coworkers (1993) reported results of 430 patients treated with HDR ^{60}Co and LCR ^{137}Cs. The 5-year cause-specific survival rates in patients having stage I (85% versus 93%), stage II (73% versus 78%), and stage III (53% versus 47%) disease were not different. Ten percent of patients undergoing HDR and 4.7% of patients undergoing LDR developed moderate to severe complications.

TABLE 8-6
High Dose–Rate Versus Low Dose–Rate Brachytherapy: Bladder Complications

STUDY	YEAR	HDR/LDR (N)	COMPLICATION RATE (%)	
			HDR	**LDR**
Vahrson	1988	147/835	3.0 (late, severe)	2.0 (late, severe)
Cikaric	1988	140/187	5.0	9.6
Akine	1988	84/372	1.2 (moderate) 0 (severe)	11 (moderate) 0.5 (severe)
Kuipers	1980	111/145	3.5 (grade III)	3.3 (grade III)
Sato	1984	87/147	9.2	7.5
Shigematsu	1983	143/106	2.0	7.0
Rotte	1980	112/237	0.8	2.5

HDR, high dose rate; *LDR*, low dose rate.

Modified from Fu KK, Phillips TL. High dose rate versus low dose rate intracavitary brachytherapy for carcinoma of the cervix. Int J Radiat Oncol Biol Phys 1990;19:791.

TABLE 8-7
High Dose–Rate Versus Low Dose–Rate Brachytherapy: Rectal Complications

			COMPLICATION RATE (%)	
STUDY	YEAR	HDR/LDR (N)	HDR	LDR
Vahrson	1988	147/835	3.0 (late, severe)	2.0 (late, severe)
Cikaric	1988	140/187	7.1	16.6
Akine	1988	84/372	24.0 (moderate) 2.4 (severe)	36.0 (moderate) 4.0 (severe)
Kuipers	1980	111/145	7.0 (grade III)	6.6 (grade III)
Sato	1984	87/147	14.9	13.6
Shigematsu	1983	143/106	36.0*	25.0*
Rotte	1980	112/237	2.6	10.5

*Rectal bleeding.
HDR, high dose rate; LDR, low dose rate.

Modified from Fu KK, Phillips TL. High dose rate versus low dose rate intracavitary brachytherapy for carcinoma of the cervix. Int J Radiat Oncol Biol Phys 1990;19:791.

Although many opponents and proponents claim importance, it appears that clinical survival is equal and the risk of late complications is not significantly different in those series reporting comparison data (Stitt 1992; Stitt et al 1992a). The theoretic increase in the incidence of late complications can be resolved if normal tissues are kept further from high-dose sources, so that doses are 20% less than that with LDR geometry (Stitt et al 1992a).

Dosimetry

Dosimetry calculations after placement of an intracavitary device have historically been determined by obtaining anteroposterior and lateral pelvic films after placing radio-opaque material in the bladder and rectum to correlate the spatial relation between the cervix, bladder, and rectum (see Fig. 8-9).

Early reports indicating the value of other methods such as ultrasound or CT (Lee et al 1980) to increase the accuracy of three-dimensional dosimetry (Goitein 1985) have been substantiated by newer data (Kapp et al 1992), which reveal the superiority of CT-assisted dosimetry in the determination of maximal normal tissue doses for intracavitary placement. In specific situations, CT simulation may decrease dose to specific organs (spine, large bowel, and kidneys; Munzenrider et al 1991). Computed tomography is likely superior in the determination of maximal normal tissue dose (Kapp 1992) and potentially improves the delivery of directed tumoricidal irradiation (Lichter et al 1994).

Computed tomography dosimetry allows calculation of the 6000-cGy isodose volume, as proposed by the International Commission on Radiological Units (ICRU; Lanciano et al 1992b). Serial magnetic reso-

nance imaging may predict tumor sensitivity and allow continued follow-up of late responders (Flueckiger et al 1992).

Although differences in institutional treatment planning exist, a single reference point taken at the bladder neck (as proposed by ICRU report 38) appears to be inadequate for the evaluation of bladder dose (Kapp 1992). When using a bladder chain to determine bladder dose, bladder base dose exceeded the calculated bladder neck dose in 63% of placements. These bladder base doses were twice as high as expected in 17.5% of intracavitary placements.

Using CT-based multidimensional dose distributions, Schoeppel (1990) indicated a maximal rectal dose 1.6 times that calculated from orthogonal films. In many situations, this dose was higher than that of point A, with a maximal rectal dose delivered at a mean 2.5 cm above the vaginal fornix (range, 0.9 to 3.5 cm).

Regardless of the method of treatment or calculation, appropriate placement, packing, and stabilization of the intracavitary device is important. Central pelvic failure in patients with early-stage (I and II) cervical cancer can often be retrospectively related to applicator malplacement (Jampolis et al 1975). Appropriate vaginal gauze packing results in a 12% reduction in the anterior rectal wall dose (Kapp 1992). Slight displacement or malposition can result in a marked alteration of tumor dose (Fig. 8-10). Corn and coworkers (1993) carefully evaluated the positional changes associated with LDR brachytherapy. Detailed analysis indicated that overall median dose (external plus brachytherapy) varied little (1.4% at point A, 1.7% at point B, 0.9% at point P) and should have little effect on cure or complication. The short duration of HDR therapy

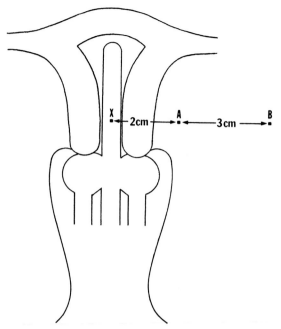

FIGURE 8-10. The dose at a particular point from the radiation source varies with the inverse of the distance squared. For example, if the dose above is 150 Gy at point X, the dose at point A ($\frac{1}{4}$ of X) would be 37.5 Gy and the dose at point B ($\frac{1}{125}$ of X) would be 6 Gy. With a 1-cm displacement to the left, the dose at point A ($\frac{1}{9}$ of X) would fall to 16.66 Gy. Because the intracavitary sources include the tandem and the vaginal ovoids, malposition or slippage result in marked alteration of dosimetry. (Shingleton HM, Orr JW Jr. Cancer of the cervix: diagnosis and treatment. New York, Churchill Livingstone, 1987:183.)

demands extreme attention because there is little opportunity to correct treatment errors.

It is important to minimize the delay when using LDR brachytherapy because prolonged intervals (more than 14 days) may allow tumor regrowth and possibly increase the risk of treatment failure (Bosch et al 1967). As previously noted, treatment delay is not encouraged but is less harmful than therapy interruption because many tumors alter their growth-kinetic profiles after 1 to 3 weeks of treatment. Volume doubling may be shortened from 100 days to 3 days (Fowler et al 1993) as the spontaneous tumor cell loss (which may average 95% before treatment) falls toward zero (Fowler et al 1993).

Neutron Therapy

The development of newer sources for brachytherapy using high linear energy transfer (LET) particles or neutrons (e.g., californium 252) may potentially be cost-saving because treatment time can be reduced from days to hours and bulky hypoxic tumors can be initially treated with brachytherapy. The radiobiologic effectiveness, dose rate, and fractionation effects for californium neutrons require a sophisticated model and is clearly not equivalent to cesium or other HDR therapy (Maruyama et al 1990a). Fast-neutron brachytherapy using ^{252}Cf has been used extensively in some institutions (Maruyama et al 1993). This high LET irradiation has a higher radiobiologic effectiveness and a lower oxygen-enhancement ratio. Fast neutrons also inhibit sublethal or potentially lethal repair. The rationale for the "early" use of fast neutrons is related to their ability to immediately affect large hypoxic or radioresistant tumors, without relying on the slow process of tumor reoxygenation. When using fast neutrons, late repeat implants may increase local complication rates 12-fold because associated rapid tumor regression may increase actual radiation delivery to normal tissues (Maruyama et al 1993). Although many potential combinations exist, neutron therapy with short-course (hours) intracavitary therapy before external therapy is superior (Maruyama et al 1991b). In this treatment schema, the need for three-dimensional tumor localization becomes even more important. Gallion and associates (1987) reported the effects of outpatient neutron brachytherapy, suggesting a cost-effectiveness and patient tolerance, whereas survival was not different when compared with LDR controls.

Interstitial Therapy

Other methods of brachytherapy have been proposed to better encompass tumor volume with a more homogenous dose while maintaining flexibility in dose distribution. Interstitial therapy allows delivery of locally high doses with rapid fall-off (Murray 1990). Afterloading perineal templates (Fig. 8-11), allowing placement of interstitial sources (^{192}Ir), have been developed to individualize cervical and parametrial dosage, particularly in tumors with altered anatomy or in tumors that have not regressed during teletherapy. Although the total clinical experience is small, advocates (Martinez et al 1984, Surwit et al 1983) report excellent pelvic control; however, others (Ampuero et al 1983) report significant morbidity. The final place of interstitial brachytherapy remains to be determined. Significant survival data and undocumented benefit that warrant routine use are not available; however, its use in specific situations (i.e., asymmetric parametrial involvement, recurrent disease) may be beneficial. Transabdominal ultrasound, CT scan, laparoscopy, or even laparotomy may assist in placement and localization of the interstitial needles.

Specific circumstances may allow altered therapy to conserve fertility. Reports using ^{125}I (Baughan 1992) and other tailor-made therapies describe successfully but conservatively treated early invasive dis-

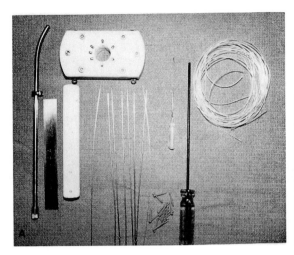

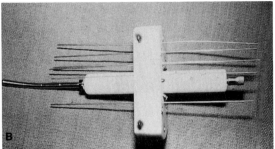

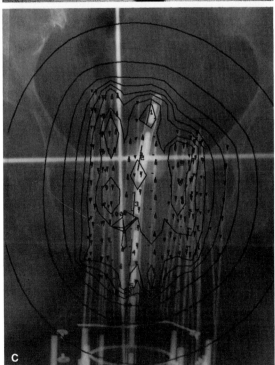

FIGURE 8-11. Interstitial perineal implants disassembled (**A**) and assembled (**B**). After placement of the needles (**C**), radioactive sources can be inserted to alter dosimetry and treat tumors with altered configuration or parametrial involvement. (Shingleton HM, Orr JW Jr. Cancer of the cervix: diagnosis and treatment. New York, Churchill Livingstone, 1987:184.)

ease. It appears that a later vaginal delivery may have catastrophic or lethal results.

SPECIFIC CLINICAL CONSIDERATIONS

Lanciano and colleagues (1991b), reporting the results from the Patterns of Care Study data, indicated that pretreatment factors associated with improved pelvic control included higher performance status, older age, unilateral parametrial involvement in women having stage I or II disease, and unilateral side wall involvement in those having stage IIIB disease. The use of intracavitary sources was the single most important factor for pelvic control in stage I, II, or III disease.

Results from evaluation of prognostic variables from pooled GOG data (626 patients) in women treated from 1977 to 1985 indicated that the significant prognostic variables for progression-free interval or survival were:

1. Patient age
2. Performance status
3. Tumor size
4. Clinical stage
5. Paraaortic node status
6. Pelvic node status
7. Bilateral parametrial extension (Stehman et al 1991)

Interestingly, cell type, histologic grade, pretreatment hematocrit, and peritoneal washings were not significant (Stehman et al 1991).

Effect of Cell Type

Conflicting reports (Wentz 1959, Finck et al 1970, Beecham et al 1978, Gauthier et al 1985) concerning the prognostic significance of cell type may be partially explained by a preradiation-biopsy histologic diagnosis not being representative of the major tumor cell type.

Adenocarcinoma (and particularly mixed adenosquamous carcinoma) has been reported to be radioresistant, with a worse stage-related prognosis than squamous cell carcinoma (Julian et al 1977, Wheeless et al 1970). Eifel and coworkers (1991) reported a comparative increase in pelvic control for stage IB adenocarcinomas (3 to 4 cm) that were treated with radiation therapy (11% failure), in contrast to those treated with radical hysterectomy (45% failure). Moberg and associates (1986) suggested that patients having stage IIIB adenocarcinoma had a lower (9%) rate of 5-year survival when compared with those having squamous cell cancer. Kovalic and colleagues (1991b) found no survival difference related to histology.

Eifel and associates (1991) evaluated the effects of irradiation, radical surgery, or combined therapy in 160 patients having stage I adenocarcinoma. This retrospective analysis suggested that when used alone, radiation therapy decreased the risk of pelvic recurrence in patients with tumors greater than 3 cm. Radiation offered no survival benefit in patients with adenocarcinomas less than 3 cm.

In a matched controlled study (Shingleton et al 1981), we were unable to demonstrate any difference in the curability of both of these tumor types when the effect of tumor volume was controlled. The excellent cure rates reported by Rutledge and colleagues (1975), using radiation therapy alone or in combination with conservative hysterectomy for adenocarcinomas, suggest that the cell type or histology is relatively unimportant and that tumor volume is more important in predicting cure. The pooled data from GOG trials suggested no effect of histologic type or grade in surgically staged patients (Stehman et al 1991). Davidson and coworkers (1989) reported no histologic effect in survival by tissue type in 1878 patients having

cervical cancer treated with radical irradiation, regardless of stage. Goodman and associates (1989) suggested an excellent response of adenocarcinoma to radiation therapy, with 100% pelvic control in patients with stage IB disease and no difference in pelvic control or survival when stage-compared with squamous cell cancers. Survival was reported to be significantly decreased in patients with poorly differentiated tumors.

Hopkins and colleagues (1987) also suggested that histology played little role in the treatment selection in patients having stage I endocervical adenocarcinoma. In a matched-pair analysis (144 patients), Kleine and coworkers (1989) suggested a lessened treatment-related survival in patients having stage I adenocarcinoma treated with radiation therapy (58% versus 86%).

Tumor Ploidy

Most cervical tumors are aneuploid, with near-diploid DNA reported in 20% to 40% of patients. Data suggest that aneuploid tumors may be more radiosensitive and have a higher complete response rate (Braley 1992). Intratreatment alteration from aneuploid to diploid has been associated with increased pelvic control. Unfortunately, tumor heterogeneity may necessitate tumor tissue sample evaluation to achieve a consistent determination of tumor ploidy to determine its potential role on prognosis.

Patient Age

Although numerous opinions exist, the effect of patient age on survival and complications after radiation treatment of cervical cancer remains controversial. Many authors suggest a decreased normal-tissue tolerance in older patients, particularly those having vascular disease. Several authors have reported a shift in DNA patterns from diploid to tetraploid to aneuploid in older women (Braley 1992).

Some have advocated a decreased fraction dose (less than 160 cGy) to decrease the risks of serious complications. Mann and colleagues' (1980) report on stage I patients indicated that survival was not different in patients younger or older than 40 years treated with irradiation or radical surgery. In a radiation therapy series, Mendenhall and associates (1984) failed to find a significant influence of age when using pelvic control as a measurable end point. The final report from the 1973 and 1978 Patterns of Care studies did not associate young age (younger than 50) with decreased survival in a multivariate analysis but did demonstrate a significant decrease in pelvic control for younger patients having stage I and II disease (Lanciano et al 1991a). Treatment-related complications were also increased in younger (younger than 40) women (Lanciano et al 1992a). The pooled results from three clinical GOG trials of 626 patients evaluated surgically suggested a favorable effect of age (older than 40 years), regardless of paraaortic lymph node status (Stehman et al 1991). When evaluating tumor size (more than 6 or less than 6 cm), Lowery and coworkers (1992) reported that pelvic control and relapse-free interval was improved in women older than 50 years and in those with hematocrits of more than 40%. In a multivariate analysis, they found young patients (younger than 30) to be at higher risk for recurrence.

Grant and colleagues (1989) indicated that the risk of irradiation-related complications were dramatically increased in patients older than 75. As many as 32% of these patients fail to complete therapy, and fatal treatment-related complications are increased (13%). In this report, complications were related to performance status. Unfortunately, most of these studies fail to control for tumor volume or other high-risk factors; because clinically it appears that younger women do not fare well, a controlled study is necessary to answer this question.

Anemia

There is no doubt that the incidence of pretreatment anemia increases with advanced-stage disease. Hemoglobin levels of less than 12 g/dl are encountered in 25% of patients who have stage I, 33% of patients who have stage II, and 45% of patients who have stage III disease (Dische 1991). Additionally, anemia is more common in patients who have larger volume tumors and parametrial involvement.

The incidence of failed radiation therapy may be increased in anemic patients (Dische 1991). One review evaluated 16 papers indicating an adverse effect of anemia and was unable to quote any report suggesting no effect or a benefit of anemia (Table 8-8). Gyne-

cologic Oncology Group data of surgically staged patients could not demonstrate an adverse effect of pretreatment hematocrit in a multivariate analysis (Stehman et al 1991). Unfortunately, patients with increased blood loss (usually associated with advanced disease) requiring transfusion do not necessarily fare well (Dische 1991). Although maintaining hemoglobin levels at 10 g% may be too low, correction above this level may contribute little to tumor control.

Pretreatment evaluation of associated medical problems is essential. It has been observed that anemia may contribute to increased tumor hypoxia. For this reason, we consider pretreatment transfusion and appropriate supplementation of those vitamins or minerals necessary to correct severe anemia. The role of additional medications such as erythropoietin is undetermined.

Other reported predictive hematologic parameters includes thrombocytosis (more than 400,000/mL), which has been associated with a poor prognosis even when adjusted for cell type, stage, and age (Hernandez et al 1992).

Malnutrition

A significant portion of the small intestine is treated during pelvic teletherapy, and some degree of irradiation enteritis occurs in most patients. Acute irradiation ileitis may cause a patient to ingest less food and lessen intestinal ability to absorb those nutrients. Although patients with advanced-stage disease appear to be at increased risk for pretreatment nutritional deficits (Orr et al 1985), the addition of irradiation may worsen nutritional status (Bandy et al 1984, Lantz et al 1984) or have an overall deleterious effect on the patient's nutritional status. Some degree of malnutrition may be expected during therapy and can become disabling. The risk of irradiation-related complications are reportedly increased in thin women (Coia et al 1990). Although the acute irradiation reaction usually sub-

TABLE 8-8
Local and Distant Relapse in Patients With Stage IIB and III. Carcinoma of Cervix According to Average Hemoglobin During Radiation Therapy

HEMOGLOBIN (G%)	PATIENTS (N)	LOCAL FAILURE	DISTANT METASTASES
<10	29	0.46	0.18
10–11.9	319	0.29	0.24
12–13.9	578	0.20	0.16
>14	129	0.20	0.18
p Value		0.002	0.1

Modified from Dische S. Radiotherapy and anaemia—the clinical experience. Radiother Oncol Suppl 1991;20:35.

radiation therapy in 48 patients having stage IVA disease. Although overall long-term survival was only 18%, it was increased in those patients who were treated with combined teletherapy and brachytherapy (23% versus 0%). Importantly, the extent of parametrial disease also correlated with survival, decreasing dramatically with pelvic side wall involvement or hydronephrosis (46% versus 5%).

Isolated rectal involvement is rare, with or without fistulas; however, if present, colostomy with fecal diversion to avoid sepsis should be considered before treatment. This patient subset may be candidates for large fraction–dose irradiation.

Large-Volume Central Tumor

Large-volume and late-stage disease is associated with poor survival. The specific definition of "bulky" cervical cancer varies, as does its inclusion in specific protocols (Grigsby 1992). In a retrospective study of 635 patients having stage IIB and IIIB cancer, central bulkiness (more than 5 cm) significantly decreased disease-free survival and increased the pelvic failure rate by 11%. Pelvic failure rates were also increased with bilateral parametrial involvement (stage IIIB) and lateral parametrial involvement (stage IIB; Kovalic et al 1991b). Perez and coworkers (1992) also reported increased pelvic failures in patients having stage IIB disease when the lateral parametrium was involved (30% versus 17%). In a multivariate analysis, Lowery and associates (1992) suggested a significant disease-free survival and pelvic control difference in larger (more than 6 cm) tumors, regardless of stage, age, or pretreatment hematocrit. In evaluating patients having stage I and II disease, Lowery and colleagues reiterated the importance of tumor volume but reported a more than 20% decrease in pelvic control and disease-free survival in women having central disease of more than 6 cm when compared with those having disease less than 3 cm. Effective pelvic control is important not only for cure but may decrease the likelihood of subsequent distal metastatic disease (Anderson et al 1981). Cervical tumors that fail locally after conventional radiation therapy do not necessarily have established distant metastasis at the time of local therapy (Fagundes et al 1992).

Cervical Stump

Carcinoma of the cervical stump is less commonly encountered than it was earlier in this century when supracervical hysterectomy was a frequently performed operation. One report (Miller et al 1984) from a referral institution, however, indicated that cervical stump cancer represented 4.5% of all patients treated during a 12-year interval ending in 1975. Although treatment

schemes may be altered, an intracavitary tandem can be used when the endocervical canal is at least 2 cm long; unless severe anatomic distortion exists, vaginal ovoids can be used (Berek et al 1988).

Rousseau and associates (1972) and Miller and coworkers (1984) have reported equal survival, stage for stage, in patients with squamous cell cervical stump cancers. Goodman and colleagues (1989) reported the outcome in 16 women having adenocarcinoma of the cervical stump. The median survival in stage I (40 months) and stage II or III (17 months) was significantly worse than that of women having cervical adenocarcinoma of an intact uterus. In contrast, Kovalic and coworkers (1991a) reviewed the therapeutic results of 70 patients having cervical stump cancer. Interestingly, these patients were 8.5 years older than women with an intact reproductive system. Cure rates were 70% (IB), 100% (IIA), 66% (IIB), and 39% (IIIB). Although prognosis was adversely affected by histologic differentiation and prolonged treatment interval, actual histology (squamous cell versus adenocarcinoma–mixed) made no difference.

Although Kovalic and associates indicated few complications occurred in their series, one patient died and 8% required surgical intervention for urinary and intestinal tract problems. Petersen and coworkers (1992) reported a retrospective review of 46 patients having cervical stump cancer. The 5-year survival rate was 62% but 7% of women had severe urinary complications (necrosis, fistulas); 31% had severe intestinal complications (proctitis, stenosis, fistula); and 18% had severe vault necrosis. It would appear that significant urinary and intestinal tract complications are a major risk for this patient subset (Kovalic et al 1991a, Miller et al 1984). Actually, Miller and associates' report (1984) of an irradiation-related death rate of 3.7% suggests that pretherapy radiologic evaluation of the upper gastrointestinal tract anatomy (to allow altered treatment planning) may be beneficial in decreasing complications.

After Total Hysterectomy

The unexpected finding of invasive cervical cancer (Table 8-10) in a total-hysterectomy surgical specimen should prompt immediate consultation and referral because these patients can be successfully treated with radiation therapy (Table 8-11). In this situation, overall results of early postoperative radiation therapy compare favorably with radiation treatment alone for similar volume disease with the uterus in place. Although the most appropriate scheme of adjunctive irradiation remains to be determined, reports from Andras and colleagues (1973) and Davy and associates (1977) indicate an excellent survival rate (85%) in patients having clear surgical margins who were promptly treated

TABLE 8-10
Unsuspected Invasive Cancer in a Standard
Hysterectomy Specimen—Reasons for Occurrence

REASONS	ROMAN 1992 (N = 146)	HOPKINS 1990 (N = 92)
Inadequate evaluation of abnormal Pap smear	21%	14%
Failure to do conization	12%	—
Pathology misread	12%	18%
No Pap smear taken	7%	—
Bleeding	29%	17%
Suspicion of endocervical carcinoma	—	10%

*33 patients with normal-appearing cervices had no investigation of abnormal bleeding.

with irradiation. These reports suggest that survival is decreased if the surgical margins are microscopically involved with residual cancer (20% to 45%) or after a prolonged delay (6 months) between hysterectomy and radiation therapy (20%). Additionally, survival is significantly decreased (8%) if a palpable recurrent tumor is present (Ito et al 1991).

A review from Anderson retrospectively evaluated 120 patients in this clinical situation treated with megavoltage therapy (Roman et al 1993). The reported 5-year survival in women without clinical disease who were treated immediately after surgery (75%) was almost twice that of women with clinical persis-

tence or recurrence (39%) at the time initial radiation therapy was begun. Other factors affecting survival included retrospective clinical stage and lymphangiogram status. Cell type (adenocarcinoma or squamous) did not influence treatment results. Locoregional recurrence was the most common site of treatment failure. Therapy complications occurred in 18% of these women; 7% experienced serious morbidity.

Hopkins and coworkers (1988) suggested that adenocarcinoma portended a worsened prognosis after total hysterectomy and radiation therapy. The 5-year survival rate was 80% in patients having squamous cell carcinoma and only 41% in women with adenocarcinoma. Others have not confirmed this finding.

Perez and associates (1992) established guidelines for delivering radiation therapy to patients in whom invasive epidermoid cancer is incidentally found at conventional (total) hysterectomy (Table 8-12). Individuals who meet criteria for microinvasion (less than 3 mm invasion) ordinarily require no additional treatment. For the remainder, treatment varies according to the size of the invasive lesion, depth of stromal invasion, and presence or absence of lymphatic vessel invasion.

When faced with this clinical situation, the same pretreatment considerations apply, and patients should be carefully evaluated because a surgical approach can be used successfully (Orr 1986, Chapman et al 1992).

Coexisting Malignancy

A coexisting second malignancy may mandate treatment modification. In many cases, it is justified to treat the cervical cancer aggressively, except in those

TABLE 8-11
Standard Hysterectomy and Invasive Cervical Cancer*: Survival by Residual Tumor
Status at Onset of Postoperative Irradiation[†]

STUDY	YEAR	NO CLINICAL RESIDUAL TUMOR		KNOWN RESIDUAL TUMOR[‡]	
		Patients (n)	5-Year Survival (%)	Patients (n)	5-Year Survival (%)
Cosbie	1963	56	71	30	30
Durrance, et al	1969	42	90	—	—
Andras, et al[§]	1973	65	89[3]	53	58
Davy, et al	1977	48	77	16	38
Edinger	1984	85	84	31	3.2
Perkins	1984	21	81	15	47
Roman, et al	1992	90	75	30	39
Fang, et al	1993	32	81	23	56

*Predominantly squamous cell cancer
[†]In a timely fashion, not exceeding 6 months.
[‡]Surgical margins involved or residual cancer clinically apparent.
[§]Includes 27 patients with microscopic disease.

TABLE 8-12
Recommended Treatment Radiation for Invasive Epidermoid Carcinoma of the Cervix
Incidentally Found at Simple (Total) Hysterectomy

	EXTERNAL RADIATION (CGY)		INTRACAVITARY OVOIDS (SURFACE DOSE)
TUMOR EXTENT	Whole Pelvis	Split Fields	
Microinvasion (<3 mm), margins clear	0	0	None or Ovoids (6500–7000)
Fully invasive (>3 mm), margins clear	2000	3000	6500
Microscopic residual (+ margins) or lymphatic permeation in stages I–II	3000	2000	7500–8000
Gross residual cut-across tumor	5000	1000–2000	7500

*Modified from Perez CA. Uterine cervix. In Perez CA, Brady LW (eds). Principles and practice of
radiation oncology, 2nd ed. Philadelphia, JB Lippincott, 1992.*

cases wherein the second malignancy has an extremely poor prognosis, in which case therapy for the cervical cancer should be directed toward palliation of symptoms. Vaginal bleeding, the most common symptom associated with advanced disease, may be effectively palliated by intracavitary irradiation. An alternate treatment program may include a reduced teletherapy field, high-dose fractions, short-duration teletherapy, or transvaginal teletherapy.

In these instances, the delivery of high-dose fractions (10 Gy) offers an excellent palliative alternative (Chafe et al 1984, Hodson et al 1983) that minimizes treatment time. Repeat therapy at weekly or monthly intervals can be offered to continue pelvic control. Additionally, selected localized radiation treatment to sites of distant metastases may assist in controlling pain.

EXTENDED-FIELD THERAPY

Review of previously published data suggests the clinical importance of out-of-field disease. The Patterns of Care Study (Coia et al 1990) indicated in-field failure rates (stage I, 12%; stage II, 27%; stage III, 51%) to be markedly different from survival rates (74%, 56%, 33% respectively). The recognition of a high incidence of extrapelvic disease (particularly paraaortic node spread; see Table 8-12) in patients having cervical cancer has created a new problem for the radiotherapist (i.e., designing an extended-field therapy regimen; see Fig. 8-6). Potish (1990a) indicated that methods to increase distal control would offer the greatest survival advantage. Local control and survival of paraaortic node disease relate to tumor burden at the initiation of

treatment (Vigliotti et al 1992). Hughes and associates (1980) found no long-term survivors when the metastases in the paraaortic nodes were not encompassed in the irradiation field.

Patients having involved paraaortic nodes have a higher risk of distal failure, even with pelvic control (Stehman et al 1991). Most reports indicate a significant increase in survival with treatment. Cunningham and colleagues (1991) reported a 43% no evidence of disease (NED) survival rate and a 19% major morbidity rate in patients having stage IB–IIA disease and paraaortic metastasis. In his review, Hacker (1988) suggested that 27% (of 170 patients) could be salvaged with extended-field therapy. More than 40% failed distally, however, and 25% failed locoregionally. Many authors have confirmed a significant survival in treated patients (see Table 8-13). DiSaia and coworkers (1987) reported a 19% 3-year survival rate in patients having paraaortic node metastasis, and Berek and associates (1988) indicated that the 5-year survival rate of patients undergoing extended-field radiation therapy with involved paraaortic nodes was 26%. Cunningham and associates (1991) reported a 48% 5-year survival rate in patients having early-stage disease and paraaortic node metastasis; however, patients having a glandular component, early-stage disease, and paraaortic metastasis had a significantly decreased survival. Cunningham and co-workers (1991) suggested the need for radiation therapy–chemotherapy in patients having adenocarcinoma and involved paraaortic nodes because these patients had a poorer outcome when compared with those having other histology.

At the time of the discovery of paraaortic node metastases, consideration should be given to a thorough chest evaluation (preferably with CT) to evaluate

TABLE 8-13
Extended-Field Radiation for Paraortic Node Metastases

Study	Year	Patients (N)	Dose (Gy)	Complications (%)	Survival (%)
Guthrie, et al	1974	10	54	—	44*
Schellhas	1975	9	60	0	—
Berman, et al	1977	4	40–52	25	—
		7	40–52	0	—
Nelson, et al	1977	48	60	48	45*
Wharton, et al	1977	24	55	42	13
Sudarsanam, et al	1978	21	40–43.2	—	20
Averette, et al	1979	29	44–50	14	—
Bonanno, et al	1980	18	60	26	21
Hughes, et al	1980	22	45–51	9	29
Ballon, et al	1981	19	43.2–51.2	0	23†
Buchsbaum	1979	23	47.5–55.4	—	22
Piver, et al	1981	21	60	62	—
		10	44–50	10	10
Welander, et al	1981	31	44	20	26
Shah, et al	1982	4	45	—	50†
Tewfik, et al	1982	23	50–55	28†	33
Komaki, et al	1983	15	50	—	40§
Berman, et al	1984	98	40	—	27*,¶
Brookland, et al	1984	15	40–50	7	40‖
Rubin	1984	14	—	—	43§
Potish, et al	1985	21	45–50	7	45‖
Nori	1985	27	—	—	29§
LaPolla	1986	13	40–50	9**	30§
Blythe	1986	11	45–60	—	25
Crawford, et al	1987	29	—	—	38
Inoue	1988	14	39.6	—	67§
Lovecchio	1989	36	45	—	50§
Gasper, et al	1989	18	45–50	25	17#
Podczaski, et al	1990	33	45	14	31
Cunningham	1991	—	—	19	43

*2-year survival.
†Projected 5-year survival.
‡Intestinal complication.
§5-year survival.
‖3-year survival.
¶Common iliac, paraaortic nodes.
#48-month survival.
**All injuries in transperitoneal incisions.

the pulmonary parenchyma and the thoracic nodes. The finding of disseminated intrathoracic disease affects therapy. Before a patient is selected for extended radiation therapy, one should consider performing chest CT and perhaps supraclavicular (scalene) node biopsies because the risk of finding metastases in supraclavicular nodes is significant (Buchsbaum 1979), and their presence precludes radiotherapeutic cure. The incidence of involved supraclavicular nodes is higher with macroscopic paraaortic node involvement (30%) than with microscopic (5%) involvement (Berek et al 1988). These patients become candidates for chemotherapy, perhaps combined with radiation ther-

apy. Additionally, the larger treatment fields that are necessary to encompass larger volume tumor may require a reduction in total dose, adding to the risk of pelvic failure. Before initiating extended-field radiation therapy, investigation of the upper gastrointestinal tract should be performed to detect active gastric or duodenal ulcers, which may be adversely affected by radiation dosages of 4500 cGy or higher (Roswit et al 1972). The concurrent administration of cimetidine decreased intestinal complaints during paraaortic irradiation (Teshima et al 1990). Inoue (1988, 1990) reported the largest node metastasis to be smaller than 20 mm in 61% of women, larger than 20 mm in 24%

of women, and extremely large and unresectable in 11% of women. His data suggest that 60% of nodes are sterilized with 6300 cGy but 40% of node metastases require higher doses (more than 7500 cGy).

The information obtained from these investigations is difficult to compare but it indicates that few patients who have macroscopic disease in aortic nodes survive; the chance of cure is decreased in the presence of bulky or advanced-stage pelvic disease because 33% to 50% of treatment failures are in the irradiation field. As may be expected, survival is improved (30% to 50%) in patients having microscopic paraaortic node metastasis and small-volume pelvic disease (Berek et al 1988). Hacker (1988) indicated the importance of both total dose and the operative approach (transperitoneal versus extraperitoneal) in the risk of irradiation complications after extended-field therapy. A total dose exceeding 4500 cGy to the paraaortic node area is associated with an increased risk of serious gastrointestinal complications, and paraaortic node biopsy or dissection by a retroperitoneal approach reduced the risk of small bowel adhesions and was associated with fewer treatment-related complications (Table 8-14). Vigliotti and associates (1992) also indicated that bowel complications are significantly lowered with extraperitoneal dissection. Potish and coworkers (1990a) suggested that as many as 33% of patients who are surgically staged (extraperitoneal) later require major surgery.

Prophylactic Paraaortic Radiation

Surgical resection of macroscopically involved nodes may increase local control (Downey et al 1989), and node resection is possible in 84% of patients who have microscopic metastasis (Potish et al 1989). Although no patient who had 10 or more pelvic nodes and involved paraaortic nodes survived, the overall 5-year survival for patients who had resected and clinically positive pelvic nodes and paraaortic nodes was 33% (Downey et al 1989). This information prompted Potish and associates (1989) to advocate node debulking. In 159 women, survival was equal in women having microscopic (56%) and completely resected macroscopic node disease (57%). Unresectable pelvic node disease was associated with higher pelvic failure and decreased survival.

The rationale for prophylactic paraaortic node irradiation relates to (1) the lack of acceptable and accurate nonsurgical methods for the detection of subclinical paraaortic node disease, (2) the documented increase in morbidity related to radiation therapy after intraabdominal staging, and (3) the potential numbers of women who develop out-of-field failure who may potentially benefit.

Because extended portal irradiation has little morbidity in the absence of surgical staging (Potish et al 1983, Crawford et al 1987), the scheme offering the best therapeutic ratio may include elective paraaortic

TABLE 8-14
Complication Rates for Extended-Field Radiation Therapy for Pan Metastases

STUDY	YEAR	PATIENTS (N)	DOSE	COMPLICATIONS (%)
TRANSPERITONEAL ROUTE				
Nelson, et al	1977	48	60	48
Wharton, et al	1977	24	55	42
Bonanno, et al	1980	18	60	26
Hughes, et al	1980	22	45–51	9
Piver, et al	1981	21	60	62
		10	44–45	10
Welander, et al	1981	31	44	20
Tewfik, et al	1982	23	50–55	28
Brookland, et al	1984	15	40–50	7
Potish, et al	1984	21	45–50	7
Gasper, et al	1989	10	45–50	50
EXTRAPERITONEAL ROUTE				
Schellhas	1975	9	60	0
Ballon, et al	1981	19	43–51	0
Potish, et al	1984	21	45–50	7
Gasper, et al	1989	8	45–50	25

PAN, paraaortic node.

irradiation for those patients having a high risk of metastases and few factors predisposing to enteric damage (i.e., pelvic inflammatory disease, diabetes mellitus, hypertension, thin physique, or previous abdominal surgery). Boronow (1991) defends the role of routine extended-field radiation therapy in high-risk patients.

The European Oncology Radiation Therapy Council (EORTC) prospective trial evaluating patients with stage I, II, and III disease was unable to detect a survival benefit of prophylactic paraaortic radiation therapy (Haie et al 1988). The rate of distal metastasis with local control was 2.4 times higher and the incidence of paraaortic nodal metastasis was 2.8 times higher in those women who received pelvic irradiation alone. Patients having stage II disease had a significant reduction in clinically evident paraaortic metastasis but no difference in survival without disease at 4 years. The incidence of severe complications was increased (2.3 times) in the extended-field–treatment group.

Rotman and colleagues (1990) reported the results from a randomized RTOG study that compared the effect of pelvic versus pelvic–paraaortic therapy (4500 cGy) in patients having large IB and IIA (more than 4 cm) or IIB cervical cancer. Those patients having surgically documented or clinically apparent paraaortic node metastasis were excluded. In 330 suitable patients, 5-year survival rates were clinically and statistically improved (66% versus 55%) in those patients who received extended-field therapy. Additionally, patients treated with pelvic irradiation alone were at higher risk to experience distal failure (32% versus 25%). Severe gastrointestinal complications were more common in those patients receiving extended-field therapy; however, this excess morbidity was mainly attributable to those patients who had prior abdominal surgery.

Intraoperative Therapy

The place for adjunctive radiosensitizers or intraoperative electron beam therapy (Delgado et al 1984) to aortic node metastases requires further investigation. Intraoperative irradiation with electrons has been used by investigators at the Mayo Clinic (Garton et al 1993). Local control and disease-free status was good; however, response was significantly improved in those women who had microscopic disease.

Some authors consider the presence of metastases in paraaortic nodes to signify the existence of systemic disease and propose the use of adjunctive chemotherapy. The impact of local tumor control on outcome has important implications. Although eradication of the primary tumor is paramount, some argue that covert but incurable micrometastases from spread before diagnosis represent the most important determinant of survival, particularly in early-stage disease. Although little prospective work has been performed in cervical cancer (Belloni et al 1983; Thomas et al 1984a, 1984b; Blake et al 1984), experimental data, theoretic considerations, and initial clinical results from other tumors (Tubiana et al 1985) suggest that some alternating or combination scheme of chemotherapy and radiation therapy may be successful.

COMPLICATIONS

All cancer therapies involve some inherent risks, and it is imperative that the patient, therapist, gynecologic oncologist, and practitioner understand that radiotherapeutic cure is associated with potential complications. Although modern techniques have reduced the overall incidence of irradiation-associated complications, the patient's risk is related to the presence or absence of the previously described technical and clinical factors. Additionally, the ultimate goal of cure may push radiation delivery to a point that increases the risk of normal tissue injury.

Although individual doses have been correlated, the risk of treatment complications may be better correlated to the volume of treatment calculations rather than rectal, bladder, or dose at point A (VanLancker et al 1991). The usual curative radiation doses approach or exceed the risk of 5% injury (see Table 8-13) in most instances.

Prospective evaluations reveal an increased risk of major complications when compared with retrospective studies (Lambin 1993). Lanciano and coworkers (1992a) evaluated complications in the Patterns of Care Study and found that major complications requiring hospitalization occurred in 14% of women during the first 5 years and were increased in those women having (1) prior laparotomy (twofold increase); (2) a high fraction dose (more than 200 cGy); (3) large field size (twofold increase); (4) high paracentral doses (more than 7500 cGy); and (5) younger age (younger than 40 years). Bowel problems were three times more common and occurred earlier (mean, 13.5 months) than bladder (mean, 23.2 months) or vaginal complications (mean, 17.4 months). Major irradiation-associated injury occurred in a stage-related fashion (Lanciano et al 1991a) and was associated with PCS point A doses of 8500 or more cGy or PCS point P dose of 5000 or more cGy.

Radiation complications are logically divided into those occurring during or shortly after therapy, secondary to irradiation reaction, and those occurring later, related to the continued irradiation effects of arteritis and fibrosis. Although acute complications are usually managed by medications or short interruption of the radiation therapy, long-term complications are usually more serious. Although the risk of long-term complications may be increased in those patients who have acute reactions, most patients can be reassured that acute irradiation effects do not herald the onset of late complications (Bourne et al 1983). Most patients with late complications do not have acute problems. Unfortunately, comparison of different treatment schemes is difficult because many papers (more than half) do not classify irradiation complications by type, time of onset, or severity (Sismondi et al 1989).

Intracavitary Complications

Acute complications of patients undergoing intracavitary therapy are rare. Psychologically, patients appear to tolerate immobilization better when placed on scheduled doses of a tranquilizer. The benefit of prophylactic antibiotics to patients who have urinary catheters or intracavitary radiation therapy devices is not clear. We previously used prophylactic subcutaneous heparin; however, we use antiembolic calf compression (Farquharson et al 1984) to decrease these risks.

Uterine Perforation

Additionally, uterine perforation occurs in at least 10% of intracavitary placements (Matsuyama et al 1986). Uterine perforation during the placement of the intracavitary apparatus should not discourage efforts for a second attempt. If necessary, CT scan or ultrasound can be used to determine applicator placement (Wong et al 1990). In Kim and associates' report (1983), 64% of patients with perforation later underwent successful placement with excellent results. In those patients discovered to have a pyometra during intracavitary placement (ICP), adequate drainage (i.e., dilation) should be established. Antibiotic therapy should be considered but therapy is usually continued with teletherapy (Shierholz et al 1977).

Febrile Complications

The development of fever during treatment is a serious problem. Van Herik (1965) reported 260 patients having fever, usually associated with intracavitary therapy. The survival in patients with fever was lessened, stage for stage, when compared with those without. Survival of those patients with fevers of long duration was less than that of those with fevers of short duration. Davy (1974) confirmed the bad prognostic significance of fever and reported only a 14% survival rate for patients having stage I or II cervical cancer if the fever had a genital origin. Kapp and Lawrence (1984) confirmed these findings; patients with a maximum

temperature of 38.3°C (101°F) during intracavitary treatment had a significant decrease in survival and an increased frequency of distant metastasis. Solberger and Sorbe (1990) reported 5-year survival (63.6% versus 31.8%) and crude survival (53.5% versus 27.3%) to be decreased by 50% in those women experiencing fever during treatment. These treatment failures may be related to (1) hypoxia in a necrotic tumor, (2) uterine perforation and tumor dissemination during intracavitary placement, (3) a delay in initiating treatment or alteration of the treatment scheme if the intracavitary source is removed, (4) altered host resistance, or (5) enhancement of distal metastases with hyperthermia.

To and colleagues (1993) evaluated febrile morbidity in patients undergoing intracavitary irradiation and reported the use of cefoxitin (3 g/24 hours) during therapy to significantly decrease the risk of fever of more than 37.5°C (99.5°F) and to decrease the need for additional antibiotics. This benefit occurred regardless of tumor size, stage, or insertion (1st or 2nd application).

We would hesitate to use an intracavitary source in the presence of a proved pyometra but would effect uterine drainage and proceed with external teletherapy. If fever develops during the intracavitary brachytherapy treatment phase, the patient is evaluated for extrapelvic causes of fever. If none are found, antibiotic coverage for gram-negative and anaerobic bacteria is begun. It is rarely necessary to remove the intracavitary system.

Cutaneous Complications

The introduction of megavoltage teletherapy has made serious skin problems less frequent. When present, however, particularly in the intertriginous areas, drying agents such as cornstarch may be helpful. Acute panniculitis or significant subcutaneous fibrosis are rare when the skin dose is 5000 cGy or less. Acute vulvitis is common in those situations requiring a low treatment field or a perineal port. Roberts and coworkers (1991) reported 12 patients with severe radionecrosis of the vulva or vagina. Radical surgical treatment, with or without flaps, was successful in the long-term treatment of these women.

Vaginal Complications

The loss of ovarian function and distortion of the vagina are concerns, especially in young women who have early-stage disease. Abitbol and Davenport (1974a, b) indicated that the triad of significant vaginal narrowing, marked pelvic fibrosis, and pelvic pain were present in most patients after irradiation for cervical cancer. Although the efficacy of estrogen therapy and vaginal dilation is unproved, we advocate the two modalities in an effort to maintain vaginal caliber and pliability. It must be remembered, however, that estrogen is freely absorbed from the irradiated vagina. Guidelines for estrogen administration should be the same as those for women who are not being treated for cervical cancer. Long-term estrogen administration probably should be coupled with progesterone supplementation to protect against physiologic stimulation of the endometrium. Additionally, psychological counseling is appropriate.

Hematologic Effects

Some concern exists over the possible acute irradiation effects on the hematologic or immunologic systems. Studies of natural killer cells (Pulay et al 1982), complement levels (Pulay et al 1980), and other immunologic markers (Hancock et al 1984) failed to demonstrate any consistent adverse effect of irradiation. Pillai and colleagues (1991) suggested the possible monitoring benefit of lymphocyte subsets during and after irradiation. The DC4[+] cell counts and the DC4 to CD8 ratio differed (lower) in those patients who were later found to have recurrent disease. Although extended-field teletherapy may have an adverse effect on hematopoietic cells, only rarely is the bone marrow suppressed to a clinically relevant point. Bone marrow suppression is usually associated with other factors, such as prior or concurrent chemotherapy and in older patients.

Acute Gastrointestinal Complications

Gastrointestinal complaints are common during therapy. Although the acute effects of irradiation begin within hours of the commencement of therapy, most patients do not experience acute symptoms until 2000 to 3000 cGy have been delivered. The incidence of grade III or IV intestinal complication is increased 2.3 times in those receiving paraaortic ports (Haie et al 1988). Erickson and associates (1994) suggest that acute intestinal toxicities are related to altered motility and precede the appearance of histopathologic lesions of the intestinal tract. Nausea and vomiting may be relieved by dietary modification, using a low-gluten, low-protein, low-lactose diet. Phenothiazines or other antiemetics should be used as necessary. Diarrhea secondary to acute ileitis can be treated symptomatically with such medications as diphenoxylate hydrochloride with atropine (Lomotil or Imodium); however, if the diarrhea is severe and unresponsive to medical therapy, treatment interruption may be necessary. Decreasing the daily dose by 10% or decreasing treated volume may suffice to decrease symptoms (Otchy et al 1993). Some authors have advocated salicylates to treat diarrhea because these decrease local prostaglandin synthesis and thereby alleviate the symptoms. Acute irradiation changes, especially diarrhea, may be related to altered absorption of bile salts. These patients may benefit from the administration of cholestyramine. Chronic diarrhea can be treated with a low-residue diet and occasionally responds to daily long-term psyllium (Metamucil). The risk of injury is increased in patients who have bowel adhesions after a previous abdominal surgical procedure or in those who have significant vascular disease (Coia et al 1990). Cramping may be associated with adhesions and is minimized by a low-residue diet.

Late Gastrointestinal Complications

Although individual risks vary, serious late gastrointestinal complications occur in as many as 12% of patients after irradiation therapy, and as many as 8% require operative intervention (Covens et al 1991). Radiologic intestinal and urinary tract changes associated with irradiation may be difficult to distinguish from recurrent disease or a new primary tumor (Taylor et al 1990).

Proctosigmoiditis (often associated with persistent rectal bleeding) may respond to a low-residue diet and steroid enemas. Topical anesthetics may constrict vessels and reduce bleeding. The risk and severity of proctitis is dose-related. Montana and coworkers (1989) indicated a small risk (2%) in patients receiving less than 5000 cGy but a high risk (18%) in women receiving more than 8000 cGy. When prospectively evaluated, sucralfate enemas (2 g) resulted in a 95% clinical improvement rate, superior to steroid enemas and oral sulfasalazine (Otchy et al 1993). If refractory to conservative measures, a diverting colostomy may be beneficial; however, persistent symptoms are common, and as many as 50% of patients continue to bleed after diversion and require bowel resection. Another acceptable alternative involves use of the Nd:YAG laser for photocoagulation of the telangiectatic rectal vessels. Although small series suggest a significant benefit, recurrent bleeding often occurs (Otchy et al 1993).

Small Bowel Complications

The terminal ileum, with its relatively fixed position and tenuous blood supply, is the segment of small bowel most commonly involved in late complications. In a study of 57 patients requiring surgery, when evaluating all types (perforation, stricture, obstruction) and sites of irradiation injury, Covens and coworkers (1991) indicated that ileal injury was associated with the worst prognosis of any site of injury and was responsible for the poor prognosis in those women with multiple sites of irradiation injury.

Van Nagell and associates (1974a) and Coia and colleagues (1990) reported those individuals with a small body habitus to be particularly prone to small bowel complications. Small bowel obstruction occurs in 1% to 4% of patients after radiation therapy. Irradiation-induced strictures and adhesions, however, comprise nearly 17% of all small bowel obstructions (Alvarez 1988). These patients usually have a long history of symptoms that are suggestive of partial small bowel obstruction. Before surgical intervention, which should be undertaken to avoid a catastrophic event (i.e., perforation), the surgeon must aggressively treat vascular volume deficits and metabolic abnormalities. Partial small bowel obstruction is more likely to respond to gastrointestinal suction than is complete obstruction. As many as 70% of women with postoperative small bowel obstruction can be successfully treated with intestinal intubation (Alvarez 1988); however, a previous history of radiation therapy decreases the success of nonoperative intervention. Unfortunately, alterations in peritoneal sensation secondary to previous irradiation may mask the usual signs or symptoms of strangulation or an early perforation.

The most appropriate surgical procedure to treat irradiation-associated small bowel obstruction is controversial (Cochrane et al 1981). Wheeless (1973) and Smith and coworkers (1966) recommended simple bypass procedures such as an ileal ascending colostomy. Schmitt and Symmonds (1981) and Smith and associates (1985) indicated that intestinal resection may be the procedure of choice because fewer patients would require further surgical procedures to treat complications of the bypassed segment. Wilkinson (1990) suggested the possible role of longitudinal serotomy to manage early postradiation small bowel obstruction. We tend to perform the simplest procedure (i.e., a bypass) unless bowel necrosis is evident.

Regardless of the procedure that is selected, meticulous surgical technique (including sharp dissection, gentle handling of irradiated tissues, and careful packing of the intraabdominal contents) should be used. Important principles in the treatment of the infected irradiated pelvis include wide drainage and irrigation of infected tissues, creation of an abdominopelvic partition (mesh or omentum), wide excision of infected irradiated tissues, and transfer of vascularized tissue—both to promote healing and fill dead space (Edington et al 1988). An inadvertent or undetected enterotomy may have catastrophic results. Additionally, new blood supply may be transferred to the irradiated anastomosis with an omental J flap to enhance healing (Alvarez 1988).

Small Bowel Fistulas

The development of a postradiation small bowel fistula is serious (Coutsoftides et al 1979) and requires immediate medical therapy and support directed at fluid and calorie replacement and control of sepsis. During this time of resuscitation, attention should be directed to skin protection. Despite the use of parenteral hyperalimentation and antibiotics, few irradiation-associated small bowel fistulas close spontaneously. Before surgical intervention, a fistulogram, small bowel, and even large bowel series should be performed to determine the presence or absence of complex (i.e., large and small bowel) fistulas or associated distal small bowel obstruction (Palmer et al 1976). A simple bypass procedure is not recommended because it predisposes the patient to a second operation, often made necessary because of an incompetent ileocecal valve and continued fistulous drainage. We prefer to resect the involved segment and to avoid a primary anastomosis in irradiated bowel. This also allows histologic evaluation to rule out recurrence. Although the best procedure to manage postradiation intestinal fistulas remains to be determined, some (Edington et al 1988) advocate the use of resection (not bypass), suggesting a significant difference in later intestinal fistulization. After surgery, hyperalimentation allows bowel rest and continued correction of nutritional deficits.

Levenback and colleagues (1994) reported the surgical outcome for irradiation-induced complex (enterovesical) fistulas in the absence of recurrent tumor. Although their series was small (14 patients), their results strongly suggested the benefit of surgical procedures that resected necrotic small bowel with complete separation of the intestinal and urinary tracts. Complete urinary diversion may be necessary.

Rectovaginal Fistulas

Rectovaginal fistulas or rectal strictures are infrequent (about 2% or less). If a fistula occurs, biopsies should be performed at the fistulous site to determine the presence or absence of cancer. Additionally, because the development of one complication is often associated with others, the entire gastrointestinal tract should be evaluated before any surgical bypass or repair. Primary surgical repair of rectovaginal fistulas is difficult to achieve and is successful only if a new blood supply (such as with use of a bulbocavernosus flap) is transposed into the area of injury. Bricker and Johnston (1979) reported successful closure of such fistulas by sigmoid colon transposition. Despite these operative possibilities, many of these patients require a permanent diverting colostomy.

The seriousness of an operation for gastrointestinal complications after irradiation is evident in Smith and associates' (1966) report, in which postoperative deaths occurred in 11% of patients after the first operation, 27% of patients after a second operation, and 43% after a third operation. Serious postoperative complications occur in 30% of first operations (Covens et al 1991). Modern mortality rates remain at 10% (Covens et al 1991). Thirty-nine percent of first-surgery survivors require another procedure and 40% require a third procedure (Covens et al 1991). As many as 25% die of irradiation-associated complications. With the institution of hyperalimentation, broad-spectrum antibiotics, and other intensive care measures, these high complication rates probably can be lowered; however, surgical procedures on patients who have irradiated bowel are still fraught with complications. Evidence of recurrent or persistent cancer should be actively sought because it may alter the treatment plan.

In addition to the serious surgical complications, evidence (Yeoh et al 1993) indicates a significant life-long risk of irradiation-induced gastrointestinal dysfunction. In a study of 30 randomly selected patients, 29 had at least one abnormality. Significant increases in stool frequency, shortened small bowel transit times, and less absorption of bile acid, vitamin B_{12}, and lactose were present after radiation therapy. These findings suggest the important therapeutic role of dietary intervention for the treatment of irradiation enteritis.

Urinary Complications

Acute hemorrhagic cystitis is rare (slightly more than 3%) and usually self-limiting. Symptoms of urgency or frequency, however, may require investigation. Clinical infection and bacteriuria should be treated with antibiotics. Bladder fistulas and hydronephrosis are thought to be more common in women who have cystitis during therapy. Montana and associates (1989), evaluating 527 women treated with irradiation for squamous cell cancer, reported a nonsignificant relation between cystitis (and degree) and a significant dose-related risk of proctitis. The latter ranged from 2% (2000-cGy external therapy) to 14% (4000-cGy external therapy). Montana and colleagues (1989) reported the risk of cystitis to range from 2% in patients receiving a bladder dose of less than 5000 cGy to 18% in women receiving a bladder dose of more than 8000 cGy. There was an apparent dose relation to the severity of cystitis.

Levenback and coworkers (1994) reported hemorrhagic cystitis in 7.1% of 1638 patients having stage IB disease. A significant proportion (34.8%) had positive urine cultures. Most were minor; however, 19.8% required admission for medical management (grade III) and 4.3% (5 patients) required major surgery (grade IV). There was one death. Their cystoscopic and clinical findings suggested little benefit of cystoscopic biopsy unless there was suspicion of tumor.

Bladder dysfunction after radiation therapy is common. Farquharson and associates (1987) reported

incontinence (requiring protection) to develop in 23% of patients after irradiation and in 63% of patients after post–radical irradiation. A dose-related decrease in bladder compliance was also noted. Urodynamic studies after irradiation suggest detrusor instability to be a potential problem rather than changes in capacity. Incontinence may occur in 23% of patients (Parkin 1989).

The incidence of serious urinary complications ranges from 1% to 5% and increases markedly in patients who are receiving more than 8000 cGy to the base of the bladder (Burns et al 1966). Seow Choen and colleagues (1993) described the successful use of formalin in the treatment of severe hemorrhage cystitis. Hemal (1989) reported the successful use of intravesical 15MF2 prostaglandins. The presence of hydronephrosis or ureteral stricture should prompt investigation for recurrent cancer. As many as 3% of women treated with curative irradiation develop obstructive uropathy related to benign fibrosis (Parliament et al 1989). Occasionally (20%), this may be bilateral. The role of percutaneous diversion in this clinical situation remains to be determined. If cancer is present and the patient is not a candidate for exenteration, no surgical therapy is indicated. If no cancer is present, therapeutic alternatives include (1) no therapy, (2) transvesical or percutaneous ureteral stents, (3) ureterolysis, (4) transureteroureterostomy, (5) ureteral reimplantation, or (6) conduit diversion (Kirkinen et al 1980). In these instances, we determine kidney function with an isotope scan. Patients with poor unilateral renal perfusion may be observed without treatment if the remaining kidney has adequate function; however, if the obstructed kidney has good perfusion, a transureteroureterostomy (performed outside of the irradiation field) or a ureterointestinal interposition may be beneficial. In patients with bilateral obstruction due to irradiation, we recommend a continent or transverse colon conduit because attempts to reimplant the ureters into the radiated bladder are fraught with high complication rates.

Radiation-related vesicovaginal fistulas require a new source of blood supply with a matins, gracilis, or omental J flap (Parkin 1989). Some patients with irradiation-induced vesicovaginal fistulas have had primary repair using a vulvar pedicle graft or interposed omentum to provide a new blood supply (Boronow 1971a, Boronow et al 1971b, Kiricuta et al 1972). Although some fistulas can be successfully managed in this manner, most patients require permanent urinary diversion.

Bone Injury

With low-energy teletherapy, radionecrosis of the femoral head was formerly a potential complication. The introduction of supervoltage equipment has reduced the incidence of radionecrosis of bone to a negligible level. If fractured, however, previously irradiated bone heals poorly (Rubin et al 1961). A combination of sacroiliac joint fractures, leading to pubic fractures, has been described on CT after pelvic irradiation (Rafii et al 1988).

Nerve Injury

Saphner and coworkers (1989) reported an 8% risk of neurologic complications in patients having invasive cervical cancer. Lumbosacral plexopathy was the most common. Radiation myelitis is a rare but serious irradiation complication when the treatment field involves the spinal cord. Generally, 4500 to 5000 cGy delivered in 25 fractions over 33 days to a field of 10 or fewer centimeters is considered to be a safe dose. Although risks of nerve injury are related to dose, fractionation, and treatment volume, one study (Bloss et al 1991) suggested the possibility of an increased risk with concomitant 5-FU/cisplatin radiation treatment. Sacral plexus radiculopathy is a rare complication of irradiation (Stryker et al 1990). Georgiou and associates (1993) reported lumbosacral plexopathy to occur in 4 of 2410 patients treated.

Carcinogenesis

The potential risk of inducing secondary cancers in patients receiving pelvic radiation therapy has created debate and is an important potential complication. Most information (Pizzarello et al 1984) suggests that radiation therapy is only weakly carcinogenic. The risk of leukemia after irradiation may be slightly increased but not dramatically (Boice et al 1980). Arai and colleagues (1991), evaluating 11,855 irradiated patients, reported no increased incidence when all second primary sites were evaluated. The incidence of rectal cancer, bladder cancer, and leukemia were increased, however. As may be expected, the incidence of lung cancer was increased in patients having cervical cancer, regardless of treatment, because cigarette abuse is a risk factor for both primary sites. In a review, Hoffman and coworkers (1985) indicated no irradiation-related increase in colorectal cancer, leukemia, or ovarian or uterine cancer. Other forms of tumors, however, such as uterine sarcomas or carcinomas, occur in irradiated pelvic fields. Fehr and Prem (1973) indicated that the risk for the later development of sarcoma of the bony pelvis was low with megavoltage therapy. Pettersson (1990) evaluated a cancer registry cohort of 16,704 cases of invasive cervical cancer and reported an increased incidence of in-field second primaries of the rectum and bladder. The incidence of lymphosarcoma and nonlymphatic leukemia was also increased. We

have observed several such uterine fundal tumors, soft part sarcomas in a pelvic (posterior) irradiation field. One may speculate that even the squamous cell carcinomas occurring in the pelvis many years after irradiation for cancer of the cervix are irradiation-induced second primary tumors and not recurrences.

References

Abitbol MM, Davenport JH. Sexual dysfunction after therapy for cervical carcinoma. Am J Obstet Gynecol 1974a;119:181.

Abitbol MM, Davenport JH. The irradiated vagina. Obstet Gynecol 1974b;44:249.

Akine Y, Arimoto H, Ogino T, et al. High-dose-rate intracavitary irradiation in the treatment of carcinoma of the uterine cervix: early experience with 84 patients. Int J Radiat Oncol Biol Phys 1988;14:893.

Alfert HJ, Gillenwater JY. The consequences of ureteral irradiation with special reference to subsequent ureteral injury. J Urol 1972;107:369.

Allen WE Jr, Reddi RP. Simplified irradiation dosimetry in carcinoma of the cervix (external irradiation and one radium insertion). J Natl Med Assoc 1980;72:361.

Alvarez RD. Gastrointestinal complications in gynecologic surgery: a review for the general gynecologist. Obstet Gynecol 1988;72(3):533.

Alvarez RD, Potter ME, Soong SJ, et al. Rationale for using pathologic tumor dimensions and nodal status to subclassify surgically treated stage IB cervical cancer paients. Gynecol Oncol 1991;43(2):108.

Ampuero F, Doss LL, Khan M, Skipper B, Hilgers RD. The Syed-Neblett interstitial template in locally advanced gynecological malignancies. Int J Radiat Oncol Biol Phys 1983;9:1897.

Anderson B, LaPolla J, Turner D, et al. Ovarian transposition in cervical cancer. Gynecol Oncol 1993;49:206.

Anderson P, Dische S. Local tumor control and the subsequent incidence of distant metastatic disease. Int J Radiat Oncol Biol Phys 1981;7:1645.

Andras EJ, Fletcher GH, Rutledge F. Radiotherapy of carcinoma of the cervix following simple hysterectomy. Am J Radiol Oncol Biol Phys 1973;115:647.

Ang KK, Peters LJ. Altered fractionation in radiation oncology. Principles and practice of oncology, vol 8. Philadelphia: JB Lippincott, 1994.

Arai T, Nakano T, Fukuhisa K, et al. Second cancer after radiation therapy for cancer of the uterine cervix. Cancer 1991;67:398.

Arai T, Nakano T, Morita S, et al. High-dose-rate remote afterloading intracavitary radiation therapy for cancer of the uterine cervix. Cancer 1992;69:175.

Arimoto T. Significance of computed tomography-measured volume in the prognosis of cervical carcinoma. Cancer 1993;72:2383.

Averette HE, Jobson VW. The role of exploratory laparotomy in the staging and treatment of invasive cervical carcinoma. Int J Radiat Oncol Biol Phys 1979;5:2137.

Baker VV, Dudzinski MR, Fowler WC, Currie JL, Walton

LA. Percutaneous nephrostomy in gynecologic oncology. Am J Obstet Gynecol 1984;149:772.

Ballon SC, Berman ML, Lagasse LD, Petrilli ES, Castaldo TW. Survival after extraperitoneal pelvic and para-aortic lymphadenectomy and radiation therapy in cervical carcinoma. Obstet Gynecol 1981;57:90.

Bandy LC, Clarke-Pearson DL, Creasman WT. Vitamin B-12 deficiency following therapy in gynecologic oncology. Gynecol Oncol 1984;17:370.

Bastin K, Buchler D, Stitt J, et al. Resource utilization. High dose rate versus low dose rate brachytherapy for gynecologic cancer. Am J Clin Oncol 1993;16(3):256.

Bedford JS. Sublethal damage, potentially lethal damage, and chromoscomal aberrations in mammalian cells exposed to ionizing radiations. Int J Radiat Oncol Biol Phys 1991;21:1457.

Beecham JB, Halvorsen T, Kolbenstvedt A. Histologic classification, lymph node metastases and patient survival in stage IB cervical carcinoma. Gynecol Oncol 1978;6:95.

Belloni C, Mantioni C, Bortolozzi G, et al. ICRF 159 plus radiation versus radiation therapy alone in cervical carcinoma. A double-blind study. Oncology 1983;40:191.

Berek JS, Hacker NF, Hatch KD, Young RC. Uterine corpus and cervical cancer. Curr Probl Cancer 1988;XII(2):65.

Berman ML, Lagasse LD, Watring WG, et al. The operative evaluation of patients with cervical carcinoma by an extraperitoneal approach. Obstet Gynecol 1977;50:658.

Berman ML, Keys H, Creasman W, et al. Survival and patterns of recurrence in cervical cancer metastatic to periaortic lymph nodes (a gynecologic oncololgy group study). Gynecol Oncol 1984;19:8.

Blake PR, Lambert HE, MacGregor WG, et al. Surgery following chemotherapy and radiotherapy for advanced carcinoma of the cervix. Gynecol Oncol 1984;19:198.

Bloomer WD, Hellman S. Normal tissue responses to radiation therapy. N Engl J Med 1975;293:80.

Bloss JD, DiSaia PJ, Mannel RS, et al. Radiation myelitis: a complication of concurrent cisplatin and 5-fluorouracil chemotherapy with extended field radiotherapy for carcinoma of the uterine cervix. Gynecol Oncol 1991; 43:305.

Blythe JG, Hodel KA, Wahl TP, et al. Paraaortic node biopsy in cervical and endometrial cancers: does it affect survival? Am J Obstet Gynecol 1986;155:306.

Boice JD, Hutchinson GB. Leukemia in women following radiotherapy for cervical cancer, ten-year follow-up of an international study. J Natl Cancer Inst 1980;65:115.

Bonanno JP, Boyce J, Fruchter R, et al. Involvement of paraaortic lymph nodes in carcinoma of the cervix. J Am Osteopath Assoc 1980;79:567.

Boronow RC. Should whole pelvic radiation therapy become past history? A case for the routine use of extended field therapy and multimodality therapy. Gynecol Oncol 1991;43:71.

Boronow RC. Management of radiation induced vaginal fistulas. Am J Obstet Gynecol 1971a;110:1.

Boronow RC, Rutledge F. Vesicovaginal fistula, radiation, and gynecologic cancer. Am J Obstet Gynecol 1971b; 11:85.

Bosch A, Marcial VA. Evaluation of the time interval between external irradiation and intracavitary curietherapy in carcinoma of the uterine cervix: influence on curability. Radiology 1967;88:563.

Bounous G, Gentile JM, Hugon J. Elemental diet in the management of the intestinal lesion produced by 5-fluorouracil in man. Can J Surg 1971;14:312.

Bourne RG, Kearsley JH, Grove WD, Roberts SJ. The relationship between early and late gastrointestinal complications of radiation therapy for carcinoma of the cervix. Int J Radiat Oncol Biol Phys 1983;9:1445.

Brady LW, Perez CA, eds. Principals and practice of radiation oncology, 2nd ed. Philadelphia: JB Lippincott, 1992: 1162.

Braley PS. The current status of flow cytometry in gynecologic oncology. Oncology 1992;6(1):23.

Brenner DJ, Huang Y, Hall EJ. Fractionated high dose rate versus low dose rate regimens for intracavitary brachytherapy of the cervix: equivalent regimens for combined brachytherapy and external irradiation. Int J Rad Oncol Biol Phys 1991;21:1415.

Bricker EM, Johnston WD. Repair of postirradiation rectovaginal fistula and stricture. Surg Gynecol Obstet 1979;148:499.

Brookland RK, Rubin S, Danoff BF. Extended field irradiation in the treatment of patients with cervical carcinoma involving biopsy proven para-aortic nodes. Int J Radiat Oncol Biol Phys 1984;10:1875.

Browde S, Nissenbaum M, DeMoor NG. High dose weekly fractionation radiotherapy in advanced cancer of the uterine cervix. South Afr Med J 1984;66:11.

Brown JM. Sensitizers and protectors in radiotherapy. Cancer 1985;55:2222.

Buchsbaum HJ. Extrapelvic lymph node metastases in cervical carcinoma. Am J Obstet Gynecol 1979;133:814.

Burns BC, Upton RT. Management of urinary tract complications of treatment for carcinoma of the uterine cervix. In Clinical Conference on Cancer, MD Anderson Hospital and Tumor Institute, Houston. Cancer of the uterus and ovary: a collection of papers. Chicago: Year Book Medical Publishers, 1966:257.

Calais G, LeFloch O, Chauvet B, et al. Carcinoma of the uterine cervix stage IB and early stage II. Prognostic value of the histological tumor regression after initial brachytherapy. Int J Radiat Oncol Biol Phys 1989; 17:1231.

Cardinale JG, Peschel RE, Gutierrez E, et al. Stage IIIA carcinoma of the uterine cervix. Gynecol Oncol 1986; 23:199.

Chafe W, Fowler WC, Currie JL, et al. Single-fraction palliative pelvic radiation therapy in gynecologic oncology: 1000 rads. Am J Obstet Gynecol 1984;148:701.

Chambers SK, Chambers JT, Kier R, Peschel RE. Sequelae of lateral ovarian transposition in irradiated cervical cancer patients. Int J Radiat Oncol Biol Phys 1991;20:1305.

Chapman JA, Mannel RS, DiSaia PJ, Walker JL, Berman ML. Surgical treatment of unexpected invasive cervical cancer found at total hysterectomy. Obstet Gynecol 1992; 80:931.

Chen MS, Lin FJ, Hong CH, et al. High-dose-rate afterloading technique in the radiation treatment of uterine cervical cancer: 399 cases and 9 years experience in Taiwan. Int J Radiat Oncol Biol Phys 1991;20:915.

Choo YC, Hsu C, Ma HK. The assessment of radio-response of cervical carcinoma by colposcopy. Gynecol Oncol 1984;18:28.

Cikaric S. Radiation therapy of cervical carcinoma using either HDR or LDR afterloading: comparison of 5-year results and complications. Strahlenther Onkol 1988; 82(suppl):119.

Cochrane JP, Yarnold JR, Slack WW. The surgical treatment of radiation injuries after radiotherapy for uterine carcinoma. Br J Surg 1981;68:25.

Cohen L, Hendrickson FR, Kurup ID, et al. Clinical evaluation of neutron beam therapy. Cancer 1985;55:10.

Coia L, Won M, Lanciano R, Marcial VA, Martz K, Hanks G. The patterns of care outcome study for cancer of the uterine cervix. Results of the second national practice survey. Cancer 1990;66:2451.

Copeland EM. Intravenous hyperalimentation as an adjunct to cancer patient management. CA Cancer J Clin 1978;28: 322.

Corn BW, Galvin JM, Soffen EM, et al. Positional stability of sources during low dose rate brachytherapy for cervical carcinoma. Int J Radiat Oncol Biol Phys 1993; 26(3): 513.

Corn BW, Hanlon AL, Pajak TF, et al. Technically accurate intracavitary insertions improve pelvic control and survival among patients with locally advanced carcinoma of the uterine cervix. Gynecol Oncol 1994;53:294.

Cosbie WG. Radiotherapy following hysterectomy performed for or in the presence of cancer of the cervix. Am J Obstet Gynecol 1963;85:332.

Coutsoftides T, Fazio VW. Small intestine cutaneous fistulas. Surg Gynecol Obstet 1979;149:333.

Covens A, Thomas G, DePetrillo A, et al. The prognostic importance of site and type of radiation-induced bowel injury in patients requiring surgical management. Gynecol Oncol 1991;43:270.

Cox JD. Large dose fractionation (hypofractionation). Cancer 1985;55:2105.

Crawford JS, Harisiadis L, McGowan L, Rogers CC. Para-aortic lymph node irradiation in cervical carcinoma without prior lymphadenectomy. Radiology 1987; 164:255.

Cunningham MJ, Dunton CJ, Corn B, et al. Extended field radiation therapy in early stage cervical carcinoma: survival and complications. Gynecol Oncol 1991;43:51.

Daly JM. Nutritional support. In DeVita VT, Hellman S, Rosenberg SA, eds. Cancer, principles and practice of Oncology, 4th ed. Philadelphia: JB Lippincott, 1993: 2480.

Davidson SE, Symonds RP, Lamont D, et al. Does adenocarcinoma of uterine cervix have a worse prognosis than squamous carcinoma when treated by radiotherapy? Gynecol Oncol 1989;33:23.

Davy M. The prognosis of carcinoma of the cervix with particular reference to infection. Aust NZ J Obstet Gynaecol 1974;14:1.

Davy M, Bentzen H, Jahren R. Simple hysterectomy in the presence of invasive cervical cancer. Acta Obstet Gynecol Scand 1977;56:105.

Delgado G, Goldson AL, Ashayeri E, et al. Intraoperative radiation in the treatment of advanced cervical cancer. Obstet Gynecol 1984;63:246.

Deore SM, Viswanathan PS, Shrivastava SK, et al. Predictive role of TDF values in late rectal recto-sigmoid complications in irradiation treatment of cervix cancer. Int J Radiat Oncol Biol Phys 1992;24:217.

DiSaia PJ, Bundy BN, Curry SL, et al. Phase III study on the treatment of women with cervical cancer, stage IIB, IIIB, and IVA (confined to the pelvis and/or periaortic nodes), with radiotherapy alone versus radiotherapy plus immunotherapy with intravenous *Corynebacterium parvum*: a gynecologic oncology group study. Gynecol Oncol 1987;26:386.

Dische S. Radiotherapy and anaemia—the clinical experience. Radiother Oncol 1991;20(Suppl):35.

Dische S. The clinical use of hyperbaric oxygen and chemical hypoxic cell sensitizers. In Steel GG, Adams GE, Peckham MJ, eds. The biological basis of radiotherapy. Amsterdam, Elsevier, y1983a:225.

Dische S, Anderson PJ, Sealy R, Watson ER. Carcinoma of the cervix—anaemia, radiotherapy and hyperbaric oxygen. Br J Radiol 1983b;56:251.

Donaldson SS, Wesley MN, Ghavimi S, et al. A prospective randomized clinical trial of the value of total parenteral nutrition in children with cancer. Med Pediatr Oncol 1982;10:129.

Downey GO, Potish RA, Adcock LL, Prem KA, Twiggs LB. Pretreatment surgical staging in cervical carcinoma: therapeutic efficacy of pelvic lymph node resection. Obstet Gynecol 1989;160:1055.

Durrance FY, Fletcher GH, Rutledge F. Analysis of central recurrent disease in stage I and II squamous cell carcinomas of the cervix on intact uterus. Am J Roentgenol 1969;106:831.

Dusenberry KE, Carson LF, Potish RA. Perioperative morbidity and mortality of gynecologic brachytherapy. Cancer 1991;67:2786.

Edinger DD Jr, Watring WG, Anderson B, Mitchell GW Jr. Residual tumor following radiotherapy for locally advanced carcinomas of the uterine cervix: prognostic significance. Eur J Gynaecol Oncol 1984;5:90.

Edington HD, Sugarbaker PH, McDonald HD. Management of the surgically traumatized, irradiated, and infected pelvis. Surgery 1988;103(6):690.

Eifel PJ, Burke TW, Delclos L, Wharton JT, Oswald MJ. Early stage I adenocarcinoma of the uterine cervix: treatment results in patients with tumor ≤ 4 cm in diameter. Gynecol Oncol 1991;41:199.

Eifel PJ. High dose rate brachytherapy for carcinoma of the cervix: high tech or high risk? Int J Radiat Oncol Biol Phys 1992;24:383.

Erickson BA, Otterson MF, Moulder JE, Sarna WK. Altered motility causes the early gastrointestinal toxicity of radiation. Int J Radiat Oncol Biol Phys 1994;28(4):905.

Fagundes H, Perez CA, Grigsby PW, Lockett MA. Distant metastases after irradiation alone in carcinoma of the uterine cervix. Int J Radiat Oncol Biol Phys 1992; 24:197.

Fang FM, Yeh CY, Lai YL, Choiu JF, Change KH. Radiotherapy following simple hysterectomyy in patients with invasive carcinoma of the uterine cervix. J Formosa Med Assoc 1993;92(5):420.

Farquharson DIM, Orr JW Jr. Thromboembolic complications in gynecology. J Reprod Med 1984;29:845.

Farquharson DIM, Singleton HM, Soong SJ, et al. The adverse effects of cervical cancer treatment on bladder function. Gynecol Oncol 1987;27:15.

Fehr PE, Prem KA. Postirradiation sarcoma of the pelvic girdle following therapy for squamous cell carcinoma of the cervix. Am J Obstet Gynecol 1973;116:192.

Finck FM, Denk M. Cervical carcinoma: relationship between histology and survival following radiation therapy. Obstet Gynecol 1970;35:339.

Fletcher GH. Clinical dose response curves of human malignant epithelial tumours. Br J Radiol 1973;46:1.

Flueckiger F, Ebner F, Poschauko H, et al. Cervical cancer: serial MR imaging before and after primary radiation therapy—a 2-year follow-up study. Radiology 1992; 184:89.

Fowler JF, Harari PM. Hyperfractionation's promise in cancer treatment. Contemp Oncol 1993;3:14.

Fu KK, Phillips TL. High dose rate versus low dose rate intracavitary brachytherapy for carcinoma of the cervix. Int J Radiat Oncol Biol Phys 1990;19:791.

Fyles A, Keane TJ, Barton M, Simm J. The effect of treatment duration in the local control of cervix cancer. Radiother Oncol 1992;25:273.

Gallion HH, Maruyama Y, van Nagell JR, et al. Treatment of stage IIIB cervical cancer with californium-252 fast-neutron brachytherapy and external photon therapy. Cancer 1987;59:1709.

Garton GR, Gunderson LL, Webb MJ, et al. Intraoperative radiation therapy in gynecologic cancer: the Mayo Clinic experience. Gynecol Oncol 1993;48:328.

Gasper LE, Cheung AYC, Allen HH. Cervical carcinoma: treatment results and complications of extended field irradiation. Radiology 1989;172:271.

Gauthier P, Gore I, Shingleton HM, Soong S-J, Orr JW Jr, Hatch KD. Identification of histopathologic risk groups in stage IB squamous cell carcinoma of the cervix. Obstet Gynecol 1985;66:569.

Georgiou A, Grigsby PW, Perez CA. Radiation induced lumbosacral plexopathy in gynecologic tumors: clinical findings and dosimetric analysis. Int J Radiat Oncol Biol Phys 1993;26:479.

Goitein M. Future prospects in planning radiation therapy. Cancer 1985;55:2234.

Goodman HM, Niloff JM, Buttlar CA, et al. Adenocarcinoma of the cervical stump. Gynecol Oncol 1989; 35:188.

Grant PT, Jeffrey JF, Fraser RC, et al. Pelvic radiation therapy for gynecologic malignancy in geriatric patients. Gynecol Oncol 1989;33:185.

Greer BE, Koh W-J, Figge DC, et al. Gynecologic radiotherapy fields defined by intraoperative measurements. Gynecol Oncol 1990;38:421.

Grigsby PW. Treatment selection for "bulky" carcinoma of the endocervix. Int J Radiat Oncol Biol Phys 1992; 23:673.

Grigsby PW, Perez CA. Radiotherapy alone for medically

inoperable carcinoma of the cervix: stage IA and carcinoma in situ. Int J Radiat Oncol Biol Phys 1991; 21:375.

Gronroos M, Klemi P, Piiroinen O, et al. Ovarian function during and after curative intracavitary high dose rate irradiation: steroidal output and morphology. Eur J Obstet Gynaecol Reprod Biol 1982;14:13.

Guthrie RT, Buchsbaum HJ, White AJ, Latourette HB. Paraaortic lymph node irradiation in carcinoma of the uterine cervix. Cancer 1974;34:166.

Hacker NF. Clinical and operative staging of cervical cancer. Baillieres Clin Obstet Gynaecol 1988;2(4):747.

Haie C, Pejovic MH, Gerbaulet A, et al. Is prophylactic paraaortic irradiation worthwhile in the treatment of advanced cervical carcinoma? Results of a controlled clinical trial of the EORTC radiotherapy group. Radiother Oncol 1988;11:101.

Hall EJ. Radiobiology for the radiologist. Hagerstown MD, Harper Row, 1978.

Hall EJ. Radiation biology. Cancer 1985;55:2051.

Hamberger AD, Fletcher GH, Wharton JT. Results of treatment of early stage I carcinoma of the uterine cervix with intracavitary radium alone. Cancer 1978;41:980.

Hamberger AD. Long term results of radium therapy in cervical cancer. Int J Radiat Oncol Biol Phys 1980;6:647.

Hancock BW, Bruce L, Whitham MD, Ward AM. The effects of radiotherapy on immunity in patients with cured localized carcinoma of the cervix uteri. Cancer 1984; 53:884.

Hanks GE, Herring DF, Kramer S. Patterns of care outcome studies: results of the national practice in cancer of the cervix. Cancer 1983;51:959.

Hemal AK, Praveen BV, San Karanara Yanan A, Vaidyanathan S. Control of persistent vesical bleeding due to radiation cystitis by intravesical application of 15 (S) 15–methyl prostaglandin F2–alpha. Indian J Cancer 1989;26:99.

Herbert SH, Curran WJ Jr, Solin LJ, et al. Decreasing gastrointestinal morbidity with the use of small bowel contrast during treatment planning for pelvic irradiation. Int J Radiat Oncol Biol Phys 1991;20:835.

Hernandez E, Lavine M, Dunton CJ, Gracely E, Parker J. Poor prognosis associated with thrombocytosis in patients with cervical cancer. Cancer 1992;69:2975.

Hilesmaa VK, Vesterinen E, Nieminen U, Grohn P. Carcinoma of the uterine cervix stage III: a report of 311 cases. Gynecol Oncol 1981;12:99.

Hintz BL, Kagan AR, Gilbert HA, et al. Systemic absorption of conjugated estrogenic cream by the irradiated vagina. Gynecol Oncol 1981;12:75.

Hodson DI, Krepart GV. Once monthly radiotherapy for the palliation of pelvic gynecological malignancy. Gynecol Oncol 1983;16:112.

Hoffman M, Roberts WS, Cavanagh D. Second pelvic malignancies following radiation therapy for cervical cancer. Obstet Gynecol Surv 1985;40(10):611.

Hong JH, Chen MS, Lin FJ, Tang SG. Prognostic assessment of tumor regression after external irradiation for cervical cancer. Int J Radiat Oncol Biol Phys 1992; 22:913.

Hopkins MP, Sutton P, Roberts JA. Prognostic features and treatment of endocervical adenocarcinoma of the cervix. Gynecol Oncol 1987;27:68.

Hopkins MP, Peters WA, Anderson W, Morley GW. Invasive cervical cancer treated initially by standard hysterectomy. Gynecol Oncol 1990;36:7.

Hopkins MP, Schmidt RW, Roberts JA, Morley GW. The prognosis and treatment of stage I adenocarcinoma of the cervix. Obstet Gynecol 1988;72:915.

Horiot J, Pigneux J, Pourquier H, et al. Radiotherapy alone in carcinoma of the intact uterine cervix according to GH Fletcher guidelines: a French cooperative study of 1383 cases. Int J Radiat Oncol Biol Phys 1988;14:605.

Hornback NB, Shupe RE, Shidnia H, et al. Advanced stage IIIB cancer of the cervix treatment by hyperthermia and radiation. Gynecol Oncol 1986;23:160.

Hughes RR, Brewington KC, Hanjani P, et al. Extended field irradiation for cervical cancer based on surgical staging. Gynecol Oncol 1980;9:153.

Inoue T, Morita K. 5-year results of postoperative extended-field irradiation on 76 patients with nodal metastases from cervical carcinoma stages IB to IIIB. Cancer 1988; 61:2009.

Inoue T, Morita K. The prognostic significance of number of positive nodes in cervical carcinoma stages IB, IIA, and IIB. Cancer 1990;65:1923.

Ito H, Kumagaya H, Shigematsu N, et al. High dose rate intracavitary brachytherapy for recurrent cervical cancer of the vaginal stump following hysterectomy. Int J Radiat Oncol Biol Phys 1991;20:927.

Jacobs AJ, Faris C, Perez CA, et al. Short-term persistence of carcinoma of the uterine cervix after radiation: An indicator of long-term prognosis. Cancer 1986;57:944.

Jampolis S, Andras EJ, Fletcher GH. Analysis of sites and causes of failures of irradiation in invasive squamous cell carcinoma of the intact uterine cervix. Radiology 1975; 115:681.

Janson PO, Jansson I, Skryten A, et al. Ovarian endocrine function in young women undergoing radiotherapy for carcinoma of the cervix. Gynecol Oncol 1981;11:218.

Johns HE. Optimization of energy and equipment. In Kramer S, Sunthralingam N, Zinninger GF, eds. High-energy photons and electrons. New York: John Wiley & Sons, 1976:33.

Jones RD, Symonds RP, et al. A comparison of remote afterloading and manually inserted cesium in the treatment of carcinoma of the cervix. Clin Oncol (R Coll Radiol) 1990;2:193.

Joslin CAF. Brachytherapy: a clinical dilemma. Int J Radiat Oncol Biol Phys 1990;19:801.

Julian CG, Kaikoku NH, Gillespie A. Adenoepidermoid and adenosquamous carcinoma of the uterus. Am J Obstet Gynecol 1977;128:106.

Kapp DS. The role of the radiation oncologist in the management of gynecologic cancer. Cancer 1983a;51:2485.

Kapp DS, Fischer D, Gutierrez G, Kohorn EI, Schwartz PE. Pretreatment prognostic factors in carcinoma of the uterine cervix: a multivariable analysis of the effect of age, stage, histology and blood counts on survival. Int J Radiat Oncol Biol Phys 1983b;9:445.

Kapp DS, Lawrence R. Temperature elevation during brachytherapy for carcinoma of the uterine cervix: adverse effect on survival and enhancement of distant metastasis. Int J Radiat Oncol Biol Phys 1984;10:2281.

Katz HJ, Davies JNP. Death from cervix uteri carcinoma: the changing pattern. Gynecol Oncol 1980;9:86.

Kavadi VS, Eifel PJ. FIGO stage IIIA carcinoma of the uterine cervix. Int J Radiat Oncol Biol Phys 1992;24:211.

Kim RY, Levy DS, Brascho DJ, Hatch KD. Uterine perforation during intracavitary application. Prognostic significance in carcinoma of the cervix. Radiology 1983; 147:249.

Kim RY, Salter MM, Weppelmann B, Brascho DJ. Analysis of treatment modalities and their failures in stage IB cancer of the cervix. Int J Radiat Oncol Biol Phys 1988; 15:831.

Kinsella TJ, Bloomer WD. New therapeutic strategies in radiation therapy. JAMA 1981;245:1669.

Kiricuta I, Goldstein AMB. The repair of extensive vesico-vaginal fistulas with pedicled omentum: a review of 27 cases. J Urol 1972;108:724.

Kirkinen P, Kauppila A, Kontturi M. Treatment of ureteral strictures after therapy for carcinoma of the uterus. Surgery Gynecol Obstet 1980;151:487.

Kleine W, Rau K, Schwoeorer D, et al. Prognosis of the adenocarcinoma of the cervix uteri. A comparative study. Gynecol Oncol 1989;35:145.

Kolstad P. Followup study of 232 patients with stage IAa and 411 patients with stage IA2 squamous cell carcinoma of the cervix (microinvasive cardinoma). Gynecol Oncol 1989;33:265.

Komaki R, Mattingly RF, Hoffman RG, et al. Irradiation of para-aortic lymph node metastases from carcinoma of the cervix or endometrium. Preliminary results. Radiology 1983;147:245.

Komaki R, Pajak TF, Marcial VA, et al. Twice-daily fractionation of external irradiation with brachytherapy in bulky carcinoma of the cervix. Cancer 1994;73:2619.

Kovalic JJ, Perez CA, Grigsby PW, Lockett MA. The effect of volume of disease in patients with carcinoma of the uterine cervix. Int J Radiat Oncol Biol Phys 1991b;21:905-10.

Kraiphibul P, Srisupundit S, et al. Results of treatment in stage IIB squamous cell carcinoma of the uterine cervix: comparison between two and one cavitary insertion. Gynecol Oncol 1992;45:160.

Kramer C, Peschel RE, Goldberg N, et al. Radiation treatment of FIGO stage IVA carcinoma of the cervix. Gynecol Oncol 1989;32:323.

Kucera H, Enzelsberger H, Eppel W, Weghaut K. The influence of nicotine abuse and diabetes mellitus on the results of primary irradiation in the treatment of carcinoma of the cervix. Cancer 1987;60:1.

Kuipers T. Dosimetry and complication rate in the treatment of cervix carcinoma with external irradiation and brachytherapy. Strahlenther Onkol 1980;82(suppl):127.

Kurohara SS, DiSaia P, Kurohara J, et al. Uterine cervical cancer: treatment with megavoltage radiation results and afterloading intracavitary techniques. Am J Radiol 1979;133:293.

Lanciano RM, Pajak TF, Martz K, Hanks GE. The influence of treatment time on outcome for squamous cell cancer of the cervix treated with radiation: a patterns-of-care study. Int J Radiat Oncol Biol Phys 1993;25:391.

Lanciano RM, Martz K, Montana GS, Hanks GE. Influence of age, prior abdominal surgery, fraction size, and dose on complications after radiation therapy for squamous cell cancer of the uterine cervix. A patterns of care study. Cancer 1992a;69:2124.

Lanciano RM, Corn BW. Radiotherapy for gynecologic malignancies. Curr Opin Oncol 1992b;4:930.

Lanciano RM, Won M, Coia LR, Hanks GE. Pretreatment and treatment factors associated with improved outcome in squamous cell carcinoma of the uterine cervix: a final report of the 1973 and 1978 patterns of care studies. Int J Radiat Oncol Biol Phys 1991a;20:667.

Lanciano RM, Martz K, Coia LR, Hanks GE. Tumor and treatment factors improving outcome in stage IIIB cervic cancer. Int J Radiat Oncol Biol Phys 1991b;20:95.

Lantz B, Einhorn N. Intestinal damage and malabsorption after treatment for cervical carcinoma. Acta Radiol Oncol 1984;23:33.

LaPolla JP, Schlaerth JB, Gaddis O, Morrow CP. The influence of surgical staging on the evaluation and treatment of patients with cervical carcinoma. Gynecol Oncol 1986;24:194.

Larson JE, Whitney CW, Zaino R, et al. Case report: endometrial response to endogenous hormones after pelvic irradiation for genital malignancies. Gynecol Oncol 1990;36:106.

Lee KR, Mansfield CM, Dwyer SJ III, et al. CT for intracavitary radiotherapy planning. Am J Radiol 1980;135:809.

Levenback C, Gershenson DM, McGehee R, et al. Enterovesical fistula following radiotherapy for gynecologic cancer 1994;52:296.

Levenback C, Eifel P, Turke T, Morris M, Gershenson D. Hemorrhagic cystitis following radiotherapy for stage IB cancer of the cervix (abstract). 25th Annual Meeting of the Society of Gynecologic Oncologists, Orlando, Florida, February 6, 1994.

Lichter AS, Ten Haken RK. Three-dimensional treatment planning and conformal radiation dose delivery. Principles and practice of oncology updates, vol 8(5). Philadelphia: JB Lippincott, 1994.

Lovecchio JL, Averette HE, Donato D, Bell J. 5-year survival of patients with periaortic nodal metastases in clinical stage IB and IIA cervical carcinoma. Gynecol Oncol 1989;34:43.

Lowery GC, Mendenhall WM, Million RR. Stage IB or IIA-B carcinoma of the intact uterine cervix treated with irradiation: a multivariate analysis. Int J Radiat Oncol Biol Phys 1992;24:205.

Mann WJ Jr, Levy D, Hatch KD, Shingleton HM, Soong S-J. Prognostic significance of age in stage I carcinoma of the cervix. South Med J 1980;73:1186.

Mann WJ Jr, Hatch KD, Taylor PT, Partridge EM, Orr JW Jr, Singleton HM. The role of percutaneous nephrostomy in gynecologic oncology. Gynecol Oncol 1983; 16:393.

Marcial VA, Bosch A. Fractionation in radiation therapy of carcinoma of the uterine cervix. Results of a prospective study of 3 vs. 5 fractions per week. Front Radiat Ther Oncol 1968;3:238.

Marcial VA, Amato DA, Marks RD, et al. Split course versus continuous pelvic irradiation in carcinoma of the uterine cervix: a prospective randomized clinical trial of the radiation therapy oncology group. Int J Radiat Oncol Biol Phys 1983;9:431.

Marcial LV, Marcial VA, Krall JM, et al. Comparison of 1 vs. 2 or more intracavitary brachytherapy applications in the management of carcinoma of the cervix, with irradiation alone. Int J Radiat Oncol Biol Phys 1991;20:81.

Martinez A, Cox RS, Edmundson GK. A multiple-site perineal applicator (MUPIT) for treatment of prostatic, anorectal and gynecologic malignancies. Int J Radiat Oncol Biol Phys 1984;10:297.

Maruyama Y, Yoneda J, van Nagell JR, et al. Tumor regression and histologic clearance after neutron brachytherapy for bulky localized cervical carcinoma. Cancer 1982;50:2802.

Maruyama Y, Feola JM, Wierzbicki J, et al. Clinical study of relative biological effectiveness for cervical carcinoma treated by ^{252}Cf neutrons and assessed by histological tumour eradication. Br J Radiol 1990a;63:270.

Maruyama Y, Feola JM, Wierzbicki J. Evaluation of time-dose and fractionation for ^{252}Cf neutrons in preoperative bulky-barrel cervix carcinoma radiotherapy. Int J Radiat Oncol Biol Phys 1990b;19:1561.

Maruyama Y, van Nagell JR, Yoneda J, et al. A review of californium-252 neutron brachytherapy for cervical cancer. Cancer 1991a;68:1189.

Maruyama Y, Van Nagell JR, Yoneda J, et al. Specimen findings and survival after preoperative Cf-252 neutron brachytherapy for stage II cervical carcinoma. Gynecol Oncol 1991b;43:252.

Maruyama Y, Yoneda J, Coffey C, Wierzbicki J. Tandem-vaginal cylinder applicator for radiation therapy of uterine adenocracinoma. Radiother Oncol 1992;25:140.

Maruyama Y, van Nagell JR, Yoneda J, et al. Schedule of Cf-252 neutron brachytherapy: complications after delayed implant therapy for cervical cancer in a phase II trial. Am J Clin Oncol 1993;16(2):168.

Matsuyama T, Tsukamoto N, Matsukuma K, et al. Uterine perforation at the time of brachytherapy for the carcinoma of the uterine cervix. Gynecol Oncol 1986; 23:205.

McKay MJ, Bull CA, Houghton CR, Langlands AO. Letter to the editor. Gynecol Oncol 1990;39:236.

Mendenhall WM, Thar TL, Bova FJ, et al. Prognostic and treatment factors affecting pelvic control of stage IB and IIA-B carcinoma of the intact uterine cervix treated with radiation therapy alone. Cancer 1984;53:2649.

Miller BE, Copeland LJ, Hamberger AD, et al. Carcinoma of the cervical stump. Gynecol Oncol 1984;18:100.

Million RR, Rutledge F, Fletcher GH. Stage IV carcinoma of the cervix with bladder invasion. Am J Obstet Gynecol 1972;113:239.

Milsom I, Friberg LB. Primary adenocarcinoma of the uterine cervix. A clinical study. Cancer 1983;52:942.

Moberg PJ, Einhorn N, Sifversward C, Soderberg G. Adenocarcinoma of the uterine cervix. Cancer 1986;57:407.

Montana GS, Fowler WC, Varia MA, et al. Carcinoma of the cervix, stage III: results of radiation therapy. Cancer 1986;57:148.

Montana GS, Fowler WC, Varia MA, et al. Analysis of results of radiation therapy for stage IB carcinoma of the cervix. Cancer 1989;60:2195.

Munzenrider JE, Coppke KP, et al. Three-dimensional treatment planning for paraaortic node irradiation in patients with cervical cancer. Int J Radiat Oncol Biol Phys 1991;21:229.

Murray MJ. New techniques in radiation therapy for cervical cancer. Clin Obstet Gynecol 1990;33(4):889.

Nahhas WA, Nisce LZ, D'Angio CJ, Lewis JL Jr. Lateral ovarian transposition. Obstet Gynecol 1971;38:785.

Nelson JH Jr, Boyce J, Macasaet M, et al. Incidence, significance and follow-up of para-aortic lymph node metastases in late invasive carcinoma of the cervix. Am J Obstet Gynecol 1977;128:336.

Nordqvist SRB, Jaramillo B, Sudarsanam A, et al. Selective therapy for early cancer of the cervix. II. Surgically non-explored cases. Gynecol Oncol 1979;7:257.

Nori D, Valentine E, Hilaris BS. The role of paraaortic node irradiation in the treatment of cancer of the cervix. Int J Radiat Oncol Biol Phys 1985;11:1469.

Orr JW Jr, Ball GC, Soong SJ, et al. Surgical treatment of women found to have invasive cervical cancer at the time of total hysterectomy. Obstet Gynecol 1986;68:353.

Orr JW Jr, Barrett JM, Holloway RW. Neoplasia in pregnancy. In Moore TR, Reiter RC, Reban RW, Baker VV (eds). Gynecology and obstetrics: a longitudinal approach. New York: Churchill Livingstone 1993.

Orr JW Jr, Brown KF. Cardiovascular complications. In Orr JW Jr, Shingleton HM (eds). Complications in gynecologic surgery: prevention, recognition, and management. Philadelphia: JB Lippincott 1994.

Orr JW Jr, Holloway RW. Surgical aspects of cervical cancer. Surg Clin North Am 1991;71:1067.

Orr JW Jr, Shingleton HM. Nutritional assessment and support: importance in surgical and cancer patients. J Reprod Med 1984;29:635.

Orr JW Jr, Wilson K, Bodiford C, et al. Nutritional status of patients with untreated cervical cancer. Am J Obstet Gynecol 1985;151:625.

Orton CG, Seyedsadr M, Somnay A. Comparison of high and low dose rate remote afterloading for cervix cancer and the importance of fractionation. Int J Radiat Oncol Biol Phys 1991;21:1425.

Orton CG. Fractionation is important for HDR cervix cancer brachytherapy. Int J Radiat Oncol Biol Phys 1992a;22:222.

Orton CG. Letter to the editor. Int J Radiat Oncol Biol Phys 1992b;24:387.

Otchy DP, Nelson H. Radiation injuries of the colon and rectum. Surg Clin North Am 1993;73(5):1017.

Palmer JA, Busch RS. Radiation injuries to the bowel associated with the treatment of carcinoma of the cervix. Surgery 1976;80:458.

Parker M, Bosscher J, Barnhill D, Park R. Ovarian management during radical hysterectomy in the premenopausal patient. Obstet Gynecol 1993;82(2):187.

Parkin DE. Lower urinary tract complications of the treatment of cervical carcinoma. Obstet Gynecol Surv 1989;44(7):523.

Parliament M, Genest P, Girard A, et al. Obstructive ureteropathy following radiation therapy for carcinoma of the cervix. Gynecol Oncol 1989;33:237.

Perez CA, Camel RM, Kuske RR, et al. Radiation therapy alone in the treatment of carcinoma of the uterine cervix: a 20-year experience. Gynecol Oncol 1986;23:127.

Perez CA, Grigsby PW, Nene SM, et al. Effect of tumor size on the prognosis of carcinoma of the uterine cervix treated with irradiation alone. Cancer 1992;69:2796.

Perez CA. Part I. Radiation therapy in the management of cancer of the cervix. Oncology 1993;7(2):89.

Perkins PL, Chu AM, Jose B, et al. Posthysterectomy megavoltage irradiation in the treatment of cervical carcinoma. Gynecol Oncol 1984;17:340.

Petersen LK, Mamsen A, Jakobsen A. Carcinoma of the cervical stump. Gynecol Oncol 1992;46:199.

Pettersson F, Ryberg M, Malker B. Second primary cancer after treatment of invasive carcinoma of the uterine cervix, compared with those arriving after treatment for in situ carcinomas: an effect of irradiation? Acta Obstet Gynaecol Scand 1990;69:161.

Pillai R, Balaram P, Nair BS, et al. Lymphocyte subset distribution after radiation therapy for cancer of the uterine cervix. Cancer 1991;67:2071.

Pitkin RM, VanVoorhis LW. Postirradiation vaginitis: an evaluation of prophylaxis with topical estrogen. Radiology 1971;99:417.

Piver MS, Lele S. Enterovaginal and enterocutaneous fistulae in women with gynecologic malignancies. Obstet Gynecol 1976;48:560.

Piver MS, Barlow JJ, Krishnamsetty R. Five-year survival (with no evidence of disease) in patients with biopsy-confirmed aortic node metastasis from cervical carcinoma. Am J Obstet Gynecol 1981;139:575.

Pizzarello DJ, Roses DF, Newall J, Barish RJ. The carcinogenicity of radiation therapy. Surgery Gynecol Obstet 1984;159:189.

Podczaski E, Stryker JA, Kaminski P, et al. Extended-field radiation therapy for carcinoma of the cervix. Cancer 1990;66:251.

Potish RA, Twiggs LB, Prem KA, et al. The impact of extraperitoneal surgical staging on morbidity and tumor recurrence following radiotherapy for cervical carcinoma. Am J Clin Oncol 1984;7:245.

Potish RA, Twiggs LB, Adcock LL, et al. Para-aortic lymph node radiotherapy in cancer of the uterine corpus. Obstet Gynecol 1985;65:251.

Potish RA, Downey GO, Adcock LL, Prem KA, Twiggs LB. The role of surgical debulking in cancer of the uterine cervix. Int J Radiat Oncol Biol Phys 1989;17:979.

Potish RA, Twiggs LB, Prem KA, Carson LF, Adcock LL. Surgical intervention following multimodality therapy for advanced cervical cancer. Gynecol Oncol 1990a;38:175.

Pulay AT, Fust G, Caomor A. Serum complement levels in patients with cancer of the uterine cervix before and after radiation therapy. Neoplasma 1980;27:211.

Pulay AT, Benczur M, Varga M. Natural killer lymphocyte function in cervical cancer patients. Neoplasma 1982;29:237.

Rafii M, Firooznia H, Golimbu C, Horner N. Radiation induced fractures of sacrum: CT diagnosis. J Comput Assist Tomogr 1988;12(2):231.

Richter MP, Laramore GE, Griffin TW, Goodman RL. Current status of high linear energy transfer irradiation. Cancer 1984;54:2814.

Roberts WS, Hoffman MS, et al. Management of radionecrosis of the vulva and distal vagina. Am J Obstet Gynecol 1991;164:1235.

Rogers CC, Levitt SY, Crosby WC, Brandt EN Jr. Effect of hypertension and arteriosclerosis on response to radiation therapy of carcinoma of the cervix: a retrospective clinical study. Radiology 1967;89:733.

Roh HD, Boucher Y, Kalnicki S, et al. Interstitial hypertension in carcinoma of uterine cervix in patients; possible correlation with tumor oxygenation and radiation response. Cancer Res 1991;51:6695.

Roman LD, Morris M, Eifel PJ, et al. Reasons for inappropriate simple hysterectomy in the presence of invasive cancer of the cervix. Obstet Gynecol 1992;79:485.

Roman LD, Morris M, Mitchell MF, Eifel PJ, Burke TW, Atkinson EN. Prognostic factors for patients undergoing simple hysterectomy in the presence of invasive cancer of the cervix. Gynecol Oncol 1993;50:179.

Roswit B, Malsky T, Reid CB. Severe radiation injuries of the stomach, small intestine, colon and rectum. Am J Roentgenol Radium Ther Nucl Med 1972;114:460.

Rotman M, Choi K, Guze C, Marcial V, Hornback N, John M. Prophylactic irradiation of the para-aortic lymph node chain in stage IIB and bulky stage IB carcinoma of the cervix, initial treatment results of RTOG 7920. Int J Radiat Oncol Biol Phys 1990;19:513.

Rotte K. A randomized clinical trial comparing a high dose rate with a conventional dose-rate technique. In Bates TD, Berry RJ, eds. High dose rate afterloading in the treatment of cancer of the uterus. Br J Radiol Special Report 1980;17:75.

Rousseau J, Fenton J, Debertrand P, Mathieu G. Carcinoma of the cervix. Radiology 1972;103:413.

Rubin S. Which patients can have their para-aortic node metastases controlled by para-aortic radiation. (Letter) Int J Radiat Oncol Biol Phys 1984;10:2167.

Rubin P, Casarett GW. Clinical radiation pathology, vol II. Philadelphia: WB Saunders, 1968:919.

Rubin P, Prabhasawat D. Characteristic bone lesions in post-irradiated carcinoma of the cervix: metastases versus osteonecrosis. Radiology 1961;76:703.

Rutledge FN, Galakatos AE, Warton JT, Smith JP. Adenocarcinoma of the uterine cervix. Am J Obstet Gynecol 1975;122:236.

Saphner T, Gallion HH, van Nagell JR, et al. Neurologic complications of cervical cancer: a review of 2261 cases. Cancer 1989;64:1147.

Sato S, Yajima A, Suzuki M. Therapeutic results using high-dose-rate intracavitary irradiation in cases of cervical cancer. Gynecol Oncol 1984;19:143.

Schellhas HG. Extraperitoneal para-aortic node dissection through an upper abdominal incision. Obstet Gynecol 1975;46:444.

Schmitt EH III, Symmonds RE. Surgical treatment of radiation induced injuries of the intestine. Surgery Gynecol Obstet 1981;153:896.

Schoeppel SL, LaVigne ML, McShan D, et al. 3-D treatment planning of intracavitary gynecologic implants: analysis of ten cases and implications for dose specification. Int J. Radiat Oncol Biol Phys 1990;19(suppl):129.

Seow Choen F, Goh HS, Eu KW, Ho YH, Tay SK. A simple and effective treatment for hemorrhagic radiation proctitis using formalin. Dis Colon Rectum 1993;36:135.

Shah K, Olson MH, Dillard EA. Carcinoma of the cervix: surgical staging and radiotherapy with 32 MeV betatron. Int J Radiat Oncol Biol Phys 1982;8:1601.

Shanahan TG, Mehta MP, Gehring MA, et al. Minimization of small bowel volume utilizing customized "belly board" mold. Int J Radiat Oncol Biol Phys 1989; 17:187.

Shierholz JD, Buchsbaum HJ, Lifshitz S, Latourette HB. Pyometra complicating radiation therapy of uterine malignancy. J Reprod Med 1977;19:100.

Shigematsu Y, Nishiyama K, Masaki N, et al. Treatment of carcinoma of the uterine cervix by remotely controlled afterloading intracavitary radiotherapy with high dose rate: a comparative study with a low-dose rate system. Int J Radiat Oncol Biol Phys 1983;9:351.

Shingleton HM, Gore H, Soong S-J, Bradley D. Adenocarcinoma of the cervix: I. Clinical evaluation and pathological features. Am J Obstet Gynecol 1981;138:799.

Sismondi P, Sinistrero G, Zola P, et al. Complications of uterine cervix carcinoma treatments: the problem of a uniform classification. Radiother Oncol 1989;14:9.

Smit BM. Prospects for proton therapy in carcinoma of the cervix. Int J Radiat Oncol Biol Phys 1991;22:349.

Smith JP, Golden PE, Rutledge FN. Surgical management of intestinal injuries following irradiation for carcinoma of the cervix. In Clinical Conference on Cancer, MD Anderson Hospital and Tumor Institute, Houston. Cancer of the uterus and ovary: a collection of papers. Chicago: Year Book Medical Publishers, 1966:241.

Smith ST, Seski JC, Copeland LJ, et al. The surgical management of irradiation induced small bowel damage. Obstet Gynecol 1985;65:563.

Solberger O, Sorbe B. Fever, haemoglobin and smoking as prognostic factors during the treatment of cervical carcinoma by radiotherapy. Eur J Gynaecol Oncol 1990; XI(2):97.

Souhami L, Melo JAC, Pareja V. The treatment of stage III carcinoma of the uterine cervix with telecobalt irradiation. Gynecol Oncol 1987;28:262.

Stehman FB, Bundy BN, DiSaia PJ, et al. Carcinoma of the cervix treated with radiation therapy I. Cancer 1991;67:2776.

Stehman FB, Bundy BN. Carcinoma of the cervix treated with chemotherapy and radiation therapy. Cooperative studies in the gynecologic oncology group. Cancer 1993;71:1697.

Stitt JA. High-dose-rate intracavitary brachytherapy for gynecologic malignancies. Oncology 1992;6(1):59.

Stitt JA, Fowler JF, Thomadsen BR, et al. High dose rate intracavitary brachytherapy for carcinoma of the cervix: the Madison system: I. Clinical and radiobiological considerations. Int J Radiat Oncol Biol Phys 1992a; 24:335.

Stitt JA, Fowler JF, Thomadsen BR. High dose rate brachytherapy for cervical carcinoma. Int J Radiat Oncol Biol Phys 1992b;24:574. Letter.

Stryker JA, Sommerville K, Perez R, Velkley DE. Sacral plexus injury after radiotherapy for carcinoma of cervix. Cancer 1990;66:1488.

Sudarsanam A, Charyulu K, Belinson J, et al. Influence of exploratory celiotomy on the management of carcinoma of the cervix. Cancer 1978;41:1049.

Suresh UR, Smith VJ, Lupton EW, Haboubi NY. Radiation disease of the urinary tract: histological features of 18 cases. J Clin Pathol 1993;46:228.

Surwit EA, Alberts DS, Aristizabel S, et al. Treatment of primary and recurrent, advanced squamous cell cancer of the cervix with mitomycin-C + vincristine + bleomycin (MOB) plus cisplatin (PLAT). In Proceedings of the American Society of Clinical Oncologists, 1983. Abstract C-496.

Sutton G, Bundy B, Delgado G, et al. Ovarian metastases in stage IB carcinoma of the cervix: a Gynecologic Oncology Group study. Am J Obstet Gynecol 1992;166:50.

Sutton G, Bundy B, Delgado G, et al. Evaluation of the role of radiotherapy following radical hysterectomy in patients with clinical stage IB squamous carcinoma of the cervix: a study of the gynecologic oncology group. 24th Annual Meeting, Society of Gynecologic Oncologists, Palm Desert, California, February 7–10, 1993.

Taylor PT, Andersen WA. Untreated cervical cancer complicated by obstructive uropathy and oliguric renal failure. Gynecol Oncol 1981;11:162.

Taylor PM, Johnson RJ, et al. Radiological changes in the gastrointestinal and genitourinary tract following radiotherapy for carcinoma of the cervix. Clin Radiol 1990;41:165.

Teshima T, Inoue T, Chatani M, et al. Radiation therapy of the para-aortic lymph nodes in carcinoma of the uterine cervix: the concurrent use of cimetidine to reduce acute and subacute side effects from radiation. Clin Ther 1990;12:71.

Teshima T, Inoue T, Ikeda H, et al. High-dose rate and low-dose rate intracavitary therapy for carcinoma of the uterine cervix. Cancer 1993;72:2409.

Tewfik H, Buchsbaum HJ, Lifshitz S, Latourette HB. Para-aortic lymph node irradiation in carcinoma of the cervix after exploratory laparotomy and biopsy-proven positive aortic nodes. Int J Radiat Oncol Biol Phys 1982;8:13.

Thomadsen BR, Shahabi S, Stitt JA, et al. High dose rate intracavitary brachytherapy for carcinoma of the cervix: the Madison system: II. Procedural and physical considerations. Int J Radiat Oncol Biol Phys 1992;24:349.

Thomas G, Dembo A, Beale F, et al. A phase I-II study of mitomycin C (MIT), 5-fluorouracil (5FU) and radiation therapy (RT) in poor prognosis carcinoma of cervix. Proceedings of the American Society of Clinical Oncologists. Int Radiat Oncol Biol Phys 1984;10:1785.

Thomas G, Dembo A, Beale F, et al. Concurrent radiation, mitomycin C and 5-fluorouracil in poor prognosis carcinoma of cervix: preliminary results of a phase I-II study. Int J Radiat Oncol Biol Phys 1984b;10:1785.

To WWK, Ngan Hys, Wong LC, Choy DTK, Ma HK. Use of prophylactic antibiotics in patients with carcinoma of the cervix receiving intracavitary radium insertion. Eur J Gynaec Oncol 1993;XIV(3):197.

Toki N, Tsukamoto N, Kaku T, et al. Microscopic ovarian metastasis of the uterine cervical cancer. Gynecol Oncol 1991;41:46.

Tubiana M, Arriagada R, Cosset JM. Sequencing of drugs and radiation: the integrated alternating regimen. Cancer 1985;55:2131.

Vahrson G, Romer G. 5-year results with HDR afterloading in cervix cancer: dependence on fractionation and dose. Strahlenther Onkol 1988;82(suppl):139.

Valerio D, Overett L, Malcolm A, et al. Nutritional support for cancer patients receiving abdominal and pelvic radiotherapy: a randomized preoperative clinical experiment of intravenous versus oral feeding. Surg Forum 1978; 29:145.

Van Herik M. Fever as a complication of radiation therapy for carcinoma of the cervix. Am J Roentgenol Rad Ther Nucl Med 1965;93:104.

VanLancker M, Storme G. Prediction of severe late complications in fractionated, high dose raet brachytherapy in gynecological applications. Int J Radiat Oncol Biol Phys 1991;20:1125.

van Nagell JR Jr, Maruyama Y, Parker JC Jr, Dalton WL. Small bowel injury following radiation therapy for cervical cancer. Am J Obstet Gynecol 1974a;118:163.

van Nagell JR Jr, Parker JC Jr, Maruyama Y, et al. The effect of pelvic inflammatory disease on enteric complications following radiation therapy for cervical cancer. Am J Obstet Gynecol 1977;128:767.

van Nagell JR Jr, Kieler R, Donaldson ES, et al. Correlation between retinal and pelvic vascular status: a determinant factor in patients undergoing pelvic irradiation for gynecologic malignancy. Am J Obstet Gynecol 1979; 134:551.

van Nagell JR Jr, Barber HRK, eds. Modern concepts of gynecologic oncology. Boston, John Wright-PSG, 1982.

Varghese CV, Rangad F, Jose CC, et al. Hyperfractionation in advanced carcinoma of the uterine cervix: a preliminary report. Int J Radiat Oncol Biol Phys 1992;23:393.

Vigliotti AP, Wen B-C, Hussey DH, et al. Extended field irradiation for carcinoma of the uterine cervix with positive periaortic nodes. Int J Radiat Oncol Biol Phys 1992;22:501.

Welander CE, Pierce VK, Nori D, et al. Pretreatment laparotomy in carcinoma of the cervix. Gynecol Oncol 1981;12:336.

Wentz WB, Reagan JW. Survival in cervical cancer with respect to cell type. Cancer 1959;12(2):384.

West CM, Davidson SE, Hendry JH, Hunter RD. Prediction of cervical carcinoma response to radiotherapy. Lancet 1991;338:818. Letter.

Wharton JT, Jones HW III, Day TG Jr, et al. Pre-irradiation celiotomy and extended field irradiation for invasive carcinoma of the cervix. Obstet Gynecol 1977;49:333.

Wheeless CR Jr, Graham R, Graham JB. Prognosis and treatment of adenoepidermoid carcinoma of the cervix. Obstet Gynecol 1970;35:928.

Wheeless CR Jr. Small bowel bypass for complications related to pelvic malignancy. Obstet Gynecol 1973;42:661.

White AC. An atlas of radiation histopathology. Washington

DC: Technical Information Center, U.S. Energy Research and Developmental Administration, 1975.

Whitmore GF. Summary of conference in time and dose relationships in radiation biology as applied to radiotherapy. Brookhaven National Laboratory Report 50203 1969; (C-57):353:8.

Wilkinson S. Early post-irradiation bowel obstruction managed by longitudinal serotomy. Aust NZ J Surg 1990; 60:136.

Withers HR. Biologic basis for altered fractionation schemes. Cancer 1985;55:2086.

Wong F, Bhimji S. The usefulness of ultrasonography in intracavitary radiotherapy using selectron applicators. Int J Radiat Oncol Biol Phys 1990;19:477.

Yeoh E, Horowitz M, Russo A, et al. A retrospective study of the effects of pelvic irradiation for carcinoma of the cervix on gastrointestinal function. Int J Radiat Oncol Biol Phys 1993;26:229.

Cancer of the Cervix by Hugh M. Shingleton and James W. Orr, Jr.
J. B. Lippincott Company, Philadelphia, © 1995.

9

Other Treatments

The treatment of choice for early-stage nonbulky cervical cancer is radical surgery, whereas radiation therapy is appropriate therapy for the remaining patients, including those with bulky pelvic disease and advanced-stage tumors. The literature, however, describes many combinations of therapy involving surgery, radiation therapy, and chemotherapy and in some cases, immunotherapy. Additionally, oncologists are responsible for the treatment of women having rare tissue types such as sarcoma, melanoma, lymphoma, and small cell (neuroendocrine) cervical tumors. Many of these tumors are treated by combinations of therapy. This chapter addresses multimodality therapy as a planned approach to certain clinical situations.

ADJUVANT HYSTERECTOMY AFTER RADIATION

Little rationale exists for the planned combination of irradiation followed by adjuvant total abdominal hysterectomy (Marcial et al 1993) because the combination of extrafascial hysterectomy and radiation therapy significantly increases intestinal and urinary complications. Residual postradiation microscopic disease in the hysterectomy specimen (even in the presence of negative pelvic nodes) is associated with a significant decrease in survival (Davidson 1989). Maruyama (1991), reporting on 27 patients having operable International Federation of Gynecology and Obstetrics (FIGO) stage II disease, indicated a statistically adverse effect on survival (93% versus 46%) when residual tumor was discovered at the time of extrafascial hysterectomy and abdominal staging after intracavitary and whole-pelvis irradiation. It has not been shown that this combination improves survival, and we do not advocate it.

PREOPERATIVE IRRADIATION AND EXTRAFASCIAL HYSTERECTOMY FOR BULKY LESIONS

Advocacy of preoperative irradiation and extrafascial hysterectomy for bulky or barrel-shaped stage IB or stage II disease originated with publications from the M.D. Anderson Hospital (Nelson et al 1975, Fletcher 1979). Barrel-shaped tumors are those that expand the lower uterine segment, such that the lateral extension of the tumor mass may extend beyond the usual isodose curves of brachytherapy (Fig. 9-1). Heightened concerns regarding central pelvic recurrence prompted many centers to adopt Fletcher's approach and to deliver whole-pelvis teletherapy (40 to 50 Gy) and a single intracavitary application of cesium before conservative hysterectomy. This treatment was found to decrease the rate of central pelvic recurrence, although significant improvement in long-term survival has not been demonstrated in most series (Table 9-1). Edinger and associates (1984) observed that prognosis depended on the ability of radiation therapy to sterilize the central lesion. In their series, none of the patients whose primary lesions were sterilized by radiation therapy before hysterectomy died of disease, whereas more than 50% of patients whose primary lesions were incompletely sterilized were found to be at significant risk of recurrent (and distant) metastatic disease. These findings confirmed an earlier observation by Nelson and coworkers (1975) that recurrences after a combined treatment plan of irradiation–extrafascial hysterectomy are more likely at distant sites and not within the irradiation field. For this reason, Edinger and colleagues also suggested that adjunctive hysterectomy may in effect be used as a directed biopsy after radiation therapy to identify patients for adjunctive chemotherapy or exenterative surgery.

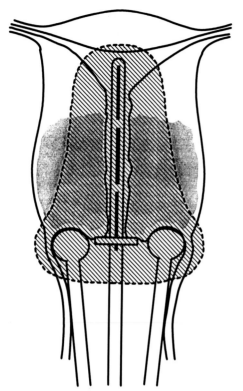

FIGURE 9-1. Stage IB "barrel-shaped" tumor with intra-cavitary implant in place. Note that the tumor border is beyond the curative isodose curve. (Modified from Gallion HH, van Nagell JR Jr, Donaldson ES, et al. Combined radiation therapy and extrafascial hysterectomy in the treatment of stage IB barrel-shaped cervical cancer. Cancer 1985,56:262, with permission.)

Perez and associates (1985, 1987), in retrospective analyses of 128 patients with barrel-shaped or expanded cervical lesions (more than 5 cm), failed to document a survival benefit of use of postradiation hysterectomy over complete radiation therapy alone. Overall complications were increased (21% versus 7%) in those patients having large lesions (more than 5 cm) undergoing combined surgery and irradiation, as compared with those treated by irradiation alone.

Although more recurrences were apparent in women who had bulky central tumors, Mendenhall (1991), evaluating the role of adjuvant hysterectomy in 150 patients having large (≥6 cm) tumors, indicated no difference in cause-specific (62% versus 55%) or absolute 5-year survival (54% versus 52%). However, overall complications were increased threefold (16% versus 5%) in patients undergoing combined therapy.

Thoms and coworkers (1992) reviewed the M. D. Anderson experience with bulky cervical tumors (6 or more cm); whereas survival was significantly decreased in those women with 8-cm tumors, they reported no

survival advantage of postradiation hysterectomy in patients who had no pretreatment lymph node involvement and no posttreatment palpable parametrial disease. Pelvic control rates were not different. Treatment-related deaths in patients with such bulky disease were high (3.6%).

In our practice, we have treated barrel-shaped tumors with curative doses of radiation therapy and only intervened surgically in the event of lack of tumor shrinkage on completion of the irradiation; in this case, we have at times selected anterior pelvic exenteration to complete the therapy. Thus, we have never advocated combined irradiation and extrafascial hysterectomy as routine treatment.

Prempree and colleagues (1985) and Eifel and associates (1991) studied patients having bulky stage IB, stage II, or barrel-shaped adenocarcinoma treated by radiation and extrafascial hysterectomy (see Table 9-1). Prempree and coworkers observed an advantage for combined therapy only in large (4 or more cm) stage IB or stage II tumors but not for the smaller adenocarcinomas. Eifel and associates reported no advantage of combined therapy over irradiation therapy alone but noted that those patients treated only by radical hysterectomy had a higher recurrence rate than those treated by combined therapy or irradiation alone. Eifel and coworkers (1990) reported no survival advantage of irradiation plus surgery over irradiation alone in patients who had bulky early-stage adenocarcinoma.

Combined preoperative irradiation–extrafascial hysterectomy (Table 9-2) is associated with more complications than the use of either modality alone. The incidence of bowel and urologic complications seems to exceed that of surgery or irradiation used alone. Some authors reported a high rate of vaginal vault necrosis or vaginal strictures (Perkins et al 1984, Weems et al 1985). In contrast, Thoms and colleagues (1992) reported no significant differences when comparing complications from irradiation alone and irradiation followed by surgery. The potential for increased complications should thus be a consideration in selecting combined irradiation–surgery for patients having bulky stage I and II disease of either major tissue type.

Bachaud and associates (1991), reporting a retrospective analysis of 252 combined-therapy patients, could not demonstrate a survival benefit of adjuvant surgery but indicated a 2.5% mortality rate in patients having stage IB or early IIB disease who were subjected to such therapy.

The value of extrafascial hysterectomy after irradiation is controversial. Although pelvic recurrence may be lessened by the addition of the adjunctive hysterectomy after radiation therapy, a long-term survival advantage is not apparent and complications, including treatment-associated mortality, are higher with the combined approach.

TABLE 9-1
Value of Extrafascial Hysterectomy After Irradiation

STUDY	YEAR	PATIENTS (N)	HISTOLOGY	STAGE	SURVIVAL ADVANTAGE OVER SINGLE MODALITY?
Gallion, et al	1985	79	Predominantly SCC	Bulky/barrel stage IB	Pelvic recurrence decreased from 19% to 2%; Increased survival (no figures quoted)
Maruyama, et al	1989	80	"	Bulky/barrel stage IB	No Controls; 84% 5-year survival not shown to be superior to single modality therapy
Abayomi, et al	1990	24	"	Bulky stage II	Hysterectomy did not improve therapy results
Coleman, et al	1992	43	"	Bulky/barrel stage IB, II	"
Thoms, et al	1992	134	"	IB	No significant differences in survival (p=.46) in comparing radiation alone and radiation followed by hysterectomy
Prempree, et al	1985	29	Adenocarcinoma	IB, II	Radical surgery or radiation equal to combined RT/TAH for stage IB; improved survival in large IB ($\geq$4 cm) or II with radiation/TAH
Eifel, et al	1991	20	"	IB	RT/TAH pelvic recurrence rates identical to those treated by radiotherapy alone but for less (11% vs 45%) than those greated by RHPND alone

R*T/TAH*, radiotherapy/total abdominal hysterectomy; *RHPND*, radical hysterectomy, pelvic node dissection.

PREOPERATIVE IRRADIATION AND RADICAL HYSTERECTOMY

Some investigators have advocated use of preoperative irradiation combined with radical hysterectomy (Table 9-3). Such treatment may have originally been a compromise; after the establishment of radium and x-ray therapy as the dominant treatment of cervical cancer in the earlier part of this century, those who reintroduced radical surgical treatment may have wished to accommodate and not directly challenge their radiology colleagues. A stated theoretic value of preoperative irradiation includes "sterilization" of the parauterine tissues, supposedly lessening the risk of spread of cancer cells during the subsequent radical operation. Some suggested that by using preoperative irradiation, the ureteral and paracervical dissection need not be so extensive; however, this view never gained wide acceptance. Most American gynecologic oncologists prefer irradiation *or* surgery in individual cases. In a large national American College of Surgeons Patterns of Care Study of invasive cervical cancer, only 10% of hysterectomies performed in the year 1990 for this disease were preceded by radiation therapy (Shingleton et al

1994). In reported series of patients having squamous cell carcinoma and adenocarcinoma (stages IB and II), no author reports a survival advantage of preoperative irradiation radical hysterectomy and pelvic node dissection (RHPND), compared with either radiation therapy or radical surgery alone (see Table 9-3).

In Kjorstad and coworkers' (1984) large series of women having stage IB disease, patients with adenocarcinoma enjoyed a high (88%) 5-year survival; however, because there were no controls, one cannot determine whether there was any improvement by using combined therapy. Pozzi and associates (1991), treating more advanced disease, also advocated combined irradiation and surgery; without controls, however, no firm conclusions can be drawn as to its value.

Complications of Preoperative Irradiation and Radical Hysterectomy

Urologic complications are appreciably higher in patients who are subjected to preoperative intracavitary irradiation before extended radical hysterectomy (Talbert 1965, Shingleton et al 1968). If preoperative whole-pelvis irradiation also is added, bowel complica-

TABLE 9-2
Complications of Preoperative Radiation and Extrafascial Hysterectomy

Study	Year	Patients (N)	Stage	Type Radiation	Bowel Fistula (%)	Bowel Obstruction Stricture (%)	Ureteral Stricture (%)	Urologic Fistula (%)	Vaginal Necrosis or Stricture (%)	Overall Complications (%)
O'Quinn, et al	1980	155	I, II	IC, WP	3.9*	3.9	—	6.5	0.6	12.3[†]
Blake, et al[‡]	1984	10	I–IV	IC, WP	30	10	—	10	—	50
Edinger, et al	1984	120	I–III	IC, WP	—	—	—	0.8	—	0.8
Perkins, et al	1984	36	I, II	IC, WP	5.6	2.8	2.8	2.8	5.6	19.6
Gallion, et al	1985	43	I	IC, WP	—	—	—	—	—	9.3
Weems, et al	1985	53	I, II	IC, WP	1.9	—	3.8	—	7.5	32.0
Coleman, et al	1992	43	I, II	IC, WP	2.3	7	—	7	7	23.3
Gerbaulet, et al	1992	442	I, II	IC, WP		1.3		3.4		5.3[§]

IC, intracavitary radiation; *WP,* whole-pelvis radiation.
*Adjunctive.
[†]Includes 2.6% multiple fistulas.
[‡]Chemotherapy (avg, five courses).
[§]Severe = 3.4%.

tions increase, as do overall complication rates (Table 9-4). These rates vary widely from series to series and are most likely radiation dose–related. One may conclude that the overall risk of complications is increased but there is not universal agreement on this point. The occurrence of multiple fistulas in some patients merits mention because this particular type of complication is not expected to any degree in patients who are receiving single-modality therapy.

De Graaff (1980) reported 270 women who were treated with intracavitary irradiation followed by extraperitoneal lymphadenectomy and radical *vaginal* hysterectomy. Crude survival rates were 83.9% for stage IB, 72.2% for stage IIA, and 68.9% for stage IIB. Although the authors reported low morbidity in their patients, their reported survival rates are modest, compared with historical controls, and thus suggest no obvious advantage of using this combination of therapy.

IRRADIATION AFTER RADICAL HYSTERECTOMY

Whole-pelvis irradiation has been used commonly after radical hysterectomy and pelvic node dissection to treat such findings as pelvic node metastases, deep cer-

vical stromal invasion, lymphvascular space invasion, parametrial involvement by tumor, and close or involved surgical margins (Table 9-5). Although it is recognized that such postoperative whole-pelvis irradiation increases pelvic control, it has not been demonstrated that it invariably improves long-term survival rates.

Two studies address the interesting question of the role of adjuvant radiation therapy in stage IB cervical cancer patients having negative or only microscopically positive lymph nodes. Fallo and colleagues (1993) produced 36 pairs of patients having negative nodes matched according to depth of stromal involvement and lymphvascular invasion, half of whom underwent adjuvant radiation therapy while the others were observed without additional treatment. The 5-year disease-free survival rate was identical in the two groups (89%). Eisner and coworkers (1993) studied 25 women who were found to have microscopically positive pelvic nodes (three or fewer). Of this group, 18 received pelvic irradiation postoperatively, whereas 7 did not. The 5-year survival rates of the two groups were 88.8% and 83.9%; however, this was not statistically different. Eisner and associates concluded that there is no evidence of a survival benefit from postoperative pelvic irradiation in individuals with three or fewer microscopic pelvic lymph nodes discovered at

TABLE 9-3
Value of Radiotherapy Before Radical Hysterectomy

STUDY	YEAR	PATIENTS (N)	HISTOLOGY	STAGE	RADIATION THERAPY PRE-OP	COMMENT/ CONCLUSIONS
Gynning, et al	1983	274	Predominantly SCC	IB	IC/WP	No survival advantage, compared with radiation alone
Rabin, et al	1984	92	"	IB, IIA	IC	No survival advantage, compared with RT alone
Perez, et al	1985	49	"	IB, IIA	IC/WP	Not superior to radiation alone
Alcock, et al	1987	181	"	IB, II	IC	Survival by stage not superior to single modality therapy
Pearcey, et al	1988	113	"	IB, II	IC	No survival advantage, compared with radical surgery alone
Tinga, et al	1990	23	"	IB	IC	No survival advantage, compared with radical surgery alone
Kjorstad, et al	1984	149	Predominantly adenocarcinoma	IB	IC/WP*	88% 5-year survival; no controls
Pozzi, et al	1991	70	"	IB–III	IC/WP*	82% (stage IB); 35% (stage II); 0% (stage III) 5-year survival; no controls

*Whole-pelvis radiation given for positive pelvic lymph nodes.
IC, intracavitary radiation; *WP,* whole-pelvis radiation; *RT,* radiation therapy.

TABLE 9-4
Complications of Preoperative Radiation and Radical Hysterectomy

STUDY	YEAR	PATIENTS (N)	STAGE	TYPE RADIATION	BOWEL FISTULA (%)	BOWEL OBSTRUCTION (%)	URETERAL STRICTURE	UROLOGIC FISTULA (%)	OVERALL COMPLICATIONS (%)
Surwit, et al	1976	58	I	IC	—	2	6.8	5	19
Einhorn, et al	1980	74	I, II	IC	1.4	1.4	—	2.7	5.4
Bonar, et al	1980	96	I, II	IC	—	2	—	5.2	13.4
Iversen, et al	1982	560	I	IC	0.5	—	—	1.2	2
Timmer, et al	1984	119	I–III	IC	—	—	6	2	13.1*
Adcock, et al	1979	43	I, II	IC/WP	2.3	—	27.9	7	41.9†
Perez, et al	1980	41	I, II	IC/WP	—	—	4.9	—	4.1
Kjorstad, et al	1983	612	IB	IC/WP	1	0.3	1.1	1.3	3.3
Jacobs, et al	1985	102	I, II	IC/WP	1	3	4	1	16
Crawford, et al	1965	137	I, II	IC/WP‡	6.6	8	5.1	5.1	25.5
Rampone, et al	1973	537		IC/WP‡	—	—	0.9	1.5	2.8
Weed, et al	1967	156	I, II	IC/WP‡	0.6	—	1.3	3.2	5.1

IC, preoperative intracavitary radiation; *WP,* whole-pelvis radiation.
*Includes three operative deaths (1.5%)
†4.7% multiple fistulae
‡WP delivered postoperatively in high risk patients

TABLE 9-5
Pelvic Irradiation After Radical Hysterectomy for High Risk Factors*

STUDY	PATIENTS (N)	STAGE	CONCLUSIONS
11 reports†—data from 15 institutions	1163	IB, IIA	May increase pelvic control No significant differences in survival

*Node metastases, close margins, parametrial extension, deep stromal invasion, lymphvascular space involvement.

†Morrow 1980, Hogan et al 1982, Larson et al 1987, Baltzer et al 1988, Gonzalez et al 1989, Kinney et al 1989, Berman et al 1990, Remy et al 1990, Soisson et al 1990, Bloss et al 1992, Sutton et al 1993.

time of radical hysterectomy for stage IB cancer of the cervix.

Although consensus seems to have been reached regarding the lack of proved effectiveness of postoperative adjunctive pelvic irradiation, its use persists in many centers, perhaps because the patients are often young women and most oncologic surgeons wish to reduce the chance of pelvic recurrence and the chance for cure. Thomas and colleagues (1991) developed an algorithm for treatment by pelvic irradiation based on numbers of positive nodes and presence or absence of unfavorable tumor factors. Individuals judged to have low relapse risk receive no further treatment; those thought to have mainly pelvic relapse risk receive

pelvic irradiation, whereas those at risk for extrapelvic and pelvic relapse receive pelvic and systemic therapy (Fig. 9-2).

In one retrospective multi-institutional study that matched stage, tumor size, number, and location of node metastases, the authors could not demonstrate an overall or cancer-specific increased survival for those patients receiving pelvic radiation therapy (Kinney et al 1989). The adjuvant postoperative pelvic radiation therapy (median, 5000 cGy) statistically decreased the risk of isolated pelvic recurrences, however ($p =.01$).

Two surgical studies demonstrate the relation of tumor volume to end results. Alvarez and coworkers

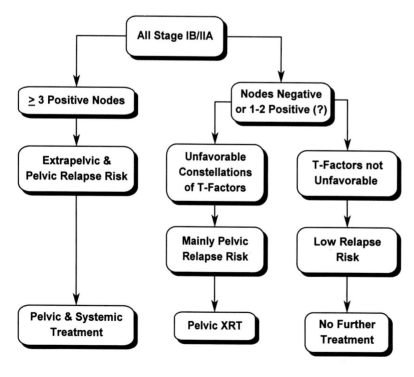

FIGURE 9-2. Algorithm of possible management of patients with cervical cancer after radical hysterectomy and pelvic lymphadenectomy. T-factors, tumor factors, eg, large tumor size, deep stromal invasion, lymphvascular space involvement, and tumor de-differentiation; XRT, radiotherapy. (Modified from Thomas GM, Dembo AJ. Is there a role for adjuvant pelvic radiotherapy after radical hysterectomy in early stage cervical cancer? Int J Gynecol Cancer 1991;1:1, with permission.)

(1991) reported the results of 57 stage IB patients treated with adjunctive irradiation after radical hysterectomy. Overall 5-year survival was 85% but was less than 30% for those patients having large-volume cervical tumors (more than 3 cm) and regional node metastases. Of interest is that women having tumors more than 3 cm and negative nodes had 5-year survival rates almost the same as those having smaller lesions and positive nodes (Fig. 9-3). Soisson and associates (1990) reported 72 patients receiving post–radical hysterectomy irradiation, indicating that radiation therapy was not beneficial to those women with large-volume cervical tumors, even though they were shown to have negative pelvic nodes and adequate surgical margins. Although pelvic control seemingly was improved by the irradiation, 84% of recurrences presented as distant metastases.

It appears that gynecologic oncologists request post–radical hysterectomy pelvic irradiation when the number of risk factors increase (Sutton et al 1993). They evaluated the Gynecologic Oncology Group (GOG) experience of post–radical hysterectomy adjuvant radiation therapy. In their review of 731 patients having clinical stage IB disease—151 of whom (20.6%) underwent postoperative radiation therapy—the radiation therapy was more frequently prescribed for (1) older women, (2) those having deep stromal invasion, and (3) those having vascular space, parametrial, and margin involvement. In a multiple regression analysis, radiation therapy was thought to be of value only in patients having gross node disease or extrapelvic spread. Overall, there was no apparent advantage in the recurrence-free interval for irradiated patients, compared with surgery-only controls.

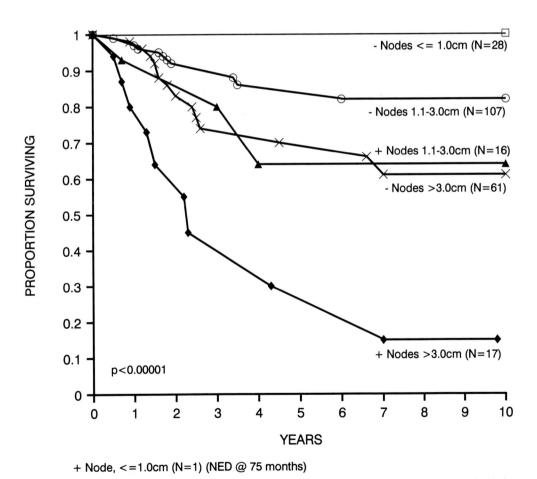

+ Node, <=1.0cm (N=1) (NED @ 75 months)

FIGURE 9-3. Radical surgery and postoperative pelvic radiation therapy for positive nodes and high risk factors. Survival by pathologic tumor diameter and node status. (Alvarez RD, Potter ME, Soong SJ, et al. Rationale for using pathologic tumor dimensions and nodal status to subclassify surgically treated stage IB cervical cancer patients. Gynecol Oncol 1991;43:108, with permission.)

ADENOCARCINOMA AND POSTOPERATIVE RADIATION THERAPY

Some (Kamura et al 1992) believe that patients who have adenocarcinomas and node metastases have a worse prognosis than patients who have squamous cell lesions and node metastasis. Several authors, including us, have noted considerably increased recurrence rates (see Table 7-17 in Chap. 7) and in some cases decreased survival rates in adenocarcinoma patients, when comparing stage IB surgically treated patients of the two major tissue types. Even using meta-analysis, because of the few cases involved, the patients with adenocarcinoma cannot be shown to have significantly increased recurrence rates, although a strong trend is apparent. Small numbers preclude an adequate study of the value of postoperative radiation therapy for adenocarcinoma patients who have node metastases.

COMPLICATIONS OF RADICAL HYSTERECTOMY AND POSTOPERATIVE RADIATION THERAPY

Many authors have compared the complications of patients undergoing radical hysterectomy and postoperative pelvic irradiation with those treated by surgery alone. Increased bowel complications, urologic fistulas, and overall complications have been reported for this combination of therapy (Fuller et al 1982, Gonzalez et al 1989). Some studies have control groups of nonirradiated patients for comparison (Table 9-6). In the series with high overall complications rates (Bilek 1982, Barter et al 1989) whole-pelvis dosages exceeding 50 Gy had been administered; when lesser dosages were used, lower overall complication rates were noted, thus demonstrating that the complications are dose-related.

In a report of 50 patients undergoing radical hysterectomy and pelvic radiation therapy (mean, 4700 cGy), Fiorica and colleagues (1990) indicated a 14% rate of intestinal morbidity and a 10% risk of major gastrointestinal complications, all occurring within 12 months. He suggested that such gastrointestinal and genitourinary morbidity was acceptable in high-risk situations. Hopkins and associates (1991) reported the need for surgical intervention in 6.3% of patients in the postoperative irradiation group and in 2.8% of patients undergoing surgery alone for stage IB squamous cell cancer of the cervix. Remy and coworkers (1986) reported acceptable minimal complications of irradiation after radical surgery when delivered at 180 cGy, whereas a higher post–radical irradiation-related gastrointestinal (9%) and genitourinary (14%) complication rate occurred when daily radiation dose was equal to or exceeded 400 cGy.

Because of the increased rate of complications associated with pelvic irradiation after radical hysterectomy, we advocate its use only in patients who have three or more nodes containing metastases or those who have more than one node group containing metastases (e.g., those having bilaterally positive nodes) because these patients are at increased risk for recurrence. Irradiation should also be considered in those having involved surgical margins, possibly in the form of both vaginal cuff brachytherapy and whole-pelvis teletherapy.

COMBINED TREATMENT AND THE URINARY TRACT

Farquharson and colleagues (1987) performed a prospective study of three groups of 30 women who were treated by (1) radical hysterectomy alone, (2) radiation therapy alone, or (3) radical hysterectomy followed by postoperative whole-pelvis radiation therapy. They observed that altered bladder sensation and voiding problems were associated more with surgery or combined therapy than with radiation therapy alone.

Urinary incontinence was present in 13% of Farquharson and associates' patients before therapy. After treatment, incontinence requiring protection developed in 23% of patients who were treated with radiation therapy alone, in 26% of patients who were treated with radical hysterectomy alone, and in 63% of those who received combined treatment. The severity of the incontinence was also greater in the combined-treatment patients, an observation that seems to be supported by Kadar and Nelson's (1984) report. Bladder neck and urethral function was similar in all patient groups in Farquharson and coworkers' study; however, bladder compliance was reduced in radiation therapy patients and significantly reduced in the combined-treatment group. These observations were not confirmed by Kristensen and colleagues (1984) nor by Petri (1984).

Ralph and associates (1990) performed postoperative urodynamic studies on 116 patients after radical hysterectomy with or without adjuvant radiation therapy. They reported that 78% of patients who were treated with surgery only had no urologic complications in long-term follow-up. Only half the patients treated by surgery and adjuvant radiation therapy were asymptomatic long-term; however, their complaints mostly involved impaired bladder sensation, frequency, and nocturia. There seems to be enough evidence by literature review to conclude that bladder function is

TABLE 9-6
Complications of Radical Hysterectomy and Postoperative Whole-Pelvis Radiation

	STUDY	YEAR	PATIENTS (N)	STAGE	TYPE RADIATION	BOWEL FISTULA OR OBSTRUCTION (%)	URETERAL STRICTURE (%)	UROLOGIC FISTULA (%)	OVERALL COMPLICATIONS (%)
Without controls	Fuller, et al	1982	32	I, II	40 Gy (mean)	3.1	0	6.2	12.5*
	Hogan, et al	1982	21	I, II	40–60 Gy	4.8	4.8	4.8	33.3
	Kucera, et al	1984	176	I, II	57 Gy	4.5	0	2.8	7.3
	Gonzalez, et al	1989	89	I, II	40–45 Gy in 4–5 wks +2000mgh radium (23 pts)	4.5	4.5	7.9	29.2†
With controls	Morrow	1980	49	I	40–60 Gy	4	2.0	2.0	12.2
			146	I	Controls	1.4	1.4	3.4	6.2
	Bilek, et al	1982	60	I	52 Gy	5	3	0	28*
			60	I	Controls	0	1.5	0	10
	Barter, et al	1989	50	I, II	53 Gy	20	2	4	28‡
			200	I, II	Controls	0.5	0.3	1.3	3.1
	Rettenmaier, et al	1989	32	I	50, 4 Gy + 45 Gy PAN (4 pts)	6.3	0	0	9.4
			60		Controls	1.6	0	1.6	3.2
	Bloss, et al	1992	42	I	50, 4 Gy + 45 Gy PAN (4 pts)	13.9	0	2.4	16.3
			42		Controls	4.8	0	0	13.7

PAN, paraaortic nodes
*One death, operative or postoperative.
†12.3% long-term bladder atony.
‡Needing at least one operation: 14%.

adversely affected by the combination of pelvic surgery and irradiation.

DEBULKING LYMPHADENECTOMY BEFORE IRRADIATION

Downey and coworkers (1989) reported a series of patients who had surgical staging before radiation therapy. One hundred fifty-six patients were divided by pelvic node status after surgical staging and pelvic lymphadenectomy. One group had negative nodes; the second group had microscopic metastases only; a third group had macroscopic but resected node metastases, whereas the last group had unresectable node metastases. The groups were matched by FIGO stage, grade, histology, and incidence of paraaortic metastases. The 5-year recurrence-free survival in the macroscopic but resected group of 48 patients was not different from that of the group (18 patients) with only microscopic node metastases (51% versus 57%). In contrast, those having unresectable disease had no survivors (Fig. 9-4). Inoue and Morita (1988) also reported an improved 5-year survival rate in patients having resected macroscopically involved common iliac nodes (67%) when compared with nonresected common iliac nodes (44%). Hacker and colleagues (1993), reporting 31 patients having bulky positive nodes, concluded that resection can be performed safely and that such resections appear to improve disease-free survival for this group of women.

PELVIC IRRADIATION AND POSTTHERAPY LYMPHADENECTOMY

A trial over a 10-year period of pelvic lymphadenectomy after full-dosage external beam therapy and radium implants was conducted at M.D. Anderson Hospital (Rutledge et al 1965). The intent of the study was to cure more patients having node metastases and to study the effectiveness of supervoltage irradiation on positive pelvic lymph nodes. No survival advantages were shown by this technique, although it was associated with many complications, likely related to the high radiation dose used in the early days of the new supervoltage equipment. Somewhat later, Lagasse and associates (1974) reported 118 patients having stage I cervical cancer treated by pelvic radiation therapy, either before or after transperitoneal pelvic lymphadenectomy. There was a 50% reduction in expected rates of positive pelvic nodes after irradiation (5000 cGy to point B). There were no operative deaths, no operative urinary tract injuries, nor were other complications more frequent or more severe in the group undergoing surgery after irradiation. The study suggested that irradiation can eradicate metastatic carcinoma from nodes in a significant proportion of

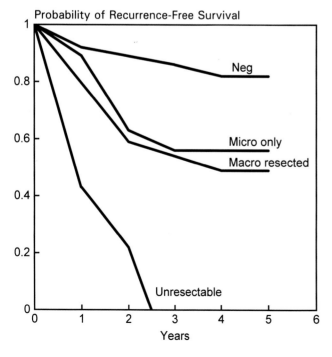

FIGURE 9-4. Recurrence-free survival by pelvic node status. (Downey GO, Potish RA, Adcock LL, Prem KA, Twiggs LB. Pretreatment surgical staging in cervical carcinoma: therapeutic efficacy of pelvic lymph node resection. Am J Obstet Gynecol 1989;160:1055, with permission.)

the cases. No authors have advocated this approach and it is unlikely to gain a place in the routine management of women who have cervical cancer.

INTRAOPERATIVE RADIATION THERAPY

Yordan (1988) reviewed the status of intraoperative irradiation therapy. In concept, local control of advanced pelvic tumors, especially when complete surgical resection is not possible, is often impeded by the intolerance to irradiation of normal tissues adjacent to the residual tumor, limiting deliverance of tumoricidal dosages to the target area. Ordain reported 15 patients having gynecologic malignancies (5 patients having cancer of the cervix) who were considered to be at high risk for local failure. Intraoperative irradiation therapy was administered at a dosage range of 10 to 26 Gy directly to the tumor with the abdomen open, the bowel displaced, and the tumor area directly exposed. The authors concluded that probability of local control improved when the tumor was at least partially resectable and when local dosages (given as a combination of intraoperative irradiation and external beam irradiation) exceeded 70 Gy. Thus, intraoperative radiation therapy may be viewed as a modality that is capable of delivering an irradiation therapy boost in patients having incomplete surgical resection. The drawbacks of extending this therapy to more patients include the expense and the logistic problem of facilities that allow abdominal surgery in the same room with supervoltage radiation therapy equipment, as well as the inability to provide more than one therapy boost without a subsequent laparotomy.

CHEMOTHERAPY, IRRADIATION, AND SURGERY COMBINATIONS

Chemotherapy and Surgery

An appreciable volume of literature has evolved on the subject of adjuvant chemotherapy (presurgery chemotherapy, postsurgery chemotherapy) for patients who have high-risk factors; pre-irradiation chemotherapy (systemic, intraarterial); and concomitant irradiation and chemotherapy (Table 9-7). Runowicz (1993) addressed all of these subjects in a review article. She concludes that neoadjuvant and concomitant chemotherapy in patients having locally advanced cervical cancer is feasible; therefore, no further pilot studies are needed. Regarding neoadjuvant chemotherapy and surgery combinations, the literature demonstrates the chemosensitivity of cervical cancer, allowing more pa-

tients to be eligible for surgical resection. Prospective randomized trials are suggested to determine whether single-agent or combination chemotherapy should be used and the number of cycles required before the surgical therapy. Improved study design and longer follow-up in the neoadjuvant groups are needed to answer the question of overall usefulness. Thomas (1993), in an editorial that reviewed the literature and specifically discussed Sardi and associates' 1993 study (with its short follow-up period), concluded that it is doubtful, given the available chemotherapeutic agents, that neoadjuvant chemotherapy before surgery yields significant survival benefits. The GOG plans to conduct a prospective randomized study soon.

Chemotherapy and Irradiation

CHEMOTHERAPY BEFORE RADIATION THERAPY

The primary rationale of combining irradiation with chemotherapy is to increase local control, decrease distal metastasis, and improve survival. Significant theoretic limitations in the use of neoadjuvant therapy include cross-resistance (chemotherapy versus radiation therapy); accelerated tumor growth, which may occur with protracted treatment; and the potential limitations to the delay of additional definitive radiation therapy (Thomas 1993).

Clinical studies for the delivery of radiation therapy and chemotherapy have evolved independently. Unfortunately, the underlying therapeutic strategy for delivering chemotherapy (large doses at distinct intervals) and radiation therapy (small fractions given daily) have not been integrated in many situations. Alternating dose, dosage, and fraction allows many potential combinations or permutations. Clinical, experimental, and theoretic data suggest the need to intensify both modalities during induction therapy of high-risk cervical cancer (Looney 1991).

Regarding chemotherapy delivered before irradiation therapy, randomized trials by Souhami and coworkers (1991) and Cardenas and associates (1992), in addition to some previous reports (Table 9-8), reveal that 2- and 5-year survival is not enhanced by using this treatment approach for stages III and IV cervical cancer.

Concomitant Chemotherapy–Radiation Therapy

The concept of concurrent chemoradiation therapy offers several advantages over neoadjuvant therapy, primarily no delay or no prolongation of radiation therapy. The use of weekly cisplatin (mg/kg maximum, 60

TABLE 9-7
Adjuvant Chemotherapy and Surgery

STUDY	YEAR	PATIENTS (N)	STAGE	AGENTS	CONCLUSIONS
PRESURGERY					
Giaroli, et al	1990	169	IB–III	VBP	↓ LN metastases
Sardi, et al	1990	151	107 IIB 44 IIIB	VBP "	Critical treatment volume 84 cm³; for larger tumors, surgery better than RT
Deppe, et al	1991	17	IB–IIIB Diam >5cm	Mit C Platinol	76.5% initial response; 2 complete, 8 partial path. response
Dottino, et al	1991	28	Loc. adv. IB-IVA	VBP Mit C	35% CR; 65% PR; 4 complete path. response
Panici, et al	1991	75	Loc. adv. IB–III	PBM	15% CR; 68% PR; responders ↑ 3-year survival
Parham, et al	1993	15	Loc. adv. IIB–IIIB	Platinol	Concur. chemo. radiation before surgery; 67% CR, high complete path. response (90%)
Sardi, et al	1993	151	IB bulky	VBP	Improved operability; decrease in histopathologic risk factors. NS improvement in survival (short follow-up)
Jones	1993		IB bulky loc. adv.		71.2% operability, 16.5 CR
POSTSURGERY FOR HIGH-RISK FACTORS*					
Lahousen, et al	1988	27	IB–IIB	VBP Mit C	↓ Rec, ↑ survival
Lai, et al	1989	40	IB–IIB	VBP	↑ 3-year survival
Lewis, et al	1989	60	IB–IIA	Platinol/ bleomycin	↑ 5-year survival
Ng, et al	1992	96	IB–IIIA	VBP	↓ Recurrence rates 34% vs 65% ($p<.01$)
Zanetta, et al	1993	24	Loc. adv.	CVB	33% 3-year survival

Mit C, mitomycin C; *VBP,* vincristine, bleomycin, platinol; *PBM,* platinol, bleomycin, methotrexate; *CR,* complete response; *PR,* partial response; *CVB,* cisplatin, vinblastine, bleomycin; *LN,* lymph node; *RT,* radiation therapy; *loc. adv.,* locally advanced (tumor).
*Positive nodes, close margins, lymph vascular space involvement.

mg) administered during radiation therapy did not diminish radiation dose in Malfetano's (1993) study.

In their review of concomitant irradiation and chemotherapy, Runowicz and colleagues (1989) concluded that therapy trials have demonstrated the feasibility of combining standard pelvic radiation therapy and chemotherapy. Although the initial response rates are encouraging, the impact on overall survival is unclear, particularly in stages III and IV. Studies have not shown the advantage of combination chemotherapy over single-agent therapy. In Runowicz's own studies (1991, 1993), she reported improvement in disease-free survival and overall survival in women who have stage I and II disease. Clearly, randomized prospective trials of concomitant chemoradiation ther-

apy versus pelvic radiation therapy alone are needed. The Radiotherapy Oncology Group (RTOG) has in progress a phase III study of pelvic irradiation with concomitant chemotherapy, comparing this with pelvic and paraaortic irradiation for high-risk cervical cancer. The value or role of chemoradiation therapy thus remains undetermined. Marcial and Marcial (1993) believe that if it gains use, the chemotherapy will probably be administered concurrently and not sequentially. Varia and coworkers (1986), reporting the results of GOG protocol 59, found prohibitive toxicity of extended-field irradiation and cisplatin treatment. Several other investigators (see Table 9-8) did not confirm this finding and stated that the toxicity is manageable.

TABLE 9-8
Adjuvant Chemotherapy and Irradiation

STUDY	YEAR	PATIENTS (N)	STAGE	AGENTS	CONCLUSIONS
BEFORE RADIATION THERAPY					
Symonds, et al	1989	55	III–IVA	VBP	All 27 responders also CR to radiotherapy; ↑2-year survival
Soeters, et al	1989	9	Advanced	VBP	No CR, 11% PR
Sardi, et al	1990	57	II–III	VBP	Improved 2-year survivals in chemotherapy group, compared with controls ($p < .01$)
Park, et al	1991	113	III, IV	SCC: Platinol, 5-FU; adenocarcinoma, CAP	Effective preradiation adjunct; toxicity requires altering doses 61%
Patton, et al	1991	44	IIIB, IVA	Intraarterial PBM + vincristine	24% CR, 52% PR
Souhami, et al	1991	52	IIIB	BOMP	Severe toxicity, no survival advantage
CONCOMITANT WITH RADIATION THERAPY					
Haie, et al	1988	36	III–IV	Platinol, cyclophosphamide	Feasibility study—35% 4-year survival; Low complications
Roberts, et al	1989	23	Advanced	Platinol, 5-FU	87% CR, 9% PR; responses often not sustained
Runowicz, et al	1989	43	Loc. adv. IB–IVA	Platinol	Well-tolerated; 91% CR
Heaton, et al	1990	29	Bulky, >8 cm	Cisplatin	66% CR, 65% 5-year survival rate
Thomas, et al	1990	200	Loc. adv.	Phase I, II 5-FU, Mit C	Acceptable toxicity—phase III study of 5-FU planned
Malfetano, et al	1991	13	PAN mets	Platinol and ext-field RT (phase I, II)	Encouraging results; acceptable toxicity
Chang, et al	1992	20	IIB–IVA	VBP	65% CR, 25% PR; enhances local control; toxicity tolerable
Park, et al	1993	37	I–II	Cisplatin, 5-FU	100% 30-month survival rate; manageable toxicity; superior to radiation alone

Mit C, mitomycin C; *BOMP,* VBP, Mit C; *VBP,* vincristine, bleomycin, platinol; *PBM,* platinol, bleomycin, methotrexate; *RT,* radiation therapy; *CR,* complete response; *PR,* partial response; *SCC,* squamous cell carcinoma, *loc. adv.,* locally advanced.

Three-Modality Therapy

Zanetta and colleagues (1993) reported discouraging 3-year follow-up results in 24 patients having locally advanced (node-positive) cervical cancer that was treated with neoadjuvant chemotherapy (cisplatin, vincristine, bleomycin [VBP]); radical surgery; and postoperative radiation therapy. Three-year survival was 33% (8 of 24). Sardi and associates (1990, 1993) reported a prospective randomized trial of neoadjuvant chemotherapy (quick VBP), before radi-

cal surgery followed by 5000 cGy to the whole pelvis or before irradiation alone. Their results suggested a possible benefit in bulky tumors (those 60 or more cm³) but no benefit in smaller tumors. Although Sardi and coworkers did not comment on morbidity related to the radical surgery–irradiation combination, it is our belief that extended surgery and pelvic irradiation results in increased morbidity (see Table 9-6). It has not been shown that multimodality therapy results in improved long-term survival.

RADIATION SENSITIZERS

A significant portion of patients have tumor that is confined to the pelvis. Those patients who have a large hypoxic tumor component may benefit from the use of radiosensitizing agents that eliminate the adverse or poor cell kill effects that are associated with low tissue levels of oxygen. These sensitizers may benefit the patient by increasing the effective dose of radiation to the tumor, recognizing that the tolerance of the surrounding normal tissue limits the actual radiation dose that can be given.

Stehman (1993) addressed the subject of concurrent chemoradiation and radiosensitizers in cancer of the cervix. Some enthusiasm has been generated for use of such agents during radiation therapy in an attempt to enhance the irradiation effect (Table 9-9). Patients treated with hydroxyurea have been shown in several studies (Piver et al 1977, Hreshchyshyn et al 1979) to have longer progression-free intervals and improved survival, especially those patients who have bulky stage III and IV tumors. Hreshchyshyn and coworkers (1979) reported the randomized prospective evaluation of the GOG using hydroxyurea in patients having stage IIIB or IV disease. Complete tumor regression, progression-free interval, and survival probability were all increased in patients who received hydroxyurea. Long-term follow-up from GOG protocol 56 suggests an advantage of hydroxyurea over misonidazole in progression-free interval and survival, particularly in women who have stage II or IVA disease (Stehman et al 1993). Excellent survival rates (stage IIB, 94%; stage IIIB, 90%) in patients having disease known to be confined to the pelvis have been previously reported (Piver et al 1983). With the exception of an increased risk of leukopenia (less than 2500/mL), no other significant irradiation side effects appear to be increased. Gynecologic Oncology Group protocol 59 evaluated the use of hydroxyurea and extended-field therapy (proved paraaortic node metastases); however, it was not well-tolerated (Stehman et al 1993). Some investigators have tried cisplatin and 5-fluorouracil as radiosensitizers but phase III data confirming any advantage in terms of local control, disease-free survival, or overall survival have been published only for hydroxyurea. Further studies are required for agents other than hydroxyurea to gain their use as part of standard therapy for locally advanced carcinoma of the cervix. Hydroxyurea inhibits ribonucleoside diphosphate reductase, an enzyme necessary for DNA synthesis and repair. This drug, which specifically inhibits DNA, kills cells during the S phase, a time of relative radioresistance. Additionally, hydroxyurea blocks G_1 cells at the S-phase interface, ren-

TABLE 9-9
Chemosensitizers in Cervical Cancer

STUDY	YEAR	PATIENTS (N)	STAGE	AGENTS	CONCLUSIONS
Piver, et al	1977	130	IIB, IIIB	Hydroxyurea	Significant improvement in survival in stage IIB pts; trend towards longer survival in stage IIIB pts; significant improvement in survival in IIIB pts with neg. paraaortic nodes and continuous-course RT
Hreshchyshyn, et al	1979	104	IIIB, IVA	Hydroxyurea	Significant increase in tumor regression; improvement in survival and progression-free interval
Piver, et al	1983	40	IIB	Hydroxyurea	Improved 5-year survival (94% vs 53% for placebo)
Noda, et al	1993	292	II, III	Sizofiran	Complete response rate improved—stage II, 91% vs 79.1% (control); stage III, 77.9% vs 61.2% (control)
Dische	1993	184	II, III	Pimonidazole Ro 03-8799	No benefit—poorer local tumor control and survival
Stehman, et al	1993	294	IIB–IVA	Hydroxyurea Misonidazole	Improved progression-free interval and survival; hydroxyurea superior to misonidazole

RT, radiation therapy.

dering those cells remaining in G_1 more radiosensitive than those progressing to the S phase, thereby increasing the number of cells that are vulnerable during radiation therapy. The optimal dose or schedule has not been determined; however, it is thought that synchronizing the G_1–S phase and potentiation should be related to its administration in proximity of the irradiation (Stehman 1992, Stehman 1993).

The use of LC9018 (a biologic-response modifier) combined with radiation therapy significantly enhanced tumor regression and relapse-free interval, and prolonged survival in a randomized prospective study of 228 patients having stage IIIB disease (Okawa et al 1993). Radiation-induced leukopenia was less severe and side effects (fever and injection-site lesions) were tolerable. A randomized controlled trial of RO03-8799 (pimonidazole) in 183 patients having stage II or III disease suggests a potential adverse effect on survival of this radiosensitizer (Dische 1993). A collaborative randomized study of 315 patients from 52 institutions (Noda et al 1993), evaluating the biologic-response modifier sizofiran, indicated a significant increase in complete response for stages II and III dis-ease. Treated patients had a more rapid lymphocyte recovery.

Phase II and III trials of newer radiosensitizers such as SR2508, which have higher tumor concentrations and lower risk of toxicity, are underway. Additionally, drugs such as buthionine sulfoximine, which deplete specific intracellular nonprotein sulfhydrals and enhance the radiosensitizing potentials of other drugs, will soon be tested. Radioprotective drugs such as WR2721 may play a future role in the chemomodification of radiation therapy (Brady et al 1985). The radiosensitizer WR2721 is an organothiophosphate that selectively protects against the toxicities of cisplatin and alkylating agents (Wadler et al 1993). Its use results in hypocalcemia, mediated partly by a direct inhibition of parathyroid hormone.

ADJUVANT IMMUNOTHERAPY

Several immunotherapy trials have been conducted in conjunction with irradiation or surgery for all stages of cancer of the cervix (Table 9-10). These trials employ

TABLE 9-10
Adjuvant Immunotherapy Trials

STUDY	YEAR	PATIENTS (N)	STAGE	AGENTS	CONCLUSIONS
PROSPECTIVE RANDOMIZED STUDIES					
Cervical Cancer Immunotherapy Study Group	1987	221	I–IV	OK 432, radiation w/wo surgery	Significant increase in recurrence-free rate at 36 mo (p =.01)
DiSaia,* et al	1987	283	IIB–IV	C-Parvan and radiation (vs radiation alone)	No therapeutic value demonstrated
Noda, et al	1989	382	II–III	OK 432, radiation w/wo surgery	Increase in recurrence-free interval and survival for stage II; not effective for stage III
Okamura, et al	1989	195	II–III	Sizofuran and radiation	Increased survival, both stages
Okawa, et al	1993	228	III	LC 9018 and radiation	Significantly reduced tumor volume; prolonged survival and relapse-free interval (p <.05)
CLINICAL TRIALS (NO CONTROLS)					
Welander, et al	1991	21	Advanced or recurrent	Alpha interferon and doxorubicin	35% partial responses; two 5-year survivors
PILOT STUDY OF INTERFERON-SYSTEM PARAMETERS					
Chadha, et al	1991	53	Advanced	Alpha interferon and radiation	Changes in the interferon system, induced by advanced carcinoma, normalize after successful radiation treatment and/or chemotherapy

*Gynecologic Oncology Group study.

a variety of agents; whereas some studies suggest a benefit, the use of immunotherapy in conjunction with the standard treatment modalities has not gained a role in the treatment of this disease.

Concurrent administration of immunostimulants has not been beneficial. Interferons, a family of cytokines, exhibit a direct antitumor effect by modulating tumor cell sensitivity and an indirect antitumor effect, possibly by protecting the host antineoplastic lymphocytes from irradiation. Interferon, which may directly modulate cellular cytotoxicity or the immune system, has shown in vitro activity when combined with irradiation in an in vitro session but has not been demonstrated to be clinically active in patients who have cervical cancer (Angioli et al 1992). DiSaia and colleagues (1987), reporting on GOG protocol 24 (evaluating *Corynebacterium parvum*), indicated no difference in survival or disease-free interval in patients having stage IIB, IIIB, or IVA disease treated with radiation therapy. Although possibly offering an advantage when combined with irradiation, therapeutic trials are needed. In vitro data (Herzog et al 1992) suggest the possible synergistic effect of tumor necrosis factor and irradiation.

TREATMENT OF RARE TUMORS

Cervical Sarcoma

Sarcoma is one of the least common primary neoplasms of the cervix. In a review article, Rotmensch and coworkers (1983) quoted the instance to be 0.5% of cervical cancers. There are a variety of histologic types and because of their rarity, there is no agreed histologic classification. Some pathologists have suggested modification of the classification of uterine sarcomas to include cervical tumors. The lack of a classification makes the critical evaluation of treatment results difficult.

Abell and associates (1973) reviewed the treatment of cervical sarcoma and carcinosarcoma. Independent of treatment, most patients with leiomyosarcomas, carcinosarcomas, or endocervical stromal sarcomas died within 2 years.

In Rotmensch and colleagues' (1983) series, 96 sarcoma cases of various tissue types were included. A variety of treatment was used, including hysterectomy, irradiation, and chemotherapy, singly or in combination. Results of treatment were generally poor but lack of criteria for diagnosis and the small number of patients with each tissue type precluded evaluation of individual therapies. Montag and associates (1986) reported 6 patients who had embryonal rhabdomyosarcoma of the uterus or cervix who were treated with combination chemotherapy and in one or two cases,

radical hysterectomy and pelvic lymphadenectomy; pelvic radiation therapy was advocated for involved surgical margins or positive nodes. Using these combinations of treatment, most patients achieved long-term survival. Montag and coworkers also compiled 28 additional patients with embryonal rhabdomyosarcoma from the literature. Of these, 19 of 24 patients (79%) who were treated with combination therapy were alive a median of 61 months after diagnosis.

Brand and associates (1987) reviewed 21 cases of sarcoma botryoides, including four that were previously unreported. Ages ranged from 5 months to 48 years (peak incidence, 14 to 18 months). The prognosis was considered to be similar to that of other genital tract rhabdomyosarcomas and recommended therapy was vincristine–dactinomycin and conservative surgery, with an attempt to conserve the bladder, rectum, vagina, and ovaries. Müllerian adenosarcomas have also been reported (Gast 1989).

Lymphoma

Lymphomas involving the cervix and other parts of the female reproductive tract are quite rare. It is more likely to find lymphomatous involvement of the cervix in generalized disease rather than as a primary cervical lesion. We have seen primary lymphoma only six times in a series of cervical cancer exceeding 3400 invasive tumors. The treatment is varied because of the rarity and the lack of agreement regarding the effectiveness of various modalities. Chorlton and coworkers (1974) reported that lymphoma patients having FIGO stage I tumors have a 5-year survival rate of 60%. Young and colleagues (1985) added a note of caution from the viewpoint of the pathologist, stating that microscopic differential diagnosis of malignant lymphoma and benign lymphoid infiltrates in the lower genital tract may be difficult. Before therapy for cervical lymphoma is undertaken, consultation with a pathologist who is familiar with lymphomas is mandatory.

In the English literature, Khoury and Robinson (1989) located only 21 well-documented cases of cervical lymphoma in which disease was localized to the genital tract. Muntz and associates (1991) accumulated a total of 38 previously reported cases in addition to the five included in his report. Such tumors are said to be typically of large size. The stage distribution that is listed in Muntz and coworkers' report was 44% stage I, 42% stage II, 12% stage III, and 2% stage IV. Most (70%) were of the diffuse large cell type. Most patients were treated with external beam radiation therapy; there was only one treatment failure among 28 patients whose treatment included radiation therapy. Muntz and colleagues concluded that most primary lymphoma of the cervix can be cured with combinations of hysterectomy and irradiation therapy. Johnston and associates (1989) reported an 8-cm stage IIIB lymphoma in a young nulliparous woman who was treated with combination chemotherapy (methotrexate, doxorubicin, cyclophosphamide, vincristine, prednisone, and bleomycin). This was selected to preserve her reproductive potential. A 4-cm left parametrial mass was excised as part of her treatment but otherwise, she received only chemotherapy. Menses resumed after 6 months and the patient was clinically disease-free at 33 months. In another review of 70 patients having non-Hodgkins lymphoma, Perren and coworkers (1992) suggested the benefit of chemotherapy in patients having bulky, advanced pelvic disease. Awwad and colleagues (1994) questioned the role of radical irradiation, suggesting that combination chemotherapy offers excellent survival and potentially preserves reproductive function.

In summary, treatment of lymphoma may involve irradiation therapy alone, irradiation combined with hysterectomy, or chemotherapy alone if reproductive potential conservation is desired.

Melanoma

Mordel and associates (1989) and Santoso and coworkers (1990) reported two cases and reviewed the literature on the subject of primary malignant melanoma of the cervix. To make this diagnosis, one must have histologic confirmation of melanoma in the cervix in the absence of distal metastases. Because of the extreme rarity of this tumor and lack of a standard treatment approach, reported cases were treated in a variety of ways, ranging from simple excision to radical hysterectomy with pelvic lymphadenectomy to whole pelvis irradiation therapy. Rarely have patients been treated with modern chemotherapy and none have been treated with immunotherapy. Historically, the patients did not respond well and most died of their disease within 2 years, although a few have experienced long-term survival. Most gynecologic oncologists select treatment for such a patient based on the size and distribution of the primary tumor, appreciating the virulent nature of these tumors. Such treatment likely would include extended surgery, with or without regional lymphadenectomy and pelvic irradiation therapy.

Verrucous Carcinoma

Biopsies of verrucous carcinoma are commonly misinterpreted as being condyloma acuminata; this confusion often results in a prolonged delay of appropriate treatment. Conveyance to the pathologist of the extent and clinical behavior of the lesion may facilitate early recognition (i.e., if the clinical features suggest malignant disease, one should not accept a biopsy di-

agnosis of benign condyloma). Degefu and associates (1986) accumulated reports of 27 cases of verrucous carcinoma in the world literature. To these they added two other cases. The treatment approaches have usually been surgical, ranging from total hysterectomy to radical hysterectomy to exenteration, whereas irradiation therapy is not thought to be effective—indeed, is thought possibly to induce malignant transformation. Lymphadenectomy is not recommended because this is a local expanding tumor and rarely metastasizes to nodes. Partridge and coworkers (1980) and Kawagoe and colleagues (1984) also reported this disease entity.

Small Cell Neuroendocrine Tumors

Neuroendocrine small cell carcinomas of the cervix are virulent tumors that are associated with a poor prognosis. Tumors of small cell pattern represent about 10% of all cervical carcinomas (Shingleton et al 1987), and a subset of these tumors falls into the amine precursor uptake and decarboxylation (APUD) cell system category. Such argyrophilic (APUD) tumors are thought to have a worse prognosis than those without such cells. Many authors have reported on these tumors (Jones et al 1974, van Nagell et al 1977, Matsuyama et al 1979, Habib et al 1979, Mackay et al 1979, Inoue et al 1984, Yamasaki et al 1984, Silva et al 1984, Yoshida et al 1984, O'Hanlan et al 1991, Lewandowski et al 1993). Treatment follows that (stage by stage) for other cervical malignancies. Surgery and adjunctive postoperative irradiation have been commonly used in an attempt to achieve local control, although many have advocated systemic chemotherapy in addition to employing regimens with documented activity against small cell carcinoma of the lung of neuroendocrine origin, such as etoposide and cisplatin (Turrisi et al 1988, Lewandowski et al 1993).

Multiple Primary Tumors

Axelrod and coworkers (1984) reported 78 synchronous or metachronous tumors among 2362 patients in the Downstate University Gynecologic Tumor Registry. Second primary tumors were found in 1.7% of patients having carcinoma in situ of the cervix (70% synchronous), whereas 3.9% of those having invasive cervical cancer had second primaries (31% synchronous). Significant synchronous tumor pairs included cervix (invasive and in situ)–ovary, cervix (in situ)–endometrial, cervix–upper alimentary tract, and cervix–rectosigmoid. The synchronous tumors (ovary, endometrium, gastrointestinal tract) and breast cancers are likely to be discovered at the time of initial evaluation or in the case of the ovary and endometrium, included in the treatment fields for the cervical cancer.

Other Rare Tumors

Germ cell tumors of the cervix, including mature teratoma (dermoid; Hanai et al 1981) and cervical endodermal sinus tumors, have been described (Copeland et al 1985). The latter group responds to combination chemotherapy (vincristine, actinomycin D, cytoxan [VAC]) and surgery and may survive long-term.

References

Abayomi O, Chun M, Ball H. Stage II carcinoma of the cervix: analysis of the value of pretreatment extraperitoneal lymph node sampling and adjunctive surgery following irradiation. Radiother Oncol 1990;19:43.

Abell MR, Ramirez JA. Sarcomas and carcinosarcomas of the uterine cervix. Cancer 1973;31:1176.

Adcock LL. Radical hysterectomy preceded by pelvic irradiation. Gynecol Oncol 1979;8:152.

Alcock CJ, Toplis PJ. The influence of pelvic lymph node disease on survival for stage I and II carcinoma of the cervix. Clin Radiol 1987;38:13.

Alvarez RD, Potter ME, Soong SJ, et al. Rationale for using pathologic tumor dimensions and nodal status to subclassify surgically treated stage IB cervical cancer patients. Gynecol Oncol 1991;43:108.

Angioli R, Sevin B, Perras J, et al. Rationale for combining radiation and interferon for the treatment of cervical cancer. Oncology 1992;49:445.

Awwad JT, Khalil AM, Shamseddine AI, Mufarrij AA. Primary malignannt lymphoma of the uterine cervix: is radiotherapy the best therapeutic choice for stage IE. Gynecol Oncol 1994;52:91.

Axelrod JH, Fruchter R, Boyce JG. Multiple primaries among gynecologic malignancies. Gynecol Oncol 1984;18:359.

Bachaud JM, Fu RC, Dellanes M, et al. Non-randomized comparative study of irradiation alone or in combination with surgery in stage IB, IIA and "proximal" IIB carcinoma of the cervix. Radiother Oncol 1991;22:104.

Baltzer J, Ober KG, Zander J. Adjuvant radiotherapy in patients undergoing surgical treatment for carcinoma of the cervix. Baillieres Clin Obstet Gynaecol 1988;2:999.

Barter JF, Soong SJ, Shingleton HM, Hatch KD, Orr JW Jr. Complications of combined radical hysterectomy-postoperative radiation therapy in women with early stage cervical cancer. Gynecol Oncol 1989;32:292.

Berman ML, Bergen S, Salazar H. Influence of histological features and treatment on the prognosis of patients with cervical cancer metastatic to pelvic lymph nodes. Gynecol Oncol 1990;39:127.

Bilek K, Eveling K, Leitsmann H, Seidel G. Radical pelvic surgery versus radical surgery plus radiotherapy for stage IB carcinoma of the cervix uteri. Preliminary results of a prospective randomized clinical study. Arch für Geschwulstforschung 1982;52:223.

Blake PR, Lambert HE, MacGregor WG, O'Sullivan JC, Dowdell JW, Anderson T. Surgery following chemotherapy and radiotherapy for advanced carcinoma of the cervix. Gynecol Oncol 1984;19:198.

Bloss JD, Berman ML, Mukherjee J, Manetta A, Rettenamier ED, DiSaia PJ. Bulky stage IB cervical carcinoma managed by primary radical hysterectomy followed by tailored radiotherapy. Gynecol Oncol 1992;47:21.

Bonar LD. Results of radical surgical procedures after radiation for treatment of invasive carcinoma of the uterine cervix in a private practice. Am J Obstet Gynecol 1980;136:1006.

Brady LW, Markoe AM, Sheline GE, et al. Radiation oncology: programs for the present and future. Cancer 1985;55:1445.

Brand E, Berek JS, Nieberg RK, Hacker NF. Rhabdomyosarcoma of the uterine cervix: sarcoma botryoides. Cancer 1987;60:1552.

Cardenas J, Olguin A, Figueroa F, Pena J, Huizar R, Becerra F. Neoadjuvant chemotherapy and radiotherapy versus radiotherapy alone in stage IIIB cervical carcinoma. Preliminary results. Proc Am Soc Clin Oncol 1992;11:232.

Cervical Cancer Immunotherapy Study Group. Immunotherapy using the streptococcal preparation OK-432 for the treatment of uterine cervical cancer. Cancer 1987;60:2394.

Chadha KC, Ambrus JL, et al. The interferon system in carcinoma of the cervix. Cancer 1991;67:87.

Chang HC, Lai CH, Chen MS, Chao AS, Chen LH, Soong YK. Preliminary results of concurrent radiotherapy and chemotherapy with cis-platinum, vincristine, and bleomycin in bulky, advanced cervical carcinoma: a pilot study. Gynecol Oncol 1992;44:182.

Chorlton I, Karnei RF, Norris HJ. Primary malignant reticuloendothelial disease involving the vagina, cervix and corpus uteri. Obstet Gynecol 1974;44:735.

Coleman DL, Gallup DG, Wolcott HD, Otken LB, Stock RJ. Patterns of failure of bulky-barrel carcinomas of the cervix. Am J Obstet Gynecol 1992;166:916.

Copeland LJ, Sneige N, Ordonez NG. Endodermal sinus tumor of the vagina and cervix. Cancer 1985;55:2558.

Crawford ER Jr, Robinson LS, Vaught J. Carcinoma of the cervix. Results of treatment by radiation alone and by combined radiation and surgical therapy in 335 patients. Am J Obstet Gynecol 1965;91:480.

de Graaff J. The Mitra Schauta operation in combination with pre-operative irradiation as treatment for carcinoma of the cervix. Gynecol Oncol 1980;10:267.

Degefu S, O'Quinn AG, Lacey CG, Merkel M, Barnard DE. Verrucous carcinoma of the cervix: a report of two cases and literature review. Gynecol Oncol 1986;25:37.

Deppe G, Malviya VK, Han I, et al. A preliminary report of combination chemotherapy with cisplatin and mitomycin-C followed by radical hysterectomy or radiation therapy in patients with locally advanced cervical cancer. Gynecol Oncol 1991;42:178.

DiSaia PJ, Bundy BN, Curry SL, Schlaerth J, Thigpen JT. Phase III study on the treatment of women with cervical cancer, stage IIB, IIIB and IVA (confined to the pelvis and/or periaortic nodes), with radiotherapy alone versus radiotherapy plus immunotherapy with intravenous *Corynebacterium parvum*. A gynecologic oncology group study. Gynecol Oncol 1987;26:386.

Dische S. A trial of RO 03-8799 (pimonidazole) in carcinoma of the uterine cervix: an interim report from the

Medical Research Council Working Party on advanced carcinoma of the cervix. Radiother Oncol 1993;26:93.

Dottino PR, Plaxe SC, Beddoe AM, Johnston C, Cohen CJ. Induction chemotherapy followed by radical surgery in cervical cancer. Gynecol Oncol 1991;40:7.

Downey GO, Potsh RA, Adcock LL, Prem KA, Twiggs LB. Pretreatment surgical staging in cervical carcinoma: therapeutic efficacy of pelvic lymph node resection. Am J Obstet Gynecol 1989;160:1055.

Edinger DD Jr, Watring WG, Anderson B, Mitchell GW Jr. Residual tumor following radiotherapy for locally advanced carcinomas of the uterine cervix: prognostic significance. Eur J Gynaecol Oncol 1984;5:90.

Eifel PJ, Burke TW, Delclos L, Wharton JT, Oswald MJ. Early stage I adenocarcinoma of the uterine cervix: treatment results in patients with tumors ≤4 cm in diameter. Gynecol Oncol 1991;41:199.

Eifel PJ, Morris M, Oswald MJ, Wharton JT, Delclos L. Adenocarcinoma of the uterine cervix. Cancer 1990; 65:2508.

Einhorn N, Bygdeman M, Sjoberg B. Combined radiation and surgical treatment for carcinoma of the uterine cervix. Cancer 1980;45:720.

Eisner RF, Cirisano F, Berek JS. Adjuvant radiation therapy for microscopic positive pelvic lymph nodes following radical hysterectomy for stage IB cervical cancer (abstract). Fourth Biennial Meeting of the International Gynecologic Cancer Society, Stockholm, Sweden, 1993. Int J Gynecol Cancer 1993;3:14.

Fallo L, Sartori E, La Face B, Gambino A, Pecorelli S, Bianchi UA. Adjuvant radiotherapy in stage IB cervix cancer with negative lymph nodes: a matched-control study (abstract). Fourth Biennial Meeting of the International Gynecologic Cancer Society, Stockholm, Sweden, 1993. Int J Gynecol Cancer 1993;3:13.

Farquharson DIM, Shingleton HM, Soong S-J. The adverse effects of cervical cancer treatment on bladder function. Gynecol Oncol 1987;27:15.

Fiorica JV, Roberts WS, Greenberg H, et al. Morbidity and survival patterns in patients after radical hysterectomy and postoperative adjuvant pelvic radiotherapy. Gynecol Oncol 1990;36:343.

Fletcher GH. Predominant parameters in the planning of radiation therapy of carcinoma of the cervix. Bull Cancer (Paris) 1979;66:561.

Fuller AF, Elliott N, Kosloff C, Lewis JL Jr. Lymph node metastases from carcinoma of the cervix, stages IB and IIA: implications for prognosis and treatment. Gynecol Oncol 1982;13:165.

Gallion HH, van Nagell JR Jr, Donaldson ES. Combined radiation therapy and extrafascial hysterectomy in the treatment of stage IB barrel-shaped cervical cancer. Cancer 1985;56:262.

Gast MJ, Radkins LV, Jacobs AJ, Bersell D. Müllerian adenosarcoma of the cervix with heterologous elements: diagnostic and therapeutic approach. Gynecol Oncol 1989;32:381.

Gerbaulet AL, Kunkler IH, Kerr GR, et al. Combined radiotherapy and surgery: local control and complications in early carcinoma of the uterine cervix—Villejuif experience, 1975–1984. Radiother Oncol 1992;23:66.

Giaroli A, Sananes C, Sardi JE, et al. Lymph node metastases in carcinoma of the cervix uteri: response to neoadjuvant chemotherapy and its impact on survival. Gynecol Oncol 1990;39:34.

Gonzalez DG, Ketting BW, van Bunningen B, van Dijk JDP. Carcinoma of the uterine cervix stage IB and IIA: results of postoperative irradiation in patients with microscopic infiltration in the parametrium and/or lymph node metastasis. Int J Radiat Oncol Biol Phys 1989;16:389.

Gynning I, Johnsson JE, Alm P, Trope C. Age and prognosis in stage IB squamous cell carcinoma of the uterine cervix. Gynecol Oncol 1983;15:18.

Habib A, Kaneko M, Cohen CJ, Walker G. Carcinoid of the uterine cervix. Cancer 1979;43:535.

Hacker NF, Wain GV, Nicklin J. Resection of bulky positive lymph nodes in cervical cancer. Int J Gynecol Cancer 1993;3:2.

Haie C, George M, Pejovic MH, et al. Feasibility study of an alternating schedule of radiotherapy and chemotherapy in advanced uterine carvical carcinoma. Radiother Oncol 1988;12:121.

Hanai J, Tsuji M. Uterine teratoma with lymphoid hyperplasia. Acta Pathol Jpn 1981;31:153.

Heaton D, Yordan E, Reddy SA, et al. Treatment of 29 patients with bulky squamous cell carcinoma of the cervix with simultaneous cisplatin, 5-fluorouracil, and split-course hyperfractionated radiation therapy. Gynecol Oncol 1990;38:323.

Herzog TJ, Nelson PK, Mutch DG, Wright WD, Collins JL. Effects of radiation on TNFα-mediated cytolysis of cell lines derived from cervical carcinomas. Gynecol Oncol 1992;47:196.

Hogan WM, Littman P, Griner L, Miller CL, Mikuta JJ. Results of radiation therapy given after radical hysterectomy. Cancer 1982;49:1278.

Hopkins MP, Morley GW. Radical hysterectomy versus radiation therapy for stage IB squamous cell cancer of the cervix. Cancer 1991;68:272.

Hreshchyshyn MM, Aron BS, Boronow RC, Franklin EW III, Shingleton HM, Blessing JA. Hydroxyurea or placebo combined with radiation to treat stages IIB and IV cervical cancer comfined to the pelvis. Int J Radiat Oncol Biol Phys 1979;3:317.

Inoue T, Morita K. Five-year results of postoperative extended field irradiation on 76 patients with nodal metastases from cervical carcinoma stage IB to IIIB. Cancer 1988;61:2009.

Inoue T, Yamaguchi K, Suzuki H, Abe K, Chihara T. Production of immunoreactive-polypeptide hormones in cervical carcinoma. Cancer 1984;53:1509.

Iversen T, Kjorstad KE, Martimbeau PW. Treatment results in carcinoma of the cervix stage IB in a total population. Gynecol Oncol 1982;14:1.

Jacobs AJ, Perez CA, Camel HM, Kao M-S. 1985 Complications in patients receiving both irradiation and radical hysterectomy for carcinoma of the uterine cervix. Gynecol Oncol 1985;22:273.

Johnston C, Senekjian EK, Ratain MJ, Talerman A. Conservative management of primary cervical lymphoma using combination chemotherapy: a case report. Gynecol Oncol 1989;35:391.

Jones HW III, Plymate S, Gluck FB, Miles PA, Greene JF Jr. Small cell nonkeratinizing carcinoma of the cervix associated with ACTH production. Cancer 1974;38:1629.

Jones WB. New approaches to high risk cervical cancer. Cancer 1993;71:1451.

Kadar N, Nelson JH. Treatment of urinary incontinence after radical hysterectomy. Obstet Gynecol 1984;64:400.

Kamura T, Tsukamoto N, Tsuruchi N, et al. Multivariate analysis of the histopathologic prognostic factors of cervical cancer in patients undergoing radical hysterectomy. Cancer 1992;69:181.

Kawagoe K, Yoshikawa H, Kawana T, Mizuno M, Sakamoto S. Verrucous carcinoma of the uterine cervix. Nippon Sanka Fujinka Gakkai Zasshi 1984;36:617.

Khoury GG, Robinson A. Lymphoma of uterine cervix. Eur J Surg Oncol 1989;15:65.

Kinney WK, Alvarez RD, Reid GC, et al. Value of adjuvant whole-pelvis irradiation after Wertheim hysterectomy for early-stage squamous carcinoma of the cervix with pelvic nodal metastasis: a matched-control study. Gynecol Oncol 1989;34:258.

Kjorstad KE, Kolbenstvedt A, Strickert T. The value of complete lymphadenectomy in radical treatment of cancer of the cervix, stage IB. Cancer 1984;54:2215.

Kjorstad KE, Martimbeau PW, Iversen T. Stage IB carcinoma of the cervix, the Norwegian Radium Hospital: results and complications. Gynecol Oncol 1983;15:42.

Kristensen GB, Frimodt-Moller PC, Poulsen HK, Ulbak S. Persistent bladder dysfunction after surgical and combination therapy of cancer of the cervix uteri stages IB and IIA. Gynecol Oncol 1984;18:38.

Kucera H, Skodler W, Weghaup K. Postoperative radiotherapy of cervical cancer: complications and implications for the surgical indications. Wein Klin Wochenschr 1984;96:451.

Lagasse L, Smith M, Moore J, Morton D, Jacobs M, Johnson G. The effect of radiation therpay on pelvic lymph node involvement in stage I carcinoma of the cervix. Am J Obstet Gynecol 1974;119:328.

Lahousen M, Pickel H, Haas J. Adjuvant chemotherapy after hysterectomy for cervical cancer. Baillieres Clin Obstet Gynaecol 1988;2:1049.

Lai C-H, Lin T-S, Soong Y-K, Chen H-F. Adjuvant chemotherapy after radical hysterectomy for cervical carcinoma. Gynecol Oncol 1989;35:193.

Larson DM, Stringer CA, Copeland LJ, Gershenson DV, Malone JM Jr, Rutledge FN. Stage IB cervical carcinoma treated with radical hysterectomy and pelvic lymphadenectomy: role of adjuvant radio-therapy. Obstet Gynecol 1987;69:378.

Lewandowski GS, Copeland JL. The potential role for intensive chemotherapy in the treatment of small cell neuroendocrine tumors of the cervix (review). Gynecol Oncol 1993;48:127.

Lewis JL, Nori D, Hoskins W, et al. Adjuvant cisplatin/bleomycin and radiation in patients at high risk of recurrence after radical surgery for stage IB/IIA cervix carcinoma (abstract). 2nd Annual Meeting, International Gynecologic Cancer Society, Toronto, Ontario, Canada, October 9–13, 1989.

Looney WB, Hopkins HA. Rationale for different chemotherapeutic and radiation therapy strategies in cancer management (review). Cancer 1991;67:1471.

Mackay B, Osborne BM, Wharton JT. Small cell tumor of cervix with neuroepithelial features. Cancer 1979; 43:1138.

Malfetano JH, Keys H. Aggressive multimodality treatment for cervical cancer with paraaortic lymph node metastases. Gynecol Oncol 1991;42:44.

Malfetano JH, Keys H, Kredentser D, et al. Weekly cisplatin and radical radiation therapy for advanced, recurrent, and poor prognosis cervical carcinoma. Cancer 1993; 71:3703.

Marcial VA, Marcial LV. Radiation therapy of cervical cancer. New developments. Cancer 1993;71:1438.

Maruyama Y, Donaldson E, van Nagell JR, et al. Specimen findings and survival after preoperative 252Cf neutron brachytherapy for stage II cervical carcinoma. Gynecol Oncol 1991;43:252.

Maruyama Y, van Nagell JR, Yoneda J, et al. Dose-response and failure pattern for bulky or barrel-shaped stage IB cervical cancer treated by combined photon irradiation and extrafascial hysterectomy. Cancer 1989;63:70.

Matsuyama M, Inoue T, Arivoshi Y, et al. Argyrophil cell carcinoma of the uterine cervix with ectopic production of ACTH, β-MSH, serotonin, histamine and amylase. Cancer 1979;44:1813.

Mendenhall WM, McCarty PJ, Morgan LS, Chafe WE, Million RR. Stage IB or IIA-B carcinoma of the intact uterine cervix greater than or equal to 6 cm in diameter: is adjuvant extrafascial hysterectomy beneficial? Int J Rad Oncol Biol Phys 1991;21:899.

Montag TW, D'Ablaing G, Schlaerth JB, Gaddis O Jr, Morrow CP. Embryonal rhabdomyosarcoma of the uterine corpus and cervix. Gynecol Oncol 1986;25:171.

Mordel N, Mor-Yosef S, Ben-Baruch N, Anteby S. Malignant melanoma of the uterine cervix: case report and review of the literature. Gynecol Oncol 1989;32:375.

Morrow CP. Is pelvic radiation beneficial in the postoperative management of stage IB squamous cell carcinoma of the cervix with pelvic node metastasis treated by radical hysterectomy and pelvic lymphadenectomy? Gynecol Oncol 1980;10:105.

Muntz HG, Ferry JA, Flynn D, Fuller AR Jr, Tarraza HM. Stage IE primary malignant lymphomas of the uterine cervix. Cancer 1991;68:2023.

Nelson AJ, Fletcher GH, Wharton JT. Indications for adjunctive conservative extrafascial hysterectomy in selected cases of carcinoma of the uterine cervix. Am J Radiol 1975;123:91.

Ng GT, Shyu SK, Chen YK, Yuan CC, Chao KC, Kan YY. A scoring system for predicting recurrence of cervical cancer. Int J Gynecol Cancer 1992;2:75.

Noda K, Teshima K, TeKeuti K, et al. Immunotherapy using the streptococcal preparation OK-432 for the treatment of uterine cervical cancer: cervical cancer immunotherapy study group. Gynecol Oncol 1989;35:367.

Noda K, Takeuchi S, Yajima A, et al. Clinical effect of sizofiran combined with irradiation in cervical cancer patients: a randomized controlled study. Cooperative study group on SPG for gynecological cancer. Jpn J Clin Oncol 1993;22:17.

O'Hanlan KA, Goldberg GL, Jones JG, et al. Adjuvant therapy for neuroendocrine small cell carcinoma of the cervix: review of the literature. Gynecol Oncol 1991;43:167.

O'Quinn AG, Fletcher GH, Wharton JT. Guidelines for conservative hysterectomy, after irradiation. Gynecol Oncol 1980;9:68.

Okamura K, Hamazaki Y, et al. Adjuvant immunotherapy: two randomized controlled studies of patients with cervical cancer. Biomed Pharmacother 1989;43:177.

Okawa T, Niibe H, Arai T, et al. Effect of LC9018 combined with radiation therapy on carcinoma of the uterine cervix. Cancer 1993;72:1949.

Panici PB, Greggi S, Scambia G, et al. High-dose cisplatin and bleomycin neoadjuvant chemotherapy plus radical surgery in locally advanced cervical carcinoma: a preliminary report. Gynecol Oncol 1991;41:212.

Parham G, Syed S, Savage E. Concurrent chemoradiation followed by modified abdominal hysterectomy, pelvic and retroperitoneal para-aortic lymphadenectomy: effective multimodality treatment for advance, bulky cervical cancer (abstract). Gynecol Oncol 1993;49:112.

Park TK, Choi DH, Kim SN, et al. Role of induction chemotherapy in invasive cervical cancer. Gynecol Oncol 1991;41:107.

Park TK, Lee SK, Kim SN, et al. Combined chemotherapy and radiation for bulky stages I–II cervical cancer: comparison of concurrent and sequential regimens. Gynecol Oncol 1993;50:196.

Partridge EE, Murad T, Shingleton HM, Austin JM, Hatch KD. Verrucous lesions of the female genitalia. II. Verrucous carcinoma. Am J Obstet Gynecol 1980;137:412.

Patton TJ, Kavanagh JJ, Delclos L, et al. Five-year survival in patients given intra-arterial chemotherapy prior to radiotherapy for advanced squamous carcinoma of the cervix and vagina. Gynecol Oncol 1991;42:54.

Pearcey RG, Peel KR, Thorogood J, Walker K. The value of pre-operative intracavitary radio-therapy in patients treated by radical hysterectomy and pelvic lymphadenectomy for invasive carcinoma of the cervix. Clin Radiol 1988;39;95.

Perez CA, Camel HM, Kao MS, Askin F. Randomized study of preoperative radiation and surgery or irradiation alone in the treatment of stage IB and IIA carcinoma of the uterine cervix: preliminary analysis of failures and complications. Cancer 1980;45:2759.

Perez CA, Camel HM, Kuske RR, et al. Randomized study of preoperative radiation and surgery or irradiation alone in the treatment of stage IB and IIA carcinoma of the uterine cervix: final report. Gynecol Oncol 1987;27:129.

Perez CA, Kao M-S. Radiation therapy alone or combined with surgery in the treatment of barrel-shaped carcinoma of the uterine cervix (stages IB, IIA, IIB). Int J Radiat Oncol Biol Phys 1985;11:1903.

Perkins PL, Chu AM, Jose B, Achino E, Tobin DA. Posthysterectomy megavoltage irradiation in the treatment of cervical carcinoma. Gynecol Oncol 1984;17:340.

Perren T, Farrant M, McCarthy K, Harper P, Wiltshaw E. Lymphomas of the cervix and upper vagina: a report of five cases and a review of the literature. Gynecol Oncol 1992;44:87.

Petri E. Bladder after radical pelvic surgery. In Stanton SL (ed). Clinical gynecologic urology. St. Louis, CV Mosby, 1984:220.

Piver MS, Barlow JJ, Vongtama V, Blumenson L. Hydroxurea as a radiation sensitizer in women with carcinoma of the uterine cervix. Am J Obstet Gynecol 1977; 129:379.

Piver MS, Barlow JJ, Vongtama V, Blumenson L. Hydroxyurea: a radiation potentiator in carcinoma of the uterine cervix. Am J Obstet Gynecol 1983;147:803.

Pozzi M, Iacovelli A, Diotallevi FF, Giovagnoli A, Castagnola D, Vincenzoni C. Adenocarcinoma del canale cervicale: considerazioni clinico-statistiche. Rivista di Ostetricia e Ginecologia 1991;IV:3.

Prempree T, Amornmarn R, Wizenberg MJ. A therapeutic approach to primary adenocarcinoma of the cervix. Cancer 1985;56:1264.

Rabin S, Browde S, Nissenbaum M, Koller AB, De Moor NG. Radiotherapy and surgery in the management of stage IB and IIA carcinoma of the cervix. South Afr Med J 1984;65:374.

Ralph G, Tamussino K, Lichtenegger W. Urological complications after radical hysterectomy with or without radiotherapy for cervical cancer. Arch Gynecol Oncol 1990;248:61.

Rampone JF, Klem V, Kolstad P. Combined treatment of stage IB carcinoma of the cervix. Obstet Gynecol 1973;41:163.

Remy JC, DiMaio T, Fruchter RG, et al. Adjunctive radiation after radical hysterectomy in stage IB squamous cell carcinoma of the cervix. Gynecol Oncol 1990;38:161.

Remy JC, Fruchter RG, Choi K, Rotman M, Boyce JG. Complications of combined radical hysterectomy and pelvic radiation. Gynecol Oncol 1986;24:317.

Rettenmaier MA, Casanova DM, Micha JP, et al. Radical hysterectomy and tailored postoperative radiation therapy in the management of bulky stage IB cervical cancer. Cancer 1989;63:2220.

Roberts WD, Kavanagh JJ, Greenberg H, et al. Concomitant radiation therapy and chemotherapy in the treatment of advanced squamous carcinoma of the lower female genital tract. Gynecol Oncol 1989;34:183.

Rotmensch J, Rosenshein NB, Woodruff JD. Cervical sarcoma: a review. Obstet Gynecol Surv 1983;38:456.

Runowicz CD, Smith HO, Goldberg GL. Multimodality therapy in locally advanced cervical cancer (review). Curr Opin Obstet Gynecol 1993;5:92.

Runowicz CD, Wadler S, Rodriguez-Rodriguez L, et al. Concomitant cisplatin and radiotherapy in locally advanced cervical carcinoma. Gynecol Oncol 1989;34: 395.

Rutledge FN, Fletcher GH, McDonald EJ. Pelvic lymphadenectomy as an adjunct to radiation therapy in treatment for cancer of the cervix. Am J Roentgenol 1965;93;607.

Santoso JT, Kucera PR, Ray J. Primary malignant melanoma of the uterine cervix: two case reports and a century's review. Obstet Gynecol Surv 1990;45:733.

Sardi J, Sananes C, et al. Neoadjuvant chemotherapy in locally advanced carcinoma cervix uteri. Gynecol Oncol 1990;38:486.

Sardi J, Sananes C, Giaroli A, et al. Results of a prospective randomized trial with neoadjuvant chemotherapy in stage IB, bulky, squamous carcinoma of the cervis. Gynecol Oncol 1993;49:156.

Shingleton HM, Jones WB, Russell AH. American College of Surgeons invasive cervical cancer patterns of care study. 1995. In preparation.

Shingleton HM, Palumbo L Jr. Ureteral complications of radical hysterectomy: effects of preoperative radium and ureteral catheters. Surg Forum 1968;19:410.

Silva EG, Kott MM, Ordonez NG. Endocrine carcinoma intermediate cell type of the uterine cervix. Cancer 1984;54:1705.

Soeters R, Bloch B, Levin W, Dehaeck CMD, Goldberg G. Combined chemotherapy and radiotherapy in patients with advanced squamous carcinoma of the cervix (cisplatinum-bleomycin-vinblastine). Gynecol Oncol 1989;33:44.

Soisson AP, Soper JT, Clarke-Pearson DL, Berchuck A, Montana G, Creasman WT. Adjuvant radiotherapy following radical hysterectomy for patients with stage IB and IIA cervical cancer. Gynecol Oncol 1990;37:390.

Souhami L, Gil RA, Allan SE, et al. A randomized trial of chemotherapy followed by pelvic radiation therapy in stage IIIB carcinoma of the cervix. J Clin Oncol 1991;9:970.

Stehman FB, Bundy BN, Thomas G, et al. Hydroxyurea versus misoidazole with radiation in cervical carcinoma: long term follow-up of a gynecologic oncology group trial. J Clin Oncol 1993;11:1523.

Surwit E, Fowler WC Jr, Palumbo P, Koch G, Gjertsen W. Radical hysterectomy with or without preoperative radium for stage IB squamous cell carcinoma of the cervix. Obstet Gynecol 1976;48:130.

Sutton G, Bundy B, Delgado G, et al. Evaluation of pelvic radiotherapy following radical hysterectomy in patients with clinical stage IB squamous carcinoma of the cervix: a study of the gynecologic oncology group (abstract). Gynecol Oncol 1993;49:112.

Symonds RP, Burnett RA, Habeshaw T, Kaye SB, Snee MP, Watson ER. The prognostic value of a response to chemotherapy given before radiotherapy in advanced cancer of the cervix. Br J Cancer 1989;59:473.

Talbert LM, Palumbo L, Shingleton HM, Bream CA, McGee J. Urologic complications of radical hysterectomy for carcinoma of the cervix. South Med J 1965;58:11.

Thomas G, Dembo A, Fyles A, et al. Concurrent chemoradiation in advanced cervical cancer. Gynecol Oncol 1990;38:446.

Thomas GM, Dembo AJ. Is there a role for adjuvant pelvic radiotherapy after radical hysterectomy in early stage cervical cancer? Int J Gynecol Cancer 1991;1:1.

Thomas GM. Is neoadjuvant chemotherapy a useful strategy for the treatment of stage IB cervix cancer? Gynecol Oncol 1993;49:153. Editorial.

Thoms WW Jr, Eifel PJ, Smith TL, et al. Bulky endocervical carcinoma: a 23 year experience. Int J Radiat Oncol Biol Phys 1992;23:491.

Timmer PR, Aalders JG, Bouma J. Radical surgery after preoperative intracavitary radiotherapy for stage IB and IIA carcinoma of the cervix. Gynecol Oncol 1984;18:206.

Tinga DJ, Bouma J, Hollema H, Aalders JG. Radical surgery compared with intracavitary cesium followed by radical surgery in cervical carcinoma stage IB. Acta Obstet Gynecol Scand 1990;69:239.

Turrisi AT, Glover DJ, Mason B, Tester W. Concurrent twice daily multi-field radiotherapy (2X/DX RT) and platinum-etoposide chemotherapy (P/E) for limited small cell lung cancer. Lung Cancer 1988;7:211.

van Nagell JR, Donaldson ES, Parker JC, van Dyke AH, Wood EG. The prognostic significance of cell type and lesion size in patients with cervical cancer treated by radical surgery (abstract). Gynecol Oncol 1977;5:142.

Varia MA, Stehman F, Hanjani P, Bunby B. Metastatic cervical carcinoma to para-aortic nodes: results of extended field radiation therapy with hydroxurea—a GOG study (abstract). 72nd scientific assembly and annual meeting, Radiologic Society of North America, Chicago, November 30–December 5, 1986.

Wadler S, Haynes H, Beitler JJ, et al. Management of hypocalcemic effects of WR2721 administered on a daily times five schedule with cisplatin and radiation therapy. J Clin Oncol 1993;11:1517.

Weed JC, Holland JB. Combined irradiation and extensive operations in the treatment of stages I and II carcinoma of the cervix uteri. Surg Gynaecol Obstet 1977;144:869.

Weems DH, Mendenhall WM, Bova FJ, Marcus RB Jr, Morgan LS, Million RR. Carcinoma of the intact uterine cervix, stage IB–IIA-B greater than or equal to 6cm in diameter: irradiation alone vs. preoperative irradiation and surgery. Int J Radiat Oncol Biol Phys 1985;11:1911.

Welander CE, Pierce VK, Nori D, et al. Pretreatment laparotomy in carcinoma of the cervix. Gynecol Oncol 1981;12:336.

Yamasaki M, Tateishi R, Hongo J, Ozaki Y, Inoue M, Ueda G. Argyrophil small cell carcinomas of the uterine cervix. Int J Gynecol Pathol 1984;3:146.

Yordan EL, Jurado M, Kiel K, et al. Intraoperative radiation therapy in the treatment of pelvic malignancies: a preliminary report. Bailliere's Clinical Obstetrics and Gynecology 1988;2:1023.

Yoshida A, Yoshida H, Fukunishi R, Inohara T. Carcinoid tumor of the uterine cervix. A light and electron microscopic study. Virchows Arch A Pathol Anat Histopathol 1984;402:331.

Young RH, Harris NL, Scully RE. Lymphoma-like lesions of the lower female genital tract: a report of 16 cases. Int J Gynecol Pathol 1985;4:289.

Zanetta G, Landoni F, Colombo A, et al. Three-year results after neoadjuvant chemotherapy, radical surgery and radiotherapy in locally advanced cervical carcinoma. Obstet Gynecol 1993;82:447.

Cancer of the Cervix by Hugh M. Shingleton and James W. Orr, Jr.
J. B. Lippincott Company, Philadelphia, © 1995.

10

Cervical Cancer Complicating Pregnancy

The diagnosis of invasive cervical cancer during pregnancy creates uncertainty and anxiety for the patient, her family, the physician, and others. Diagnostic and therapeutic decisions, which potentially jeopardize the mother and fetus, become complex and may assume emotional, religious, and ethical overtones. Additional clinical problems occur when physicians must weigh existing diverse and sometimes conflicting opinions regarding the possible effect of pregnancy and delivery on the biology of the cervical cancer or the potential adverse effects of the disease, evaluation, or treatment on the fetus. Unfortunately, no reported experience at any one institution allows the determination of an optimal therapeutic approach in every clinical situation.

The reported incidence of abnormal cervical cytology during pregnancy varies considerably, depending on risk factors of the screened population. In addition to screening and evaluation of abnormal cytology, the practicing obstetrician must address the question of pregnancy in women who have been previously treated for cervical dysplasia. Although the extent of cervical removal or destruction may alter cervical function (Jones et al 1979, Larsson et al 1982), prior treatment for malignant precursors (almost regardless of method) generally has little effect on future fertility or pregnancy outcome (Harris 1982, Moinian et al 1982, Hemmingson 1982, Hollyock et al 1983, Luesley et al 1985, Bigrigg et al 1991, Keijser et al 1992).

Abitbol and coworkers (1973), in a retrospective review of 13,000 pregnant patients, reported an incidence of abnormal cervical smears of 2.2%. Lurain and associates (1979) reported an incidence of 1.3%. The risk of carcinoma in situ (CIS) is lower, with an incidence as low as 0.025% (Wanless 1971); however, in a

review, Hacker and colleagues (1982) reported a prevalence for CIS of 1.3 in 1000 pregnancies, suggesting a trend toward an increased incidence. Prospective evaluations of pregnant women using abrasive cytology indicates a 1.8% risk of abnormal smears in a private practice population (Orr et al 1992) and an 8.5% risk in a university population (Rivlin et al 1993). Additionally, the incidence of human papillomavirus–associated cytologic abnormalities discovered during pregnancy may be as high as 28% (Hannigan 1990, Patsner et al 1990).

The determination of risk should be a simple mathematic exercise in joint probability; however, the true incidence of pregnancy and coexisting invasive cervical cancer is difficult to establish. Clearly, a significant proportion (30% or more) of patients diagnosed with cervical cancer are reproductive-aged women (younger than 35 years old; Clark et al 1991). Most reports detail patients treated at referral institutions, which may or may not have an obstetric service representative of the local area. Additionally, most reports include results from patients treated both antepartum and 2 to 18 months postpartum (Table 10-1). Depending on the patient's socioeconomic status, the hospital's referral base, and the duration of the study, 0.02% to 0.9% of pregnancies are complicated by coexisting invasive cervical cancer (i.e., the chance of finding an invasive cervical cancer in the pregnant woman ranges from 1 in 110 to 1 in 5000). Conversely, between 0.1% to 7.6% of cervical cancer patients are pregnant at the time of diagnosis. In an American College of Surgeons Patterns of Care Study that included 11,717 invasive cancers in the years 1984 and 1990, 161 (1.4%) were apparent at initial diagnosis (Shingle-

TABLE 10-1
Invasive Cervical Cancer Associated with Pregnancy

STUDY	YEAR	FOUND ANTEPARTUM (N)	PREGNANT PATIENTS (%)	CERVICAL CANCER PATIENTS (%)	FOUND POSTPARTUM (%)	CERVICAL CANCER PATIENTS (%)
Stander, et al	1960	27	—	0.1	6	0.03
Lash	1961	18	—	—	—	—
Gustafsson, et al	1962	82	—	1.1	157§	2.2
Cromer, et al	1963	16	—	1.9	—	—
Waldrop, et al	1963	48	—	0.8	132§	2.2
Williams, et al	1964	12	0.02	0.7	12†	0.7
Van Praagh, et al	1965	41	0.9	—	43	1.0
Bosch, et al	1966	26	—	0.9	40§	1.5
Prem, et al	1966	22	—	0.2	78**	6.9
O'Leary, et al	1966	18	0.02	—	0	—
Herold	1967	24	—	0.7	39§	1.2
Mikuta	1967	18	0.03	2.0	12¶	1.3
Shaffer, et al	1969	32	0.4	7.6	12#	2.9
Creasman, et al	1970	48	—	3.4*	65†	4.6*
Wanless	1971	11	0.03	—	—	—
Fogh	1972	65	—	0.8	16¶	0.2
Dudan, et al	1973	23	0.05	—	—	—
Sall, et al	1974	23	0.04	—	11¶	0.03
Thompson, et al	1975	41	0.05	6.0	1‡	0.1
Sablinska, et al	1977	63	—	0.8	264§	3.2
Lutz, et al	1977	23	0.2	1.0	7†	0.3
Funnell, et al	1980	10	—	3.8	7‡	2.6
Lee, et al	1981	21	—	2.4	20†	2.2
Fay, et al	1982	6	—	5.0	6	5.0
Bokhman, et al	1989	1	0.17	—	—	—
Baltzer, et al	1990	24	—	2.1	16	1.5
Zemlickis, et al	1991	23	—	1.2	17	0.9
Sivanesaratnam, et al	1993	16	0.02	—	4‡‡	0.1
Duggan, et al	1993	27	0.01	—	—	—

*Percentage of patients age 19–49 with cervical cancer.
†Within 6 months.
‡Within 3 months.
§Within 6 months.
¶Within 2 months.
#Within 4 months.
**Within 18 months.
††Within 5 months.
‡‡<20 weeks.

ton 1994). Fay and coworkers (1982) called attention to the importance of screening the pregnant woman because of the apparently increasing risk of invasive cancer in younger women. Depending on the definition of the postpartum state, it appears that postpartum patients comprise 0.03% to 6.9% of women with cervical cancer. As expected, reports that include a shorter postpartum interval indicate a lower incidence than those including longer postpartum follow-up.

DIAGNOSIS

Cytologic Screening

Pregnancy represents an ideal time to screen for cervical cancer because most women receive prenatal care. The safety, acceptance, and routine use of antenatal cervical cytologic screening is responsible for increasing the number of cervical cancers detected antepartum and the percentage of patients having early stage invasive disease (Zemlickis et al 1991).

A vaginal speculum and bimanual pelvic examination are accepted standards of routine prenatal care. The addition of cervical cytology, sampling both the exocervix and endocervical canal, lessens the risk of an occult lesion escaping detection. Although physiologic basal cell hyperactivity of the ectocervical epithelium or the presence of decidual, trophoblastic, or Arias-Stella cells are commonly present and may cause confusion, cytologic interpretation of cervical neoplasia is as accurate during pregnancy as in the nonpregnant woman. Prospective evaluations comparing the value of using a cotton-tipped swab or abrasive cervical cytology (Orr et al 1992, Rivlin et al 1993) indicate a clinically and statistically significant increase in cytologic specimen adequacy without an associated increase in adverse pregnancy events when using the Cytobrush (Orr et al 1992). Regardless of cytologic results, visible suspicious cervical lesions should be evaluated and biopsies obtained when deemed necessary. Palpable parametrial induration or a markedly enlarged nodular cervix should increase clinical suspicion of underlying invasive cancer.

Symptoms

Associated symptoms of cervical cancer do not necessarily differ from "normal" pregnancy symptoms (Table 10-2). Although not always present, vaginal bleeding is the most common symptom. Vaginal discharge and pain are less frequent but may coexist. The frequency of asymptomatic patients (up to 70% in some series) establishes the importance of prenatal cervical cytology and careful pelvic examination. When a pregnant woman complains of excessive symptoms such as bleeding or discharge, obstetricians should perform cervical inspection and palpation to exclude the presence of a clinical cervical cancer, regardless of the stage of the patient's pregnancy. Occasionally, some pregnancy complications such as placenta previa may limit the extent and reliability of antenatal examination. Additionally, the cervix of asymptomatic and symptomatic women should be carefully examined during the puerperium. In the United States, a cytologic smear is usually performed at the first postpartum visit. Cervical ectropion after delivery may be misleading; however, regardless of antenatal cytology results, directed biopsies should be considered when a lesion suspicious for cervical cancer is present, even

TABLE 10-2
Symptoms in Patients with Pregnancy Coexisting with Cervical Cancer

STUDY	YEAR	PATIENTS (N)	ASYMPTO-MATIC (%)	BLEEDING (%)	DISCHARGE (%)	PAIN (%)
Stander, et al	1960	30	13.0	87.0	—	—
Lash	1961	18	22.2	77.8	—	—
Waldrop, et al	1963	170	7.2	—	—	—
Williams, et al	1964	24	20.8	58.3	8.3	4.2
Bosch, et al	1966	66	9.0	80.0	5.0	6.0
Prem, et al	1966	100	12.0	69.0	—	—
O'Leary, et al	1966	18	44.4	27.8	27.8	—
Mikuta	1967	30	70.0	30.0	—	—
Shaffer, et al	1969	11	18.2	81.8	—	—
Creasman, et al	1970	113	3.0	5.4	13.0	—
Fogh	1972	81	1.0	77.0	21.0	1.0
Dudan, et al	1973	23	95.0	5.0	—	—
Lutz, et al	1977	30	†	26.7	—	—
Lee, et al	1981	41	36.1	55.6*	—	—
Baltzer	1990	40	20.0	55.0	—	—
Hopkins, et al	1992	53	69.0‡	41.0	—	—
Sivanesaratnam, et al	1993	20	55.0	15.0	—	—

*Bleeding and discharge.
†Most patients.
‡Positive cytology leading to diagnosis.

when cytology is negative or only atypical (Lurie et al 1991).

It is uncommon for a pregnant woman to have cervical cancer, and most practicing obstetricians only make this diagnosis once or twice during their career. Given the rarity of this occurrence, physicians tend to be less suspicious of specific symptoms, with a resultant delay in diagnosis and treatment. Unfortunately, the average duration of symptoms of cervical cancer associated with pregnancy is 4.5 months (Hacker et al 1982) and can be longer when a thorough postpartum examination is not performed. Sablinska and associates' (1977) report of an increased rate of postpartum discovery of cervical cancer in women younger than 30 emphasizes this problem.

Evaluation of Precursor Lesions in Pregnancy

Prenatal cytologic screening has been associated with an increased rate of detection of invasive and preinvasive cervical disease in asymptomatic pregnant women. Before the 1960s, the evaluation of abnormal cervical cytology during pregnancy included iodine staining, random punch biopsies, or conization. The first two procedures, considered to be inadequate because of false-negative rates of 40% (Roberts 1983), and the latter, fraught with maternal and fetal risks, have been replaced by colposcopically directed biopsy. Although concern that pregnant patients might have an increased risk of complications after directed cervical biopsy, the reported experience at the University of Alabama at Birmingham, where 230 pregnant women underwent diagnostic cervical biopsies during a 10-year study period, indicates that although vaginal bleeding may occur, bleeding that requires transfusion is exceedingly rare (Orr et al 1983). Patient anxiety can be decreased when patients are instructed that limited vaginal bleeding is likely to occur after cervical biopsy. Several reports (Creasman et al 1970, DePetrillo et al 1975, Lurain et al 1979, Fowler et al 1980, Yoonessi et al 1982, Benedet et al 1987, LaPolla et al 1988) substantiate this information and indicate that cervical biopsy does not increase the risk of abortion. The risk of biopsy-related complications is 0.6% (Hacker et al 1982).

Colposcopy

Pregnancy-associated cervical hypertrophy and dilation usually facilitates adequate visualization of the squamocolumnar junction and satisfactory colposcopic examination (Campion et al 1993). Displacement of the hyperemic redundant vaginal mucosa of pregnancy, especially the lateral vaginal walls, can be facilitated with a tongue blade, vaginal retractors, or a condom-covered speculum (Orr et al 1993). When adequate visualization is obscured or invasion is suspected, referral to a gynecologic oncologist may be appropriate. Although decidual transformation of the cervix may mimic the colposcopic appearance of precursor lesions (Madej et al 1992) and pregnancy may exaggerate the colposcopic appearance of squamous intraepithelial lesion (SIL), many reports (Ortiz et al 1971, Stafl 1973, DePetrillo et al 1975, Tunca et al 1976, Talebian et al 1976, Trombetta 1976, Lurain et al 1979, Ostergard et al 1979, Fowler et al 1980, Yoonessi et al 1982, Benedet et al 1987, LaPolla et al 1988, and Economos et al 1993) indicate that in experienced hands, the colposcopic evaluation of a pregnant woman who has abnormal cervical cytology can effectively limit the risk of an invasive carcinoma remaining undetected. In these authors' combined series of 2466 patients, the incidence of undetected or unsuspected invasive cancer during the antepartum period was less than 0.1% when the colposcopic examination was adequate. The necessity of cervical conization ranged from 1% (DePetrillo et al 1975) to 12% (Fowler et al 1980). The colposcopic evaluation of persistent squamous cytologic atypia during pregnancy (Kaminski et al 1992) results in the diagnosis of SIL in 21% of patients. Obviously, a rare invasive cancer can escape detection with cervical cytology and colposcopy (Bakri et al 1990); however, only an expert colposcopist should omit cervical biopsy, particularly when only one antepartum examination is planned (Hannigan 1990). Atypical glandular cells in the cervical smear require specific evaluation; the diagnosis of adenocarcinoma may present a difficult clinical problem in the pregnant woman because endocervical evaluation may be limited (Edinger et al 1982, Lurie et al 1991).

Our current scheme for the evaluation of abnormal cytology in pregnant women (Fig. 10-1) has been satisfactory. In evaluating 230 patients over a 10-year period, not a single patient with invasive cancer escaped antepartum detection. Only 2 patients (0.9%) have required cervical conization (Orr, unpublished data).

Conization

Although there is little role for therapeutic conization during pregnancy, the indications for diagnostic conization are essentially the same as those for the nonpregnant woman. Conization should be considered in any patient whose biopsy or cytologic smear suggests invasive carcinoma when an invasive diagnosis may result in a treatment or delivery modification. We do not favor the use of diagnostic cervical conization for evaluation of an inadequate colposcopic examina-

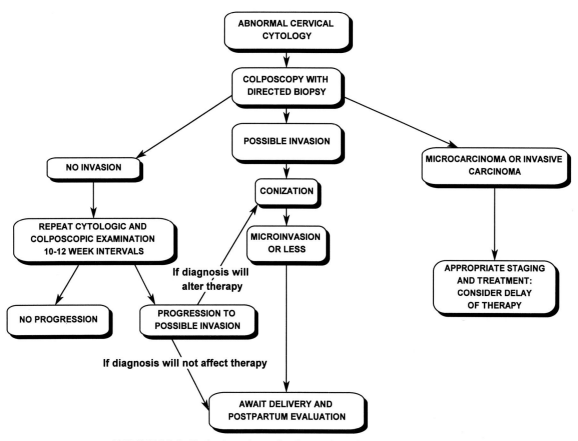

FIGURE 10-1. Evaluation scheme for abnormal cytology in pregnant women.

tion unless the cytology after review was highly suspicious for the presence of an invasive cancer.

Conization increases the risk of maternal and fetal complications (Table 10-3) and should be performed only after a thorough review of all previous cytologic and biopsy specimens. Perioperative hemorrhage is a major risk of conization performed during pregnancy. In one tabulated review, Hannigan (1990) indicated immediate excessive blood loss in 8.9% (40 of 448) of pregnant patients, with a risk of delayed cervical bleeding of 3.3% (15 of 448). Averette and colleagues' (1970) report indicated that this risk was negligible during the first trimester, 5% in the second trimester, and 10% after conization during the third trimester. Goldberg and associates (1991) reported a method of cone cerclage in 17 patients, with no transfusion or other hemorrhagic complications. Cervical stenosis follows conization in 3% of pregnant patients, whereas cervical lacerations have been noted in 3% to 18% of patients having a later vaginal delivery. Concerns regarding induced abortion or premature delivery are justified. The risk of postconization abortion varies from 3% to 8%; however, when performed during the first trimester, abortion rates are 17.7% to 50% (Nebel et al 1967, Hannigan 1990). When indicated, diagnostic conization should not be unduly delayed; however, it seems prudent to avoid conization during the first trimester in those women who desire to maintain their pregnancy. Other complications, such as inadvertent rupture of the chorioamnion or intrauterine infections, are rarely reported. In those situations wherein diagnosis of an invasive lesion may modify therapy, we endorse Hacker and coworkers' (1982) suggestion of a "segmental" wedge resection of the abnormal colposcopic area. There is no significant experience that suggests that the use of diagnostic loop diathermy conization or segmental resection alters these risks. Despite associated risks with conization, term infants are delivered in about 80% of pregnancies that are complicated by the necessity of antepartum conization. Overall, fetal salvage rates approach 95% (Hannigan 1990).

In contrast to cervical conization performed in the nonpregnant woman, residual intraepithelial disease is probably more common after the procedure performed during pregnancy (Hacker et al 1982);

TABLE 10-3
Complications Related to Cervical Conization During Pregnancy

Study	Year	Patients (N)	Hemorrhage (%)	Stenosis (%)	Lacerations (%)	Infants (%)	Abortion (%)	Immature (%)	Premature Rate (%)	Fetal Salvage (%)
O'Leary, et al	1966	39	2.6	—	7.7	—	7.7	—	—	—
Moore, et al	1966	29	6.9	—	6.9	—	6.9	—	8.3	—
Rogers, et al	1967	72	13.8	2.8	5.6	80.6	4.2	2.8	55.0	—
Smith, et al	1968	47	8.5	—	—	—	4.5	—	4.3	—
Daskal, et al	1968	77	10.4	—	2.6	78.4	8.1	—	12.2§	87.0
Stromme	1969	28	7.1	—	—	—	7.1	—	3.6	—
Shaffer, et al	1969	20	10.0	—	—	—	—	—	—	—
Bolognese, et al	1969	33	0	—	3.0	79.0	3.0	—	15.0	—
Averette, et al	1970	180	7.2*	2.2	7.2	76.0	4.4	1.1†	13.0‡	89.0
Fowler, et al	1980	13	0	—	—	—	—	—	12.5	88.0
Hannigan, et al	1982	82	12.4*	—	18.0	—	3.6	4.2	11.1	—

*500 mL.
†Related to conization (total of 2.2%).
‡79% of prematures survived.
§67% of those premature survived.

residual dysplasia may be present in more than 50% of hysterectomy specimens after a conization during pregnancy (Hannigan et al 1982). This problem is likely related to the surgeon's conservative approach to minimize cervical trauma in order to minimize fetal or maternal risk or avoid promoting premature labor. It is therefore especially important that patients who are found to have high-grade preinvasive or even focal microinvasive lesions early in pregnancy undergo repeat cytology and colposcopic evaluation later in the pregnancy; in the absence of progressive disease, further testing and treatment can be deferred until the postpartum period. The timing of postpartum reevaluation is related to the expected extent of disease.

TREATMENT: PRECURSOR LESIONS

Although conservative treatments, including cryotherapy (Matanyi 1989), have been used without event during pregnancy, the natural history of intraepithelial neoplasia, the unlikelihood of progression to invasive disease, the relatively high incidence of regression, and the possible side effects of therapy prompt us to recommend no antepartum therapy to patients with SIL (Anderson 1991). The reported rate of progression to CIS or invasive cancer (Richart et al 1969) is longer than most gestations. Cytologic and colposcopic examination (with or without biopsy) in each trimester of pregnancy allows the physician to diagnose progression if it occurs (Jolles 1989). Repeat evaluation should certainly be considered in those patients having CIS because 4% of nonpregnant patients may progress to invasion during a year of observation (Petersen 1956). The necessity of multiple colposcopic examinations in pregnant women with histologically documented low-grade SIL has been questioned. One report (Patsner et al 1990) detailed 55 patients who were evaluated by a gynecologic oncologist, with biopsy and satisfactory colposcopic evaluation indicating cervical intraepithelial neoplasia (CIN) I. None had progression to CIS or invasive cancer during pregnancy. It is our contention that colposcopic evaluation during pregnancy need not be performed by a gynecologic oncologist; however, the ability to colposcopically detect early invasive cancer is increased with frequent examinations by those having good colposcopic skills and experience.

A postpartum colposcopic reevaluation should be performed before treatment because regression has been reported to occur in as many as 77% of pregnant patients with CIN I or II (Roberts 1983, Patsner et al 1990). Postpartum treatment of persistent SIL (see Chap. 4) is indicated for those women who have high-grade precursor lesions or in the few women whose low-grade SIL lesions have progressed.

EVALUATION AND TREATMENT: INVASIVE CANCER

When the diagnosis of invasive cervical carcinoma is established, pretreatment evaluation should be performed commensurate with the clinical stage of disease, fetal gestational age, and the patient's wishes regarding preservation of the pregnancy.

In those patients having clinically staged IA2 or small IB cervical lesions, there is little benefit of multiple pretreatment radiologic studies because they rarely contribute to important therapeutic decisions. Irradia-

tion effects must also be considered in those patients who are undergoing radioisotope diagnostic scans or radiographic studies during their pretreatment evaluation. Prenatal development, with intensive cell proliferation, differentiation, and migration, render the fetus susceptible to the direct effects of ionization of essential molecules and cellular components. The fetus is at risk for damage when the mother is receiving therapeutic radiation therapy. When extracervical disease is suspected and additional radiologic diagnostic studies are necessary, the treating physician must be cognizant of potential fetal radiation exposure of these studies (Table 10-4). Although no absolutely "safe" fetal radiation dose has been determined, the incidence of dangerous exposure can be limited. Appropriate recommendations for the diagnostic evaluation and treatment of cancer during pregnancy requires knowledge of fetal irradiation effects. This information should be discussed with the patient and her family before any diagnostic or therapeutic decisions are made.

Although serum tumor markers such as TA-4 may assist in the evaluation and surveillance of invasive squamous cell cancer, their role during pregnancy is undefined (Holloway et al 1989). Furthermore, 0.9%

TABLE 10-4
Estimated Dose of Fetal Radiation

STUDY	FETAL DOSE (MRAD)
Isotope	
Thyroid (Na^{131}I)	15*
Renal (Hypuran ^{131}I)	0.3
Radiologic	
Abdomen	290
Barium enema	800
Cervical spine	2
Chest radiograph	8
Cholecystography	200
Computed tomography (abdomen)	≤5000
Extremity	1
Hip	300
Lymphangiogram	1100
Lumbar spine	275
Magnetic resonance imaging	0
Mammogram	<1
Pelvis	40
Pyelography	400
Shoulder	1
Skull	4
Upper GI series	560

*Concentrates in fetal thyroid (5000 cGy).

Modified from Orr JW Jr, Barrett JR, Holloway RW: Neoplasia in pregnancy. In Moore, Reiter, Rebar, Baker (eds). Gynecology and obstetrics: a longitudinal approach. New York: Churchill Livingstone, 1993:385.

of pregnant women with normal cytology had an elevated serum squamous cell antigen.

Fetal Risk From Irradiation

The projected fetal risk of irradiation-induced injury is determined by a complex formula related to gestational age, radiation dose, field size, energy source, and dose rate. The most commonly reported adverse fetal effects of radiation exposure include growth retardation, malformation, and fetal death. Before and immediately after implantation, the developing embryo is highly susceptible to the lethal effects of irradiation. This risk apparently is not related to an alteration in maternal or placental circulation but to direct fetal injury, primarily the developing central nervous system (Orr et al 1983). Embryonic cell multipotentiality allows repair of sublethal damage during early gestation because few patients deliver a malformed infant after low-level exposure of irradiation during this time. Although most organ systems become less susceptible after organogenesis (2- to 12-week gestational age), some organ systems (e.g., central nervous, hematopoietic, and respiratory) remain susceptible even to low levels of radiation therapy beyond that time. The overall maximum fetal risk of an in utero exposure of 1 cGy has been calculated to be 0.003% (Brent 1986). Small head size and severe mental retardation have been reported at low-dose exposure (9 cGy or less); however, the risks are dramatically increased with intrauterine exposure of 10 or more cGy (Orr et al 1983). More than 50% of infants exposed in utero to 250 cGy at 3 to 10 weeks gestation age have low birth weight, microcephaly, mental retardation, retinal degeneration, cataracts, genital or skeletal malformations (Orr et al 1983). The risk of severe mental retardation during the eighth to fifteenth postconceptional week is about 0.4%/cGy. Deficits in scholastic achievement have been reported with lesser in utero radiation exposure during this sensitive period (Michel 1989). Later radiation exposure (after 20 weeks) results in less severe anomalies consisting of anemia, pigmentation changes, and erythema. Actual fetal dose, although related to gestational age, is a vital factor in ultimate pregnancy outcome. The lethal dose at which 50% (LD_{50}) of gestations abort or result in stillbirth is 70 cGy at day 1, increases to 150 cGy at day 18, and to 300 to 400 cGy after the first trimester (Orr et al 1983). Fetal growth retardation may be the most sensitive indicator of intrauterine radiation exposure, and later radiation exposure results in the greatest degree of postnatal growth retardation; infants who receive less than 25 cGy in utero rarely exhibit growth retardation.

Radiation exposure less than 10 cGy (five times the recommended dose prescribed by the National Council on Radiation Protection and Management) result in subtle pathologic effects but not in gross fetal malformation or fetal growth retardation. Although isolated reports of "normal" infants receiving in utero radiation exposure exist, therapeutic abortion should be considered and discussed when the sum of any diagnostic or therapeutic fetal radiation exposure exceeds 10 cGy. When radiographic evaluation is indicated to evaluate maternal status during pregnancy, it should be performed with the minimal number of films required to adequately evaluate the clinical situation.

Pretreatment Evaluation

The recommended pretreatment metastatic evaluation does not differ from the nonpregnant woman. Pregnancy is associated with upper urinary tract dilation, beginning at 6 to 7 weeks gestational age and persisting as late as the third postpartum month. These physiologic changes may mimic obstructive uropathy and when present do not demand clinical upstaging of the patient. Because bimanual examination may be difficult, we consider the use of computerized tomography or magnetic resonance imaging (MRI) when necessary to aid in delineating extracervical disease (Fig. 10-2). The risks and benefits of fetal radiation exposure with tomography (1 cGy/section) and other radiologic procedures should be evaluated when delayed therapy and fetal salvage is a strong consideration. The substi-

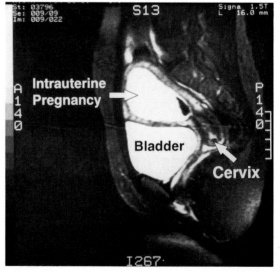

Figure 10-2. An MRI scan of the pelvis in a woman with an eight-week uterine pregnancy. The cervix, bladder, and intrauterine contents are clearly delineated. There was no evidence of paracervical distention on sagittal or transverse views. The study resulted in negligible radiation exposure and allowed continuation of the pregnancy to term.

tution of MRI eliminates radiation exposure and there is little evidence to suggest that the electric fields associated with MRI interfere with human development (Hannigan 1990).

Therapy Delays During Pregnancy

Obviously, the decision to initiate or delay cancer therapy during pregnancy is difficult because the emotional, religious, and moral needs of the mother and family become extremely important. Most pregnant women with cervical cancer have children (mean parity, four); however, the decision to treat immediately (disregarding the pregnancy) or to delay cancer therapy may become more complex in the primigravida patient. Any delay in the institution of therapy that would be detrimental to the patient is difficult to accept; however, in specific situations (i.e., advanced, incurable maternal disease), the delivery of a viable fetus may take precedence over maternal well-being.

Several reports assess the effect of a planned delay in therapy. It appears that therapy of microinvasive or early cervical cancer can be safely delayed with apparently little risk of disease progression. Prem and coworkers (1966) first reported 5 women followed-up who had early invasive asymptomatic stage I disease, discovered between 20 and 34 weeks gestation. A planned therapy delay of 11 to 17 weeks did not adversely affect pregnancy outcome or cancer therapy. All of these women survived. Boutselis (1972) allowed 9 patients who had microinvasive cancer (less than 5 mm of stromal invasion) discovered during the first, second, or third trimester to complete their pregnancies. This delay was not detrimental and all patients later underwent successful cancer therapy. Thompson and associates (1975) reported 7 patients having stage IA disease (less than 3 mm of invasion) who had a mean therapy delay of 12 weeks (range, 5 to 28 weeks). All mothers were successfully treated after delivery. Lee and colleagues (1981) detailed 8 patients (1 with stage IA, 2 with stage IB, and 5 with stage II) who delivered after planned therapy delays of 1 to 11 weeks (mean, 5 weeks). This delay allowed the birth of eight live infants and none of the women experienced a progression in her clinical stage. Greer and associates (1989) had 5 patients with stage IB cancer whose therapy was delayed for 6 to 17 weeks without apparent maternal morbidity. Monk and Montz (1992) reported the results of delayed therapy in 7 additional patients having clinical stage I cervical cancer diagnosed during pregnancy. Three patients who were diagnosed during the second trimester had an average therapy delay of 13 weeks (range, 10 to 16 weeks). Three patients who were diagnosed in the third trimester had a 3-week delay. One patient underwent conization (IA2 disease) in the first trimester and was treated after a term delivery. There was no apparent adverse effect on maternal survival associated with therapy delay; however, the authors used postsurgical pelvic radiation therapy for 33% of their patients who had "high-risk" lesions. Duggan and coworkers (1993) reported 8 patients having stage IA or IB disease, with a mean treatment delay of 20.6 weeks (range, 7.6 to 30.1 weeks) to reach a mean gestational age of 37 weeks. Fetal outcome, when compared with that of 19 patients who elected immediate cancer therapy, was superior and all patients with a planned therapy delay are free of disease at a mean follow-up of 23 months. Sivanesaratnam and associates (1993) delayed therapy for 14 weeks in 1 patient having stage IA2 disease, without maternal or fetal sequelae. Two additional patients who were diagnosed in the third trimester had uneventful therapy delay for 4 and 2 weeks.

In contrast to those studies suggesting no ill effect of planned therapy delay, Dudan and colleagues (1973) reported a delay-associated clinical stage disease progression in 8 pregnant patients. Three patients had apparent progression with prolonged therapy delays (less than 1 year); however, 3 other patients progressed from CIS to invasive carcinoma after a therapy delay of only 2 to 5 months. Two additional patients having initial stage IB disease experienced a progression to clinical stage IIA and IIIB after 2- and 6-month delays. Nisker and colleagues (1983) reported the cancer-related death of 1 woman who had stage IB disease who had a therapy delay of 24 weeks. Lee and associates (1981) reported 1 patient with a conization diagnosis of CIS who was found to have microinvasive disease after an 8-month delay and another patient whose invasive carcinoma was discovered in a postpartum hysterectomy specimen after a second-trimester conization that had been interpreted as being negative. Giuntoli and coworkers (1991) reported a case of apparent progression of CIN II to microinvasion during a 6-month antepartum surveillance in a women who had previously (2 years before) been treated with cryotherapy. These reports certainly emphasize the importance of accurate initial histologic and clinical evaluation of patients having high-grade lesions and invasive disease but also report a rapidly progressive disease that might be considered unusual in nonpregnant women and raise questions about a potential problem with "underdiagnosis" of the original abnormality.

After evaluation of these reports, it seems reasonable in patients having stage IA1, IA2, and IB disease (less than 3 cm) to discuss the options of therapy delay in an attempt to improve fetal viability; neonatal care in a modern intensive-care nursery allows the salvage of about 80% of infants delivered at 28 weeks and nearly 98% of those delivered at 32 weeks gestational age (Bowes et al 1979, Philip et al 1981, Kopelman

1978, Stewart et al 1981, Greer et al 1989). As importantly, Greer and coworkers (1989) indicated that the risk of hyaline membrane disease, bronchopulmonary dysplasia, and intraventricular hemorrhage decreases dramatically between 28 weeks (72%, 34%, 34%, respectively) and 32 weeks gestational age (33%, 2%, 2%, respectively). In those surviving infants delivered at less than 1500 g, 54% require specialized or resource help at age 7 years (Greer et al 1989). Although there are no existing guidelines, this information suggests that for every 2-week delay, there is a significant decrease in the mortality and morbidity of prematurity (Greer et al 1989). We believe that therapy delays in an attempt to reach fetal viability are justified in those women who have early-stage disease and desire to maintain their pregnancy. The use of antepartum steroid administration should be considered when delivery is contemplated without documented fetal pulmonary maturity.

In patients having large-volume cervical cancer (bulky stage IB or more advanced stages), a delay in therapy in excess of 6 weeks seems to be potentially detrimental to the mother's chances of survival. Although delivery after 32 weeks gestational age is ideal, infants older than 26 weeks are potentially viable; one should develop a management plan according to the patient's desires and the stage (volume) of disease.

Other than the problems associated with possible premature delivery, the fetus is apparently unaffected by the presence of cervical cancer. We have reported a squamous cell cancer of the head and neck metastatic to the placenta (Orr et al 1982); however, there have been no reports of placental or fetal metastasis from cervical cancer.

Effect of Gestational Age at Diagnosis

Some authors indicate decreased survival when cancer is detected or treatment is begun in the third trimester or after delivery. Cited literature (Table 10-5) suggests that clinical stage is the most important prognostic factor. Five-year survival is not significantly different when women with stage I disease are treated in the first trimester (84% survival), second trimester (89% survival), third trimester (77% survival), or postpartum (77% survival) (Table 10-6). The same is true of patients with stage II disease. Unfortunately, it appears that the third trimester or postpartum discovery of cervical cancer is associated with a more advanced clinical stage, with a corresponding decrease in survival rate. Pregnancy, however, does not have any adverse survival effects on the ultimate prognosis of cervical cancer (Zemlickis et al 1991, Hopkins et al 1992).

Mode of Delivery and Survival

Regardless of the decision to continue or interrupt the pregnancy, the appropriate mode of delivery must be considered. Kinch (1961), reviewing previous literature, postulated that vaginal delivery should be avoided because of the potential of disseminating tumor cells. Problems of excessive bleeding or obstructed labor have also been reported. Hemorrhage is a significant or even lethal risk of vaginal delivery in patients having large cervical cancers (Hacker et al 1982). Other authors have indicated that the mode of delivery has little effect on maternal survival. Considering patients with all stages of cervical cancer, survival after vaginal delivery (52.9% of 419 patients) is not different from that after abdominal delivery (46.1% of 115 patients; Table 10-7). In women having stage I disease, this collected series indicates that after vaginal delivery, 80.5% of treated patients survive, whereas 71.6% of treated patients survive after abdominal delivery. Although these data are not adjusted for gestational age or tumor volume, it suggests that the risk of widespread dissemination of cancer after vaginal delivery may be more theoretic than real.

Postdelivery surveillance must consider unusual metastatic sites because squamous cell cancer (Gordon et al 1989) and adenocarcinoma (Copeland et al; 1987; Hopkins et al 1992) have recurred in the episiotomy site.

Although extremely rare, pregnancy has been reported in women after radiation therapy for cervical cancer (Baughan et al 1991, Browde et al 1986). The irradiation-induced upper vaginal and cervical changes make vaginal delivery hazardous in this situation because reported maternal mortality rates approach 50% (Browde et al 1986).

Treatment of Early Cancer

Patients who have early invasive carcinoma (IA1) can be treated by cesarean section combined with concomitant total hysterectomy. Although feasible, the authors believe that there are certain disadvantages to this type of treatment. The more conservative diagnostic conization often performed during pregnancy may not be predictive of the true extent of invasion (Hacker et al 1982). In those women having stage IA1 or even IA2 disease diagnosed with conization, a postdelivery delay of 4 to 6 weeks allows further evaluation before a final therapy decision is made. This delay may allow more conservative therapy (i.e., conization alone) in specific situations (i.e., stage IA1 disease) but may indicate the need for more extensive therapy (i.e., lymphadenectomy) in specific patient

TABLE 10-5
Survival Related to Trimester of Discovery and Treatment

Study	Year	Stage	First Trimester		Second Trimester		Third Trimester		Postpartum	
			Patients (n)	Survival (%)	Patients (n)	Survival (%)	Patients (n)	Survival (%)	Patients (n)	Survival (%)
Kinch	1961	All Stages	10	60	10	50	6	67	49	37
Lash*	1961	I	4	100	6	83	2	50	1	100
Barber, et al	1963	All Stages	2	100	2	100	1	0	27	37
Van Praagh, et al	1965	I	71	86	4	—	4	50	15	67
		II	3	67	1	50	3	33	11	27
		III	—	—	—	0	—	—	3	0
		IV	—	—	—	—	2	6	6	17
Prem, et al	1966	All Stages	6	83	9	78	5	100	60	57
O'Leary, et al	1966	I	2	50	1	100	3	33	1	100
		II	1	0	1	100	—	—	—	—
		III	1	0	—	—	—	—	—	—
Herold	1967	I	11	73	5	60	2	50	15	47
		II	1	0	2	50	1	0	9	33
		III	—	—	—	—	2	0	12	0
		IV	—	—	—	—	—	—	2	0
Smith, et al	1968	I	3	100	—	—	2	100	1	100
Mikuta	1968	All Stages	3	67	9	100	2	50	12	50
Creasman, et al	1970	I	9	100	8	100	5	100	25	84
		II	5	80	9	88	2	50	21	67
Wanless	1971	All Stages	4	100	2	50	4	75	—	—
Fogh	1972	I	23	80	—	—	5	80	8	100
		II	14	43	—	—	4	100	5	40
		III	2	0	—	—	3	33	2	0
		IV	1	0	—	—	—	—	1	0
Sall, et al	1974	IB	5	100	6	100	12	92	6	100
Sablinska, et al	1977	All Stages	41	73	22	50	—	—	181	37
Lutz, et al	1977	IB	2	100	3	100	2	0	3	100
		IIA	—	—	2	0	1	0	—	—
		IIB	—	—	—	—	1	0	—	—
		III	—	—	—	—	1	0	—	—
		IV	—	—	—	—	2	0	—	—
Nisker, et al	1983	IB	7	86	6	67	5	60	25	68
Baltzer, et al	1990	I	—	84	—	89	—	77	—	77
Hopkins, et al	1992	I	—	—	11	91	5	80	17	65

*Actual survival data not given but no statistical difference between semesters ($p = .68$).

TABLE 10-6
Survival of Patients with Stage IB Cervical Cancer Related to the Mode of Therapy

		SURGICAL		RADIATION		COMBINED	
STUDY	YEAR	Patients (n)	Survival (%)	Patients (n)	Survival (%)	Patients (n)	Survival (%)
Stander, et al	1960	—	—	24	83	—	—
Kinch	1961	—	—	19	68	4	50
Lash*	1961	12	92	1	0	2	100
Waldrop, et al	1963	—	—	40	78	—	—
Van Praagh, et al	1965	5	60	14	71	7	71
Bosch, et al	1966	2	0	7	71	—	—
Prem, et al	1966	—	—	58	83	—	—
O'Leary, et al	1966	3	100	4	25	—	—
Smith, et al	1968	5	100	1	100	—	—
Wanless	1971	3	100	2	100	—	—
Sall, et al	1974	23	95	—	—	—	—
Thompson, et al	1974	9	89	5	100	—	—
Lutz, et al	1977	3	67	6	67	2	50
Funnell, et al	1980	—	—	—	—	12	100
Lee, et al	1981	17	93	4	80	1	100
Nisker, et al	1983	11	64	25	76	5	80
Baltzer, et al	1990	—	89	—	87	—	82
Zemlickis, et al†	1991	12	—	13	—	—	—
Hopkins, et al	1992	21	86	12	58(7)	—	—
Monk, et al	1992	14	100	—	—	7	86
Sivanesaratnam, et al	1993	18	78	—	—	—	—

*2-year survival.
†No significant difference.

subsets (i.e., stage IA2 disease). The risks of genitourinary injury, bleeding, and loss of ovarian function after cesarean hysterectomy are higher than those of an interval therapeutic conization or total hysterectomy. Additionally, the increased cervical size and pliability may render complete cervical removal more difficult in the pregnant woman (Park et al 1980). Given these factors, we prefer to await vaginal delivery, reevaluate these patients within 4 to 6 weeks, and then institute appropriate therapy (Table 10-8) for women who have early invasive disease. We consider cesarean hysterectomy if the patient is unlikely to return for postpartum treatment, however. When this operation is performed, delivery is accomplished through a vertical uterine incision, leaving the lower uterine segment and cervix undisturbed for later pathologic study. Elective cesarean hysterectomy is not indicated for high-grade SIL because this precursor can be treated with less morbidity after delivery.

Treatment of Clinical Invasive Cancer: Surgical

Treatment of the pregnant woman having a clinically invasive cervical cancer may involve radical surgery or radiation therapy. When radical surgery is performed, specific attention must be devoted to the cardiac, pulmonary, and hematologic physiologic changes of pregnancy that may affect anesthesia and perioperative care (Orr et al 1993). Unfortunately, the evaluation of the merits of these two modalities as treatment of pregnant women has been inadequate; most studies include few patients, and investigators have failed to stratify their results according to the size of the cervical lesion. Advocates of primary surgical therapy promote the potential of ovarian and vaginal conservation, the aspects of surgical staging, and the information gained by expeditious therapy that avoids the potential long-term complications of irradiation in

TABLE 10-7
Effect of Mode of Delivery on Cervical Cancer in Pregnancy

STUDY	YEAR	STAGE	ABDOMINAL DELIVERY		VAGINAL DELIVERY	
			Patients (n)	Surviving (%)	Patients (n)	Surviving (%)
Kinch	1961	All Stages	10	20	61	44
Barber, et al	1963	All Stages	2	100	28	36
Waldrop, et al	1963	I	8	75	47	70
		II	7	0	48	44
		III	12	25	40	20
		IV	7	0	13	15
Van Praagh, et al	1965	All Stages	12	17	74	55
Bosch, et al	1966	I	2	50	11	45
		II	4	0	13	38
		III	—	—	8	25
		IV	—	—	2	0
Prem, et al	1966	I	3	67	8	63
		II	1	0	2	0
		III	1	0	2	100
O'Leary, et al	1966	I	4	50	3	67
		II	1	100	1	0
Mikuta	1967	All Stages	5	80	11	55
Shaffer, et al	1969	All Stages	3	67	3	100
Creasman, et al	1970	I	9	89	15	87
		II	4	50	14	64
Lee, et al	1981	IA	2	100	1	100
		IB	10	90	10	90
		II	5	40	4	43
Nisker, et al	1983	I	14	64	17	65
Baltzer, et al	1990	I		80.5		71.5
		All Stages		46.1		52.9
Zemlickis, et al*	1991	All Stages	13	*	8	*

*No significant difference.

TABLE 10-8
Management of Patients with Stage I Cervical Cancer

HISTOLOGIC DIAGNOSIS	GESTATIONAL AGE		
	0–12 Weeks	13–26 Weeks	27–40 Weeks
Focal microinvasion	Institute therapy; delay to viability	Consider therapy or delay to viability	Delay to viability
Microcarcinoma	Institute therapy; delay may increase maternal risks	Consider therapy or delay to viability	Delay to viability; deliver and institute therapy
Carcinoma*	Institute therapy; delay increases maternal risks	Institute therapy; consider delay to viability	Consider delay to viability; deliver and institute therapy

*Avoid prolonged delays in patients with large (>30cm) clinical lesions.

these young women. Sall and coworkers (1974) reported 23 surgically treated pregnant patients having early carcinoma of the cervix; 95% of these patients were 5-year survivors. Funnell and associates (1980), operating on 17 pregnant patients, suggested that the associated pregnancy changes facilitated the surgical dissection. Mikuta and colleagues (1977) reported fewer postoperative complications in pregnant patients when compared with nonpregnant patients. Monk and Montz (1992) described the perioperative morbidity of radical hysterectomy in 13 patients who were treated during pregnancy. The mean operative time was 281 minutes; as expected, mean blood loss was statistically greater (1750 mL) with cesarean delivery than with radical hysterectomy alone (777 mL); 62% of pregnant patients were transfused. One patient developed a vesicovaginal fistula after inadvertent cystotomy; however, there were no significant vascular, ureteral, or intestinal injuries. Average hospital stay was 10 days. Although most authors describe better planes of surgical dissection, the operative time (usually 5 hours) and blood loss (Sivanesaratnam et al 1993) is increased over procedures performed in nonpregnant women (Orr et al 1990).

Although data relating tumor volume is scarce, Nisker and associates (1983) and Hopkins and coworkers (1992) suggest a high rate (25% and 33%) of node metastases in pregnant patients. Others have reported no difference; for example, Sivanesaratnam and colleagues (1993) reported node metastasis in 16% of women. Baltzer and associates (1990) carefully evaluated the histologic findings of 21 pregnant and 16 postpartum women who were treated with radical surgery. The risk of vascular space involvement and macroscopic node metastasis were higher but not significantly different from controls. Care should be exercised intraoperatively to not abandon surgical therapy solely with the finding of enlarged pelvic or paraaortic nodes because node hypertrophy can occur with pregnancy alone. Decidual changes in nodes can be confusing during histologic evaluation (Covell et al 1977, Ashraf et al 1984) and must be properly distinguished from cancer metastases.

There is no apparent difference in survival (see Table 10-6) in pregnant patients having stage IB disease treated surgically when compared with patients treated with irradiation or with combined therapy. Once the decision is made to initiate therapy, we prefer primary surgical treatment for those women who are acceptable operative candidates. Careful pretreatment histologic evaluation is important because rare cervical tumor types such as neuroendocrine tumors (Turner et al 1986) or even metastasis to the cervix from other primary tumors have been encountered (Sommerville et al 1991) and may require different treatment.

Radiation Therapy

Radiation is appropriate therapy for patients who have stage IB cancer who are poor surgical risks and for patients having advanced stage disease. When viable, the fetus is usually delivered by cesarean section, with teletherapy instituted postoperatively. When the fetus is not considered to be viable or when delay is not considered to be an option, teletherapy may be started. Creasman and colleagues (1970) indicated that more than 70% of abortions occurred before the delivery of 4000 cGy. Bosch and Marcial (1966) reported that 16 of 17 patients aborted spontaneously within 3 to 6 weeks of initiation of radiation therapy. Prem and associates (1966) indicated that the time from initiation of therapy to spontaneous abortion was shorter in pregnancies that were treated during the first trimester (29 days) than in those treated in the second trimester (38 days). These findings suggest little benefit of therapeutic pregnancy termination by hysterotomy or hysterectomy before the initiation of radiation therapy.

The possibility of altered tissue tolerance during pregnancy has been expressed by Dudan and coworkers (1973), Thompson and colleagues (1975), and Nisker and associates (1983), whose reports suggest a significant rate of gastrointestinal and urinary fistulas in pregnant patients receiving radiation therapy. Nisker and associates (1983) encountered an excessive (28.8%) risk of complications in pregnant patients having stage I cervical cancer treated with irradiation, a rate that was statistically greater than that experienced by nonpregnant patients having stage I cancer treated with irradiation at his institution. Reports from other institutions using radiation therapy as the primary method of treatment of pregnant women do not confirm this hypothesis (Hacker et al 1982).

Interestingly, Baltzer and coworkers (1990) also reported a statistically significant increased need for adjunctive irradiation after radical hysterectomy during pregnancy. In his series of 40 patients, 55% received postsurgical adjunctive radiation therapy (compared with 41% of nonpregnant women treated with radical surgery). Unfortunately, he presented no benefit of adjuvant irradiation.

References

Abitbol MM, Benjamin FI, Gastillo N. Management of the abnormal smear and carcinoma in situ of the cervix during pregnancy. Am J Obstet Gynecol 1973;117:904.

Anderson M. Should conization by hot loop or laser replace cervical biopsy? J Gynecol Surg 1991;7:191.

Ashraf H, Boyd CB, Beresford WA. Ectopic decidual cell reaction in para-aortic and pelvic lymph nodes in the presence of cervical squamous cell carcinoma during pregnancy. J Surg Oncol 1984;26:6.

Averette HE, Nasser N, Yankow SL, Little WA. Cervical conization in pregnancy. Am J Obstet Gynecol 1970; 106:543.

Bakri YN, Akhtar M, Al-Amri A. Case report. Carcinoma of the cervix in a pregnant woman with negative pap smears and colposcopic examination. Acta Obstet Gynecol Scand 1990;69:657.

Baltzer J, Regenbrecht ME, Kopcke W, et al. Carcinoma of the cervix and pregnancy. Int J Gynaecol Obstet 1990;31:317.

Barber HRK, Brunschwig A. Gynecologic cancer complicating pregnancy. Am J Obstet Gynecol 1963;85:156.

Baughan CA, Ryall RDH, Pope RA. Case report. Successful pregnancy following tailor-made intracavitary radiotherapy for microinvasive adenocarcinoma of the endocervix. Clin Oncol Feb 1992;4:192.

Benedet JL, Selke PA, Nickerson KG. Colposcopic evaluation of abnormal Papanicolaou smears in pregnancy. Am J Obstet Gynecol 1987;157:932.

Bigrigg MA, Codling BW, et al. Pregnancy after cervical loop diathermy. Lancet 1991;337:119.

Bokhman JV, Urmancheyeva AF. Cervix uteri cancer and pregnancy. Eur J Gynaecol Oncol 1989;X:6.

Bolognese RJ, Corson SL. Cervical conization in pregnancy. Surg Gynecol Obstet 1969;128:1244.

Bosch A, Marcial VA. Carcinoma of the uterine cervix associated with pregnancy. Am J Roentgenol Radium Therapy Nucl Med 1966;96:92.

Boutselis JG. Intraepithelial carcinoma of the cervix associated with pregnancy. Obstet Gynecol 1972;40:657.

Bowes WA, Halgrimson M, Simmons MA. Results of intensive perinatal management of very low birth weight infants (501 to 1500 grams). J Reprod Med 1979;23:245.

Brent RL. The effects of embryonic and fetal exposure to x-ray, microwaves, and ultrasound. Clin Perinatol 1986;13(3):615.

Browde S, Friedman M, Nissenbaum M. Pregnancy after radiation therapy for carcinoma of the cervix. Eur J Gynaecol Oncol 1986;7(2):63.

Campion MJ, Sedlacek TV. Colposcopy in pregnancy. Contemp Colposcopy 1993;20(1):153.

Clark MA, Naahas W, et al. Cervical cancer: women aged 35 and younger compared to women aged 36 and older. Am J Clin Oncol 1991;14(4):352.

Copeland LJ, Saul PB, Sneige N. Cervical adenocarcinoma: tumor implantation in the episiotomy sites of two patients. Gynecol Oncol 1987;28:230.

Covell LM, Disciullu AJ, Knapp RC. Decidual change in pelvic lymph nodes in the presence of cervical squamous cell carcinoma during pregnancy. Am J Obstet Gynecol 1977;127:674.

Creasman WT, Rutledge FN, Fletcher GH. Carcinoma of the cervix associated with pregnancy. Obstet Gynecol 1970;36:495.

Cromer JK, Hawken SW. Cancer of the cervix and pregnancy. Obstet Gynecol 1963;22:346.

Daskal JL, Pitkin RM. Cone biopsy of the cervix during pregnancy. Obstet Gynecol 1968;32:1.

DePetrillo AD, Townsend DE, Morrow CP, et al. Colposcopic evaluation of the abnormal Papanicolaou test in pregnancy. Am J Obstet Gynecol 1975;121:441.

Dudan RC, Yon JL Jr, Ford JH Jr, Averette HE. Carcinoma of the cervix and pregnancy. Gynecol Oncol 1973;1:283.

Duggan B, Muderspach LI, Roman LD, et al. Cervical cancer in pregnancy: reporting on planned delay in therapy. Obstet Gynecol 1993;82:598.

Economos K, Veridiano NP, Delke I, Collado ML, Tancer ML. Abnormal cervical cytology in pregnancy: a 17-year experience. Obstet Gynecol 1993;81:915.

Edinger DD, Louis FJ. Adenocarcinoma in situ of the endocervix with coexistent intrauterine pregnancy: report of a case and review of the literature. Clinical and Experimental Obstetrics and Gynecology 1982;9:223.

Fay RA, Crandon AJ, Hudson CN, et al. Cervical carcinoma associated with pregnancy. Lancet 1982;2:1213. Letter.

Fogh I. Cancer colli uteri and pregnancy. Cancer 1972; 29:114.

Fowler WC Jr, Walton LA, Edelman DA. Cervical intraepithelial neoplasia during pregnancy. South Med J 1980;73:1180.

Funnell JD, Puckett TG, Strebel GF, Kelso JW. Carcinoma of the cervix complicating pregnancy. South Med J 1980;73:1308.

Giuntoli R, Tien Yeh I, Bhuett N, et al. Case report. Conservative management of cervical intraepithelial neoplasia during pregnancy. Gynecol Oncol 1991;42:68.

Goldberg GL, Altaras MM, Bloch B. Cone cerclage in pregnancy. Obstet Gynecol 1991;77:315.

Gordon AN, Jensen R, Jones HW III. Squamous carcinoma of the cervix complicating pregnancy: recurrence in episiotomy after vaginal delivery. Obstet Gynecol 1989;73:850.

Greer BE, Easterling TR, McLennan DA, et al. Fetal and maternal considerations in the management of stage I-B cervical cancer during pregnancy. Gynecol Oncol 1989;34:61.

Gustafsson DC, Kottmeier HL. carcinoma of the cervix associated with pregnancy. Acta Obstet Gynecol Scand 1962;41:1.

Hacker NF, Berek JS, Lagasse LD, et al. Carcinoma of the cervix associated with pregnancy. Obstet Gynecol 1982;59:735.

Hannigan EV. Cervical cancer in pregnancy. Clin Obstet Gynecol 1990;33(4):8387.

Hannigan EV, Whitehouse HH, Atkinson WD, Becker SN. Cone biopsy during pregnancy. Obstet Gynecol 1982;60:450.

Harris JW. Pre-pregnancy counseling of premalignant and malignant disease. Clin Obstet Gynaecol 1982;9:171.

Hemmingson E. Outcome of third trimester pregnancies after cryotherapy of the uterine cervix. Br J Obstet Gynaecol 1982;89:657.

Herold J. Cancer of the uterine cervix in pregnancy, after delivery, and after miscarriage. Acta Univ Carolinae Medica 1967;13:189.

Holloway RW, To A, Moradi M, et al. Monitoring the course of cervical carcinoma with the squamous cell carcinoma serum radioimmunoassay. Obstet Gynecol 1989;74:944.

Hollyock VW, Chanen W, Wein R. Cervical function following treatment of intraepithelial neoplasia by electrocoagulation diathermy. Obstet Gynecol 1983;61:79.

Hopkins MP, Morley GW. The prognosis and management of cervical cancer associated with pregnancy. Obstet Gynecol 1992;80:9.

Jolles CJ. Gynecologic cancer associated with pregnancy. Semin Oncol 1989;16(5):417.

Jones JM, Sweetnam P, Hibbard BM. The outcome of pregnancy after cone biopsy of the cervix: a case-control study. Br J Obstet Gynaecol 1979;86(12):913.

Kaminski PF, Lyon DS, Sorosky JI, et al. Significance of atypical cervical cytology in pregnancy. Am J Perinatol 1992;9(5-6):340.

Keijser KGG, Kenemans P, et al. Diathermy loop excision in the management of cervical intraepithelial neoplasia; diagnosis and treatment in one procedure. Am J Obstet Gynecol 1992;166:1281.

Kinch RAH. Factors affecting the prognosis of cancer of the cervix in pregnancy. Am J Obstet Gynecol 1961;82:45.

Kopelman AE. The smallest preterm infants. Am J Dis Child 1978;132:461.

LaPolla JP, O'Neill C, Wetrich D. Colposcopic management of abnormal cytology in pregnancy. J Reprod Med 1988;33:301.

Larsson G, Grundsell H, et al. Outcome of pregnancy after conization. Acta Obstet Gynecol Scand 1982;61:461.

Lash AF. Management of carcinoma of the cervix in pregnancy. Obstet Gynecol 1961;17:41.

Lee RB, Neglia W, Park RC. Cervical carcinoma in pregnancy. Obstet Gynecol 1981;58:584.

Luesley CM, McCrum A, Terry PB, et al. Complications of cone biopsy related to the dimensions of the cone and the influence of prior colposcopic assessment. Br J Obstet Gynaecol 1985;92:158.

Lurain JR, Underwood PB Jr, Rozier JC, Putney FW. Genital malignancy in pregnancy. Am J Obstet Gynecol 1979;129:536.

Lurie S, Dgani R, et al. Invasive papillary serous adenocarcinoma of the endocervix in pregnancy; a case report. Eur J Obstet Gynecol Reprod Biol 1991;40:79.

Lutz MH, Underwood PB Jr, Rozier JC, Putney FW. Genital malignancy in pregnancy. Am J Obstet Gynecol 1977;129:536.

Madej JG Jr, Szczudrawa A, Pitynski D. Colposcopy findings of CIN and cancer-like lesions of the cervix in pregnancy. Clin Exper Obstet Gynecol 1992;19:168.

Matanyi S. Cryotherapy during pregnancy. Acta Chir Hung 1989;30(4):325.

Michel C. Radiation embryology. Experientia 1989;45:69.

Mikuta JJ. Invasive carcinoma of the cervix in pregnancy. South Med J 1967;60:843.

Mikuta JJ, Giuntoli RL, Rubin EL, Mangan CE. The "problem" radical hysterectomy. Am J Obstet Gynecol 1977;128(2):119.

Moinian M, Andersch B. Does cervix conization increase the risk of complications in subsequent pregnancies? Act Obstet Gynecol Scand 1982;61:101.

Monk BJ, Montz FJ. Invasive cervical cancer complicating intrauterine pregnancy: treatment with radical hysterectomy. Obstet Gynecol 1992;80:199.

Moore JG, Wells RG, Morton DG. Management of superficial cervical cancer in pregnancy. Obstet Gynecol 1966;27:307.

Nebel WA, Singleton HHM, Swanton MC. Cold knife conization of the cervix uteri. Surg Gynecol Obstet 1967;125:780.

Nisker JA, Shubat M. Stage IB cervical carcinoma and pregnancy: report of 49 cases. Am J Obstet Gynecol 1983;145:203.

O'Leary JA, Munnell EW, Moore JG. The changing prognosis of cervical carcinoma during pregnancy. Obstet Gynecol 1966;28:460.

Orr JW Jr, Barrett JR, Holloway RW: Neoplasia in pregnancy. In Baker VV, ed. Gynecology and obstetrics: an integrated approach. New York: Churchill Livingstone, 1993:385.

Orr JW Jr, Barrett JM, Orr PJ, et al. The safety and efficacy of the cytobrush during pregnancy. Gynecol Oncol 1992;44:260.

Orr JW Jr, Grizzle WE, Huddleston JF. Squamous cell carcinoma metastatic to placenta and ovary. Obstet Gynecol 1982;59:813.

Orr JW Jr, Shingleton HM. Cancer in pregnancy. Curr Probl Cancer 1983;8:1.

Orr JW Jr, Shingleton HM. In utero exposure to diethylstilbestrol: an update. Your Patient and Cancer, February 320R, 1986.

Orr JW Jr, Sisson PF, Patsner B, et al. Single dose antibiotic prophylaxis for patients undergoing extended pelvic surgery for gynecologic malignancy. Am J Obstet Gynecol 1990;162:718.

Ortiz R, Newton M. Colposcopy in the management of abnormal cervical smears in pregnancy. Am J Obstet Gynecol 1971;109(1):46.

Ostergard DR, Nieberg RK. Evaluation of abnormal cervical cytology during pregnancy with colposcopy. Am J Obstet Gynecol 1979;134:756.

Park RC, Duff WP. Role of cesarean hysterectomy in modern obstetric practice. Clin Obstet Gynecol 1980;23:601.

Patsner B, Baker DA, Orr JW Jr. Human papillomavirus genital tract infections during pregnancy. Clin Obstet Gynecol 1990;33(2):258.

Petersen O. Spontaneous course of cervical precancerous conditions. Am J Obstet Gynecol 1956;72:1063.

Philip AGS, Little GA, Polivy DR, Lucey JF. Neonatal mortality risk for the eighties: the importance of birth weight/gestational age groups. Pediatrics 1981;68:122.

Prem KA, Makowski EL, McKelvey JL. Carcinoma of the cervix associated with pregnancy. Am J Obstet Gynecol 1966;95:99.

Richart RM, Barton BA. A followup study of patients with cervical dysplasia. Am J Obstet Gynecol 1969;105:386.

Rivlin ME, Woodliff JM, Bowlin RB, et al. Comparison of cytobrush and cotton swab for papanicolaou smears in pregnancy. J Reprod Med 1993;38(2):147.

Roberts JA. Management of gynecologic tumors during pregnancy. Clin Perinatol 1983;10:369.

Rogers III RS, Williams JH. The impact of the suspicious Papanicolaou smear on pregnancy. Am J Obstet Gynecol 1967;98:488.

Sablinska R, Tarlowska L, Stelmachow J. Invasive carcinoma

of the cervix associated with pregnancy: correlation between patient age, advancement of cancer and gestation, and result of treatment. Gynecol Oncol 1977;5:363.

Sall S, Rini S, Pineda A. Surgical management of invasive carcinoma of the cervix in pregnancy. Am J Obstet Gynecol 1974;118:1.

Shaffer WL, Merrill JA. Carcinoma of the cervix associated with pregnancy. South Med J 1969;62:915.

Shingleton HM. American College of Surgeons Patterns of Care Study. 1995. In preparation.

Sivanesaratnam V, Jayalakshmi P, Loo C. Surgical management of early invasive cancer of the cervix associated with pregnancy. Gynecol Oncol 1993;48:68.

Smith MR, Figge DC, Bennington JL. The diagnosis of cervical cancer during pregnancy. Obstet Gynecol 1968; 31:193.

Sommerville M, Koonings PP, Durtin JP, d'Ablaing G. Gastrointestinal signet ring carcinoma metastatic to the cervix during pregnancy. A case report. J Reprod Med 1991;36(11):913.

Stafl A. Colposcopy in diagnosis of cervical neoplasia. Am J Obstet Gynecol 1973;115(2):286.

Stander RW, Lein JN. Carcinoma of the cervix and pregnancy. Am J Obstet Gynecol 1960;79:164.

Stewart AL, Reynolds EOR, Lipscomb AP. Outcome for infants of very low birth weight: survey of world literature. Lancet 1981;1(8228):1038.

Stromme WB. Preclinical carcinoma and dysplasia of the cervix associated with pregnancy. Am J Obstet Gynecol 1969;105:1008.

Talebian F, Krumholz BA, Shayan A, Mann LI. Colposcopic evaluation of patients with abnormal cytologic smears during pregnancy. Obstet Gynecol 1976;47:693.

Thompson JD, Caputo TA, Franklin EW III, Dale E. The surgical management of invasive cancer of the cervix in pregnancy. Am J Obstet Gynecol 1975;121:853.

Trombetta GC. Colposcopic evaluation of cervical neoplasia in pregnancy. J Reprod Med 1976;16(5):243.

Tunca JC, Franklin EW III, Clark JC. Colposcopic management of abnormal cervical cytology during pregnancy. South Med J 1976;69:705.

Turner WA, Gallup DG, et al. Neuroendocrine carcinoma of the uterine cervix complicated by pregnancy: case report and review of the literature. Obstet Gynecol 1986; 67:80S.

Van Praagh JHL, Harvey MH, Vernon CP. Carcinoma of the cervix associated with pregnancy. J Obstet Gynecol Br Commonwealth 1965;72:75.

Waldrop GM, Palmer JP. Carcinoma of the cervix associated with pregnancy. Am J Obstet Gynecol 1963;86:202.

Wanless JF. Carcinoma of the cervix in pregnancy. Am J Obstet Gynecol 1971;110:173.

Williams TJ, Brack CB. Carcinoma of the cervix in pregnancy. Cancer 1964;17:1486.

Yoonessi M, Wieckowska W, Mariniello D, Antkowiak J. Cervical intraepithelial neoplasia in pregnancy. Int J Gynaecol Obstet 1982;20:111.

Zemlickis D, Lishner M, Degendorfer P, et al. Maternal and fetal outcome after invasive cervical cancer in pregnancy. J Clin Oncol 1991;9(11):1956.

Cancer of the Cervix by Hugh M. Shingleton and James W. Orr, Jr.
J. B. Lippincott Company, Philadelphia, © 1995.

11

Posttreatment Surveillance and Late Complications

Posttreatment surveillance is performed primarily to detect recurrent or persistent disease. Although surveillance is universally recommended by treating physicians, the timing of visits, the duration of follow-up, and the actual gain to the patient are based on tradition rather than fact. It is arguable that surveillance has limited value because most patients who develop recurrence of their tumors fail to survive. Follow-up visits, however, can be beneficial in other ways (Table 11-1). Some women can live a more normal life if the visits reduce their anxiety concerning the status of their tumors. Physical examination, careful questioning, and appropriate testing may allow early detection and therapy for posttreatment complications, other medical problems, or subsequent primary malignancies (Table 11-2).

SITE OF RECURRENCE BY TREATMENT MODALITY

Surgically treated tumors (stages IB, IIA) recur at about a 15% rate (range, 10.8 to 20.0; Table 11-3). Although there is considerable variation among series, recurrences are almost evenly distributed between central pelvic, lateral pelvic, and extrapelvic sites. Pelvic recurrences predominate; however, 26% to 44% recur out of the pelvis. Surveillance of surgical patients should focus on the pelvis but the possibility of extrapelvic metastases are distinct and the patient must be monitored for signs or symptoms of such metas-

tases also. Pelvic recurrences may manifest before distant recurrences (Look et al 1990). It is noteworthy that risk of pelvic recurrence differs when pelvic node metastases were present at the time of the original operation (see Table 7-17 in Chap. 7). Women who have either squamous cell carcinoma or adenocarcinoma and negative pelvic nodes have recurrence rates of between 6% and 20% (depending on the individual series), whereas recurrence rates double or triple for those who originally had pelvic node metastases. Those individuals who had bulky primary tumors and close surgical margins have the highest risk for pelvic recurrence (Burke et al 1987, Alvarez et al 1989, Creasman et al 1986).

In-field failure of radiation-treated patients is a factor of clinical stage (Table 11-4, Fig. 11-1). As clinical stage (and volume) of tumor increases, so does the possibility of in-field failure. Few irradiated patients recur in the central pelvis only. Perez and coworkers (1983), for example, reported that central pelvic failure alone was observed in only 7% of patients (less than 2% in stage IB and IIA, 8.7% in stage IIB, and 14.6% in stage III). Half or more of the recurrences become clinically evident as distal metastasis. Although under ideal conditions the central pelvic failure after radiation therapy is low and pelvic exenteration plays only a minor role in treatment of recurrent disease, the considerable variation in radiation treatment techniques from center to center (and resultant marginal or inadequate central pelvic dosages) may leave some individuals at risk and thus candidates for an ultradical salvage operation (Hanks et al 1983, Coia et al 1990).

TABLE 11-1
Justification for Posttreatment Surveillance

To provide reassurance and emotional support
To detect and manage complications of therapy
To detect other medical problems
To detect recurrence at the earliest time
To detect other primary cancers

Examinations within the first 6 months after radiation therapy are important, not only to detect recurrence but also for prognosis. Hardt and associates (1982) reported only a 5% recurrence rate in patients whose tumor had completely regressed on physical examination within 1 month of completion of therapy. Those having an intermediate response had a recurrence–persistence rate of 27%, whereas those women having an obvious incomplete response at 1 month had an 85% recurrence–persistence rate. Seventy-five percent of Hardt and colleagues' patients having an incom-

plete response had pelvic recurrences. Dische and coworkers (1980) also indicated that the degree of tumor regression in patients who were examined at the end of radiation therapy correlated with survival: those patients having a 75% to 100% regression had a median survival of 77 months, whereas those having less than 25% regression had a median survival of only 17 months.

RECURRENCE RISKS RELATED TO HISTOLOGIC CELL TYPE

There is controversy regarding the possibility that adenocarcinoma or adenosquamous tumors recur at a higher rate than do squamous cell tumors. Burke and associates (1987), in a surgical series, reported a recurrence rate of 9.2% for women having squamous cell tumors, compared with a 17.4% recurrence rate in women having adenocarcinoma and adenosquamous tumors. Ng and associates (1992) found no difference

TABLE 11-2
Common Problems and Concerns Associated with Cancer Treatment

SYMPTOMS OR CONCERNS	SURGICAL	RADIATION	CHEMOTHERAPY	RECURRENCE
Anxiety	++++	+	++	+++
Depression	0	+	++	+++
Pain	++	0	0	++++
Wound infection	+	0	0	0
Catheter care	++	0	0	++
Constipation	+	0	+	++++
Diarrhea	+	+++	+	0
Urinary symptoms/infection	++	++	++	++
Body image	+++	+	++	0
Sexual dysfunction	+++	+++	++	++++
Lower extremity edema	++	+	0	+++
Menopausal symptoms	++	++	++	+
Fever/infection	+	+	++++	++++
Nausea/vomiting	+	+	++++	+++
Dehydration	0	+	+++	++++
Allergic reactions	0	0	++	0
Drug toxicity	0	0	++++	0
Debility/fatigue	++	++	+++	++++
Odor	0	++	0	++++
Ostomy care	++	0	0	++
Fistula care	++	++++	0	++++

0, not a problem; + → ++++, degree of problem(s).
From Shingleton HM, Alvarez RD. The role of the general gynecologist in cancer care. In Shingleton HM, Hurt WG, (eds). Postreproductive gynecology. New York, Churchill Livingstone, 1990:295.

TABLE 11-3
Stage IB, IIA Site of Recurrence in Patients Treated by Radical Hysterectomy

STUDY	YEAR	PATIENTS (N)	RECURRENCE (n)	RECURRENCE (%)	CP (%)	LP (%)	EP (%)
Webb, et al	1980	564	104	18.4	19.2	40.2	40.6
Krebs, et al	1982	312	40	12.8	27.5	37.5	35.0
Burke, et al	1987	274	31	11.3	35.0	39.0	26.0
Larson, et al	1988	249	27	10.8	22.2	37.0	40.7
Look, et al	1990	55	11	20.0	27.2	45.6	27.2
Potter, et al	1990	469	68	14.5	48.5	22.1	29.4
Ng, et al	1992	702	116	16.5	NS	NS	NS
TOTAL		2625	397	15.1	30.1	35.1	34.8

CP, central pelvic; *LP,* lateral pelvic; *EP,* extrapelvic; *NS,* not stated.

between recurrences of these tissue types (16.2% squamous cell carcinoma, 17.7% adenocarcinoma–adenosquamous carcinoma) in a surgical series totaling 698 patients (only 62 nonsquamous cell tumors). The Alabama at Birmingham experience (Kilgore et al 1988) failed to demonstrate any significant difference in recurrence or survival rates in surgically treated patients having adenocarcinoma when compared with women having squamous cell cancers of the same stage and tumor volume. Webb and Symmonds (1980) were unable to demonstrate a significant difference in recurrence by cell type. The radiation therapy literature is inconclusive on this problem. Although some believe that adenocarcinomas are more radioresistant and have worse 5-year survival rates (Kjorstad 1977, Berek et al 1981, Kleine et al 1989), others re-

port no significant difference when patients receive optimal therapy (Weiner et al 1975, Wang 1988, Davidson et al 1989, Goodman et al 1989, Kovalic et al 1991, Kim 1993), particularly when controlled for risk factors such as tumor volume and node status (Hopkins et al 1987, Stehman et al 1991).

TIME TO RECURRENCE

Most recurrent cervical cancers are apparent soon after treatment; 70% to 89% of tumors that recur do so within the first 2 years (Muram et al 1982, Krebs et al 1982, Chen 1984, Larson et al 1988, Kim et al 1989). Generally, the time to recurrence relates to the size of the original lesion; that is, large-volume tumors tend

TABLE 11-4
Carcinoma of the Uterine Cervix: Pelvic Failure by Stage

STUDY	YEAR	TOTAL PELVIC FAILURE* (%) IB	IIA	IIB	IIIB	IVA
Perez, et al	1983	9.1	16.9	22.6	44.6	72.0
Jamopolis, et al	1975	6.3	7.3	17.6	43.1	—
Montana, et al	1983, 1985, 1986	10.2	9.3	26.9	47.7	—
Kim, et al	1989	11.2	8.4	30.1	52.3	69.0
PCS (Coia)	1990	10.0	—	26.0	51.0	—

*Pelvic failure only plus pelvic and distant failure

Modified from Kim RY. Radiotherapeutic management in carcinoma of the uterine cervix: current status. Int J Gynecol Cancer 1993;3:337.

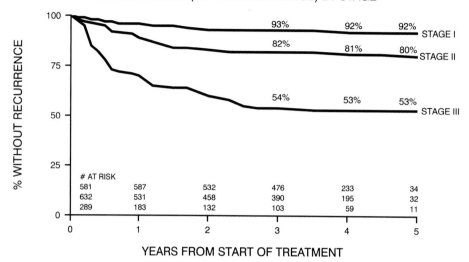

FAILURE/TOTAL: STAGE I=45/618; STAGE II=115/632; STAGE III=125/289

FIGURE 11-1. In-field failure as first recurrence by stage. (Lanciano RM, Won M, et al. Pretreatment factors associated with improved outcome in squamous cell carcinoma of the uterine cervix: a final report of the 1973 and 1978 patterns of care studies. Int J Radiat Oncol Biol Phys 1991;20;667, with permission.)

to recur earlier than small primary tumors. In a publication of the Alabama at Birmingham data, which was accumulated between 1969 and 1979 (Shingleton et al 1983), we looked at the relation of size (diameter) of stage IB tumors and treatment modality because these factors are related to time to recurrence. Tumors 2 cm or less in size recurred at a median of 1.6 years and 3-cm tumors recurred at a median of 1 year, whereas tumors larger than 3 cm that recurred did so at a median of 0.4 years. For surgically treated patients, the median time to recurrence was found to be 1 year, whereas radiation therapy patients recurred slightly later (1.3 years). It is difficult to judge lesion size in radiation therapy patients because clinical examination is unreliable for this purpose and even volumetric studies using magnetic resonance imaging (MRI) have error rates of 10% to 33% (see Table 6-7 in Chap. 6). In a publication from Alabama at Birmingham, Alvarez and colleagues (1993) reported recurrences after radical hysterectomy for bulky stage IB and IIA tumors (Table 11-5). The median time to recurrence for these tumors was 16.8 months, and it was noted that 90% of those that recurred did so within 3.5 years. Recurrences were more frequent as the tumor dimensions increased and in those individuals having poorly differentiated tumors or node metastasis.

EXAMINATION INTERVALS AFTER PRIMARY CANCER TREATMENT

An examination at the completion of radiation therapy and at least every 3 months during the first 2 years after irradiation or surgical treatment seems prudent. Patients are encouraged to return for examination at least every 6 months during the next 3 years and yearly thereafter. Some surveillance for the remainder of the patient's life may be in order because a small late risk of recurrent cancer exists many years after successful treatment, especially when the treatment was by radiation therapy. It is noteworthy that those having late central pelvic recurrences after irradiation as primary treatment are the ones most likely to be cured by pelvic exenteration (Shingleton et al 1989). Additionally, other pelvic malignancies may occur many years after therapy (Martins et al 1980). Patients who have unusual symptoms or signs (vaginal bleeding, lower extremity edema, pelvic–leg pain) are advised to see their physician immediately and not to wait for their next appointment (Tables 11-6 and 11-7).

At each visit, the physician should ask appropriate screening questions regarding symptoms and perform a thorough physical examination. Although many pa-

TABLE 11-5
Recurrence Related to Selected
Histopathologic Characteristics

	RECURRENCE	
FEATURE	(n) (total)	(%)
Maximum tumor diameter		
4.0–5.9 cm	15(39)	38.5
6.0–7.9 cm	3(7)	42.9
≥8.0 cm	1(2)	50.0
Grade		
I	0(2)	0
II	13(36)	36.1
III	6(10)	60.0
Nodal metastasis		
None	11(34)	32.4
Present	8(14)	57.1

From Alvarez RD, Gelder MS, Gore H, Soong S-J, Partridge EE. Radical hysterectomy in the treatment of patients with bulky early stage carcinoma of the cervix uteri. Surg Gynecol Obstet 1993;176:539; by permission.

TABLE 11-6
Pertinent Symptoms of Patients With Persistent
or Recurrent Disease

GENERAL

Weight loss or weight gain
Fatigue
Weakness

PULMONARY

Cough
Hemoptysis
Dyspnea
Chest pain

GASTROINTESTINAL

Abdominal pain
Nausea and vomiting
Change in bowel movements
Constipation
Diarrhea

GENITOURINARY

Dysuria
Frequency of urination
Urinary incontinence
Blood in urine
Difficulty in emptying bladder
Vaginal bleeding or discharge
Back or thigh pain
Pelvic pain or pressure
Blood in stool

MUSCULOSKELETAL

Extremity or back pain
Swelling in legs or arms

Bergen S. Surveillance of gynecologic malignancies. In Knaus JV, Isaacs JH (eds). Office gynecology: advanced management concepts. New York, Springer-Verlag, 1993:309; by permission.

tients with recurrent cervical cancer are asymptomatic, recurrence is preceded by (1) vaginal bleeding in 6% to 15% of women; (2) pain (back, sciatic, pelvic) in 20% to 50%; (3) weight loss, anorexia, or malaise in 10% to 25%; (4) leg edema in 5% to 12%; and (5) cough, dyspnea, or hemoptysis in 1% to 5% of patients (Calame 1969, Chen 1984).

VAGINAL CYTOLOGY IN FOLLOW-UP

The value of cervical smears as a predictor of recurrence is assigned varying degrees of importance by different investigators. For example, abnormal smears suggesting tumor are thought to be the first sign of recurrence in 3% to 50% of patients and may precede clinical evidence of recurrence by 3 to 24 months (Rayburn et al 1980). Of special importance is the early detection of central pelvic recurrence, which may be present in about 30% of those patients having recurrence after radical hysterectomy (see Table 11-3) and 7% of women after irradiation (Perez et al 1983). Despite contrary opinions (Adcock et al 1984), we believe that cervical cytology is such a simple, inexpensive diagnostic test that it should be used routinely to increase the opportunity for early detection of treatable pelvic recurrence. The differentiation between dysplastic cells, invasive cancer cells, and repair cells is difficult in the vaginal cytologic preparation taken after radiation therapy, particularly in the first few months (Kraus et al 1979). For this reason, care must be exer-

cised in making an early diagnosis of persistent disease in irradiated patients; adequate time must elapse to allow complete tumor response to the therapy. Reports of atypia cannot be ignored, however; when dysplastic cells are noted within 3 years of treatment, many such patients eventually develop recurrence (Wentz et al 1970).

PHYSICAL EXAMINATION

Physical examination should include supraclavicular and inguinal node palpation because this may be the initial abnormal finding in 1% to 4% of patients who

TABLE 11-7
Surveillance After Treatment for Cervical Cancer

HISTORY

Vaginal bleeding or discharge
Back, sciatic, or pelvic pain
Weight loss, anorexia
Cough, dyspnea, hemoptysis
Lower extremity swelling

PHYSICAL EXAMINATION

Weight, blood pressure
Nodal (supraclavicular and inguinal) palpation
Abdominal palpation
Vaginal speculum examination
Bimanual rectovaginal examination
Check for lower extremity edema

OTHER STUDIES

Cervicovaginal cytology
Tumor markers (optional) SCC, CA-125, CEA (see text)
Chest x-ray yearly
Intravenous pyelogram or CT scan of abdomen and pelvis
    Surgical patients: at 6 months and one year (high-risk
    patients)*; others: if symptomatic
    Radiation patients: as investigation of symptoms or abnor-
    mal pelvic findings

*High-volume tumors, positive pelvic nodes.

have recurrent disease (van Nagell et al 1979). Abdominal palpation may detect masses or hepatic enlargement. An abnormal bimanual pelvic examination is the initial evidence of recurrence in 20% to 25% of patients. Any visible cervical or vaginal lesion should undergo biopsy. The physician must be careful, however, when vaginal vault necrosis is present in the early postirradiation period; such necrosis may precede a vesicovaginal or rectovaginal fistula in many women, and overzealous use of biopsy instruments may contribute to fistula formation (Burns et al 1966).

If an abnormal bimanual examination is not accompanied by a clinical (visible) lesion, outpatient fine-needle aspiration or transvaginal cervical biopsies are indicated. Shepherd and coworkers (1981) used fine-needle aspiration of the cervix and mid-pelvis in 50 patients who had recurrent cervical cancer; the aspirate indicated the presence of tumor in 96% of patients and was more accurate than cervicovaginal exfoliative cytology or punch biopsy. Belinson and associates (1981) and Sevin and colleagues (1979) reported similar results. Fine-needle aspiration can be performed with little risk in patients who have central pelvic or parametrial lesions; however, pelvic side wall lesions should be sampled with caution because of the

proximity to major blood vessels. Fortier and coworkers (1985) also reported fine-needle aspiration to be highly accurate when used to confirm the diagnosis of extrapelvic disease. Layfield and associates (1991) reported a sensitivity of 100% and a specificity of 65% for fine-needle–aspiration cytology. Proper interpretation of the aspirate requires an experienced cytopathologist.

Selim and Beck (1984), using Vim-Silverman biopsy needles, successfully obtained a histologic specimen in 99% of patients undergoing biopsy. Correlation was excellent (97%). Lovecchio and Gal (1992) endorsed the technique using Tru-Cut or Vim-Silverman needles through various approaches (transabdominal, transvaginal, or transrectal). Careful immediate postbiopsy observation is mandatory because unintentional organ injury or concealed bleeding may result. Needle biopsies of this type are performed in the anesthetized patient and are not practical in an outpatient setting. They have been superseded by fine-needle aspiration as the initial action in most circumstances because the aspiration is simpler and less morbid than with biopsy needles.

The development of a pelvic mass (Fig. 11-2) requires careful investigation. Not all masses are malignant; patients who are treated with primary radical surgery and ovarian conservation have a small but definite risk (see Chap. 7) of requiring a second operation for ovarian extirpation because the retained ovary may degenerate and become cystic. A "benign" postsurgical pelvic lymphocyst cannot be assumed because the mass may actually represent recurrence in the pelvic node area or in the lymphocyst itself (Cantrell et al 1983). Fine-needle aspiration can be useful in such situations.

IMAGING STUDIES AND OTHER DIAGNOSTIC TESTS

Little information exists concerning the role and benefits of radiologic and other detection procedures in the early posttreatment surveillance period. Photopulos and colleagues (1977) evaluated 73 patients (surgical and radiation therapy) with a group of diagnostic tests consisting of intravenous pyelography (IVP), chest radiographs, barium enema, cystoscopy, proctoscopy, and bone scan. Overall, nine patients (12%) had an abnormal study and eight of these women died of recurrent cancer: studies were abnormal in three of 63 patients not suspected of having recurrence and in six patients out of ten who had suspected recurrence. He concluded that with the possible exception of the IVP and chest films, the other tests should not be routinely used in patients without clinical evidence of recur-

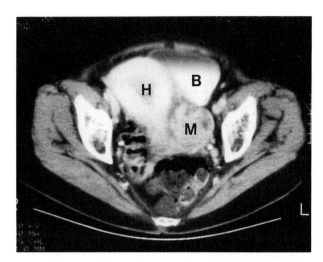

FIGURE 11-2. Computed tomography scan of a pelvic mass (*M*) displacing the bladder (*B*). Exploration revealed a benign ovarian tumor. A hydrometra (*H*) is also present. (Shingleton HM, Orr JW Jr. Cancer of the cervix: diagnosis and treatment. New York, Churchill Livingstone, 1987:213.)

rence, because most recurrences were diagnosed by physical examination.

Because chest metastases may be present in patients who have pelvic tumor recurrence, some have advocated yearly chest films as a part of routine surveillance of treated cervical cancer patients. We have not obtained them regularly because of the low yield and reserve their use for patients having pulmonary symptoms or after confirmation of pelvic recurrence. This is based on an isolated chest recurrence being unusual in cancer of the cervix. Rarely, one may encounter a solitary chest lesion, which can be resected, with control of the disease (Fig. 11-3); however, mul-

tiple chest metastases portend a poor prognosis. Perhaps as importantly, the risk of second lung primary tumors appears to be elevated in patients who have cervical cancer (Kleinerman et al 1982, Lee et al 1982, Clark et al 1984), particularly when the patient is a smoker.

Unilateral ureteral obstruction on IVP or computed tomography (CT) scan may be indicative of a pelvic side wall recurrence after radiation therapy or radical hysterectomy but such obstruction is rarely encountered in women who have a normal posttreatment pelvic examination. Ureteral obstruction after primary radiation therapy is associated with recurrence

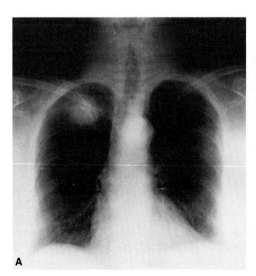

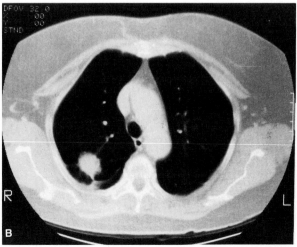

FIGURE 11-3. (**A**) An apparent isolated lesion in a 66-year-old women, 10 years after radiotherapy. She had no evidence of pelvic or intraabdominal disease. (**B**) A computed tomography chest scan indicated unresectability. (Shingleton HM, Orr JW Jr. Cancer of the cervix: diagnosis and treatment. New York, Churchill Livingstone, 1987:214.)

in more than 90% of cases. Although recommendations vary, some have suggested obtaining routine follow-up IVPs as frequently as every 6 months (Kontturi et al 1982). Because pelvic recurrence after primary surgical treatment may be cured with irradiation, we are inclined to consider an IVP at 6 months and at 1 year in those postoperative patients considered to be at high risk for failure (large lesions, pelvic node metastases). After primary treatment with irradiation, however, we do not recommend any routine schedule for IVPs but obtain them only when there are pelvic findings suggesting recurrence or symptoms suggesting ureteral obstruction. When detected, the nature of the pelvic ureteral obstruction should be confirmed by fine-needle aspiration or when necessary by laparotomy because intervention may preserve existing renal function (Fig. 11-4).

Although they have replaced IVPs in the practice of many physicians, the value of abdominal or pelvic CT scans in routine surveillance of treated cervical cancer is unproved. Although CT scans may aid in the diagnosis of pelvic recurrence, the most sensitive or useful portion of the examination may be the study of the paraaortic node chain (Bandy et al 1985). Hospitel

and coworkers (1984) confirmed the sensitivity of CT scans in extrapelvic node disease but reported its limitations in the diagnosis of active pelvic disease, an experience paralleling ours. Thus, whereas CT scaning may be used for diagnostic purposes in the posttreatment symptomatic patient, its use is not advocated on a routine basis for asymptomatic patients—if for no other reason than because of the considerable expense and lack of sensitivity and specificity (see Tables 6-4, 6-5, and 6-6 in Chap. 6).

In contrast to CT scanning, which depends on anatomic alterations, MRI is thought to have the ability to distinguish inherent differences in tissues and in anatomic changes in both transverse and longitudinal planes (Hricak 1991). Although this modality has value in cervical cancer, it has not been shown to be superior to CT scanning (see Tables 6-7, 6-8, and 6-9 in Chap. 6) and should not be routinely used for pre- or posttreatment abdominopelvic screening because it is even more expensive than CT scanning.

Other diagnostic studies (e.g., cystoscopy, proctoscopy, barium enema, and bone scans) should only be used in symptomatic women as part of an evaluation for suspected recurrence. Inevitable tissue changes within pelvic radiation fields should be kept in mind during the interpretation of these (and indeed all) imaging investigations (Meyer 1981).

TUMOR MARKERS

A large experience concerning tumor marker levels, sensitivity, specificity, and their value in posttreatment surveillance of both squamous cell carcinoma and adenocarcinoma of the cervix has been reported in the last decade. Squamous cell carcinoma (SCC)—a glycoprotein subfraction of TA-4—has a high specificity but a low sensitivity (Table 6-12 in Chap. 6). This marker varies in individual patients with volume of disease, as reflected by clinical stage. Although it may be useful for posttreatment surveillance, it is not useful for screening or diagnosis because of its low levels (17% to 50%) in stage I (low-volume) disease. SCC has not been found to be accurate for prediction of node metastasis (Patsner et al 1989). It may also vary by differentiation of tumor (Crombach et al 1989).

SCC has been evaluated for monitoring patients, regardless of initial treatment for squamous cell carcinoma (Table 11-8). At this time, however, squamous cell carcinoma is not used widely in posttreatment surveillance despite favorable reports and high accuracy rates in predicting recurrence. Rising squamous cell carcinoma levels have been found to predict recurrence, usually several months before clinical recurrence (Holloway et al 1989, Duk et al 1990, Nam et al 1990, Brioschi et al 1991, Gitsch et al 1992). In addi-

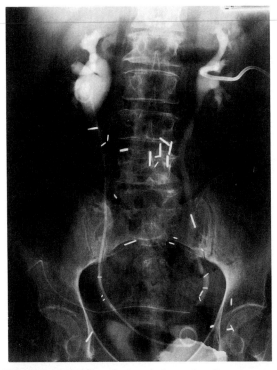

FIGURE 11-4. Bilateral ureteral obstruction. Percutaneous placement of indwelling stents allowed recovery of renal function. Indwelling "double J" stent (*right*), percutaneous stent (*left*) later internalized. (Shingleton HM, Orr JW Jr. Cancer of the Cervix: Diagnosis and Treatment. New York, Churchill Livingstone, 1987:217.)

tion to its value in postoperative patients, it has also been found to be useful in postirradiated patients (Yazigi et al 1991) and in monitoring the response to chemotherapy (see Table 11-8). There are no reports that indicate the benefit of early detection of recurrence with markers regarding subsequent treatment results or impact on survival.

Other tumor markers have been tested in the follow-up of treated squamous cell carcinoma, including carcinembryonic antigen (CEA) and CA-125 (Table 11-9). Generally, these markers and others have played little role in routine posttreatment surveillance.

Markers for Adenocarcinoma

Several markers including CA-125, CEA, and TA-4 have been evaluated in the follow-up of treated patients having cervical adenocarcinoma (Table 11-10). Marker CA-125, a high–molecular-weight glycoprotein expressed in coelomic epithelium during embryonic development, appears to have greater potential for use than does CEA (a tumor-associated glycoprotein), although CEA may be more useful in follow-up of those women who have the marker. The levels of CA-125 are thought not to be related to stage, tumor

TABLE 11-8
Squamous Cell Carcinoma Marker in Monitoring Treatment for Squamous Cell Carcinoma

STUDY	YEAR	PATIENTS (N)	TYPE OF TREATMENT	COMMENT
Dodd, et al	1989	34	All treatments	12 of 24 with recurrence had elevated and rising values before clinical evidence of disease (median, 13 mo lead time)
Holloway, et al	1989	135	All treatments	Rising SCC levels predicted recurrence in 15 of 20 women; in 10 cases, mean of 4.6 months before clinical recurrence
Maiman, et al	1989	64	All treatments	Those with recurrence had higher pretreatment titres (16.1 mg/mL vs 5.6 mg/mL); this marker has sensitivity/specificity as predictor of outcome of 63% and 90%, respectively
Neunteufel, et al	1989	91	All treatments	68% of those with recurrence had elevated titres; elevated posttreatment titres carried high risk for persistence
Duk, et al	1990	451	All treatments	Sensitivity 85.5% in predicting recurrent disease; positive predictive value, 76% (two consecutive values)
Nam, et al	1990	60	All treatments	Predicted recurrence in 4 of 7 patients with sequential titres
Brioschi, et al	1991	62	All treatments	Correlated with recurrence or progressive disease in 90% of cases; lead time of about 4 months before clinical recurrence
Tomas, et al	1991	111	All treatments	SCC levels correlate with clinical stage; clinically useful in monitoring behavior of advanced tumors
Gitsch, et al	1992	30	All treatments	7 of 14 patients with recurrence had elevated SCC values, with lead times of 3–9 months
Scambia, et al	1991	119	All treatments plus chemotherapy	Those with pretreatment levels <5mg/mL were longer survivors; predicted recurrence in 8 of 11, with lead time of 5 months
Yazigi, et al	1991	82	Radiation (18 pts)	100% accurate in predicting progression/regression
			Chemotherapy (27 pts)	96% accurate in predicting progression/regression
Ngan, et al	1989	15	Chemotherapy	Positive correlation with disease progression in 13 of 15 patients, as measured by SCC levels
Meier, et al	1990	36	Chemotherapy	Marker fell to normal in all responders after 1–2 courses
Leminen, et al	1992	23	Chemotherapy	In 91% of previously untreated patients, SCC levels decreased after chemotherapy

SCC, squamous cell carcinoma.

TABLE 11-9
Other Tumor Markers in Follow-up of Treated Squamous Cell Carcinoma

STUDY	MARKER	FINDINGS
Kjorstad, et al 1982	CEA*	Rising titre prediction of recurrence; serial values of limited value in advanced stages
te Velde, et al 1982	CEA	Elevated CEA poor prognostic indicator
Schwartz, et al 1987	CEA	Levels do not correlate with clinical status
Dodd, et al 1989	CEA	Not useful as marker
Meier, et al 1990	CEA	Useful in monitoring chemotherapy
Leminen 1992	CEA	Response to neoadjuvant chemotherapy only documented in 33% of patients
Schwartz, et al 1987	CA-125	Very low sensitivity (18.8%)
Dodd, et al 1989	CA-125	Not useful as marker
Lehtovirta, et al 1990	CA-125	Levels raised in only 26% of patients; of limited use
Goldberg, et al 1991	CA-125	Of 11 patients with pre- and posttherapy elevations, 10 died; 1 had persistent disease
Leminen, et al 1992	CA-125	Useful in demonstrating response in 83% of previously untreated women given chemotherapy
Nam, et al 1990	UGF†	More sensitive than SCC (TA-4)
Pfeiffer, et al 1989	EGF‡	High levels associated with recurrence/death, independent of stage
Schwartz, et al 1987	LSA§	Elevated in 60% of patients; sensitivity, 62.5%; specificity, 89.2%
Tomas, et al 1991	APPIII‖	As predictive of disease behavior as TA-4 commonly elevated pretreatment (40% vs 47% TA-4)
Gitsch, et al 1992	TPS¶	Sensitivity/specificity similar to SCC; useful combined with SCC in providing lead times to recurrence

*Carcinoembryonic antigen.
†Urinary gonadotropin fragment.
‡Epidermal growth factor.
§Lipid associated sialic acid.
‖Aminoterminal propeptide of type III procollagen.
¶Tissue polypeptide-specific antigen.

TABLE 11-10
Tumor Markers in Follow-up of Treated Adenocarcinoma

STUDY	YEAR	PATIENTS (N)	MARKERS	CONCLUSIONS
Leminen	1990	42	CA-125, CEA, TATI*	CA-125 (and to lesser degree) CEA + TATI useful in follow-up
Duk, et al	1990	77	CA-125, CEA, TA-4 (SCC)	CA-125 important prognostic factor and indicator of tumor virulence
Goldberg, et al	1991	9	CA 125	Levels not related to stage, tumor burden, or histologic type
Tamimi, et al	1992	55	CEA	Patients whose tumors express CEA are at increased risk for recurrence

*Tumor-associated trypsin inhibitor.

burden, or histologic type (Goldberg et al 1991). If one elected to measure CA-125 and CEA levels and found them to be elevated pretreatment, the markers may be of some prognostic value in follow-up. They have not gained general use.

SURVEILLANCE FOR DETECTION OF SECOND PRIMARY CANCER AND COEXISTENT MEDICAL DISEASE

Although all surveillance examinations are primarily intended to detect recurrent or persistent cervical cancer, it should be remembered that these women may have or may develop a second primary tumor. About 4% of women who have cervical cancer have synchronous or subsequent second primary tumors, which include uterine sarcomas, ovarian neoplasms, and other abdominal tumors (Axelrod et al 1984). The ever-present risk of breast and gastrointestinal cancer should prompt examination of the patient's breasts and she should be given instructions about breast self-examination and scheduling of mammograms. Appropriate hematologic studies and a stool specimen for occult blood should be obtained at frequent (1- to 2-year) intervals. Rectal bleeding should be investigated by appropriate endoscopic evaluation.

Although surveillance for cancer is a high priority, the opportunity exists during the visit for general medical surveillance of the patient (Table 11-11). Monitoring of weight, a cholesterol screen, dietary assistance, and discussion of the important issue of smoking cessation should be considered.

EXOGENOUS ESTROGEN

Consideration of estrogen therapy for the individuals who are menopausal as a result of ovarian ablation or removal seems appropriate. No contraindication for estrogen replacement therapy exists relative to squamous cell or adenocarcinoma of the cervix; however, other conditions may exist that affect the decision to use such therapy (Table 11-12).

ENDOMETRIAL EFFECTS

It should be noted that the irradiated endometrium can respond to hormonal stimulation (Larson et al 1990) and that almost a fourth of patients maintain endometrial sensitivity to exogenous hormones (McKay et al 1990). Unopposed estrogen administration may therefore potentially increase the risk of the development of premalignant or malignant corpus lesions. Postirradiation cervical stenosis may eliminate the biologic sign of uterine cancer (i.e., bleeding). This scenario may explain why endometrial cancers developing after irradiation are more likely to be of higher stage and carry a worse prognosis (Chen et al 1991).

TREATMENT COMPLICATIONS

Early Complications

An important part of posttreatment surveillance includes patient monitoring for the diagnosis and management of treatment complications. When considering the complications of surgical or radiation treatment (Table 11-13), it becomes evident that the most serious surgical complications often occur acutely. Attention to intraoperative technique should decrease these risks. Although surgical complications may require additional monitoring, antibiotics, drainage, or even additional surgery, they are usually amenable to some treatment and rarely result in significant long-term morbidity or in mortality.

Bladder or ureteral fistulas although rare (see Table 7-8 in Chap. 7) are serious complications that manifest in the early postoperative period. The bladder fistulas are likely to require surgical repair after general healing has occurred from the primary operation. Ureteral fistulas may heal over percutaneously placed (Mann et al 1983) or retrograde stents or when unresolved, require subsequent repair (Holley et al 1994).

Acute irradiation-induced gastrointestinal and genitourinary symptoms are common and may result in short treatment interruptions; however, they usually resolve spontaneously after completion of therapy and require minimal intervention. Rarely, patients require surgical intervention in the form of partial small bowel resection; colostomy, with or without mucous fistula formation; or combinations of the above (Tsukamoto et al 1993).

Late Complications: Surgical

In contrast to more correctable early posttreatment complications, late complications of either treatment modality are more difficult to manage. Bladder dysfunction is one of the most frequent long-term complications; the pathogenesis has been discussed (Chap. 7). Although appropriate early postoperative bladder drainage may decrease the risk, significant problems with altered bladder sensation, the inability to initiate voiding, to completely empty the bladder, or to maintain continence under stress occurs in as many as 50 % of patients after radical hysterectomy

TABLE 11-11
Recommendations for the Periodic Examination of Women Age 40 and Older

EXAMINATION	SOURCE	FREQUENCY
History and physical	a	Every 5 yr, age 40–60; every 2 yr, age 60–74; annually 75+
Blood pressure	a	Every 2 yr, age 40–50; annually age 50+
	b	Every 2 yr, age 40+
	c	Every 5 yr, age 40–45; annually age 45+
Breast examination	a	Every 2 yr, age 40–50; annually age 50+
	b	Every 2 yr, age 40–50; annually age 50+
	c	Annually age 50–59
	d	Annually
Pelvic examination	a	Every 5 yr, age 40–60; every 2 yr, age 60–74; annually 75+
	b	Every 2 yr, age 40–74
	d	Annually
Rectal examination	a	Every 5 yr, age 40–60; every 2 yr, age 60–74; annually 75+
	d	Annually
Pap smear	a	Every 2 yr, age 40–54; every 3 yr, age 55+
	b	Every 2 yr
	c	Low-risk, every 5 yr; high-risk, annually
	d	Annually
Fecal occult blood test	a	Every 3 yr, age 40–50; annually age 50+
	b	Every 2 yr, age 40–50; annually age 50+
	c	Annually age 45+
	d	Annually age 50+
Sigmoidoscopy	d	Every 3–5 yr beginning age 50 after two initial negative sigmoidoscopies 1 yr apart
Mammography	a	Annually age 50+
	c	Annually age 50–59
	d	Every 2 yr, age 40–50; annually age 50+
Hearing assessment	a	Age 50, 55, 60
VDRL	b	Age 50
	c	As clinically indicated
PPD	b	Age 50 and 60
	c	As clinically indicated
Cholesterol	a	Every 5 yr
	b	Every 5 yr
Tetanus-diphtheria booster	a	Every 10 yr
	b	Every 10 yr
Influenza immunization	a	Annually age 60+
	b	Annually age 65+

[a]Breslow L, Somers AR. The lifetime health monitoring program: a practical approach to preventive medicine. N Engl J Med 1977;296:601.
[b]Frame PS. A critical review of adult health maintenance. J Fam Pract 1986;22:341, 471, 511; 23: 29.
[c]Canadian Task Force on the Periodic Health Examination. The periodic health examination. Can Med Assoc J 1979;121:1193; 1984;130:1278; 1986;134:724; 1988;138:618.
[d]American Cancer Society. ACS report on the cancer-related health checkup. CA 1980;30:194.

From Sparks JM, Waldrop EC. Outpatient surveillance. In Shingleton HM, Hurt WG (eds). Postreproductive gynecology. New York, Churchill Livingstone, 1990:133; with permission.

(Farquharson et al 1987). If suprapubic catheter drainage does not result in effective bladder emptying and return to normal function within a few weeks, the patient should be instructed in intermittent self-catheterization. When this program is instituted, a regimen of urine acidification by vitamin C tablets or by daily intake of acid fruit juices is recommended. Only rarely are adjunctive antibiotics useful.

In those patients having chronic bladder symptomatology in the months after radical pelvic operations,

TABLE 11-12
Contraindications to Menopausal Estrogen Therapy

1. Known or suspected cancer of the breast, except in appropriately selected patients being treated for metastatic disease
2. Known or suspected estrogen-dependent neoplasia
3. Undiagnosed abnormal genital bleeding
4. Active thrombophlebitis or thromboembolic disorders
5. History of thrombophlebitis, thrombosis, or thromboembolic disorders associated with previous estrogen use
6. Active liver disease, gallbladder disease, or chronically impaired liver function

From Varner RE. Hormone replacement therapy. In Shingleton HM, Hurt WG (eds). Postreproductive gynecology. New York, Churchill Livingstone, 1990:160; with permission.

urodynamic testing is indicated (Farquharson et al 1987). Appropriate management—whether prolonged bladder drainage for voiding disorders, medication for bladder instability, surgery for anatomic defects of vesical neck support, or some combination—is instituted based on diagnosis of the specific defect.

The development of pelvic lymphocysts after radical operation is rare (see Table 7-9 in Chap. 7). Most are apparent within the first few weeks; they may be detected during surveillance examinations as asymptomatic pelvic side wall masses or may become clinically apparent because of bladder symptoms or pelvic pain.

TABLE 11-13
Potential Complications of Treatment

SURGERY	RADIATION
EARLY	
Anesthetic accidents	Anesthetic accidents
Hemorrhage	Gastrointestinal
Transfusion reactions	Diarrhea
Postoperative infection	Proctitis
Wound abscess	Genitourinary
Thromboembolic events	Hemorrhagic cystitis
Fistula of bowel, bladder, ureters	Thromboembolic events
Bladder dysfunction	Perforation of uterus, bowel bladder
Pelvic lymphocyst	
LATE	
Bladder dysfunction	Fistula of large or small bowel, bladder
Loss of sensation	Vaginal stricturing
Stress incontinence	Sexual dysfunction
Intestinal obstruction	Carcinogenic effect
Ovarian failure	Castration
Vaginal shortening	

When a pelvic mass is present in a patient whose ovary or ovaries were conserved, ultrasonography or CT scanning may help in the differentiated diagnosis of lymphocysts versus an ovarian mass. Management of lymphocysts includes percutaneous aspiration or catheter drainage (Aronowitz et al 1983, Mann et al 1989). The aspirate should be microscopically examined to rule out malignant cells. If the lymphocyst recurs after drainage, intraabdominal marsupialization, with omental interposition, may be successful in correcting the problem (Kay et al 1980).

Although gastrointestinal obstruction may occur after any abdominal procedure, it is relatively rare after radical hysterectomy (Helmkamp et al 1985). If small bowel obstruction occurs and there is no evidence of infarction, conservative management with fluid resuscitation and intestinal decompression is appropriate. The appearance of this complication remote (months) from the operation should increase the suspicion of recurrent disease, and efforts to exclude its presence with careful examination and diagnostic studies are mandatory. When surgical decompression is required, intraoperative assessment and biopsy should be performed to exclude recurrent disease.

Late ureteral obstruction, although rare, may occur after surgical treatment. This situation usually heralds recurrent disease. Seldom is it due to benign strictures (Hatch et al 1984). Fine-needle aspiration of the area of obstruction may establish the diagnosis and avoid a diagnostic surgical procedure. When malignant T cells are found, ureteral stents placed either transvesically or percutaneously may allow preservation of remaining renal function subsequent to the addition of adjuvant therapy, such as irradiation or chemotherapy (see Fig. 11-4).

LATE COMPLICATIONS: IRRADIATION

In contrast to the spontaneous resolution of most acute problems during irradiation, late irradiation complications are difficult to manage. Fortunately, modern radiation therapy techniques and dosimetry calculations minimize the risk of such sequelae. When late irradiation complications are encountered, it is important that the physician evaluate the patient for recurrent malignancy, including evaluation of all organ systems in the irradiation field. Extensive vaginal vault necrosis may herald or precede the development of a urinary or bowel fistula (Burns et al 1966). Women who develop one complication appear to be at increased risk of developing complications of other organ systems. Radiation-induced bowel obstruction and fistulas are often complex; the "obvious" recto-

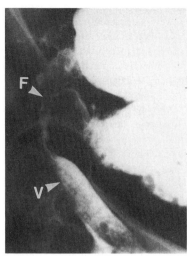

FIGURE 11-5. A 2-hour–delayed small-bowel series indicated a distal ileal vaginal fistula. Barium enema was normal. *F*, fistulous tract; *V*, vagina. (Shingleton HM, Orr JW Jr. Cancer of the cervix: diagnosis and treatment. New York, Churchill Livingstone, 1987:218.)

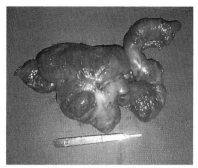

FIGURE 11-6. Marked radiation damage to small bowel in a young woman given postoperative whole-pelvis radiotherapy (50 Gy) after radical hysterectomy. Surgical resection of the matted bowel was required. Long-term hyperalimentation was necessary in this patient and a "short bowel" syndrome occurred, with permanent partial disability. (Courtesy of Dr. E.E. Partridge University of Alabama at Birmingham) See Color Figure 11-6.

vaginal fistula may have a small bowel component (Fig. 11-5). The progressive diminution of vascular supply to tissues in an irradiation field may result in severe bowel damage, resulting in long-term disability (Fig. 11-6).

POSTIRRADIATION DYSPLASIA

Postirradiation dysplasia is altered benign squamous epithelium of the cervix or vagina, occurring after a latent period of several months up to more than 10 years after successful radiation therapy, and has been thought to occur in a fifth of all surviving irradiated cervical cancer patients (Patten et al 1963, Wentz et al 1970). It is usually detected by cytology in the absence of clinically recurrent cancer. In the Papanicolaou smear, cells may occur singly or in sheets. Nuclei are enlarged, round, or oval, with coarsely granular chromatin. Nuclear–cellular ratio is slightly less than that of carcinoma in situ. Histologically, there are abnormally large nuclei in the stratified squamous epithelium and cells are somewhat smaller than in dysplasia in the nonirradiated patient. Differentiation may occur with parakeratosis (keratinization with retention of nuclei); mitoses are rare (Wentz et al 1970).

It should be noted that the changes of irradiation response described in benign squamous cells in the vaginal smear in the first few weeks postirradiation and used by some investigators in the past to determine

prognosis (Graham et al 1955) are different from those described above for postirradiation dysplasia. Although some have reported that the earlier this entity is found, the greater likelihood there is of recurrent cancer (Wentz et al 1970, Patten et al 1963, 1988); however, there is not general agreement that postirradiation dysplasia is a malignancy-associated change. Such patients should be evaluated carefully before embarking on further therapy. Should representative biopsies of the cervix and upper vagina fail to demonstrate viable tumor in the absence of any other evidence of cancer, long-term observation without therapy seems to be in order. Use of a topical estrogen cream may be considered to rule out the possibility of simple atrophy causing difficulty in cytologic diagnosis.

References

Adcock LL, Potish RA, Julian TM, et al. Carcinoma of the cervix, FIGO stage IB: treatment failures. Gynecol Oncol 1984;18:218.

Alvarez RD, Soong S-J, Kinney WK, et al. Identification of prognostic factors and risk groups in patients found to have nodal metastasis at the time of radical hysterectomy for early-stage squamous carcinoma of the cervix. Gynecol Oncol 1989;35:130.

Alvarez RD, Gelder MS, Gore H, Soong S-J, Partridge EE. Radical hysterectomy in the treatment of patients with bulky early stage carcinoma of the cervix uteri. Surg Gynecol Obstet 1993;176:539.

Aronowitz J, Kaplan AL. The management of a pelvic lymphocele by the use of a percutaneous indwelling catheter inserted with ultrasound guidance. Gynecol Oncol 1983;16:292.

Avall-Lundqvist EH, Sjovall K, Nilsson BR, Eneroth PH. Prognostic significance of pretreatment serum levels of squamous cell carcinoma antigen and CA 125 in cervical carcinoma. Eur J Cancer 1992;28A:1695.

Axelrod JH, Fruchter R, Boyce JG. Multiple primaries among gynecologic malignancies. Gynecol Oncol 1984; 18:359.

Bandy LC, Clarke-Pearson DL, Silverman PM, Creasman WT. Computed tomography in evaluation of extrapelvic lymphadenopathy in carcinoma of the cervix. Obstet Gynecol 1985;65:73.

Belinson JL, Lynn JM, Papillo JL, et al. Fine needle cytology in the management of gynecologic cancer. Am J Obstet Gynecol 1981;139:148.

Berek JS, Castaldo TW, Hacker NF, et al. Adenocarcinoma of the uterine cervix. Cancer 1981;48:2734.

Borras G, Molina R, Xercavins J, Ballesta A, Iglesias X. Squamous cell carcinoma antigen in cervical cancer. Eur J Gynaecol Oncol 1992;13:414.

Brioschi PA, Bischof P, Delafosse C, Krauer F. Squamous-cell carcinoma antigen (SCC-A) values related to clinical outcome of pre-invasive cervical carcinoma. Int J Cancer 1991;47:376.

Burke TW, Hoskins WJ, Heller PB, Shen MC, Weiser EB, Park RC. Clinical patterns of tumor recurrence after radical hysterectomy in stage IB cervical carcinoma. Obstet Gynecol 1987;69:382.

Burns BC, Upton RT. Management of urinary tract complications of treatment for carcinoma of the uterine cervix. In Cancer of the uterus and ovary. Chicago: Year Book Medical Publishers, 1966:257.

Calame RJ. Recurrent carcinoma of the cervix. Am J Obstet Gynecol 1969;105:380.

Cantrell CJ, Wilkinson EJ. Recurrent squamous cell carcinoma of the cervix within pelvic-abdominal lymphocysts. Obstet Gynecol 1983;62:530.

Chen NJ. Vagina invasion by cervical carcinoma. Acta Med Okayama 1984;38:305.

Chen MS, Lin FJ, Hong CH, et al. High-dose-rate afterloading technique in the radiation treatment of uterine cervical cancer: 399 cases and 9 years experinee in Taiwan. Int J Radiat Oncol Biol Phys 1991;20:915.

Clark EL, Kreiger N, Spengh RF. Second primary cancer following treatment for cervical cancer. Can Med Assoc J 1984;131:553.

Coia L, Won M, Lanciano R, et al. The Patterns of Care Outcome Study for cancer of the uterine cervix: results of the 2nd national practice survey. Cancer 1990; 66:2451.

Creasman WT, Soper JT, Clarke-Pearson D. Radical hysterectomy as therapy for early carcinoma of the cervix. Am J Obstet Gynecol 1986;155:964.

Crombach G, Scharl A, Vierbuchen M, Würtz H, Bolte A. Detection of squamous cell carcinoma antigen in normal squamous epithelia and in squamous cell carcinomas of the uterine cervix. Cancer 1989;63:1337.

Davidson SE, Symonds RP, Lamont D, et al. Does adenocarcinoma of uterine cervix have a worse prognosis than squamous carcinoma when treated by radiotherapy. Gynecol Oncol 1989;33:23.

Dische S, Bennett MH, Saunders MI, Anderson P. Tumour regression as a guide to prognosis: a clinical study. Br J Radiol 1980;53:454.

Dodd JK, Henry RJW, Tyler JPP, Houghton CRS. Cervical carcinoma: a comparison of four potential biochemical tumor markers. Gynecol Oncol 1989;32:248.

Duk JM, DeBruijn HWA, Groenier KH, et al. Cancer of the uterine cervix: sensitivity and specificity of serum squamous cell carcinoma antigen determinations. Gynecol Oncol 1990;39:186.

Duk JM, DeBruijn HWA, Groenier KH, Lleuren GJ, Aalders JG. Adenocarcinoma of the uterine cervix. Prognostic significance of pretreatment serum CA 125, squamous cell carcinoma antigen, and carcinoembryonic antigen levels in relation to clinical and histopathologic tumor characteristics. Cancer 1990;65:1830.

Farquharson DIM, Shingleton HM, Soong S-J, et al. The adverse effects of cervical cancer treatment on bladder function. Gynecol Oncol 1987;27:15.

Fortier KJ, Clarke-Pearson DL, Creasman WT, Johnston WW. Fine-needle aspiration in gynecology: evaluation of extrapelvic lesions in patients with gynecologic malignancy. Obstet Gynecol 1985;65:67.

Goldberg GL, Sklar A, O'Hanlan KA, Levine PA, Runowicz CD. CA-125: a potential prognostic indicator in patients with cervical cancer? Gynecol Oncol 1991; 40:222.

Goodman HM, Niloff JM, Buttlar CA, et al. Adenocarcinoma of the cervical stump. Gynecol Oncol 1989; 35:188.

Gitsch G, Kainz E, Frohlich B, Bieglmayr C, Tatra G. Squamous cell carcinoma antigen, tumor associated trypsin inhibitor and tissue polypeptide specific antigen in follow up of stage III cervical cancer. Anticancer Res 1992;12:1247.

Graham RM, Graham JB. Cytological prognosis in cancer of the uterine cervix treated radiologically. Cancer 1955;8:59.

Hanks GE, Herring DF, Kramer S. Patterns of Care Outcome Studies: results of the national practice in cancer of the cervix. Cancer 1983;51:959.

Hardt N, van Nagell JR, Hanson M, Donaldson E, Yoneda J, Maruyama Y. Radiation-induced tumor regression as a prognostic factor in patients with invasive cervical cancer. Cancer 1982;49:35.

Hatch KD, Parham G, Shingleton HM, Orr JW Jr, Austin JM Jr. Ureteral strictures and fistulae following radical hysterectomy. Gynecol Oncol 1984;19:17.

Helmkamp BF, Kimmel J. Conservative management of small bowel obstruction. Am J Obstet Gynecol 1985; 152:677.

Holley R, Kilgore L. Genitourinary considerations. In Orr JW Jr, Shingleton HM, eds. Complications in gynecologic surgery: prevention and management. Philadelphia: JB Lippincott, 1994.

Holloway RW, To A, Moradi M, Boots L, Watson N, Shingleton HM. Monitoring the course of cervical carcinoma with the squamous cell carcinoma serum radioimmunoassay. Obstet Gynecol 1989;74:944.

Hopkins MP, Sutton P, Roberts JA. Prognostic features and treatment of endocervical adenocarcinoma of the cervix. Gynecol Oncol 1987;27:68.

Hospitel S, Masselot J, Couanet D, et al. Value of x-ray computed tomography in the diagnosis and surveillance of abdominopelvic recurrence of cancers of the uterine cervix, apropos of 38 cases. J Radiol 1984;65:327.

Hricak H. Carcinoma of the female reproductive organs. Value of cross-sectional imaging. Cancer 1991;67:1209.

Hsieh CY, Chang DY, Huang SC, Yen ML, Juang GT, Ouyang PC. Serum squamous cell carcinoma antigen in gynecologic malignancies with special reference to cervical cancer. J Formos Med Assoc 1989;88:797.

Jamopolis S, Andras EJ, Fletcher GH. Analysis of sites and causes of failures of irradiation in invasive squamous cell carcinoma of the intact uterine cervix. Radiol 1975; 115:681.

Kay R, Fuchs E, Barry JM. Management of postoperative pelvic lymphoceles. Urology 1980;XV:345.

Kilgore LC, Soong S-J, Gore H, Shingleton HM, Hatch KD, Partridge EE: Analysis of prognostic features in adenocarcinoma of the cervix. Gynecol Oncol 1988;31:137.

Kim RY, Trotti A, Wu CJ, Soong SJ, Salter MM. Radiation alone in the treatment of cancer of the uterine cervix: analysis of pelvic failure and dose response relationship. Int J Radiat Oncol Biol Phys 1989;17:973.

Kim RY. Radiotherapeutic management in carcinoma of the uterine cervix: current status. Int J Gynecol Cancer 1993;3:337.

Kjorstad JE. Carcinoma of the cervix in the young patients. Obstet Gynecol 1977;50:28.

Kjorstad KE, Orjasaester H. The prognostic value of CEA determinations in the plasma of patients with squamous cell cancer of the cervix. Cancer 1982;50:283.

Kleine W, Rau K, Schwoeorer D, Pfleiderer A. Prognosis of the adenocarcinoma of the cervix uteri: a comparative study. Gynecol Oncol 1989;35:145.

Kleinerman RA, Curtis RE, Boice JD Jr, Flannery JT, Fraumeni JF Jr. Second cancers following radiotherapy for cervical cancer. J Natl Cancer Inst 1982;69:1027.

Kontturi M, Kauppila A. Ureteric complications following treatment of gynaecological cancer. Ann Chir Gynaecol 1982;71:232.

Kovalic JJ, Grigsby PW, Perez CA, Lockett MA. Cervical stump carcinoma. Int J Radiat Oncol Biol Phys 1991;20:933.

Kraus H, Schumann R. Cytologic presentation of recurrent carcinoma of the uterine cervix and corpus after radiotherapy. Acta Cytol 1979;23:114.

Krebs HB, Helmkamp BF, Sevin B-U, Nadji M, Averette HE. Recurrent cancer of the cervix following radical hysterectomy and pelvic node dissection. Obstet Gynecol 1982;59:422.

Lam CP, Yuan CC, Jeng FS, Tsai LC, Yeh SH, Ng HT. Evaluation of carcinoembryonic antigen, tissue polypeptide antigen, and squamous cell carcinoma antigen in the detection of cervical cancers. Chin Med J (Engl) 1992;50:7.

Lanciano RM, Won M, Coia LR, Hanks GE. Pretreatment and treatment factors associated with improved outcome in squamous cell carcinoma of the uterine cervix: a final report of the 1973 and 1978 patterns of care studies. Int J Radiat Oncol Biol Phys 1991;20:667.

Larson DM, Copeland LJ, Stringer CA, Gershenson DM, Malone JM Jr, Edwards CL. Recurrent cervical carcinoma after radical hysterectomy. Gynecol Oncol 1988;30:381.

Larson JE, Whitney CW, Zaino R, Kaminski P, Podczaski E, Mortel R. Endometrial response to endogenous hormones after pelvic irradiation for genital malignancies. Gynecol Oncol 1990;36:106.

Layfield LJ, Heaps JM, Berek JS. Fine-needle aspiration cytology accuracy with palpable gynecologic neoplasms. Gynecol Oncol 1991;40:70.

Lee HP, Cuello C, Singh K. Review of the epidemiology of cervical cancer in the Pacific basin. Natl Cancer Inst Monograph 1982;62:197.

Lehtovirta P, Turpeinen U, Stenman U-H. Effect of intracavitary radiotherapy on tumor-associated trypsin inhibitor (TATI) in patients with cervical and endometrial cancer. Gynecol Oncol 1990;38:110.

Leminen A. Tumor markers CA 125, carcinoembryonic antigen and tumor associated trypsin inhibitor in patients with cervical adenocarcinoma. Gynecol Oncol 1990; 39:358.

Leminen A, Alftan H, Stenman UH, Lehtovirta P. Chemotherapy as initial treatment for cervical carcinoma: clinical and tumor marker response. Acta Obstet Gynecol Scand 1992;71:293.

Look KY, Rocereto TF. Relapse patterns in FIGO stage IB carcinoma of the cervix. Gynecol Oncol 1990;38:114.

Lovecchio JL, Gal D. Diagnostic techniques in gynecologic oncology. In Hoskins WJ, Perez CA, Young RC, eds. Principles and practice of gynecologic oncology. Philadelphia: JB Lippincott, 1992:431.

Maiman M, Geuer G, Fruchter RG, Shaw N, Boyce J. Value of squamous cell carcinoma antigen levels in invasive cervical carcinoma. Gynecol Oncol 1989;34:312.

Mann WJ, Hatch KD, Taylor PT, Partridge EE, Orr JW Jr, Shingleton HM. The role of percutaneous nephrostomy in gynecologic oncology. Gynecol Oncol 1983;16:393.

Mann WJ, Vogel F, Patsner B, Chalas E. Management of lymphocysts after radical gynecologic surgery. Gynecol Oncol 1989;33:248.

Martins A, Sternberg SS, Attiveh FF. Radiation-induced carcinoma of the rectum. Dis Colon Rectum 1980;23:572.

McKay MJ, Bull CA, Houghton CR, Langlands AO. Letter to the editor. Gyncol Oncol 1990;39:296.

Meier W, Eiermann W, Stieber P, Fateh-Moghadam A, Schneider A, Hepp H. Squamous cell carcinoma antigen and carcinoembryonic antigen levels as prognostic factors for the response of cervical carcinoma to chemotherapy. Gynecol Oncol 1990;38:6.

Meyer JE. Radiography of the distal colon and rectum after irradiation of carcinoma of the cervix. Am J Radiol 1981;136:691.

Montana GS, Fowler WC, Varia MA, et al. Carcinoma of the cervix stage IB: results of treatment with radiation therapy. Int J Radiol Oncol Biol Phys 1983;9:45.

Montana GS, Fowler WC, Varia MA, et al. Analysis of results of radiation therapy for stage II carcinoma of the cervix. Cancer 1985;55:956.

Montana GS, Fowler WC, Varia MA, et al. Carcinoma of the cervix stage III. Cancer 1986;57:148.

Muram D, Curry RH, Drouin P. Cytologic follow-up of patients with invasive cervical carcinoma treated by radiotherapy. Am J Obstet Gynecol 1982;142:350.

Nam JH, Chang K-C, Chambers JT, Schwartz PE, Cole LA. Urinary gonadotropin fragment, a new tumor marker. III. Use in cervical and vulvar cancers. Gynecol Oncol 1990;38:68.

Neunteufel W, Tatra G, Bieglmayer C. Serum squamous cell carcinomaantigen levels in women with neoplasms of the lower genital tract and in healthy controls. Arch Gynecol Obstet 1989;246:243.

Ng HT, Shyu SK, Chen YK, Yuan CC, Chao KC, Kan YY. A scoring system in predicting recurrence of cervical cancer. Int J Gynecol Cancer 1992;2:75.

Ngan HY, Wong LC, Chan SY, Ma HK. Use of serum squamous cell carcinoma antigen assays in chemotherapy treatment of cervical cancer. Gynecol Oncol 1989;35:259.

Patten SF Jr, Reagan JW, Obenauf M, Ballard LA. Postirradiation dysplasia of uterine cervix and vagina: an analytical study of the cells. Cancer 1963;18:173.

Patsner B, Orr JW Jr, Allman T. Does preoperative serum squamous cell carcinoma antigen level predict occult extracervical disease in patients with stage IB invasive squamous cell carcinoma of the cervix? Obstet Gynecol 1989;74:786.

Perez CA, Breaux S, Madoc-Jones H, et al. Radiation therapy alone in the treatment of carcinoma of the uterine cervix. I. Analysis of tumor recurrence. Cancer 1983;52:1393.

Pfeiffer D, Stellwag B, Pfeiffer A, Borlinghaus P, Meier W, Scheidel P. Clinical implications of the epidermal growth factor receptor in the squamous cell carcinoma of the uterine cervix. Gynecol Oncol 1989;33:146.

Photopulos GJ, Shirley REL Jr, Ansbacher R. Evaluation of conventional diagnostic tests for detection of recurrent carcinoma of the cervix. Am J Obstet Gynecol 1977;129:533.

Potter ME, Alvarez RD, Gay FL, Shingleton HM, Soong S-J, Hatch KD. Optimal pelvic recurrence after radical hysterectomy for early-stage cervical cancer. Gynecol Oncol 1990;36:74.

Rayburn WF, van Nagell JR Jr. Cervicovaginal cytology in the diagnosis of recurrent carcinoma of the cervix uteri. Surg Gynecol Obstet 1980;151:15.

Scambia G, Panici PB, Baiocchi G, et al. The value of squamous cell carcinoma antigen in patients with locally advanced cervical cancer undergoing neoadjuvant chemotherapy. Am J Obstet Gynecol 1991;164:631.

Schwartz PE, Chambers SK, Chambers JT, Gutmann J, Katopodis N, Foemmel R. Circulating tumor markers in the monitoring of gynecologic malignancies. Cancer 1987;60:353.

Selim MA, Beck D. Parametrial needle biopsy: follow-up of pelvic malignancies. Cancer Detect Prev 1984;7:269.

Senekjian EK, Young JM, Weiser PA, Spencer CE, Magic SE, Herbst AL. An evaluation of squamous cell carcinoma antigen in patients with cervical squamous cell carcinoma. Am J Obstet Gynecol 1987;157:433.

Sevin B-U, Greening SE, Nadjii M, et al. Fine needle aspiration cytology in gynecologic oncology. I. Clinical aspects. Acta Cytol 1979;23:277.

Shepherd JH, Cavanagh D, Ruffolo E, Praphat H. The value of needle biopsy in the diagnosis of gynecologic cancer. Gynecol Oncol 1981;11:309.

Shingleton HM, Gore H, Soong S-J, et al. Tumor recurrence and survival in stage IB cancer of the cervix. Am J Clin Oncol 1983;6:265.

Shingleton HM, Soong S-J, Gelder MS, Hatch KD, Baker VV, Austin JM Jr. Clinical and histopathologic factors predicting recurrence and survival after pelvic exenteration for cancer of the cervix. Obstet Gynecol 1989;73:1027.

Sparks JM, Waldrop EC. Outpatient surveillance. In Shingleton HM, Hurt WG, eds. Postreporductive gynecology. New York: Churchill Livingstone, 1990;133.

Stehman FB, Bundy BN, DiSaia PJ, Keys HM, Larson JE, Fowler WC. Carcinoma of the cervix treated with radiation therapy. Cancer 1991;67:2776.

Tamimi HK, Gown AM, Kim-Deobold J, Figge DC, Greer BE, Cain JM. The utility of immunocytochemistry in invasive adenocarcinoma of the cervix. Am J Obstet Gynecol 1992;166:1655.

te Velde ER, Persijn JP, Ballieux RE, et al. Carcinoembryonic antigen serum levels in patients with squamous cell carcinoma of the uterine cervix: clinical significance. Cancer 1982;49:1866.

Tomas C, Risteli J, Risteli L, Vuori J, Kauppila A. Use of various epithelial tumor markers and a stromal marker in the assessment of cervical carcinoma. Obstet Gynecol 1991;77:566.

Tsukamoto N, Kinoshita H, Saito T, Tsuruchi N, Kaku T, Kamura T. Surgery for radiation enteritis in gynecologic cancer patients (abstract). Fourth Annual Meeting, International Gynecologic Cancer Society, Stockholm, Sweden, September 1993. Int J Gynecol Cancer 1993;3:48.

van Nagell JR Jr, Rayburn W, Donaldson ES, et al. Therapeutic implications of patterns of recurrence in cancer of the uterine cervix. Cancer 1979;44:2354.

Verlooy H, Devos P, Janssens J, et al. Clinical significance of squamous cell carcinoma antigen in cancer of the human uterine cervix. Comparison with CEA and CA-125. Gynecol Obstet Invest 1991;32:55.

Wang CC. Principles of radiotherapy. In Gusberg SB, Shingleton HM, Deppe G, eds. Female genital cancer. New York: Churchill Livingstone, 1988:101.

Webb MJ, Symmonds RE. Site of recurrence of cervical cancer after radical hysterectomy. Am J Obstet Gynecol 1980;138:813.

Weiner S, Wizenberg MJ. Treatment of primary adenocarcinoma of the cervix. Cancer 1975;35:1514.

Wentz WB, Reagan JW. Clinical significance of postirradiation dysplasia of the uterine cervix. Am J Obstet Gynecol 1970;106:812.

Yazigi R, Munoz AK, Richardson B, Risser R. Correlation of squamous cell carcinoma antigen levels and treatment response in cervical cancer. Gynecol Oncol 1991;41:135.

Cancer of the Cervix by Hugh M. Shingleton and James W. Orr, Jr.
J. B. Lippincott Company, Philadelphia, © 1995.

12

Recurrent Cancer: Exenterative Surgery

Early detection, modern radiation therapy techniques, and primary surgical treatment have resulted in high initial cure rates for women who have invasive cervical cancer. Despite these gratifying results, physicians treating women who have cervical cancer are frequently required to manage problems associated with persistent or recurrent disease.

Viable cancer documented within the first 6 months after therapy is often termed persistent cancer, whereas that diagnosed later is usually referred to as recurrent disease. Most gynecologic oncologists hesitate to offer additional therapy during the first 3 months after primary irradiation because tumoricidal effects of such therapy may continue for some time. A diagnosis of persistent cervical cancer should be considered if examination during or immediately after radiation therapy indicates either tumor growth or lack of tumor regression.

Persistent tumor may thus be classified as the absence of a complete clinical remission or when progressive disease is documented during or immediately after therapy, whereas recurrent cancers are those that become evident after a period of complete clinical or biochemical (tumor marker) remission. Women previously treated with radical surgery should probably be considered to have persistent disease when surgical margins are involved or when significant extrapelvic disease is detected during the operation.

DIAGNOSIS

Detecting posttreatment recurrence can be problematic. The pelvic fibrosis that is associated with radiation therapy renders the information obtained during pelvic examination less specific, even for the most experienced examiner. The problem of diagnosing a recurrence by palpation alone was exemplified by Kottmeier (1954), who reported 80 patients without a histologic diagnosis of recurrent tumor but "obvious recurrent tumor on bimanual examination"; many of these patients actually survived 15 years or more without progression. Lawhead and coworkers (1989) reported 65 patients who underwent exenteration; 3 patients (5%) had no residual carcinoma in the operative specimen despite a strong clinical impression of recurrence. Although a laparotomy may be required to confirm the diagnosis of recurrence, any form of treatment without a histologic diagnosis of recurrent cancer is unacceptable.

Disease-free interval depends on multiple factors, including the adequacy of initial treatment, tumor susceptibility, host resistance, original clinical stage, and tumor volume. More than 80% of recurrences are discovered within 2 years of initial therapy (Sommers et al 1989). Early-stage or low-volume tumors tend to recur later than those tumors that were initially of advanced stage or high volume.

Whether an early diagnosis of recurrence after irradiation increases or decreases the rate of curability has not been substantiated. Roddick and Miller (1968) reported that early diagnosis led to an increased rate of resectability; however, they failed to note an increased cure rate. Brunschwig (1967) reported an increased survival in those patients who were treated with exenterative surgery having a late recurrence (more than 6 months). Creasman and Rutledge (1972) reported increased resectability and increased 2-year survival rates, presumably based on the biologic activity of the tumor, in patients who had recurrence 2 or more years after the first treatment. Shingleton and associates (1989), reviewing a 16-year experience, reported improved survival in those patients having a disease-free interval of at least 1 year. Deckers and colleagues (1972), however, reported no survival advantage in patients undergoing exenterative surgery for late (more than 5-year disease-free interval) recurrent cervical cancer.

CHOICE OF TREATMENT

The extent and site of recurrent or persistent disease dictates the method of therapy. Patients who were initially treated with an inadequate surgical procedure (total hysterectomy) are at increased risk for pelvic recurrence. In this situation, adjunctive treatment with radiation therapy results in excellent central pelvic control.

Sommers and associates (1989) reported a retrospective analysis of 1054 patients, detailing the clinical outcome of 376 patients having recurrent disease after definitive radiation therapy. Pelvic failure alone occurred in 0.8% of patients having stage IB, in 1.7% of those having stage IIA, in 10.4% of those having stage IIB, in 15.4% of those having stage III, and in 16.7% of those having stage IV cancers. The actuarial probability of pelvic failure 5 years from initial therapy was 8% with stage I disease, 16% with stage IIA, 22% with stage IIB, 42% with stage III, and 100% for those with stage IV cervical cancer after irradiation. Sommers and colleagues reported no major difference in survival after recurrence by histologic type, initial treatment, or initial stage. The overall survival at 5 years for all untreated patients was 1%. Patients who develop disease more than 36 months after initial treatment had a median survival of 22.5 months. For those failing less than 6 months, 6 to 12 months, 13 to 24 months, and 25 to 36 months, the median survival was 12.1, 7.6, 9.4, and 9.1 months, respectively.

The incidence of distant metastases in those who experienced recurrence after irradiation may be increased when compared with those patients initially treated surgically (Paunier et al 1967, Badib et al 1968). For example, Prempree and coworkers (1983) noted a significant increase in recurrences at distant sites in young irradiation-treated women, aged 20 to 29, having stage IB disease (26% versus 5% of controls) and stage II disease (42% versus 16% of controls), with both of these differences being highly significant (p <.001). Regardless, the diagnosis of recurrent cervical cancer requires an evaluation of local, regional, and distal spread.

Most patients who have advanced and some who have early-stage disease have received radiation therapy as primary treatment, whereas others have received irradiation for treatment of a surgical recurrence. Potter and associates (1990) evaluated 48 patients having pelvic recurrence after radical hysterectomy. No patient who was treated with adjuvant irradiation after initial surgery was rendered disease-free by subsequent treatment with radiation therapy. Eleven patients initially underwent exploration for exenterative therapy; in 6 patients, exenteration was technically feasible. Three of these 6 patients remain alive without evidence of disease.

There is no curative chemotherapeutic agent or regimen for the treatment of cervical cancer; therefore, when a cure is the goal, a postirradiation recurrence usually requires a radical or ultraradical surgical approach. Most reports concerning exenterative surgery originate from the United States. When compared with salvage operations in patients having other types of cancer, pelvic exenteration ranks favorably because in most situations, long-term survival is significant, with high expectations for rehabilitation. If the disease is not amenable to surgery, the ultimate prognosis is poor. Brunschwig (1967) reported only a 3.5% 5-year survival rate when recurrent cancer is not treated. Haas and colleagues (1980) indicated that 41% of patients with unresectable cancer succumb to their cancer within 6 months and only 25% survive longer than 1 year. Ninety-five percent of patients expire within 2 years. Morley and coworkers (1989) confirmed these findings when they reported a 13% 1-year survival in patients having unresectable recurrent disease.

Operative Approaches

Total hysterectomy is inadequate therapy for patients who have a centrally recurrent cervical cancer. After therapeutic doses of megavoltage radiation therapy, this procedure carries a high risk of urinary complications and offers the least chance for cure or palliation.

A select group of patients (perhaps 15%) having a small-volume central pelvic recurrence may be successfully treated with radical hysterectomy. In selected series, 5-year survival approaches 30% to 50% (Creasman et al 1974, Jones 1987); however, the inability to accurately assess tumor volume may be associated with failure in situations in which a more radical procedure may have resulted in cure. Additionally, radical hysterectomy after tolerance doses of megavoltage radiation therapy is associated with a high rate (20% to 50%) of stricture, urinary fistulas, or other serious complications (Mattingly 1967, Bjornstahl et al 1977, Adcock 1979, Terada et al 1987).

Rubin and coworkers (1987) evaluated the role of radical hysterectomy for treatment of recurrent cervical cancer after radiation therapy. In their series of 21 patients with recurrent disease, all 11 patients having lesions of less than 2 cm were cured. Recurrence rates were 70% (7 of 10 patients) when tumor size exceeded 2 cm, however. The morbidity after radical hysterectomy in this series was significant because 10 patients (50%) developed postoperative fistulas; 9 required a urinary diversion.

Coleman and associates (1994) reported 50 patients treated with radical hysterectomy for persistent or recurrent disease. Tumor size and intravenous pyelogram (IVP) status were significant predictors of survival. Patients with tumors less than 2 cm and a normal IVP had a survival rate of 90%. Severe postoperative complications occurred in 42% of patients, however. The most common site was the urinary tract, with ureteral injuries (22%) and long-term bladder dysfunction (20%) being common. Vesicovaginal or rectovaginal fistulas occurred in 28% of patients.

Reports from the Mayo Clinic (Symmonds et al 1975) and Webb and Symmonds (1979) indicate that extended radical hysterectomy, although seeming to provide adequate treatment in central recurrence in irradiated patients, was associated with extremely high complication and failure rates and is not considered to have a place in the treatment of recurrence.

Pelvic Exenteration

Surgical techniques designed to decrease complications, including less extensive ureteral dissection, may compromise surgical margins. Because this treatment represents the last chance for cure, American gynecologic oncologists generally believe that pelvic exenteration is the surgical treatment of choice in most patients having centrally recurrent cervical cancer after radiation therapy. The magnitude and associated risks of this operative procedure should prohibit its use in institutions lacking the availability of critical care facilities or trained physicians who cannot only execute the procedure but recognize and manage potential complications. Unfortunately, the incidence of isolated central pelvic recurrence has decreased and the number of exenterative procedures performed in this country and abroad has decreased dramatically, making it difficult for surgeons to obtain or maintain their procedure-specific skills. Reports from Memorial Sloan Kettering confirm this problem: 53 exenterations were performed yearly between 1947 and 1960 (Jones 1993); only seven exenterations were performed yearly during the next decade. Other major centers perform fewer than 12 exenterations per year for recurrent cervical cancer.

Exenterative procedures (Figs. 12-1 through 12-3) may be partial (conservation of bladder or rectum) or total. Controversy exists regarding the advisability of partial exenterative procedures and early reports (Ingersoll et al 1966), indicating poor survival with partial exenteration, continue to be quoted. We

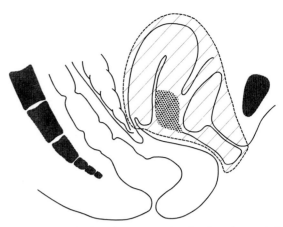

FIGURE 12-1. Anterior exenteration involves the surgical removal of the bladder, uterus, and cervix and is considered in patients with a deep cul-de-sac. It is imperative that frozen sections be obtained at the time of exploration. If tumor is present in the posterior vaginal margin, total exenteration is the preferred operation.

have demonstrated that partial exenteration can be performed successfully, with excellent survival and comparably less surgical morbidity or mortality (Table 12-1). As with radical hysterectomy, the intraoperative problem of determining the adequacy of the surgical margins with partial exenteration remains a paramount concern. Because few patients who have a positive exenteration surgical margin survive (Averette et al 1984), it is not justifiable to perform a partial exenteration unless adequate margins can be guaranteed. Patients with clear, lateral pelvic surgical margins have a significantly improved survival, compared with those whose margins are involved; after anterior exentera-

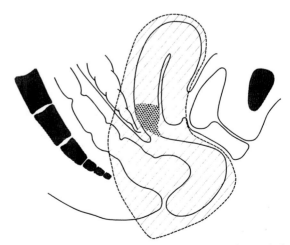

FIGURE 12-2. Posterior exenteration involves the surgical removal of the rectum, uterus, and cervix. After radiation therapy, urinary complications are high.

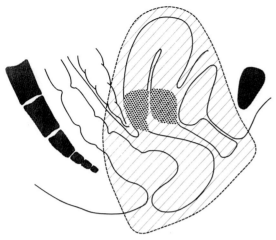

FIGURE 12-3. Total exenteration involves the removal of the bladder, urethra, cervix, uterus, vagina, and rectum. The anal canal may be preserved in some women, allowing reanastomosis of the sigmoid colon.

reduces the chances of a 5-year survival significantly (78% versus 29% [p <.001]; Shingleton et al 1989).

Hatch (1988b) focused on the problem of margins in his series of 69 patients undergoing anterior pelvic exenteration. Recurrent cancer was subsequently diagnosed in 30 of these women. The 20 patients who had pelvic recurrence were evaluated to determine whether inadequate resection could be implicated as cause of exenteration failure. Eight patients had recurrence at the pelvic floor. Of these, 2 patients had disease into the posterior margin on permanent section that was not detected on frozen section.

Given these facts, we believe that an anterior exenterative procedure may benefit those patients having small-volume central pelvic recurrence, minimal anterior vaginal or lateral pelvic extension, and a deep cul-de-sac (see Fig. 12-1). Significant vaginal extension (beyond the upper third) and posterolateral vaginal extension increases the likelihood of involvement of the margin at the rectovaginal septum, either directly or by paravaginal lymphatic extension. If extensive vaginal or parametrial involvement is present, we select total exenteration as treatment.

The proximity of the irradiated uterine cervix and the pelvic ureters and bladder increases the risk of urologic fistulas after posterior exenteration. Prolonged postoperative bladder dysfunction is common. When coupled with the impossibility of obtaining a wide anterior surgical margin (between the cervix and the

tion, this difference is 63% versus 0%; after total exenteration, the difference is 49% versus 10% (Shingleton et al 1989). The surgeon should remember that despite normal-appearing bladder or rectal mucosa, occult invasion of the submucosa of these organs may be found in some patients undergoing exenteration. Bladder invasion in an anterior exenteration specimen

TABLE 12-1
Survival and Mortality Related to the Type of Exenteration in Patients With Recurrent Cervical Cancer

STUDY	YEAR	ANTERIOR EXENTERATION			TOTAL EXENTERATION		
		Patients (n)	Surgical Mortality (%)	5-Year Survival (%)	Patients (n)	Surgical Mortality (%)	5-Year Survival (%)
Ingersoll, et al	1966	18	—	11.1	53	—	26.4
Brunschwig	1967	95	10.5	18.9	217	20.3	17.1
Ingiulla & Cosmi	1967	32	25.0	21.9	51	49.0	5.9
Ketcham, et al	1970	9	—	44.0	81	—	25.0
Creasman & Rutledge	1974	27*	—	33.3	59	—	20.3
Symmonds et al[†]	1975	59	—	42.0	36	—	41.0
Cuevas[‡]	1988	132	12.9	—	120	21.7	—
Morley[†]	1989	—	—	—	47	—	74.0
Shingleton	1989	63	1.6	63.0	78	10.3	42.0

*Partial exenteration
[†]SCC only
[‡]49.6% survival at three years

From Orr JW Jr, Shingleton HM, Hatch KD, et al. Urinary diversion in patients undergoing pelvic exenteration. Am J Obstet Gynecol 1982;142:883; Shingleton HM, Soong J-W, Gelder MS, Hatch KD, Baker VV, Austin JM Jr. Clinical and histopathologic factors predicting recurrence and survival after pelvic exenteration for cancer of the cervix. Obstet Gynecol 1989;73:1027.

bladder), this procedure should not be selected for the treatment of recurrent cervical cancer.

Total exenteration is the most commonly used surgical procedure for patients who have central recurrence.

The categorization of partial and total exenteration has been used historically to describe the extent of dissection. Magrina (1990), however, proposed an additional subgrouping of pelvic exenterations into supralevator and infralevator types, with or without vulvectomy. The practical importance of this subgrouping remains to be determined but it may find a more important role in the future as gastrointestinal reconstruction gains more widespread use.

Patients with tumor involving the lower third of the vagina may require an additional perineal resection, including a radical vulvectomy and groin dissection. Although this latter procedure may lead to an occasional cure, it is also associated with prolonged operative time, additional blood loss, and increased risk of postoperative morbidity (Cuevas et al 1988).

TUMOR VOLUME AND CURABILITY

Shingleton and colleagues (1989) performed univariate and multivariate analysis in an attempt to identify clinical and histopathologic factors predictive of prolonged postexenteration survival. Using three clinical factors (duration from initial radiation therapy to exenteration, size of central mass, and presence of preoperative side wall fixation), low-, intermediate-, and high-risk groups for recurrence were determined. The 5-year survival rates for these groups were 82%, 46%, and 0%, respectively. Inclusion of one histologic factor (margin status of the surgical specimen) added to the ability to predict 2- and 5-year survival rates. The best candidates for cure by pelvic exenteration were those having a small (less than 3 cm) mobile central tumor mass, operated a year or longer from previous primary radiation therapy.

When comparing preexenteration tumor volume, Stanhope and associates (1990) reported that the 2-year survival rate of patients having volume greater than 5 cm^3 was 56.4%, and the 5-year survival was 34.6%. In those patients with a tumor volume of less than 5 cm^3, the 2-year survival rate was 91.6% and the 5-year survival rate was 83.3%. Regardless of these risk factors, sound clinical and operative judgment is imperative when selecting the treatment that offers the best quality of life.

HISTOLOGIC SUBTYPES AND CURABILITY

Few authors have reported the effect of histologic subtype on survival. Morley and associates (1989) reported 57 patients having squamous cell carcinoma of the cervix, with a cumulative 5-year survival of 73% compared with 22% survival in patients having adenocarcinoma of the cervix. Rutledge and colleagues (1987) reported an increased risk of node metastasis in patients with adenocarcinoma (20%) when compared with those having squamous cell cancer (8.9%). There is no other effective treatment alternative for recurrent cervical adenocarcinoma.

Senekjian and coworkers (1989) reported the results of 29 pelvic exenterations performed in patients having clear cell adenocarcinoma of the vagina and cervix. The 5- and 8-year actual survival rates after exenteration (100% and 60%) were superb, and the author concluded that survival statistics after exenteration for central failure in clear cell adenocarcinoma were more favorable when compared with cases of cervical squamous cell carcinoma.

PREOPERATIVE CONSIDERATIONS

The magnitude of exenterative surgery mandates a thorough preoperative psychologic and physiologic evaluation. Surgical mortality increases with age (Table 12-2). The usual patient undergoing exenteration is in her sixth decade. Older patients are prone to have other medical conditions predisposing them to serious complications (Pierson et al 1975, Evers et al 1994, Orr et al 1994). Cardiac disease is frequent and a common cause of postoperative mortality. Additionally, older patients are more likely to have obstructive pulmonary disease, decreased renal function, increased sensitivity to temperature extremes, and altered immunologic response (Harbrecht et al 1981, Evers et al 1994).

Matthews and associates (1992) reported the effect of advanced age on the outcome of 65 patients (aged 65 years or older) undergoing pelvic exenteration between 1960 and 1991 at the M.D. Anderson Hospital. Sixty-three percent of patients had existing medical illnesses. Major or potentially life-threatening complications occurred in 38% of patients and an additional 38% experienced minor complications. Sixty percent experienced one or more infectious complications, and operative mortality was 11%, caused mostly by multisystem organ failure. The 5-year survival rate in this group of patients was 46%, however. Matthews

TABLE 12-2
Pelvic Exenteration Age-Related Operative Mortality

AGE GROUP	PATIENTS (N)	PERCENTAGE OF AGE GROUP	CUMULATIVE PERCENTAGE
< 40 years	31	0	0
41–50 years	42	4.8	2.7
51–60 years	50	10.0	5.7
> 60 years	41	12.2	7.3

From Shingleton HM, Orr JW. Cancer of the cervix: diagnosis and treatment. New York, Churchill Livingstone, 1987:227.

and coworkers indicated that age should not be considered to be a contraindication for exenteration. Although we agree that age itself is not an absolute contraindication, this procedure should rarely be considered in those patients who are older than 75 years of age.

Medical illness such as diabetes, hypertension, vascular disease, or pulmonary disease should be carefully evaluated preoperatively. Only when it appears certain that the medical disease significantly jeopardizes the patient's chances of survival should the patient not be considered a surgical candidate.

A history of recent weight loss should prompt careful evaluation for metastatic disease. Weight loss in the absence of metastatic disease is not considered to be a contraindication, but malnourished patients are subject to increased operative complications related to poor wound healing or infection and may benefit from preoperative nutritional support (Orr et al 1984a).

Obesity renders the exenterative procedure technically more difficult; however, obesity is not an absolute contraindication to an ultraradical surgical procedure. Surgical procedures in obese patients are longer and are associated with increased blood loss (Morrow et al 1977). Additionally, anesthesia in obese individuals is associated with marked cardiac dysfunction and increases the risk of postoperative pulmonary dysfunction (Orr et al 1994). Both factors may increase the risk of surgical mortality (Barber 1969). The surgeon and support staff must be aware of these risks and be willing and able to manage the specific intraoperative and postoperative complications that are associated with obesity.

An important aspect of preoperative assessment is the ability of the patient and her family to withstand the psychologic stress of the operative procedure and prolonged (3- to 4-month) recovery period. The importance of preoperative counseling of both the patient and her family cannot be overemphasized (Youngs et al 1976). Rutledge (1982), stating that the patient's emotional adequacy is an important factor to consider, included a psychosocial evaluation as an elective preoperative assessment of patients undergoing exenteration. An emotional or psychiatric disorder that significantly interferes with the patient's ability to manage her ostomy (Jones et al 1980) or contribute to her rehabilitation is a strong relative contraindication to exenterative surgery.

Because of the impact of extrapelvic disease on prognosis, each candidate should undergo extensive preoperative evaluation before exploration (Table 12-3). Historically, the combination of sciatic pain and leg edema, especially unilateral, usually contraindicates a surgical approach because few patients with these problems have a resectable tumor, and resection yields few 5-year survivors. A chest radiograph not only assists in establishing the presence or absence of pulmonary metastasis but aids in the preoperative diagnosis of coexisting pulmonary disease and serves as a baseline for postoperative surveillance. Additionally, patients who are treated for cervical cancer are reported to be at increased risk for later primary lung tumors (Clarke et al 1984, Kleinerman et al 1982, Lee et al 1982). In many situations, chest computed tomography (CT) scanning should be considered during preoperative evaluation.

Evaluation of the urinary tract is important because of its proximity to the cervix. The probability of tumor resection is directly related to the degree of abnormality on the IVP. As many as 60% of patients having unilateral obstruction and 90% of those having bilateral ureteral obstruction have unresectable tumors. Additionally, those patients with resectable tumors and abnormal pyelograms apparently have a poorer long-term prognosis when compared with those patients undergoing exenteration who have normal intravenous pyelography. Although each patient's situation must be considered individually, obstructive uropathy is a relative contraindication to exenterative surgery. The usual cause of postradiation treatment obstructive uropathy is recurrent cancer (Hatch et al 1984a); however, the burden is on the physician to prove that the obstruction is secondary to tumor and not to irradiation fibrosis or other benign causes. If an exentera-

TABLE 12-3
Preoperative Contraindication of Exenteration
in Patients With Recurrent Cervical Cancer

ABSOLUTE

Extrapelvic disease

Triad of unilateral leg edema, sciatica, and ureteral obstruction

Tumor-related pelvic side wall fixation

Bilateral ureteral obstruction (if secondary to recurrence)

Severe life-limiting medical illness

Psychosis or the inability of the patient to care for herself

Religious or other beliefs that prohibit the patient from accepting transfusion

Inability of physician or consultants to manage any or all intraoperative and postoperative complications

Inadequate hospital facilities

RELATIVE

Age older than 75

Large tumor volume (>4 cm)

Unilateral ureteral obstruction

Metastasis to the distal vagina

Adapted from Shingleton HM, Orr JW. Cancer of the cervix: diagnosis and treatment. New York, Churchill Livingstone, 1987:232.

tive procedure is planned in a patient who has high-grade unilateral ureteral obstruction, a preoperative assessment of residual function of the obstructed kidney becomes important. Because renal function may return after prolonged (months) obstruction, a short period of preoperative drainage by percutaneous nephrostomy may allow a better determination of function of an obstructed kidney. This is important information because incorporating a nonfunctioning kidney into a urinary conduit predisposes the patient to chronic infectious complications. In this situation, consideration should be given to alternatives such as nephrectomy or even permanent ureteral ligation (Magrina et al 1979).

Bladder involvement does not contraindicate a surgical approach; however, Kiselow and coworkers' (1967) and Shingleton's (1989) reports relate its prognostic significance. Although not controlled for tumor volume, Kiselow and colleagues' finding of a statistically significant decrease in survival in patients with bladder involvement (32.2%), when compared with those without (54.4%), suggests the prognostic importance of cystoscopic examination of the lower urinary tract during the preoperative evaluation, despite the fact that few exenterative procedures include bladder conservation.

Kiselow and associates (1967) also suggested that tumor invading the rectum or colon adversely affects

prognosis. Its presence was associated with a decrease in survival from 50.6% to 25.7%. Irradiation changes may make a proctoscopic examination difficult, and the finding of intact rectal mucosa does not necessarily allow the surgeon to plan rectal conservation because as many as 61% of patients may have occult tumor involvement of the muscularis of the rectum. Theoretically, patients with recurrent tumor involving the vagina may have direct extension or paravaginal lymphatic submucosal involvement of the rectum of rectovaginal septum.

Barium studies of the colon, colonoscopy, and mammograms are usually performed to establish the presence of coexisting disease, benign or malignant. Although the incidence of synchronous malignancy is small (Axelrod et al 1984), an exenterative procedure is not likely to be considered in the presence of another primary malignancy.

Although liver metastases in patients having recurrent cancer of the uterine cervix are unusual, their presence indicates disseminated disease and contraindicates a surgical approach. Serum liver function studies serve as a screen for hepatic metastases; however, CT scanning or liver ultrasonography may also be beneficial in detecting abnormalities. Any abnormality requires investigation by percutaneous or intraoperative aspiration before exenteration.

The spine is the most common site of bone metastases (Blythe et al 1975) and the previously mentioned radiographic studies are usually adequate to determine the presence or absence of metastases. Matsuyama and colleagues (1989) reported that 48 of 713 (6.7%) patients followed-up for treatment of cancer of the uterine cervix had or developed bone metastasis. This risk was clinical-stage–related and varied from 4% in stage I to 22% in stage IV disease. The most frequent site of metastasis was the vertebral column, particularly the lumbar spine (48%). Nearly two thirds of the bone lesions were detected within 1 year after completion of initial treatment and the 1-year survival rate was 7% after detection of metastasis.

Although radiation therapy is capable of sterilizing 50% of node disease (Lagasse et al 1974, Rutledge et al 1965), the possibility of lymphatic metastases (either within or outside the original treatment field) should be investigated in patients having apparent central pelvic recurrence. The most commonly involved nodes outside the primary treatment field are those in the paraaortic area. Supraclavicular and inguinal nodes may be involved later. They are more accessible to examination and biopsy, however. The latter may represent metastatic lymphatic spread by the vulvar lymphatics from disease in the lower vagina or retrograde metastasis from obstructed pelvic nodes. Diagnostic methods used in screening for intraabdominal node metastasis include CT scanning, ultrasonography, lymphangiography, and magnetic resonance imaging (MRI; Fig. 12-4).

Because of the detrimental influence of node metastasis on prognosis and because these tests are associated with little morbidity, at least one of these studies should be performed before laparotomy. The individual test is only reliable when strict criteria are used to determine the node status. Additionally, the variability in the reported false-negative and false-positive rates of these diagnostic tests suggests that the results correlate with the experience of the individual who interprets them. Because the experience may differ between institutions, it is important that physicians know which test may be most appropriate at their institution.

Ultrasonography is reputed to detect enlarged (more than 3 cm) pelvic nodes and paraaortic nodes (more than 2 cm; Brascho 1980), whereas CT may detect 1-cm nodes in both the pelvic and paraaortic space (Chen et al 1980). The resolution of the CT scanning may help identify lateral tumor extension and aid in determining resectability, including partial levator resection (Fig. 12-5); however, one must be careful in interpreting these results not to confuse fibrosis with tumor extension. Ultrasonography, CT, and MRI scans are relatively new techniques, compared with lymphangiography. Although there is a larger reported experience with CT, it should be noted that lymphangiograms are more invasive, more difficult to perform, and subject to occasional complications, such as lipoid pneumonia. Because of the lack of universal criteria, the precise incidence of false-positive results with lymphangiograms is difficult to establish (see Table 4-7 in Chap. 4); however, reports adhering to specific criteria

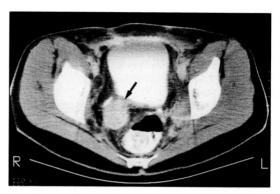

FIGURE 12-5. Recurrent mass (*arrow*) 3 months postoperatively in a 29-year-old woman with a 4-cm squamous cell tumor. Surgical margins and pelvic nodes had been negative for tumor. Needle aspirate documented recurrent cancer, which extended to the pelvic side wall.

such as node filling defects, deviation around a mass, or complete lymphatic obstruction usually result in false-positive rates greater than 15%. Importantly, Piver and Barlow (1973) reported that previous radiation therapy apparently has little effect in altering the criteria for or lymphangiographic image of metastasis or negative nodes.

Popovich and coworkers (1993) evaluated the role of MRI in determining surgical eligibility for pelvic exenteration. The accuracy of MRI in selecting patients was 83% (19 of 23), with a positive predictive value of 56% and a negative predictive value of 100%. When evaluating tumor involvement of the pelvic side wall and lymph nodes, the negative predictive values were 100% and 95%, respectively. Tumor extension to the pelvic side wall was overestimated in 4 patients, 3 of whom in which it was not possible to distinguish irradiation change from tumor on MRI. For assessing extension of these pelvic tumors in the bladder and rectum, MRI had an accuracy of 81% and 85%, respectively. It was their conclusion that irradiation changes could not be reliably distinguished from tumor involvement in patients having side wall abnormalities, especially in the first 6 to 12 months after treatment.

Regardless of the method used to evaluate the node areas, any enlarged or suspected metastasis requires histologic or cytologic confirmation before denying a surgical procedure. This may be obtained reliably by fine-needle aspiration (Tao et al 1980). When fine-needle aspiration is negative or nondiagnostic, however, exploration may still be warranted if no other contraindications exist.

Some authors perform scalene lymph node biopsies as part of their preoperative evaluation. A survey of the literature indicates that about 16% of patients with recurrence and periaortic node metastases may have subclinical metastatic disease in the scalene nodes

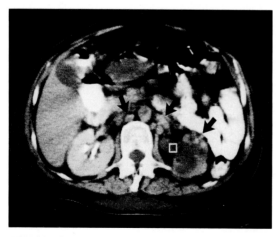

FIGURE 12-4. Computed tomography scan of a woman with recurrent squamous cell carcinoma, indicating high-grade left ureteral obstruction (*arrow*) and retroperitoneal lymphadenopathy (*arrow*).

(Table 12-4). Manetta and associates (1989), however, reported 24 patients having recurrent carcinoma of the cervix who underwent scalene node biopsy before exploration for exenteration. None had scalene node involvement. Although the procedure may be performed under local anesthesia, it should only be performed by those knowledgeable of the surgical anatomy who are willing to accept the possible complications of pneumothorax and vascular or lymphatic injury in the neck. The high sensitivity and specificity of ultrasound-guided fine-needle aspiration in the assessment of neck and node enlargement allows this modality to play an important preoperative role in detecting metastatic disease (van der Brekel et al 1991). We do not routinely advocate preoperative scalene node biopsies in patients who have a clinically negative evaluation.

Although CT or MRI scans may assist in delineating the pelvic boundaries of the tumor, examination under anesthesia should be considered to clinically confirm tumor size and mobility. Clinical pelvic side wall fixation or relative immobility that is noted preoperatively is associated with a twofold increased risk of an involved or close surgical margin after exenteration (Shingleton et al 1989). Involved margins adversely affect survival (Anthopoulos et al 1989, Shingleton et al 1989). If the nodular tumor or side wall aspirate indicates that the malignancy is fixed to the pelvic side wall, adequate surgical margins are unattainable and an exenterative procedure is contraindicated.

Morley and colleagues (1989), however, indicated that almost 50% of patients who underwent exenteration were considered preoperatively to have large lesions that were not judged to be either nonresectable or questionably resectable on preoperative assessment. Although many lesions may seem to be clinically nonresectable during examination, it is our philosophy that the operating room remains the court of last resort; in the absence of documented extracervi-cal disease, most women should be considered to be surgical candidates.

Existing data indicate that after radiation therapy, only 2% to 14% of patients have recurrent cervical cancer limited to the central pelvis. In the absence of absolute contraindications (see Table 12-3) the patient should be considered to be a candidate and prepared for curative surgery.

Preoperative Preparation

Preparation for pelvic exenteration is a traumatic experience for every patient, family, and physician. The risks involved and possible outcome create significant anxiety, particularly when the procedure has to be abandoned because of unresectable disease.

An important but difficult aspect of preoperative preparation relates to the patient's and the family's mental attitude and expectations given the circumstances. It may be impossible for the physician to explain the magnitude of this procedure or for the patient to grasp the consequences of the operation. Regardless, preoperative discussions with the patient and selected family members or support people are important. The prolonged rehabilitation period should be stressed (Dempsey et al 1975). Discussion regarding the operative algorithm, the possible need for ostomy, and the role and methods of urinary, intestinal, and vaginal reconstruction should be detailed.

All patients who are considered for exenterative surgery are candidates for nutritional assessment. Information suggests that as many as 50% of hospitalized patients have clinical or laboratory evidence of malnutrition. The incidence in patients having recurrent cancer may be higher. The prolonged period of postoperative recovery can only exacerbate potential problems. Additionally, malnourished patients are subject to increased postoperative morbidity and mortality. Although the diagnosis of a malnourished state may eas-

TABLE 12-4
Scalene Node Metastasis in Patients With Recurrent Cancer

STUDY	YEAR	PATIENTS WITH CLINICALLY NEGATIVE SUPRACLAVICULAR NODES	POSITIVE SUPRACLAVICULAR NODES (%)
Ketcham, et al	1973	22	18.2
Perez-Mesa, et al	1976	17	5.9
Lee, et al	1981	25	24.0
Burke, et al	1987	35	17.0
Manetta, et al	1989	10	0
TOTAL		109	15.6

ily be confirmed in patients who have significant recent weight loss, other nutritional parameters, such as a low serum albumin (less than 3.0 g/dL), decreased triceps skinfold thickness, low serum transferrin, or altered delayed hypersensitivity (as determined by skin testing) should be evaluated (Orr et al 1984a, 1984b). Malnourished patients may benefit from aggressive preoperative alimentation.

All exenterative procedures require an interruption of the gastrointestinal tract. Although few specific reports concerning infection after exenteration are available, a mechanical bowel preparation instituted before the procedure (Judd 1975, Parker et al 1978) decreases the risk of intraabdominal or wound infections. In our report (Orr et al 1983b), the use of a preoperative mechanical bowel preparation in patients undergoing exenteration was an important factor in reducing the risk of wound or pelvic infection by more than 50%.

Additional important preoperative studies include arterial blood gases and pulmonary function tests, as indicated. These aid in the preoperative diagnosis of subtle pulmonary disease, help predict the postoperative recovery after a long operative procedure, and allow appropriate diagnosis and management of the postoperative pulmonary complaints or complications.

Postoperative rehabilitation is greatly influenced by the patient's psychologic adjustment and her management of the urinary or fecal stoma. Preoperative discussion with the physician, stomal therapist, or another patient who has a stoma helps to allay fear and misconceptions. Preoperatively, the external stoma should be selected with extreme care. The enterostomal therapist may be helpful in selecting the appropriate site. Generally, the location should be free from skinfolds or fat creases in both standing and sitting positions. The belt line should be avoided. If possible, it should not be located close to prior abdominal scars that may interfere with proper adherence of the appliance. The stoma site should be as far lateral from the midline as possible but should always be selected to leave the bowel composing the stoma through the split rectus muscle. Failure to adhere to this latter feature promotes a high incidence of peristomal hernias (Benson et al 1992). After anesthesia, the site selected for the stoma should be marked with an "X" scratched on the abdominal wall. Ink marking should be avoided because the ink may be washed during antiseptic preparation of the skin. Because stoma care is essential to the patient undergoing conduit surgery (necessitating an appliance), the patient must be assessed for the ability to care for herself. The entire apparatus must be removed and replaced after cleansing the peristomal area on a 4-day schedule. For example, patients with multiple sclerosis, quadriplegics, and the frail or mentally impaired patient require appliance care by members of the family or visiting nurse attendants.

Preoperative hospitalization should be minimized because the rate of wound infections increases in direct proportion to the duration of preoperative hospitalization (Cruse et al 1980). Most of the preoperative evaluation can be completed in an outpatient setting. Although commonly administered, the use of perioperative parenteral antibiotics has no documented benefit in exenterative surgery. If one chooses to use antibiotics, the risk of bacterial resistance, pseudomembranous colitis, anaphylactic reactions, and fungal infection should be weighed. It is our contention that short-term broad-spectrum perioperative antibiotics should be considered and continued for at least two additional doses to counter the effects of duration or surgery, large-volume blood loss, and previous irradiation (Orr et al 1987).

The reported risk of a patient developing venous thrombosis, pulmonary emboli, or both (Fig. 12-6) after exenteration is 1% to 6%. This relatively high risk is likely related both to the duration of the operative procedure and the trauma to pelvic vessels. There is little information regarding the risks and benefits of prophylactic heparin or other methods of prophylaxis to decrease deep vein thrombosis. We no longer use perioperative heparin because it is associated with increased blood loss; however, we use pneumatic calf compression during the intraoperative and postoperative interval (Farquharson et al 1984). Some authors (Girtanner et al 1981, Morley 1984) advocate vena cava plication to decrease the risk of postoperative embolus.

THE EXENTERATIVE OPERATION

The operative procedure may be logically divided into three components: (1) determining resectability, (2) resection, and (3) reconstruction, including the construction of the urinary conduit, management of the gastrointestinal tract, vaginal reconstruction, and pelvic closure.

Resectability

In Shepherd's (1989) experience, 50% of 60 patients referred for consideration of exenteration were rejected on initial examination under anesthesia. Of the 30 patients undergoing laparotomy, exenteration was not performed in 15 patients. Therefore, only about 25% of those patients who referred were ultimately selected for the procedure. This finding is confirmed by others (Manetta et al 1989, Shingleton et al 1989, Morley et al 1989).

Our preferred incision is vertical, extended around the umbilicus as necessary. Although some authors advocate a transverse incision, reportedly to opti-

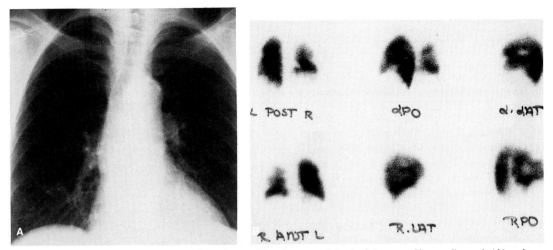

FIGURE 12-6. After exenteration, this 65-year-old patient complained of dyspnea. Chest radiograph (**A**) and cardiogram were unremarkable. A ventilation-perfusion scan (**B**) indicated the presence of multiple pulmonary emboli.

mize lateral pelvic exposure, we believe the vertical incision gives adequate exposure with a decreased risk of wound complications (Orr et al 1983b). Additionally, the vertical incision allows easy dissection of the omentum, often used to cover the pelvic basin, and allows the surgeon access to create a rectus myocutaneous flap, urinary conduit, and colostomy.

The serosal and peritoneal surfaces are carefully inspected and palpated. If intraperitoneal disease is present, the procedure is abandoned because only an occasional patient survives her disease.

Direct extension of malignancy through the pelvic peritoneum should not singularly contraindicate proceeding with the operation. Significant salvage rates have been obtained when areas of contiguous peritoneal involvement can be removed in the en bloc resection (Terada et al 1987, Averette et al 1984).

Malignant cytology is present in 10% of patients who undergo exploration for exenteration (Kilgore et al 1984); however, other poor prognostic factors are usually present when cytology is positive. In the absence of a reliable intraoperative test to determine the presence of malignant cytology, one cannot use this method; the determination of resectability is based on other factors.

The dissection of the paraaortic nodes with intraoperative histologic assessment is considered an important portion of the procedure because of the frequency of involvement of those nodes in recurrent disease and the marked difference in prognosis when metastases are present. Metastasis to aortic nodes probably contraindicates exenteration.

A pelvic lymphadenectomy after therapeutic pelvic radiation therapy is made difficult by dense ad-

hesions and tissue reaction. The technical difficulty is associated with prolonged operative time, increased blood loss, and an increased risk of postoperative lymphocysts, leg edema, and thrombophlebitis (Rutledge et al 1958). Shingleton and colleagues (1989) indicated that complete node dissection was impossible in 19% of women, secondary to extensive side wall fibrosis associated with previous radiation therapy. Although the therapeutic effect of lymphadenectomy at exenteration is not known, the prognostic significance of pelvic node metastases is well documented. The reported 5-year survival rate of patients who have negative pelvic nodes ranges between 35% and 65%, whereas only 5% to 15% of patients with node metastatic disease survive (Table 12-5). The median survival in patients having tumor metastasis to pelvic lymph nodes is 1.1 years (Shingleton et al 1989).

Some authors (Barber et al 1971, Morley 1982) believe that exenteration is contraindicated in the presence of pelvic node metastasis; others (Creasman et al 1974, Stanhope et al 1985, Rutledge et al 1987) believe that the decision to continue must be individualized. Creasman and Rutledge's (1974) report indicating no difference in survival in patients having negative nodes and those having unknown node status has prompted some surgeons to omit lymphadenectomy. These reports, however, fail to mention the possible selection process involved. Lymphadenectomy may have been performed in patients who have palpably enlarged nodes and not performed in those patients who have nonenlarged nodes. Node enlargement may be secondary to the infection that is frequently present with recurrent cervical cancer, and the procedure should not be abandoned without histologic evidence

TABLE 12-5
Survival of Patients With Recurrent Cervical Cancer Related to Lymph Node Status
at Pelvic Exenteration

STUDY	YEAR	NEGATIVE LYMPH NODES		POSITIVE LYMPH NODES	
		Patients (n)	5-Year Survival (%)	Patients (n)	5-Year Survival (%)
Ingersoll, et al	1966	39	38.5	33	6.1
Kiselow, et al	1967	88	50.0	28	21.4
Ketcham, et al	1970	69	33.0	21	11.0
Barber, et al	1971	166	17.4	97	5.1
Creasman, et al	1974	29	27.6	14	14.3
Symmonds, et al	1975	68	42.0	30	15.0
Rutledge, et al	1977	—	—	30	11.0
Averette, et al	1984	—	—	6	0.0
Rutledge, et al	1987	—	—	24	9.4
Morley, et al	1989	52	79.0	5	0.0
Shingleton, et al	1989	106	—	10	10.0*

*2-year survival.

of involvement. The clinical situation may be more complicated after a lymphangiogram, wherein reaction to dye may cause secondary node enlargement. Shingleton and coworkers (1989) reported a 48% 5-year survival in those few patients having no dissection, which was equal to that of women whose nodes were dissected. Again, the selection basis was unclear. Stanhope and Symmonds (1985) noted 2- and 5-year survival rates of 47% and 23% among 26 patients—20 of whom had only one or two microscopically positive nodes. They argued that continuation of exenterative procedures in the presence of resectable pelvic node metastasis is worthwhile. Rutledge and McGuffee (1987) reported a 33% 3-year survival and a 9.4% 5-year survival in patients having node metastasis. Interestingly, there was no apparent effect of increasing number of involved nodes. Because of its prognostic value and the possible therapeutic benefit of lymphadenectomy, we advocate extensive intraoperative pelvic node sampling and dissection, if feasible. The complication rate has been small in those procedures in which adequate pelvic drainage has been established. Based on these results, the findings of microscopically positive nodes should not necessarily be the sole reason to abandon exenteration. Metastatic disease (in multiple or bilateral pelvic nodes or in adherent nodes requiring major vessel excision), probably precludes cure (Barber et al 1971).

After intraperitoneal and retroperitoneal assessment, the avascular but occasionally fibrotic paravesical and pararectal spaces are dissected to verify resectability. Assessment of the caudal portion of the operative procedure for removing the tumor, vagina, and juxtaposed organs as they traverse the levators is important because tumor extension or skip metastases that require resection of the levator musculature are associated with a poor prognosis (Barber et al 1967, Barber 1969). If the patient's tumor is unresectable, the procedure can be stopped without a significant risk of bleeding or other serious morbidity.

Many patients who are explored have a negative intraoperative evaluation and undergo exenteration. Miller and associates (1993) detailed the effects of a positive intraoperative evaluation, which occurred in 111 of 394 (28%) patients undergoing exploration for possible pelvic exenteration for recurrent cervical cancer at the M.D. Anderson Hospital between 1970 and 1990. The median age of patients who had aborted procedures was 44. Reasons for terminating the procedure included the presence of intraperitoneal disease in 49 patients (44%); the only preoperative finding that correlated to this was the presence of a pelvic mass. Other reasons for not completing the procedure included node metastases in 45 patients (40.5%); this finding correlated to a short interval from primary radiation therapy. Parametrial fixation was present in 15 patients (13.5%) and hepatic lesions or bowel involvement were present in 5 patients (4.5%). Interestingly, peritoneal cytology was negative in 61 of 79 patients (77%) and was of predictive value only in patients who had adenocarcinoma.

In contrast, Stanhope and colleagues (1990) evaluated 72 patients undergoing exenteration for recurrent cervical cancer at the Mayo Clinic between 1977 and 1986 and reported 15 postirradiation patients who were treated with what was considered to be a palliative exenteration. The 1- and 2-year survival rates were 56% and 24%, respectively. This compared with 85%, 75%, and 52% (5-year rates) for those with a more favorable prognosis. Unfortunately, a median survival of 1 year is not dramatically different from that of patients not undergoing exenteration. Although this procedure may offer palliation in some situations, it is difficult for us to advocate a "palliative" operation of this magnitude that requires a prolonged recovery and rehabilitation.

Resection

The usual duration of the operative procedure is between 5 and 6 hours, with an anterior exenteration requiring less operative time. Prolonged operative time (more than 8 hours) is associated with decreased survival (Ketcham et al 1970) and although this may be related to increased technical difficulty or different surgical techniques, the effect on prognosis makes it important to minimize anesthesia and operative time. Although some authors have advocated a multidisciplinary team approach including general surgeons and urologists, most American gynecologic oncologists perform the procedure in its entirety. Regardless of who performs the surgery, there should be an adequate number of experienced surgeons available during the procedure to avoid fatigue as a cause of error in surgical judgment or technique.

The usual blood loss for total exenteration varies between 2000 and 4000 mL, with less occurring in subtotal procedures. The need for transfusion is 90% (Bender 1992) and as much as 24,000-mL blood loss has been reported. Ketcham and coworkers (1970) reported that mortality was increased when the procedure was associated with an intraoperative blood loss of greater than 3800 mL. Because 15% to 42% of blood loss is present on gowns and drapes, intraoperative estimates and replacement may be inadequate, predisposing the patient to hypotension; efforts should be directed to quantitating this loss. Intraoperative use of a pulmonary artery catheter allows dynamic management and appropriate maintenance of the patient's vascular volume. Our experience (Orr et al 1983a) with monitoring indicates that intraoperative fluid (crystalloid, blood, colloid) replacements in excess of 1500 mL/hour are necessary to maintain cardiovascular function. Fluid management guided by catheter measurements has been associated with a decrease in cardiovascular and pulmonary complications. Volume replacement consists of packed red blood cells, albumin, and crystalloid because whole blood offers little advantage over component therapy. Fresh frozen plasma, cryoprecipitate, and platelets are used as necessary.

Intestinal staples have been used in most recent exenterative procedures. In our hands (Orr et al 1982), their use was associated with a decrease in operative time of 20% and 28% for total and anterior exenteration, respectively (Table 12-6). Additional benefits of surgical staple use include a secure anastomosis, using a monofilament nonreactive permanent material, with less variation in surgical technique and minimal contamination. Although it has been argued that gastrointestinal staples in the urinary conduit predispose to the development of calculi, the reported incidence is small (2% to 4%). These calculi usually pass easily and are rarely responsible for decreased renal function or serious infection. Absorbable staples may eliminate this conduit problem but perform less reliably than permanent staples.

After resection, the pathologist and the surgeon should review the operative specimen together before fixation. Important surgical margins should be extensively investigated because tumor-involved margins imply recurrence and death. If an anterior exenteration is undertaken, surgical margins at Douglas' cul-de-sac should be obtained and examined intraoperatively. Although there is no evidence that adjuvant therapy benefits patients who have close margins, intraoperative or

TABLE 12-6
Operative Time Related to Type of Exenteration, Type of Intestinal Segment and Stapler Use (115 patients)

TYPE OF EXENTERATION	INTESTINAL SEGMENT	STAPLES	MEAN OPERATIVE TIME (H)
Anterior*	Ileal[†]	+	4.9 ± 0.8
	Ileal[†]	–	6.8 ± 1.3
	Transverse colon	+	5.2 ± 0.7
Total*	Ileal[†]	+	5.4 ± 0.9
	Ileal[†]	–	6.4 ± 1.3
	Transverse colon	+	5.9 ± 1.3

*Anterior exenteration significantly shorter than total exenteration (*p* <.001).
[†]Operative time when staples were used is significantly shorter in anterior
(*p* = .0001) and total (*p* = .005) exenteration.

Reprinted from Shingleton HM, Orr JW. Cancer of the cervix: diagnosis and treatment. New York, Churchill Livingstone, 1987:237.

interstitial radiation therapy may be considered for those having close or involved margins because they are at high risk for recurrence. The use of the last in these situations is untested.

Reconstruction

The ultimate goal of this customized reconstructive plan is the achievement of a primarily healed, functional restoration of the pelvic, urinary, and gastrointestinal tracts. Regardless of procedure performed, reconstruction of the urinary, intestinal, and reproductive tract is paramount to allow rehabilitation. Most serious postoperative complications, however, are related to reconstructive efforts (Orr 1983a, b, Soper et al 1989b).

Urinary Diversion

Initial attempts at urinary diversion involved a wet colostomy or a rectal bladder. Moreover, ureterosigmoidostomy may be considered to be the first successful form of continent urinary diversion. Unfortunately, problems with delayed development of malignancy in some patients with ureterosigmoidostomy have discouraged the use in most patients requiring supravesical urinary diversion. It was the serious adverse effects of fecal contamination of the urinary tract, however, that prompted the search for alternative methods. Since the first description of the urinary conduit (Butcher et al 1962), most conduits were constructed with a segment of distal ileum. Advocates of sigmoid colon conduits point out that this type of diversion avoids a primary bowel anastomosis. The effects of previous radiation therapy to these two intrapelvic bowel segments have resulted in high rates of urinary complications (Orr et al 1982, Soper et al 1989a). Although pale serosa or thickened mesentery may indicate marked irradiation effect, such changes are not always clinically apparent. The inability to judge the degree of irradiation bowel injury has prompted many surgeons to use a segment of nonirradiated transverse colon (Nelson 1969) for the urinary conduit (Fig. 12-7). We have reported its use to be associated with a decreased risk of postoperative urinary leaks (Table 12-7) and late urinary infections (Orr et al 1982). Soper and associates (1989a) confirmed these findings, reporting that patients with sigmoid or ileal conduits had a significantly higher incidence of severe surgical complications than did those with transverse colon conduits or posterior exenteration alone. The colon conduit may be peristaltic or antiperistaltic without detrimental effects on long-term function (Schmidt 1986). Avoiding an anastomosis in the irradiated ileum has also been associated with a decreased risk of small bowel obstruction or fistulas (Table 12-8). If a

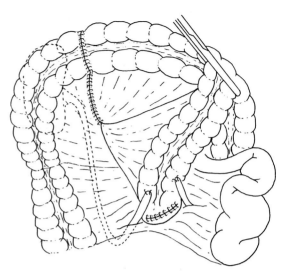

FIGURE 12-7. The segment of transverse colon has been isolated and the colon re-anastomosed. The ureters enter the peritoneal cavity through the small bowel mesentery. The conduit is then fixed to the posterior peritoneum after the single-layer ureterointestinal anastomosis.

resection or use of the ileum is necessary, an ileal ascending colostomy decreases the risk of poor healing (Lichtinger 1985).

Use of single-J ureteral stents or silastic catheters anchored to the intestinal segment or ureter by plain catgut sutures (Fig. 12-8) can decrease technical errors during conduit construction while offering protection against acute urinary strictures. Their use does not significantly increase the risk of acute postoperative pyelonephritis. Although stents preclude an antireflux anastomosis during conduit construction, there is little documentation that this type of ureterointestinal anastomosis is superior or worth the extra operating time (Bricker 1980). Appropriate stomal protrusion of a fourth to a half inch above the skin can be accomplished with a rosebud technique, which allows optimal appliance management postoperatively.

TABLE 12-7
Urinary Leaks Following Exenteration

Type of Conduit	Patients (N)	Urinary Leaks (%)
Ileal	103	9.7
Transverse colon	53	0

From Shingleton HM, Orr JW. Cancer of the cervix: diagnosis and treatment. New York, Churchill Livingstone. 1987:238.

TABLE 12-8
Gastrointestinal Complications Related to Method of Urinary Diversion

TYPE OF CONDUIT	PATIENTS (N)	SMALL BOWEL OBSTRUCTION (%)	SMALL BOWEL FISTULA (%)
Ileal	103	8.7	9.7
Transverse colon	53	0	1.9*

*Single patient required extensive ileal resection secondary to radiation damage.

From Shingleton HM, Orr JW. Cancer of the cervix: diagnosis and treatment. New York, Churchill Livingstone, 1987:239.

Continent Diversion Techniques

In 1851, Simon performed the first continent urinary diversion (ureterosigmoidostomy; Chiou et al 1993). Urinary diversion with the ileocecal segment was initially used by Berhoogen in 1908 and later described by Gilchrist in 1950. Since Kock (1982) reported his experience with the continent ileal reservoir, a resurgence of interest in continent urinary diversion has occurred, with more than 40 variants being reported worldwide. Many gynecologic oncologists have advocated its use during exenteration because patients are reported to have a better self-image, more frequent sexual activity, and a greater desire for nonsexual contact (Hogan et al 1993).

The concept of using a buttressed ileocecal valve as a dependable continence mechanism that can withstand the trauma of intermittent catheterization was first reported at Indiana University by Rowland and associates (1987). Popular alternatives include the continent ileal reservoir (Koch pouch), the Mainz pouch (1986), the Indiana pouch, the Miami pouch

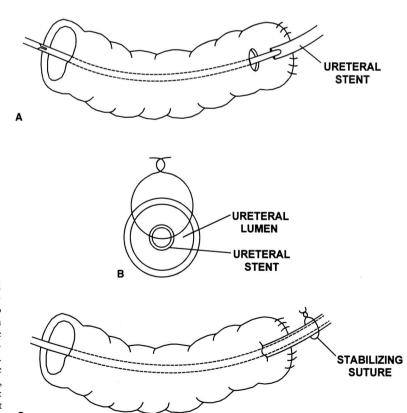

FIGURE 12-8. A silastic ureteral stent is pulled through a small incision in the bowel (**A**) and fixed to the ureter (to avoid expulsion) with a loosely tied 4–0 absorbable suture (**B**). The ureteral and intestinal mucosal surfaces are sutured (**C**). (Drawing modified from Rutledge FN, Smith JP, Wharton JT, O'Quinn AG. Pelvic exenteration: analysis of 29 patients. Am J Obstet Gynecol 1977;129:882.)

(1988), and the Penn pouch. Evaluation of neo-urethral pressure profiles indicates that the continent zone is confined to the region of the reconfigured valve. During construction, it is important to perform the imbrication while the ileocecal reservoir is still open. In this manner, one can easily observe the gradual closure of the ileocecal valve.

The goals of continent urinary diversion include (1) construction of a large-volume low-pressure reservoir with high compliance, (2) a reliable continence mechanism, (3) prevention of intestinal ureteral reflux, (4) simplicity in construction, (5) avoidance of the use of excessive length of bowel, (6) avoidance of the use of synthetic material, (7) ease of catheterization, (8) avoidance of the need for revision, and (9) good cosmetic appearance (Bissada et al 1993).

Conduit urinary diversion is the only form of diversion that should be considered in patients who have compromised renal function (Benson et al 1992). Patients undergoing construction of a catheterizable stoma are undertaking a lifelong commitment, and many patients opt for the simplicity of a conduit. It is mandatory that patients undergoing continent urinary procedures have sufficient eye–hand coordination to perform clean, intermittent catheterization.

Despite ongoing experience with numerous continent urinary diversion procedures, there is no unanimity regarding the "best" form of continent diversion (Benson et al 1992). Although continent urinary diversion is certainly appropriate in selected patients, the procedures are technically more challenging and are potentially fraught with higher complication rates than those diversions using external collecting devices. These latter procedures, with all their shortcomings, have withstood the test of time and have become part of every gynecologic oncologist's repertoire, in contrast to the newer continent diversion procedures, whose technologic demands have not been mastered by every surgeon.

It appears that continent urinary diversions require longer, more extensive surgery and have a greater inherent likelihood of surgical complications. Ahlering (1988) described a 20% risk of urine leakage and 7.5% incidence of reoperation for construction of Koch pouches in 42 highly irradiated patients. Orovan and David (1988) reported a postoperative leakage rate of 37% and a reoperative rate of 25% in 16 patients undergoing Koch pouch reconstruction after receiving 40 cGy whole-pelvis irradiation before cystectomy.

Until competence is achieved, it is likely that continent diversions will have a high risk of urine leakage and associated reoperative risk (17% versus 3% in compiled data from the literature). Importantly, conduits can be converted to a continent catheterizable stoma at a later date (Adams et al 1992).

In the gynecologic literature, Penalver and coworkers (1993) reported 33 patients undergoing continent ilealcolonic diversion for reconstruction after pelvic exenteration. Twenty-five patients were followed-up for an average of 17 months, and 23 are completely continent with intermittent catheterization at 4- to 8-hour intervals. Urodynamic studies demonstrate a mean reservoir volume of 650 mL (range, 450 to 1225 mL). Renal function deterioration occurred in 1 patient (4%). Temporary difficulties with catheterization occurred in 3 patients. One patient required percutaneous decompression. Of the 50 ureteral colonic anastomoses performed, 4 patients had partial obstruction and 1 required reoperation. Importantly, since beginning the use of ileal colonic reservoirs in February 1988, Penalver had to abandon the procedure in only 2 patients because of the technical difficulties associated with irradiation fibrosis of the ileal colonic area. Penalver and colleagues (1994) stressed the importance of the learning curve. Operative mortality rate was 16% in the first 24 patients (Bloch et al 1992).

Mannel and associates (1992) reported their experience with 37 female patients who had prior therapeutic pelvic irradiation and underwent continent urinary diversion with a detubularized right colonic segment as a urinary reservoir, plicated ileocecal valve as a continence mechanism, and a tapered distal ileum for efferent catheterization. Of the 74 implanted ureters, four had reflux (5%), two had strictures (3%), and five had mild to moderate hydronephrosis (7%). All patients achieved daytime continence with catheterization intervals of 3 to 8 hours (median, 4 hours) and capacities of 200 to 1000 mL (median, 500 mL). Nighttime continence was reported by 33 of 37 patients (89%). Reoperation was required in 3 patients (8%).

Conventionally, this portion of the surgical procedure is based on proved efficacy and safety. In most cases, however, the choice for continent urinary diversion is based primarily on "psychologic" rather than medical indications. In essence, these patients may be taking medical risks for psychologic gains. There are some complications that appear to be unique with continent diversions. For example, stone formation in the pouch is a problem that is unique in continent reservoirs and occurs at a mean postoperative interval of 2.5 years (Haddad et al 1992). Electrolyte abnormalities and metabolic acidosis potentially can develop but do not appear to be significant problems for continent diversion with short-term follow-up. Metabolic problems are apparently low (Hall et al 1991).

Ureterosigmoidostomy was widely used for urinary diversion, and it was only in the 1960s that its association with cancer was finally recognized. It is known that patients with ureterosigmoidostomies who have been followed-up for 10 years or longer have a 5% to 13% chance of carcinoma development in the vicinity of the ureteral colonic anastomosis. The risk of cancer in patients who underwent ureterosigmoidostomy for benign disease is at least 400 times greater than expected in the general population (Chiou et al 1993). The incidence of cancer development in a continent reservoir does not become clear for several years after its application. In the presence of bacteria, microbiologic and chemical investigations of the urine of patients who have an ileal reservoir show that nitrates, nitrites, and nitrosamines are formed endogenously in the ileal pouch. If the nitrosamines theory for carcinogenesis is true, patients having continent reservoirs can be expected to be at a higher risk for developing malignancy in the reservoir than is reported for ileal conduits. These patients will require periodic evaluations to assess this risk. Because continent reservoirs remain with the patients for their entire lives, long-term management must be considered. A variety of illnesses may cause impairment of hand function, dexterity, and mental capacity. Parkinson's disease, stroke, arthritis, and many other diseases can all make self-catheterization difficult or even impossible. If these patients live long enough, it is not a matter of whether they will one day become incapable of catheterizing themselves, it is only a matter of when that day will arrive.

Regardless of type, during the construction of any continent pouch, intraoperative testing for integrity is always performed (Benson et al 1992).

Pelvic Reconstruction

The raw, denuded pelvic cavity, with its dense fibrous reaction, may predispose to postoperative infections and gastrointestinal complications. Techniques consisting of grafts constructed of foreign material such as amnion or Marlex (Wheeless et al 1971), which is designed to decrease the contact of small bowel and the raw surfaces, have not proved satisfactory. Although a pedicle or free peritoneal graft (as described by Morley and Lindenauer [1976]) provides a possible alternative to cover the denuded pelvic floor, optimal closure probably involves transposing new blood supply into the pelvis, such as transposition of an omental pedicle (Powers et al 1976) into the pelvis (Fig. 12-9). The use of omental grafts has been associated with a decreased rate of major small bowel complications. If the omentum is inadequate or surgically absent, we consider using a peritoneal graft with vaginal reconstruction.

Buchsbaum and coworkers (1985) advocated the use of a polyglycolic acid mesh to protect the pelvis and allow a bed for normal healing. In an animal model, however, Montz and colleagues (1990) indicated that the placement of polyglycolic acid mesh induces significant pelvic adhesions and potentiates the formation of pelvic abscess.

Clarke-Pearson and colleagues (1988) reported the use of a polyglactin (Vicryl) mesh in 6 patients whose omentum was unsuitable for use. No gastroin-

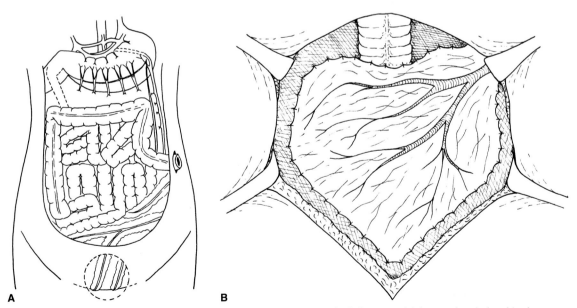

FIGURE 12-9. The omental flap has been created (conserving the left gastroepiploic artery) and placed in the gutter to completely cover the denuded pelvis. (*A* modified from Rutledge FN, Smith JP, Wharton JT, O'Quinn AG. Pelvic exenteration: analysis of 29 patients. Am J Obstet Gynecol 1977;128:882; *B* modified from Wheeless, 1981.)

testinal complications occurred; however, 4 patients developed pelvic infections that eventually resolved with surgical drainage and antibiotic therapy. There was no evidence of intraabdominal infection above the mesh. No chronic infections developed during a 24-month follow-up. Serial examination of these patients having a Vicryl mesh pelvic lid suggested that the small bowel remains suspended across the level of the pelvic inlet. This preliminary experience suggests that Vicryl mesh may be useful for the formation of a pelvic lid after exenterative surgery, even when the omentum is unavailable.

In 13 patients undergoing reconstruction of the pelvic floor using Vicryl mesh and omentum after pelvic exenteration, Hoffman and coworkers (1989) reported 1 patient who developed a conduit leak and 1 patient who developed an enterocutaneous fistula. Six patients developed significant postoperative pelvic infections, four of which manifest as abscess below the mesh. All were successfully treated with antibiotics and drainage.

We have been concerned about the potential adverse effects of Vicryl mesh pelvic floor reconstruction (Patsner et al 1990) and do not recommend routine use. In specific situations (i.e., absent omentum), an absorbable mesh may be necessary to isolate the small bowel from the denuded pelvic cavity.

Pearlman and associates (1990) suggested the benefit of using the urinary reservoir for filling the postexenterative pelvis. Their complication rate fell from 44% to 18%.

In most instances, we incorporate other methods to decrease the size of the pelvic defect and protect the small bowel after total exenteration, including methods reported by Lagasse and colleagues (1973), Berek and associates (1984a), and others.

Establishing Fecal Continence

The use of end-to-end anastomotic stapling instruments allows the mobilized sigmoid colon to be anastomosed to a short rectal stump (Griffin et al 1992, Wheeless 1993, Barter et al 1986). The neorectum is normally reconstructed using a denervated small caliber (compared with the normal rectum) colon. The anal sphincters are usually outside the field of irradiation. Functional results are likely maximized by total left colon mobilization, use of descending colon rather than sigmoid colon, and adequate length to allow "sacralization" of the colon with return of the normal anal rectal angle. Careful attention to five technical points are essential for optimal functional outcome in patients undergoing coloanal anastomosis (Paty et al 1992). These techniques include (1) complete mobilization of the left colon, (2) sharp dissection, (3) restoration of the anal–rectal right angle, (4) complete

mobilization of the transposed colonic segment, (5) meticulous pelvic hemostasis and drainage to avoid septic complications and (6) the routine use of diverting colostomy until completion of healing. This technique not only fills the posterior pelvic defect but can be of great psychologic benefit to the patient (Prudden 1971). Attention to surgical margins remains of utmost importance, however. Although problems with healing and rectal fistula are evident, the posterior pelvis is protected and 45% of patients heal adequately, allowing the diverting colostomy to be temporary. Berek and coworkers (1984a) described 11 patients who were managed in this manner, with no anastomotic leaks and with bowel continence reestablished in 63.6%. Harris and Wheeless (1986) reported 17 patients having a 12% anastomotic leak rate, with a 12.4% stricture rate. Both authors advised using a diverting colostomy in the previously irradiated patient.

Our experience has been similar. Hatch and associates (1988a) reported a series of 20 patients undergoing supralevator total pelvic exenteration with low rectal reanastomosis for radiorecurrent cancer, of whom 14 (70%) had complete healing. Three of 7 patients who had a rectal stump length of less than 6 cm healed primarily, whereas 11 of 13 who had a rectal stump length of more than 6 cm experienced complete healing. Overall, 13 of the 20 patients are clinically free of disease and 61% of those enjoy life with excellent bowel continence.

In a later report, Hatch and coworkers (1990) indicated that the use of an omental wrap facilitated healing. In the subset of patients having an omental wrap (13%), complete healing of the rectal anastomosis was 85%. Interestingly, although used in 12 patients, protective colostomies did not improve the healing rate for the low rectal reanastomosis when parenteral nutritional support and bowel rest was used. Again, the incidence of nonmalignant fistula or poor healing was high in those patients having a rectal stump of less than 6 cm·(7 of 11 patients), when compared with those patients having a longer rectal stump (8 of 20 patients). The reoperation rate in patients having pelvic exenteration and low rectal reanastomosis (23%) was higher than in those undergoing anterior exenteration (4.4%). We usually perform a protective diverting colostomy.

Although rectal reanastomosis during exenteration is technically feasible, long-term follow-up evaluation of some outcomes has revealed some bowel dysfunction. Although fecal continence is usually obtained, bowel dysfunction from loss of the normal rectal reservoir may remain problematic, even after years of adaptation. In 11 patients having recurrent carcinoma of the cervix, Trelford and colleagues (1992) reported follow-up evaluation that indicated intestinal retraining took 3 months to 1 year (average, 5 months). Although continence was achieved in all patients, several had little or no warning of evacuation.

Patients with a traditional end-to-end low anastomosis of colon and rectum (less than 3 cm) are frequently left with increased tenesmus, resulting in unacceptable fecal frequency and staining. Multiple stools, urgency, and episodic frequency are common during the first 6 months after proctectomy and coloanal or low rectal reconstruction. He suggested that construction of a rectal J pouch low-pressure reservoir diminished the symptoms. Wheeless and coworkers (1989) indicated that 42% of patients were still having four to six bowel movements per day for up to 2 years after surgery and low rectal anastomosis. Using a rectal J pouch coloproctostomy significantly reduced these symptoms of fecal frequency, with no significant increase in fecal incontinence. A statistically significant difference in the number of patients having more than four versus one to two stools per day was noted between the group with end-to-end anastomosis when compared with those who had a rectal J pouch. Sixty percent of those with a reservoir had one to two bowel movements per day versus 33% of those with end-to-end anastomosis. Cohen (1993) incorporated an 8-cm J pouch coloanal reconstruction in 23 patients and confirmed that this technique minimized early colon dysfunction.

Vaginal Reconstruction

One of the primary goals of pelvic reconstruction after radical gynecologic procedures includes creation of a pliable, durable, functional neovagina that can be used to supply potential new blood supply to aid in the recovery from radical pelvic surgery. The principal goals of reconstruction include restoring the pelvic floor and preventing herniation of intraabdominal contents, obliterating pelvic dead space, and limiting the pelvic "burn," promoting rapid wound healing and allowing uninterrupted adjuvant therapy and vaginal reconstruction. Minimizing technical difficulty, operating time, and injury to the donor sites is important (Pursell et al 1990).

Morley and associates (1973) indicated that sexual desires may increase after recovery; however, Dempsey and coworkers (1975) reported a significant loss of sexuality after exenteration. Brown and colleagues (1972) reported that whereas 73% of these women had no postoperative sexual interest, 1 patient experienced sensation in a phantom vagina and 26% had dreams with sexual content. The sexual partner's attitude is an important variable. Fear and lack of understanding of the disease, operation, and his altered perception of his partner's body image may result in him avoiding her.

Rehabilitation after a sexually mutilating surgical procedure begins preoperatively. There should be discussions regarding the desirability or necessity of constructing a neovagina at the time of exenteration because half of the patients may reject an attempt at vaginal reconstruction if a second operation is required. The most quoted objections to declining vaginal reconstruction include lack of sexual desire, advanced age, lack of a sexual partner, or a negative attitude toward a second operation by both the patient and her sexual partner.

Numerous methods of vaginal reconstruction performed initially or at an interval have been described (Table 12-9). Although spontaneous epithelialization of the vagina may occur, particularly in patients undergoing an anterior exenteration, it rarely results in a satisfactory vaginal vault. Morley and colleagues (1973) reported adequate sexual function after the placement of split-thickness skin grafts, performed as an interval procedure. Pregraft requirements include a good bed of granulation tissue. Care must be taken to not damage the gastrointestinal tract during the second operation. Beemer and coworkers (1988) reported their experience with split-thickness skin grafting for vaginal reconstruction. This procedure often requires a delay in reconstruction from 2 to 8 weeks while an adequate granulation bed forms. Prolapse of split-thickness skin graft on omentum has been reported (Koonings 1993).

Berek and colleagues (1984a) demonstrated that neocolorectal anastomosis serves as a posterior wall for proposed neovagina. The anterior lateral walls can then be made from an omental flap. By modifying the omental flap, the surgeon may create a cylinder, providing anterior, posterior, and lateral walls for the neovagina. A satisfactory functional neovagina can be created when the cylinder is sutured to the introitus, lined with split-thickness skin graft (0.35 nanometers to 12/1000 of an inch), and expanded in the postoperative period by a soft foam rubber vaginal form. The

TABLE 12-9
Methods Described for Vaginal Reconstruction After Exenteration

Spontaneous epithelialization
Split-thickness skin grafts
Sigmoid vaginostomy
Vulvovaginoplasty
Ileal vagina
Myocutaneous flaps
   Thigh pedicle
   Gluteal pedicle
   Vulvobulbocavernosus
   Rectus muscle
Amnion grafts

omentum is enervated by the vagus nerve and forms the wall of the neovagina. Normally, tugging or pulling on the omentum does not produce a sensation of pleasure that one would associate with sexual intercourse. It is of interest, however, that about 40% of patients who have undergone this operation report that they experience sexual orgasm.

Vulvovaginoplasty consists of the creation of a vaginal pouch that is constructed from vulvar or perineal tissue and can be performed as a part of or at any time after exenteration. Day and Stanhope (1977) reported the successful use of vulvovaginoplasty in 8 patients. Morbidity was minimal and 7 of 8 patients had excellent function results. They suggested that this less extensive procedure was useful after exenteration. Seven patients undergoing Williams vulvovaginoplasty after supralevator total pelvic exenteration were reported by Hoffman and associates (1991). The results of intercourse were neither negative nor positive. The authors concluded that Williams' vulvovaginoplasty appeared to be a reasonable alternative for vaginal reconstruction in patients who have had previous exenteration. The drawbacks of Williams vulvovaginoplasty include its failure to replace tissue loss or enhance pelvic support. Accomplishment of these goals is considered to be a major advantage of some of the other methods of vaginal reconstruction. Hoffman and coworkers suggested that this procedure is a reasonable alternative for vaginal reconstruction in those patients having adequate vulvar tissue. The resultant shallow vagina is usually in a vertical plane, may require a change in the coital position, and in our experience has not been a satisfactory solution to this problem.

The use of the intestinal lumen (both small bowel and large bowel) has been an intriguing concept for neovaginal reconstruction (Shiromizu et al 1989). The advantage of the use of an isolated segment of rectosigmoid colon is preservation of the integrity of the vascular supply of the colon and the superior hemorrhoid artery. Unlike small bowel, the secretions of an isolated 10- to 12-cm sigmoid colon are not so copious that they inconvenience the patient with a daily troubling discharge.

In addition, an anastomotic advantage of the rectosigmoid colon over the use of isolated segments of small bowel is the marginal artery of the colon (marginal artery of Drummond). This artery allows the surgeon to reverse the peristaltic direction of the colon to obtain greater mobility by transecting the mesentery proximal to the marginal artery with the sigmoid branches of the hemorrhoidal artery; it also allows the superior hemorrhoid artery to provide the appropriate vascular supply to the colonic segment by the marginal artery.

Nineteen patients undergoing a sigmoid segment placement of neovagina were evaluated. The anatomic result was good in 18 patients, although several reoperative procedures were necessary. Sexual adjustment was satisfactory in 12 of 19 patients and 16 were capable of achieving orgasm. These patients had not undergone exenteration. Interestingly, prolapse of the sigmoid neovagina has been reported (Freundt et al 1993).

Transposition of an ileal or sigmoid segment for use as a neovagina has been associated with an irritating discharge and coital pain and should not be chosen as a primary method of reconstruction.

Pedicle Flaps and Myocutaneous Grafts

Pedicle flaps from the vulva (Hatch 1984b), gluteal (Trelford et al 1979, Achauer et al 1984), or thigh regions have been described (see Table 12-9). Hemorrhage, infection, suture line breakdown, and prolonged hospitalization are potential complications. Becker and associates' (1979) report that 95% of neovaginas were termed adequate for sexual function is promising, despite the finding that patients with neovaginas were less orgasmic and only 65% of patients with neovaginas had subjectively normal sexual function. These grafts not only allow vaginal reconstruction but provide additional sources of blood supply to the irradiated pelvis or to a low rectal intestinal anastomosis. Experimental data confirm the enhanced ability of musculocutaneous grafts to resist bacterial infection (Kusiak 1993). These flaps also provide a conduit for the delivery of host defense components. Although individual selection of the most appropriate graft is necessary, the overall operative time can be reduced if a second team of surgeons begins the vaginal reconstruction while the urinary conduit is being performed.

The initial report on gracilis myocutaneous graft for pelvic perineal reconstruction after exenteration was published by McCraw in 1976. The short gracilis myocutaneous flap derives its blood supply from terminal branches of the obturator artery, and the vascular pedicle derived from the medial circumflex femoral artery is sacrificed.

The gracilis myocutaneous graft allows immediate pelvic reconstruction without lost time or additional blood loss when the procedure is performed using a two-team approach. This may represent a great advantage over the additional cost, anesthesia, exposure, and less satisfactory results of a delayed reconstruction and allow the blood supply to assist in pelvic healing.

Lacey and coworkers (1988) reported 18 vaginal reconstructive procedures using gracilis flaps at the time of pelvic exenteration. They suggested that there was no significant difference, when compared with patients not undergoing flap reconstruction, with respect to operative time, blood loss, or duration of postoperative hospitalization. There were, however, fewer significant serious complications in the patient receiving gracilis flaps. They reported the mean operative time to be 7.4 hours with neovaginal reconstruction and 6.8 hours with controls. They clearly indicate that the time for performing flaps in sequence operative procedure is markedly prolonged (9.5 hours). Serious complications related to the exenterative aspects of the procedure were increased in the control group (8 of 13 patients [62%]) when compared with those patients who received gracilis muscle reconstruction (4 of 18 patients [22%]). Major complications associated with gracilis flaps were infrequent; however, debridement or partial sloughing occurred in 11% of patients, infection in 6% of patients, elective revision (because of protrusion) in 17% of patients, and leg wound disruption in 6% of patients. Total complication rate was 39%.

Questionnaires were sent to 11 surviving patients after vaginal reconstruction and only 2 patients indicated that they had used the vagina for intercourse. For 1 patient, the experience was satisfactory; it was partially satisfactory for the other. Five patients stated that they were not interested in sex. The common theme found in these responses was "the comfort of knowing it is there" was important. Only 2 patients were satisfied with the leg scars. Lacey and associates believed that the low incidence of repeat laparotomy secondary to exenterative complications related to placement of the gracilis graft. Lacey and colleagues believed that even in sexually inactive patients, the combination of improved healing, postoperative rehabilitation, and improved self-image should persuade the physician and patient to decide in favor of the procedure. They believed this to be particularly the case if the low rectal reanastomosis was performed.

Soper and colleagues (1989b) reported 21 short gracilis myocutaneous flaps used for vulvovaginal reconstruction in 11 patients undergoing radical pelvic surgery. Vaginal caliber and depth were excellent in 10 patients at 1 to 22 months follow-up. There was a trend toward a decreased risk of complications in those patients undergoing gracilis flap pelvic reconstruction. Forty-one of the 69 patients had persistent or recurrent cervical carcinoma (Soper et al 1989b).

Copeland and colleagues' (1989) retrospective review compares the operative and perioperative morbidity in 107 patients, using gracilis myocutaneous vaginal reconstruction concurrent with total pelvic exenteration to 44 patients who did not have reconstruction. With incorporation of the reconstruction procedure (a two-team technique), there were no increases in operating time, blood loss, or length of hospitalization.

Before 1980, 65% of patients experienced prolapse of the neovagina; 25% were severe. The frequency of prolapse has since decreased to 16% (6% severe) because of several modifications, including the use of small flaps, anchoring the neovagina to the levator and retropubic fascia, and when necessary for mobilization, ligating the neurovascular pedicles. With these modifications, 66% of patients also remained free of wound breakdown or necrosis. The frequency of severe necrosis decreased from 24% to 13%.

Although fluorescein was first used in Copeland and coworkers' study, they found that a failure to stain was not a reliable indicator of devascularization and therefore omitted it from their technique. Omental lids were created in all but 3 patients in this series. Eighty-eight of the patients who underwent myocutaneous reconstruction had drains placed for leg wounds. One of these patients (1.1%) developed a leg wound abscess and 1 patient (1.1%) developed cellulitis. Of the 19 patients having no drain placement, 1 (5.3%) developed cellulitis at the donor site and 1 (5.3%) developed a wound abscess. The incidence of pelvic abscess was 2.3% in those undergoing concurrent myocutaneous reconstruction and 9.4% in those patients without reconstruction.

Between 1977 and 1979, the size of the flaps was usually between 18 to 23 cm in length and 6 to 8 cm in width. Between 1980 and 1983, the dimensions were decreased to 12 to 15 cm in length and 5 to 8 cm in width. Since 1983, most flaps range from 8 to 14 cm in length and 4 to 7 cm in width.

The overall duration of hospitalization for all patients having reconstruction is similar to that or slightly less than that for patients having no reconstruction.

Twenty-four patients who had concurrent gracilis myocutaneous grafts and pelvic exenteration during the period 1962 to 1986 were reported by Cain and colleagues (1989). The rate of fistula formation in the hospital was significantly less in the graft group (p =.004) but it was not different when compared with the contemporary graft patients only. The total infection rate (wound and pelvic) was decreased in the graft group when graft infections were excluded. The major problem with this graft was the significant incidence of flap necrosis that occurred in 9 of the 24 patients. There were no life-threatening complications attributed to concurrent placement of gracilis myocutaneous grafts. Only 2 patients who had grafts developed enterocutaneous fistulas that were not associated with malignancy during long-term follow-up (8.3%), whereas 8 patients without grafts developed fistulas that were not associated with malignancy in this same time interval (33%). Cain and associates (1989) reported a mean blood loss of 4160 mL with grafts and 3847 mL in patients without grafts. This is supported by others (Berek et al 1984b). Total hospital stay was

33 days with grafts and 33 days without grafts. None of these were significantly different. The early prolapse of graft in 1 patient identified the need for careful securing of the graft apex in the pelvis. Although Cain and coworkers suggested an advantage for use of the myocutaneous graft, they admitted that the overall difference may represent only the evolution of technique and perioperative support changes.

In the study reported by Berek and colleagues (1984b), there were no enterocutaneous fistulas reported in the long-term (4 years 3 months) follow-up of patients receiving concurrent grafts. They reported a blood loss for concurrent grafts of 3000 mL mean blood loss and a mean hospital stay of 21 days. Berek and coworkers reported a mean blood loss (usually nongraft patients) of 2292 mL and a mean hospital stay of 37 days.

The gracilis muscles, particularly in the obese patient, are unreliable. In addition, the limited arc of rotation of the lower pelvis makes it a second-choice flap for reconstruction of most pelvic exenterations.

Objective evidence that these grafts may further decrease postoperative complications is lacking but it appears to show promise. It increases operating time and presents certain problems and complications, primarily related to blood supply to the flap and wound breakdown of the graft site.

Pursell and colleagues (1990) described 22 patients who had undergone distally based rectus abdominis flap for reconstruction. The flap was thought to be technically easy to create, reliable, with minimal tissue loss and few donor site complications. Infectious complications at the flap site were noted in 14% of patients and one of these was associated with an enteroneovaginal fistula, which required surgical closure. A wound infection occurred in 3 (14%) abdominal incisions and a superficial wound separation occurred in 9 patients (41%). Operative time is potentially minimized because the procedure requires only unilateral mobilization. Five of 7 women have attempted intercourse and 4 of these 5 patients have been successful. Eighteen patients (82%) had no flap loss less than gracilis. Two patients (9%) lost less than 20% of their flaps. Neovaginal prolapse occurred in only 1 patient (5%). Subsequent abdominal surgery has been performed without fascial complications. The authors concur with others (Benson et al 1993) that this flap offers reconstruction that allows extensive mobilization of well-vascularized nonirradiated tissues, with minimal tissue loss or prolapse rates. The only disadvantage involves closure of the donor site, which may require a synthetic patch closure.

After reconstruction with rectus abdominis myocutaneous flap, CT findings should be carefully evaluated. The myocutaneous flap appears as a unilateral arcuate band of soft tissue, extending from the linea alba to the sacrum. Additional CT findings include symmetric thinning of the ventral abdominal wall, fluid collections, vaginal breakdown, and presacral soft-tissue thickening (Willing et al 1991).

Hatch (1984b) proposed an alternative method for vaginal reconstruction after partial exenteration using a bulbocavernosus myocutaneous flap (Figure 12–10) for posterior vaginal reconstruction, combining this with an omental carpet, and reported satisfactory results in 8 patients. The disadvantages of the bulbocavernosus flap are that it does not provide an entire vaginal tube and it does not allow sufficient tissue for neovaginal reformation after total exenteration with removal of the perineal body and anus. Additionally, the bulbocavernosus flap is not large enough to obliterate dead space in the pelvis.

Abdominal Closure

Although a running monofilament en bloc closure may save 8 to 10 minutes (Orr 1990), our method of abdominal closure is a Smead-Jones technique (Wallace et al 1980), using a permanent monofilament suture material. This internal retention suture is reported to offer optimal protection against abdominal dehiscence, which occurs with increased frequency when the incision is all or partly in an irradiation field.

POSTOPERATIVE CARE

Substantial changes have occurred during the past two decades that have lowered perioperative morbidity (Averette et al 1984, Orr et al 1983a, b, c, Cain et al 1989).

After exenteration, the patient is monitored in an intensive care unit for 48 to 72 hours because the marked fluid shifts and possibility of occult bleeding require close monitoring of the patient's volume status.

A pelvic exenteration defect is often equated with a 20% body surface area burn and can lead to massive sequestration of interstitial fluid. Routine central venous pressure monitoring has been replaced by the pulmonary artery catheter. The latter enables the physician to monitor postoperative cardiac performance and volume status, intervening with supportive pharmacologic therapies as necessary. Such a catheter is more invasive and is subject to more complications than a central venous line; however, in more than 110 patients, its use has resulted in only one major complication, a hemothorax. The physician should be aware of other potential complications of the pulmonary artery catheter, including pulmonary parenchymal damage, balloon rupture, cardiac arrhythmias, infection, thrombophlebitis, or inadvertent knotting of the

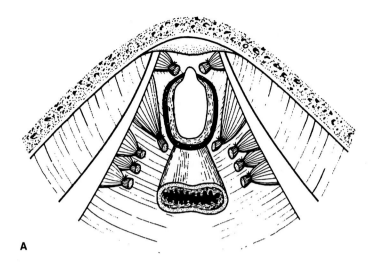

A

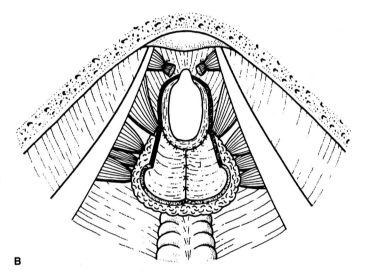

FIGURE 12-10. Pelvic reconstruction after exenteration. (**A**) The previously irradiated and denuded pelvic floor and often the lower rectum require closure. (**B**) Myocutaneous flaps (in this case, bulbocavernosus) can be placed to provide blood supply and an epithelial cover. The remainder of the pelvis can be covered with an omental flap (see Fig. 12–9*B*).

B

catheter (Orr et al 1994). Other possible complications (e.g., valvular damage or endocardial vegetations) have been reported but only after long-term use.

As many as 38% of patients have significant preoperative blood volume deficits (Hoye et al 1972). When combined with extensive intraoperative blood loss, fluid shifts, and the necessity for a prolonged anesthetic, we believe that additional monitoring with an arterial line is warranted intraoperatively and during the acute postoperative recovery period.

Large-volume blood loss may be associated with a consumptive coagulopathy. After a one-volume transfusion, however, clotting elements are reduced by 70% to 75% (Sohmer et al 1979, Orr et al 1987). Clinical bleeding may not occur until after a two-volume transfusion, when about 10% of the original blood clotting elements remain. Because stored blood is essentially devoid of platelets and is markedly depleted in factors V and VIII, we prefer to use blood-component therapy (consisting of packed red blood cells, to increase oxygen-carrying capacity) and platelets, fresh frozen plasma, and cryoprecipitate (containing factors V, VIII, XII, and fibrinogen) to correct a coagulopathy. If additional volume restoration is necessary, albumin is preferable to frozen plasma because it has a decreased risk of hepatitis. This careful attention to postoperative resuscitation has been associated with a decrease in morbidity and mortality (Girtanner et al 1981, Orr et al 1983a).

Fiorica and colleagues (1991) reported a retrospective nonrandomized study in comparable groups, evaluating the effect of a slow infusion of concentrated albumin during the immediate 16-hour postoperative period. Twenty-eight patients undergoing pelvic exenteration for gynecologic cancer (between 1986 and 1989) were managed by one of two postoperative fluid and electrolyte regimens. Patients receiving an albumin infusion were found to have a more stable postoperative course, evidenced by the need for fewer fluid boluses ($p < .01$), fewer electrolyte bolus requirements ($p < .01$), and easier management of blood pressure and urine output. There was a 50% decrease in total fluid requirements, higher mean right atrial pressure, and a lower maintenance intravenous fluid rate. As a consequence, central hyperalimentation was started earlier and the patients receiving the albumin infusion left the intensive care unit sooner than patients receiving crystalloid.

Parenteral Hyperalimentation

Most patients are unable to tolerate an adequate oral intake until the tenth to 14th postoperative day. This, coupled with the marked catabolic response to such a major surgical procedure, may predispose to the rapid development of malnutrition, with its resultant increased risk of poor wound healing or other postoperative complications. In an effort to minimize these risks, parenteral hyperalimentation with dextrose and amino acid solutions is begun immediately postoperatively. Central venous access is established with a single- or multiple-lumen catheter (Orr et al 1994). The use of an intraoperatively placed jejunostomy feeding tube allows effective long-term enteral hyperalimentation with less expense (Ballon 1982, Orr et al 1984a) and risk of complications associated with parenteral feeding. Randomized prospective studies indicate that patients who have abdominal injury have about 65% fewer infectious complications when fed enterally rather than parenterally (Alexander 1993).

Jejunal Feeding

Spirtos and Ballon (1988) reported 60 patients having gynecologic cancer who underwent immediate postoperative feeding. Only one catheter-related complication occurred. Patients in this study group received significantly more calories and were better able to maintain serum levels of transferrin than those in the control group. He concluded that an elemental diet administered through needle catheter jejunostomy effectively maintains postoperative nutrition and is associated with few complications. Newer enteral preparations using arginine, glutamine, long-chain polyunsaturated omega 3 and omega 6 fatty acids, ribonucleic acid, and vitamins E, C, and A have been designed to pharmacologically immunoenhance nutritionally deficient patients (Alexander 1993).

Hypoproteinemia or extensive retroperitoneal dissection may result in initial intolerance to jejunal feedings. Parenteral alimentation can usually be discontinued by the fourth postoperative day, however, when most patients are able to receive at least 2500 calories by the jejunostomy tube. Before using this scheme of postoperative hyperalimentation, our patients lost 10.6% of their total body weight during an average 21-day postoperative hospital stay; since its institution, this weight loss has been reduced to 1.8%. The benefits of hyperalimentation after exenteration are justified by the evidence that it reduces the risk of sepsis and promotes healing in patients who have received radiation therapy. A decrease in the production of albumin, coupled with an increased catabolism and a shift in albumin from the intravascular to the extravascular space, leads to hypoalbuminemia. Thus, in the stressed patient, hypoalbuminemia is an excellent marker for the injury response for and an imperfect marker for nutritional deficit status.

Care of Urinary Pouches and Conduits

Postoperatively, in all catheterized pouches, the larger catheter used for drainage of the pouch should be irrigated at frequent intervals to prevent mucous obstruction. This can be performed at 4-hour intervals by simple irrigation with 45 to 50 mL of saline. At about the tenth to 12th postoperative day, a contrast study is performed to ensure that there is no pouch leakage. Mannel and coworkers (1990) reported the results of a dye pouchogram and an excretory urogram performed 2 to 3 weeks after surgery. The radiographic study showed no leakage in patients who were self-catheterized every 2 to 4 hours, with continued irrigation four times daily as long as significant mucous was present. In the early postoperative weeks, the interval between catheterization should be no more than 4 hours. Brand (1991) reported early catheterization 2 weeks postoperatively. One week later, cecal rupture occurred that was not related to suture line (technical) failure. Because of the high wall tension and reduced compliance in the irradiated cecum, most authors do not recommend catheterization of the urinary reservoir for 4 to 6 weeks and then only after a pouchogram.

Postoperatively, the silastic urinary stents are expelled on the 19th to 21st day, coinciding with the resorption of the stabilizing plain catgut sutures. No manipulation of these stents should be performed before that time. When using single J stents, we prefer to leave them in situ for 2 to 3 months.

The pelvis may be examined in the early postoperative period if indicated by sepsis or bleeding. At that time, pelvic irrigations with saline may begin and may be used on a daily basis as long as they seem beneficial.

An early examination also allows inspection to detect necrosis of myocutaneous grafts.

PERIOPERATIVE COMPLICATIONS

The risk of major complications associated with exenterative surgery is significant (Tables 12-10 and 12-11). This procedure is performed in small numbers in many individual institutions, which does not allow adequate evaluation of technical modifications designed to decrease complications. Jakowatz and associates (1985), reporting on 104 patients undergoing exenteration, indicated that the overall complication rate was 77% and the reoperation rate was 35%. Patients must also be evaluated for multiple potential complications; Jakowatz and colleagues reported 2.85 complications per patient who experienced any complication, and 2.2 complications per patient at risk.

Efforts to decrease the incidence of intraoperative hypotension include careful attention to ligation of vessels, especially those small penetrating vessels over the sacrum, at the pelvic side wall, and in the periurethral area near the pubic symphysis. Additional modifications include the use of an aortic tourniquet, hypotensive anesthesia, and pelvic packs. Although serious postoperative bleeding may be managed by reoperation, newer radiologic techniques (Fig. 12-11), using arteriographic Gelfoam or coil embolization of bleeding vessels, have given excellent results. This procedure should be considered because it is likely to be associated with less morbidity than is reexploration (Mann et al 1980).

Febrile and Infectious Complications

Febrile morbidity occurs in 75% to 85% of patients after exenteration. Pulmonary atelectasis is responsible for the fever in 40% to 70% of patients. Although some authors maintain patients on a ventilator for 48 to 72 hours postoperatively, we extubate the patient when she (1) can maintain adequate arterial oxygenation, (2) is able to generate an acceptable negative inspiratory force (more than 30 cm of H_2O), and (3) has an acceptable tidal volume (more than 700 mL). Only on rare occasions has a patient required more than 6 hours of postoperative ventilation. No patient has required reintubation in the immediate postoperative period unless she required reoperation, which has occurred in 1% of patients.

Infectious pulmonary complications are reported in fewer than 10% of exenterative patients. When pneumonia develops, however, unusual or opportunistic organisms such as *Pseudomonas* or *Serratia* may be the etiology because the patient's normal defense mechanisms are likely to be suppressed.

Pelvic cellulitis is the most common cause of infectious morbidity after pelvic exenteration. Regardless of surgical technique, the denuded and irradiated pelvis is routinely contaminated during the operative procedure. Clinically, cellulitis usually presents as a low-grade fever and slowly responds to antibiotics and irrigation of the pelvic operative site. Use of the omental carpet, myocutaneous grafts, or both has resulted in a clinical reduction in the amount of postoperative pelvic cellulitis; theoretically, the new blood supply and reduction in size of the pelvic defect will increase local defense mechanisms and improve healing.

Although less frequent, the development of a pelvic abscess after exenteration is associated with major morbidity. In our experience, the overall incidence of pelvic abscess was less than 3%; however, all 3 patients developed major urinary or intestinal complications.

The reported incidence of pyelonephritis after exenteration ranges between 5% and 20% (Orr et al 1983b, Roberts et al 1987, Soper et al 1989a). After 1 postoperative week, most urinary conduits are colonized with bacteria, which makes the diagnosis of pyelonephritis difficult. The type of urinary conduit or the introduction of a ureteral stent does not appear to alter the risk of pyelonephritis. The use of perioperative antibiotics has little effect on reducing the incidence of pyelonephritis; however, it appears that urinary prophylaxis may prevent infection if administered around the time of stent removal (Morgan et al 1980). Wound infections and dehiscence are common. The overall risk of abdominal wound infection varies between 5% and 30%. In our experience, the use of gastrointestinal staplers for bowel anastomosis and a preoperative mechanical and antibiotic bowel preparation have reduced the incidence of wound infection from 16.6% to 7.3%. Superficial skin breakdown is not uncommon.

Thromboembolic Complications

Symptomatic pulmonary emboli are reported to occur in 1% to 5% of patients after exenteration and are not infrequently stated to be the cause of postoperative deaths. Our experience indicates that thromboemboli are rarely fatal unless accompanied by other major postoperative complications (e.g., gastrointestinal or urinary fistulas). During and after exenteration, the pelvic vessels are traumatized and exposed to local infection, both of which predispose to thrombus formation. Little evidence exists that perioperative subcutaneous heparin or other forms of prophylaxis (e.g., pneumatic compression stockings) decrease the risk of

(text continues on page 286)

TABLE 12-10

Acute and Intermediate Complications After Pelvic Exenteration

ACUTE AND INTERMEDIATE	KISELOW 1967, 207 PTS (%)	KETCHAM 1970, 94 PTS (%)	SYMMONDS 1975, 198 PTS (%)	KARLEN & PIVER 1975, 87 PTS (%)	RUTLEDGE 1977, 296 PTS (%)	MORGAN 1980, 56 PTS (%)	AVERETTE 1984, 92 PTS (%)	ORR 1985, 137 PTS (%)	SOPER 1989, 69 PTS (%)	ROBERTS 1987, 38 PTS (%)	MATTHEWS 1989, 63 PTS (%)	LAWHEAD 1989, 65 PTS (%)	CUEVAS 1989, 252 PTS (%)
Cardiovascular													
Cerebrovascular accident	0.5	1.1		1.1			2.1	0.1	3.0				
Coagulopathy													
Hemorrhage	3.9	20.2	1.5	10.3	11.1*		2.1						
Myocardial infarction		3.2						0.1	1.5		3.2	6	1.2
Thromboembolism		6.4	2.0	4.6			4.3	3.6	7.0		1.6	2	1.2
Thrombophlebitis	4.3	15.6	4.5					3.6			3.2	3	
Infections													
Pelvic cellulitis	18.8†	9.6	4.0	9.2		70.0‡	3.3	36.5	17.0		19.0	58	26‡‡
Pelvic abscess		17.0	3.0	2.2				2.2		2.6			
Pneumonia		10.6				5.4		2.9	3.0				
Pyelonephritis	3.9	21.3	7.1	16.1		12.5		17.5	13.0		17.5		
Wound infection		29.8	14.6	20.7§		23.2	9.8‖	13.9	12.0		6.3		
Sepsis (not defined)				4.6	20.9¶	12.5					3.2	22	
Intestinal													
Evisceration			1.0									2	
Fistula/leak	2.9#	8.5	5.1	26.4	13.9**		16.0	6.6††	9.0	23.4		5	11.9
Obstruction	11.6	18.1	6.6	13.8			5.4	3.6	1.5	21.0	4.8	6	5.9
Bleeding									1.5				9.9
Stomal necrosis		2.1											
Psychosis	1.9				1.0			4.4					
Pulmonary													
Edema/failure	1.0	5.3		2.3			11.9					3	
Urinary													
Fistula/leak	1.4	13.8	1.0	10.3				7.3	10.0	10.5		5	198
Obstruction			1.0										
Uremia (without obstruction)					5.7						4.8	6	

*Includes cerebrovascular accidents, coagulopathy, myocardial infarction, thrombophlebitis, hemorrhage.
†Includes wound infection, pelvic abscess, cellulitis.
‡Cellulitis and abscess.
§Includes wound infection, dehiscence, and hernia.
‖Dehiscence.
¶All sources.
#Urinary and gastrointestinal fistulas.
**Includes obstruction and fistulas.
††Small bowel.
‡‡All infections.

TABLE 12-11
Late Complications After Pelvic Exenteration

	KISELOW 1967, 191 PTS (%)	KETCHAM 1970, 73 PTS (%)	SYMMONDS 1975, 183 PTS (%)	KARLEN & PIVER 1975, 65 PTS (%)	RUTLEDGE 1977, 256 PTS (%)	MORGAN 1980, (%)	ORR 1985, 125 PTS (%)	SOPER 1989, 69 PTS (%)
Intestinal								
Fistula	5.8	8.2	8.2	—	—	—	1.6	10.0
Hernia	2.6	—	—	—	—	—	—	—
Stoma revision	8.4	8.2	—	4.6	4.6*	—	2.4	—
Obstruction	6.3	21.9	5.5	—	—	5.1	5.6	3.0
Urinary								
Calculi	1.0	5.5	—	—	—	—	2.4	—
Infection	6.3	24.7	3.8	21.5	12.1	—	14.4	—
Loss of renal unit or procedure to prevent same	1.6	13.7	1.6	—	—	—	3.2	—
Stoma revision	7.3	—	—	7.7	—	—	2.4	—
Fistula	—	—	3.2	—	—	—	0.8	—
Pelvic abscess or sinus	3.7	—	—	—	—	—	—	4.0

*Fecal or urinary stoma.

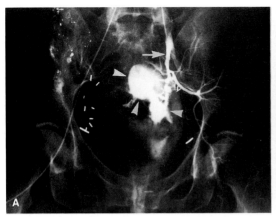
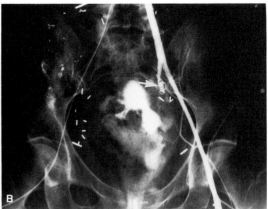

FIGURE 12-11. Postoperative hemorrhage 14 days after exenteration in a 48-year-old woman. (**A**) Bleeding from the hypogastric artery, demonstrated by arteriogram. Acute extravasation of contrast (*arrowheads*) is seen from a branch of the hypogastric artery (*arrow*). (**B**) Steel coil hypogastric artery embolization (*arrow*) stopped the hemorrhage immediately. Residual contrast from previous extravasation is still present.

embolic prophylaxis; some authors advocate intraoperative inferior vena caval occlusion (Girtanner et al 1981).

A rare but important etiology of postoperative febrile morbidity is septic pelvic thrombophlebitis (Dunn et al 1967). Patients with spiking temperatures and tachycardia that are unresponsive to antibiotics should be suspect. Systemic heparinization results in rapid defervescence.

Gastrointestinal Complications

Although the incidence of many complications (e.g., blood loss, sepsis, or cardiovascular accidents) has decreased, reports indicate that the single most life-threatening complication is the development of a gastrointestinal obstruction or fistula. Although prolonged postoperative ileus is frequent, the risk of small bowel obstruction varies between 5% and 10% and is not related to the magnitude of the surgical procedure. Attempts to decrease this risk by "stenting" the small bowel with a long intestinal tube have not proved helpful. There is still controversy concerning the optimal protective type of pelvic closure; however, most authors agree that placing the ileum or small bowel into the denuded pelvis without some type of protective covering predisposes it to a dense fibrotic reaction, increasing the risk of obstruction. In our previous report (Orr et al 1983b), the most common factor associated with obstruction was an anastomosis in the irradiated small bowel, performed after the construction of an ileal conduit. In contrast, no patient having a transverse colon conduit and adequate pelvic closure has suffered this complication. Obstruction,

abdominal distention, and postoperative nausea and vomiting require prompt management. Immediate attention to prevent electrolyte and volume depletion, sepsis, and aspiration are imperative. A small barium meal demonstrates the point of obstruction within 30 minutes and the barium usually spills into the colon within 2 hours if obstruction is not present (Han et al 1979). Initial management with a long intestinal tube may be preferable to surgery, especially considering reports in which a second operative procedure in the immediate postoperative period may carry a mortality rate of 20% to 50%. A reoperation in an irradiated pelvis may be made extremely difficult by dense adhesions and fibrosis, increasing the risk of inadvertent enterotomies and possible disruption of the urinary conduit.

If surgery is necessary, controversy exists regarding the appropriate operative procedure to relieve small bowel obstruction in previously irradiated small bowel. Some authors report less postoperative morbidity when the entire affected segment is resected; however, we usually perform a simple bypass procedure. If at least 60 cm of functional small bowel can be preserved and there is no evidence of bowel necrosis, the bypass procedure can be performed with minimal morbidity or mortality.

Rectovaginal fistulas after anterior exenteration are not uncommon. Dissection of the rectovaginal septum in the presence of progressive irradiation fibrosis and endarteritis probably leads to altered rectal blood supply, thereby predisposing the patient to a fistula. With the development of such a fistula, there may be difficulty controlling infection in the pelvis, and healing may be delayed. Even in patients undergoing colostomy for such fistulas, surgical mortality is high (33%; Orr et al 1983b).

Bowel Fistulas

Gastrointestinal fistulas involving small bowel after exenteration occur in 5% to 10% of patients and are associated with mortality in 30% to 40% of patients (Clark et al 1962, Devereux et al 1980, Orr et al 1983b). The irradiated ileum is the most common site of the fistula, and few spontaneous closures (less than 15%) occur despite the use of hyperalimentation. Although several authors (Piver et al 1976) stress the importance of obtaining a fistulogram and early operative intervention, the appropriate surgical procedure (bypass versus resection) to correct this fistula is not known. We favor a trial of hyperalimentation for 3 to 4 weeks; however, when surgery is elected, we usually favor intestinal resection rather than bypass to eliminate the risk of subsequent bowel necrosis. Postoperative gastrointestinal obstruction occurs in as many as 11% of patients (Bricker 1970). A conservative method (intestinal suction) is the preferred initial treatment. Reoperation carries a high mortality.

Curtin and coworkers (1990) reported a patient who developed an enteroneovaginal fistula after total pelvic exenteration. The patient was successfully treated with a somatostatin analogue—a tetradecapeptide that is produced by the hypothalamus and pancreas and has an inhibitory effect on gastric, biliary, pancreatic, and intestinal secretions. Additionally, somatostatin decreases intestinal motility. There have been reports that somatostatin or somatostatin analogues increase the spontaneous closure of enterocutaneous fistulas and shorten the time of spontaneous closure. Additionally, failure of somatostatin or somatostatin analogue may also aid in the early identification of patients who are not responsive to conservative management and require surgical intervention as treatment.

Urinary Tract

Postoperative complications involving the urinary tract are serious. Subclinical urinary leaks after supravesical urinary diversion probably occur and may close spontaneously. The development of a conduit-to-cutaneous or conduit-to-pelvic defect urinary fistula is serious. Possible etiologies include (1) conduit necrosis secondary to compromised blood supply, (2) disruption of one or both ureteral anastomosis (particularly in irradiated bowel segments), or (3) disruption of the closed end of the conduit. The incidence decreases with increasing operative experience (Symmonds et al 1975, Morley et al 1976). Additionally, the use of the transverse colon conduit initially described by Nelson (1969) allows the anastomosis to be made in nonirradiated bowel while displacing the ureteral anastomosis away from the pelvic defect. Reoperation to repair the urinary leak has been associated with significant (30% to 50%) mortality and should be reserved for those women having life-threatening infection, deterioration of renal function, or complex fistulas. In our reports, conservative management is associated with spontaneous closure in 30% of patients, although strictures of ureters may result in loss of some kidneys (Barber et al 1967, 1969, Orr et al 1982). This conservative approach has been challenged by some (Soper et al 1989a, Roberts et al 1987) who advocate aggressive surgical management with lower (8%) reoperative mortality rate.

Postoperative depression, disorientation, and occasionally frank psychosis may be encountered. Infectious, metabolic, or cardiac etiologies should be considered in these situations because correction of these abnormalities usually results in the return of a normal mental status.

Operative mortality is increased with age, increased in patients undergoing total exenteration, and decreased as the experience of the surgical team increases. The reported operative mortality varies between 7% and 37% (Tables 12-12 and 12-13).

TABLE 12-12
Surgical Mortality of Patients With Recurrent Cervical Cancer Treated by Exenteration

STUDY	YEAR	PATIENTS (N)	SURGICAL MORTALITY
Ingersoll, et al	1966	87	15.0
Brunschwig	1967	312	17.3
Ingiulla & Cosmi	1967	100	37.0
Kiselow, et al	1967	207	7.8
Ketcham, et al	1970	90	22.0
Creasman, et al	1972	156	16.0
Averette, et al	1984	92	23.9
Shingleton, et al	1985	156	7.7
Talledo	1985	42	23.8*
Roberts, et al	1987	38	5.3
Cuevas, et al	1988	252	17.4
Morley, et al	1989	100	2.0
Soper, et al	1989a	69	7.2
Shepherd	1989	52	6.0
Lawhead, et al	1989	65	9.2
Stanhope, et al	1990	133	6.7
Matthews, et al	1992	63	11.0

*Patients ≥65.

TABLE 12-13
Causes of Postoperative Deaths After Exenteration

	KETCHAM (%)	KARLEN (%)	MATTHEWS (%)	CUEVAS (%)	ORR (%)
Cardiac event	9.5	—	14.3	—	16.7
Cerebrovascular accident	—	8.3	—	—	—
Hemorrhage	14.3	25.0	—	11.6	8.3
Hepatitis	—	8.3	—	—	—
Ileofemoral thrombosis	—	—	—	—	8.3
Pneumonia	4.8	—	—	18.7	8.3
Pulmonary	—	8.3	—	—	—
Renal failure	9.5	—	28	—	—
Sepsis	42.9	33.3	57	55.8	33.3
Thromboembolism	19.0	8.3	—	16.3	25.0
Unknown	—	8.3	—	—	—

The most common causes of operative mortality are sepsis, pulmonary embolus, and hemorrhage. The first two causes usually constitute 50% of operative deaths, and a complicated and prolonged postoperative course associated with a fistula is the usual occurrence.

LONG-TERM POSTOPERATIVE MANAGEMENT

Psychologic and social stresses are experienced by patients after pelvic exenteration. Dempsey and associates (1975) noted the importance of the adequate preoperative contact between physician and patient and the necessity for presenting the nature of the recurrent tumor in a manner that prevents the patient from equating recurrence with death. Unrealistic expectations, denial, and high anxiety levels appear to be detrimental to postoperative adjustment. Postoperative intervention by the physicians, nurses, and stomal therapists is essential. The actual ability of the patient to accept and manage the colostomy and the conduit depends on the instructions and concerns of the healthcare team. Most (80%) return to work and are able to resume a nearly normal lifestyle within 4 to 6 months. Reports on patients followed-up for longer than 3 years indicate that their overall psychologic adjustment is good, indicating that the negative reaction of many physicians to pelvic exenteration may be unfounded.

In some series (Anthopoulos et al 1989), few patients (16%) survive without rehospitalization. Unfortunately, many serious complications (58%) requiring surgical intervention occur more than 1 year after resection and many complications that were managed conservatively (74%) occur within the first postoperative year.

Late Urinary Tract and Bowel Complications

Long-term follow-up of exenteration patients is important, not only to aid in psychologic rehabilitation but to detect and treat the late complications of ultraradical surgery. The most common non–cancer-related indication for rehospitalization is associated with problems in the urinary tract, especially pyelonephritis. Although most urinary conduits are colonized with urinary pathogens, the exact significance of asymptomatic bacteriuria of the conduit is unknown. If pyelonephritis occurs repeatedly, the urinary tract should be investigated (Fig. 12-12). As many as 10% of those patients rehospitalized require revision of the urinary conduit stoma; previously irradiated ileum is not infrequently associated with stomal stricture, leading to partial urinary obstruction.

Late unilateral ureteral obstruction or stricture in the absence of infection or deteriorating renal function does not necessarily require conduit revision. Close observation and evaluation with renal scans, intravenous pyelography, and serum creatinine testing is indicated, however. If deterioration of renal function is evident, an intervening percutaneous nephrostomy (Mann et al 1983) may be performed to better decide whether the conduit should be revised or the kidney salvaged.

Non–cancer-related gastrointestinal complications occur in 10% to 15% of patients, including colostomy prolapse that requires revision and late small bowel obstruction.

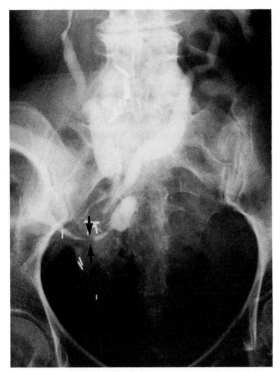

FIGURE 12-12. Investigation of the lower urinary tract 3 years after exenteration indicated a stricture in the mid-segment of the ileal conduit (*arrows*) in a woman with recurrent urinary tract infection and abdominal pain. Also note severe hydroureter bilaterally.

Observation for Recurrence: Long-Term Survival

After exenteration, bimanual examination is difficult or impossible. Pelvic-defect cytology is collected at each visit. Any unusual discharge or bleeding requires investigation because the pelvis is the site of disease in more than 50% of those having recurrence. Recurrence of tumor after exenteration is associated with a short survival. The average survival after recurrence is 5.2 months after anterior exenteration and 2.8 months after total exenteration (Shingleton et al 1989).

References

Achauer BM, Braly P, Berman ML, DiSaia PJ. Immediate vaginal reconstruction following resection for malignancy using the gluteal thigh flap. Gynecol Oncol 1984;19:79.

Adams MC, Bihrle R, Foster RS, Brito CG. Conversion of an ileal conduit to a continent catheterizable stoma. J Urol 1992;147:126.

Adcock LL. Radical hysterectomy preceded by pelvic irradiation. Gynecol Oncol 1979;8:152.

Ahlering TE, Kanellos A, Boyd SD, et al. Comparative study of perioperative complications with Kock pouch urinary diversion in highly irradiated versus nonirradiated patients. J Urol 1988;139:1202.

Alexander JW. Immunoenhancement via enteral nutrition. Arch Surg 1993;128:1242.

Anthopoulos AP, Manetta A, Larson JE, Podczaski ES, Bartholomew MJ, Mortel R. Pelvic exenteration: a morbidity and mortality analysis of a seven-year experience. Gynecol Oncol 1989;35:219.

Averette HE, Lichtinger M, Seven B-U, Girtanner RE. Pelvic exenteration: a 15-year experience in a general metropolitan hospital. Am J Obstet Gynecol 1984;150:179.

Axelrod JH, Fruchter R, Boyce JG. Multiple primaries among gynecologic malignancies. Gynecol Oncol 1984; 18:359.

Badib AO, Kurohara SS, Webster JH, Pickren JW. Metastasis to organs in carcinoma of the uterine cervix. Cancer 1968;21:434.

Ballon SC. Effective early postoperative nutrition by defined formula diet via needle catheter jejunostomy. Gynecol Oncol 1982;14:23.

Barber HRK, Brunschwig A. Excision of major blood vessels at the periphery of the pelvis in patients receiving pelvic exenteration: common and/or iliac arteries and veins. Surgery 1967;62:426.

Barber HRK, Jones W. Lymphadenectomy in pelvic exenteration for recurrent cervix cancer. JAMA 1971; 215(12):1945.

Barber HRK. Relative prognostic significance of preoperative and operative findings in pelvic exenteration. Surg Clin NA 1969;49:431.

Barter JF, Sanz LE. Staplers for gynecologic surgery—what's available. Contemp OB/GYN 1986;28:87.

Becker DW Jr, Massey FM, McCraw JB. Musculocutaneous flaps in reconstructive pelvic surgery. Obstet Gynecol 1979;54:178.

Beemer W, Hopkins MP, Morley GW. Vaginal reconstruction in gynecologic oncology. Obstet Gynecol 1988; 72:911.

Bender HG. Personal experiences with exenterations in patients with gynecologic malignancies. Clin Exp Obstet Gynecol 1992;19(4):270.

Benson C, Soisson AP, Carlson J, et al. Neovaginal reconstruction with a rectus abdominis myocutaneous flap. Obstet Gynecol 1993;81(5):871.

Benson MC, Olsson CA. Urinary diversion. Urol Clin North Am 1992;19:779.

Berek JS, Hacker NF, Lagasse LD. Rectosigmoid colectomy and reanastomosis to facilitate resection of primary and recurrent gynecologic cancer. Obstet Gynecol 1984a; 64:715.

Berek JS, Hacker NF, Lagasse LD. Vaginal reconstruction performed simultaneously with pelvic exentreation. Obstet Gynecol 1984b:63:318.

Bissada NK, Marshall IY, Kaczmarek A. Continent urinary diversion and bladder substitution. J SC Med Assoc 1993;89:435.

Bjornstahl H, Johnsson JE, Lindberg LG. Hysterectomy in central recurrence of carcinoma of the uterine cervix. Acta Obstet Gynecol Scand 1977;56:227.

Bloch WE, Bejany DE, Penalver MA, Politano VA. Complications of the Miami pouch. J Urol 1992;147:1017.

Blythe JG, Ptacek JJ, Buchsbaum HJ, Latourette HB. Bony metastases from carcinoma of the cervix. Cancer 1975;36:475.

Brand E. Cecal rupture after continent ileocecal urinary diversion during total pelvic exenteration. Obstet Gynecol 1991;78:570.

Brascho DJ. Gynecologic malignancy. In Brascho DJ, Shawker TH, eds. Abdominal ultrasound in the cancer patient. New York: John Wiley, 1980:209.

Bricker EM. Current status of urinary diversion. Cancer 1980;45:2986.

Bricker EM. Pelvic exenteration. Adv Surg 1970;4:13.

Brown RS, Haddox V, Posada A, Rubio A. Social and psychological adjustment following pelvic exenteration. Am J Obstet Gynecol 1972;114:162.

Brunschwig A. Surgical treatment of carcinoma of the cervix, recurrent after irradiation or combination of irradiation and surgery. Am J Roentgenol, Rad Ther, Nuc Med 1967;99:365.

Buchsbaum HJ, Christopherson W, Lifshitz S, Bernstein S. Vicryl mesh in pelvic floor reconstruction. Arch Surg 1985;120:1389.

Burke TW, Hoskins WJ, Heller PB, et al. Clinical patterns of tumor recurrence after radical hysterectomy in stage IB cervical carcinoma. Obstet Gynecol 1987;69:382.

Butcher HR Jr, Sugg WL, McAfee CA, Bricker EM. Ileal conduit method of ureteral urinary diversion. Ann Surg Oct 1962;156:682.

Cain JM, Diamond A, Tamimi HK, Greer BE, Figge DC. The morbidity and benefits of concurrent gracilis myocutaneous graft with pelvic exenteration. Obstet Gynecol 1989;74:185.

Chen SS, Kumari S, Lee L. Contribution of abdominal computed tomography (CT) in the management of gynecologic cancer: correlated study of CT image and gross surgical pathology. Gynecol Oncol 1980;10:162.

Chiou RK, Taylor RJ, Mays SD. Has the pendulum swung too far for continent diversion? A case for ileal conduit. Semin Urol 1993;XI(2):99.

Clark DGC, Daniel WW, Brunschwig A. Intestinal fistulae following pelvic exenteration. Am J Obstet Gynecol 1962;84:187.

Clarke EA, Kreiger N, Spengler RF. Second primary cancer following treatment for cervical cancer. Can Med Assoc J 1984;131:553.

Clarke-Pearson DL, Soper JT, Creasman WT. Absorbable synthetic mesh (polyglactin 910) for the formation of a pelvic "lid" after radical pelvic resection. Am J Obstet Gynecol 1988;258:258.

Cohen AM. Colon J-pouch rectal reconstruction after total or subtotal proctectomy. World J Surg 1993;17:267.

Coleman R, Keeney E, Freedman R, Burke T, Eifel P, Rutledge F. Radical hysterectomy for recurrent carcinoma of the uterine cervix after radiotherapy (abstract). 25th Annual Meeting, Society of Gynecologic Oncologists, Orlando, Florida, February 6 1994.

Copeland LJ, Hancock KC, Gershenson DM, et al. Gracilis myocutaneous vaginal reconstruction concurrent with total pelvic exenteration. Am J Obstet Gynecol 1989; 160:1095.

Creasman WT, Rutledge F. Is positive pelvic lymphadenopathy a contraindication to radical surgery in recurrent cervical carcinoma. Gynecol Oncol 1974;2:482.

Creasman WT, Rutledge F. Preoperative evaluation of patients with recurrent carcinoma of the cervix. Gynecol Oncol 1972;1:111.

Cruse PJ, Foord R. The epidemiology of wound infection. A 10-year prospective study of 62,939 wounds. Surg Clin North Am 1980;60:27.

Cuevas HR, Torres A, DeLaGarza M, Hernandez D, Herrera L. Pelvic exenteration for carcinoma of the cervix: analysis of 252 cases. J Surg Oncol 1988;38:121.

Curtin JP, Wheelock JP, Burt LL. Case report: successful treatment of small intestine fistula with somatostatin analog. Gynecol Oncol 1990;39:225.

Day TG, Stanhope R. Vulvovaginoplasty in gynecologic oncology. Obstet Gynecol 1977;50(3):361.

Deckers PJ, Sugarbaker EV, Pilch YH, Ketcham AS. Pelvic exenteration for late second cancers of the uterine cervix after earlier irradiation. Ann Surg 1972;175:48.

Dempsey GM, Buchsbaum HJ, Morrison J. Psychosocial adjustment to pelvic exenteration. Gynecol Oncol 1975; 3:325.

Devereux DG, Sears HG, Ketcham AS. Intestinal fistula following pelvic exenterative surgery: predisposing causes and treatment. J Surg Oncol 1980;14:227.

Dunn LJ, VanVoorhis LW. Enigmatic fever and pelvic thrombophlebitis. Response to anticoagulants. N Engl J Med 1967;276:265.

Evers BM, Townsend CM Jr, Thompson JC. Organ physiology of aging. Surg Clin North Am 1994;74(1):23.

Farquharson DIM, Orr JW Jr. Thromboembolic complications in gynecology. J Reprod Med 1984;29:845.

Filtenborg TA, Hansen HH, et al. A phase II study of ifosfamide, carboplatin and cisplatin in advanced and recurrent squamous cell carcinoma of the uterine cervix. Ann Oncol 1993;4:485.

Fiorica JV, Roberts WS, Hoffman MS, et al. Concentrated albumin infusion as an aid to postoperative recovery after pelvic exenteration. Gynecol Oncol 1991;43:265.

Freundt I, Toolenaar T, et al. Long-term psychosexual and psychosocial performance of patients with a sigmoid neovagina. Am J Obstet Gynecol 1993;169:1210.

Freundt I, Toolenaar T, Jeekel H, et al. Prolapse of the sigmoid neovagina: report of three cases. Obstet Gynecol 1994;83:876.

Gelister JSK, Woodhouse CRJ. Role of continent suprapubic diversion in pelvic cancer. Br J Urol 1991;68:176.

Girtanner RE, DeCampo T, Alleyn JN, Averette HE. Routine intensive care for pelvic exenterative operations. Surg Gynecol Obstet 1981;153:657.

Griffin FD, Knight CD Sr, Knight CD Jr. Results of the double stapling procedure in pelvic surgery. World J Surg 1992;16:866.

Haas T, Buchsbaum HJ, Lifshitz S. Nonresectable recurrent pelvic neoplasm: outcome in patients explored for pelvic exenteration. Gynecol Oncol 1980;9:177.

Haddad FS, Campbell OP. Lithiasis in the ileal conduit and

the continent urinary pouch: two cases and a review. Urol Int 1992;49:114.

Hall MC, Koch MO, McDougal WS. Metabolic consequences of urinary diversion through intestinal segments. Urol Clin North Am 1991;18:725.

Han SY, Laws HL, Aldrete JS. How and when to use barium for diagnosis of small bowel obstruction. South Med J 1979;72:1519.

Harbrecht PJ, Garrison RN, Fry DE. Surgery in elderly patients. South Med J 1981;74:594.

Harris WJ, Wheeless CR Jr. Use of the end-to-end anastomosis stapling device in low colorectal anatomosis associated with radical gynecologic surgery. Gynecol Oncol 1986;23:350.

Hatch KD. Construction of a neovagina following exenteration utilizing the vulvo-bulbocavernosus myocutaneous graft. Obstet Gynecol 1984a;63:110.

Hatch KD, Gelder MS, Soong S-J, Baker VV, Shingleton HM. Pelvic exenteration with low rectal anastomosis: survival, complications, and prognostic factors. Gynecol Oncol 1990;38:462.

Hatch KD, Parham G, Shingleton HM, Orr JW Jr, Austin JM Jr. Ureteral strictures and fistulae following radical hysterectomy. Gynecol Oncol 1984b;19:17.

Hatch KD, Shingleton HM, Potter ME, Baker VV. Low rectal resection and anastomosis at the time of pelvic exenteration. Gynecol Oncol 1988a;32:262.

Hatch KD, Shingleton HM, Song S-J, Baker VV, Gelder MS. Anterior pelvic exenteration. Gynecol Oncol 1988b;31:205.

Hoffman MS, Fiorica JV, Roberts WS, et al. Williams' vulvo-vaginoplasty after supralevator total pelvic exenteration. South Med J 1991;84(1):43.

Hoffman MS, Roberts WS, LaPolla JP, et al. Use of Vicryl mesh in the reconstruction of the pelvic floor following exenteration. Gynecol Oncol 1989;35:170.

Hogan MW, Boente MP. The role of surgery in the management of recurrent gynecologic cancer. Semin Oncol 1993;20(5):462.

Hoye RC, Bennett SH, Geelhoed GW, Gorschboth C. Fluid volume and albumin kinetics occurring with major surgery. JAMA 1972;222:1255.

Ingersoll FM, Ulfelder H. Pelvic exenteration for carcinoma of the cervix. N Engl J Med 1966;274:648.

Ingiulla W, Cosmi EV. Pelvic exenteration for advanced carcinoma of the cervix. Am J Obstet Gynecol 1967;99:1083.

Jakowatz JG, Porudominsky D, Riihimaki DU, et al. Complications of pelvic exenteration. Arch Surg 1985;120:1261.

Jones MA, Breckman B, Hendry WF. Life with an ileal conduit: results of questionnaire surveys of patients and urological surgeons. Br J Urol 1980;52:21.

Jones WB. New approaches to high-risk cervical cancer. Advanced cervical cancer. Cancer 1993;71:1451.

Jones WB. Surgical approaches for advanced or recurrent cancer of the cervix. Cancer 1987;60:2094.

Judd ES. Preoperative neomycin-tetracycline preparation of the colon for elective operations. Surg Clin North Am 1975;55:1325.

Karlen JR, Piver MS. Reduction of mortality and morbidity associated with pelvic exenteration. Gynecol Oncol 1975;3:154.

Ketcham AS, Chretien PB, Hoye RC, et al. Occult metastases to the scalene lymph nodes in patients with clinically operable carcinoma of the cervix. Cancer 1973;31:180.

Ketcham AS, Deckers PJ, Sugarbaker EV, et al. Pelvic exenteration for carcinoma of the uterine cervix, a 15-year experience. Cancer 1970;26:513.

Kilgore LC, Orr JW Jr, Hatch KD, Shingleton HM, Roberson J. Peritoneal cytology in patients with squamous cell carcinoma of the cervix. Gynecol Oncol 1984;19:24.

Kiselow M, Butcher HR Jr, Bricker EM. Results of the radical surgical treatment of advanced pelvic cancer: a 15-year study. Ann Surg 1967;166:428.

Kleinerman RA, Curtis RE, Boice JD Jr, et al. Second cancers following radiotherapy for cervical cancer. J Natl Cancer Inst 1982;69:1027.

Kock NG, Nilsson LO, Norlen LJ, et al. Urinary diversion via a continent ileal reservoir: clinical results in 12 patients. J Urol 1982;128:469.

Koonings PP. Neovaginal procidentia. Ann Plast Surg 1993;30:466.

Kottmeier HL. The treatment by fulguration of recurrent cancer of the cervix following radiation. In Meigs J, ed. The surgical treatment of cancer of the cervix. New York: Grune & Stratton, 1954:412.

Kusiak JF. Considerations for reconstruction after surgery for recurrent cancer. Semin Oncol 1993;20:430.

Lacey CG, Stern JL, Feigenbaum, et al. Vaginal construction after exenteration with use of gracilis myocutaneous flaps: the University of California, San Francisco experience. Am J Obstet Gynecol 1988;158:1278.

Lagasse LD, Johnson GH, McClure LS, et al. Use of sigmoid colon for rectal substitution following pelvic exenteration. Am J Obstet Gynecol 1973;116:106.

Lagasse LD, Smith ML, Moore JG, et al. The effect of radiation therapy on pelvic lymph node involvement in stage I carcinoma of the cervix. Am J Obstet Gynecol 1974;119:328.

Lawhead RA Jr, Clark DGC, Smith DH, et al. Pelvic exenteration for recurrent or persistent gynecologic malignancies: a 10-year review of the Memorial Sloan-Kettering Cancer Center experience (1972–1981). Gynecol Oncol 1989;33:279.

Lee HP, Cuello C, Singh K. Review of the epidemiology of cervical cancer in the Pacific Basin. NCI Monograph 1982;62:197.

Lee RB, Weisbaum GS, Heller PB, Park RC. Scalene node biopsy in primary and recurrent invasive carcinoma of the cervix. Gynecol Oncol 1981;11:200.

Lichtinger M. Small bowel complications after supravesical urinary diversion in pelvic exenteration (abstract). 16th Annual Meeting of the Society of Gynecologic Oncologists, Miami, Florida, February 3–6, 1985.

Magrina JF. Types of pelvic exenterations: a reappraisal. Gynecol Oncol 1990;37:363.

Magrina JF, Symmonds RE, Leary FJ. Intentional ureteral ligation in advanced malignant disease. Obstet Gynecol 1979;53:685.

Manetta A, Podczaski ES, Larson JE, DeGrest K, Mortel R. Scalene lymph node biopsy in the preoperative evaluation of patients with recurrent cervical cancer. Gynecol Oncol 1989;33:332.

Mann WJ Jr, Hatch KD, Taylor PT, et al. The role of percutaneous nephrostomy in gynecologic oncology. Gynecol Oncol 1983;16:393.

Mann WJ Jr, Jander HP, Orr JW Jr, et al. The use of percutaneous nephrostomy in gynecologic oncology. Gynecol Oncol 1980;10:343.

Mannel RS, Braly PS, Buller RE. Indiana pouch continent urinary reservoir in patients with previous pelvic irradiation. Obstet Gynecol 1990;75:891.

Mannel RS, Manetta A, Buller R, Braly P, Walker J, Archer S. Use of ileocecal continent urinary reservoir in patients with previous pelvic irradiation (abstract). 23rd Annual Meeting of the Society of Gynecologic Oncologists, San Antonio, Texas, March 15–18, 1992.

Matsuyama T, Tsukamoto N, Imachi M, Nakano H. Bone metastasis from cervix cancer. Gynecol Oncol 1989; 32:72.

Matthews C, Morris M, Burke T, Gershenson D, Wharton J, Rutledge P. Pelvic exenteration in the elderly patient. Obstet Gynecol 1992;79:773.

Mattingly RF. Indications, contraindications, and method of total pelvic exenteration. Oncology 1967;21:241.

McCraw JB, Massey FM, Shanklin KD, Horton CE. Vaginal reconstruction with gracilis myocutaneous flaps. Plast Reconstr Surg 1976;58:176.

McMahon MM, Farnell MB, Murray MJ. Nutritional support of critically ill patients. Mayo Clin Proc 1993; 68:911.

Miller B, Morris M, Rutledge F, Mitchell MF, et al. Aborted exenterative procedures in recurrent cervical cancer. Gynecol Oncol 1993;50:94.

Montz FJ, Wheeler JH, Lau LM. Inability of polyglycolic acid mesh to inhibit immediate post-radical pelvic surgery adhesions. Gynecol Oncol 1990;38:230.

Morgan LS, Daly JW, Monif GRG. Infectious morbidity associated with pelvic exenteration. Gynecol Oncol 1980;10:318.

Morley GW, Hopkins MP, Lindenauer SM, Roberts JA. Pelvic exenteration, University of Michigan: 100 patients at 5 years. Obstet Gynecol 1989;74:934.

Morley GW, Lindenauer SM. Pelvic exenterative therapy for gynecologic malignancy: an analysis of 70 cases. Cancer 1976;38:581.

Morley GW, Lindenauer SM, Youngs D. Vaginal reconstruction following pelvic exenteration: surgical and psychological considerations. Am J Obstet Gynecol 1973; 116:996.

Morley GW. Pelvic exenterative therapy and the treatment of recurrent carcinoma of the cervix. Semin Oncol 1982;9:331.

Morrow CP, Hernandez WL, Townsend DE, DiSaia PJ. Pelvic celiotomy in the obese patient. Am J Obstet Gynecol 1977;127:335.

Nelson JH Jr. Atlas of radical pelvic surgery. New York: Appleton-Century-Crofts, 1969:181.

Orovan WL, David IR. Urinary diversion using the Koch ileal reservoir in patients with irradiated bowel. Can J Surg 1988;31:2433.

Orr JW Jr, Cornwell A, Wilson K, et al. Nutritional status of patients with untreated cervical cancer. Am J Obstet Gynecol 1984a;151:625.

Orr JW Jr, Hatch KD, Shingleton HM, et al. Gastrointestinal complications associated with pelvic exenteration. Am J Obstet Gynecol 1983a;145:325.

Orr JW Jr, Orr PF, Barrett JM, Ellington JR, Jennings RH, Paredes K, et al. Fascial closure: continuous or interrupted? A prospective evaluation of #1 Maxon suture in 402 gynecologic procedures. Am J Obstet Gynecol 1990;163:1485.

Orr JW Jr, Shingleton HM. Choosing the best diversion in gynecological patients. Contemp Obstet Gynecol 1983b: 22:253.

Orr JW Jr, Shingleton HM, Hatch KD, et al. Urinary diversion in patients undergoing pelvic exenteration. Am J Obstet Gynecol 1982;142:883.

Orr JW Jr, Shingleton HM. Importance of nutritional support in the surgical patient. J Reprod Med 1984b; 29:635.

Orr JW Jr. Pulmonary complications. In Orr JW Jr, Shingleton HM (eds). Complications of gynecologic surgery: prevention, recognition and management. Philadelphia: JB Lippincott, 1994.

Orr JW Jr, Shingleton HM, Soong S-J, et al. Hemodynamic parameters following pelvic exenteration. Am J Obstet Gynecol 1983c;146:882.

Orr JW Jr, Taylor PT. Reducing postoperative infection in the patient with gynecologic cancer. Infect Surg 1987; 6:666.

Parker TH, O'Leary JP. Effect of preparation of the small intestine on microflora and postoperative wound infection. Surg Gynecol Obstet 1978;146:379.

Patsner B, Mann WJ, Chalas E, Orr JW Jr. Intestinal complications associated with the use of Dexon mesh sling in gynecologic surgery. Gynecol Oncol 1990;38:146.

Paty PB, Enker WE. Coloanal anastomosis following low anterior resection. J Gastroenterol 1992;39:202.

Paunier J-P, Delclos L, Fletcher GH. Causes, time of death, and sites of failure in squamous cell carcinoma of the uterine cervix on intact uterus. Radiology 1967;88: 555.

Pearlman NW, Donohue RE, Wettlaufer JN, Stiegmann GV. Continent ileocolonic urinary reservoirs for filling and lining the post-exenteration pelvis. Am J Surgery 1990;160:634.

Penalver MA, Bejany DE, Donato DM, Sevin B-U, Averette HE. Functional characteristics and follow up of the continent ileal colonic urinary reservoir. Cancer 1993;71(4):1667.

Penalver MA, Donato D, Sevin B-U, Block WE, Alvarez WJ, Averette H. Complications of the ileocolonic continent urinary reservoir (Miami Pouch). Gynecol Oncol 1994;52:360.

Perez-Mesa C, Spratt JS Jr. Scalene node biopsy in the pretreatment staging of carcinoma of the cervix uteri. Am J Obstet Gynecol 1976;125:93.

Pierson RL, Figge PK, Buchsbaum HJ. Surgery for gynecologic malignancy in the aged. Obstet Gynecol 1975; 46:523.

Piver MS, Barlow JJ. Para-aortic lymphadenectomy, aortic node biopsy, and aortic lymphangiography in staging patients with advanced cervical cancer. Cancer 1973; 32:367.

Piver MS, Lele S. Enterovaginal and enterocutaneous fistulae in women with gynecologic malignancies. Obstet Gynecol 1976;48:560.

Popovich MJ, Hricak H, Sugimura K, Stern JL. The role of MR imaging in determining surgical eligibility for pelvic exenteration. Am J Roentgenol 1993;160:525.

Potter ME, Alvarez RD, Gay FL, Shingleton HM, Soong S-J, Hatch KD. Optimal therapy for pelvic recurrence after radical hysterectomy for early-stage cervical cancer. Gynecol Oncol 1990;37:74.

Powers JC, Fitzgerald JF, McAlvanah MJ. The anatomic basis for the surgical detachment of the greater omentum from the transverse colon. Surg Gynecol Obstet 1976;143:105.

Prempree T, Patanaphan V, Sewchand W, Scott RM. The influence of patient's age and tumor grade on the progress of carcinoma of the cervix. Cancer 1983; 51:1764.

Prudden JF. Psychological problems following ileostomy and colostomy. Cancer 1971;28:236.

Pursell SH, Day TG Jr, Tobin GR. Distally based rectus abdominis flap for reconstruction in radical gynecologic procedures. Gynecol Oncol 1990;37:2348.

Roberts WS, Cavanagh D, Bryson SCP, Lyman GH, Hewitt S. Major morbidity after pelvic exenteration: a seven-year experience. Obstet Gynecol 1987;69:617.

Roddick JW, Miller DH. Factors affecting the management of recurrent cervical carcinoma. Am J Obstet Gynecol 1968;101:53.

Rowland RG, Mitchell ME, Bihrle R. Alternative techniques for a continent urinary reservoir. Urol Clin North Am 1987;14:797.

Rubin SC, Hoskins WJ, Lewis JL Jr. Radical hysterectomy for recurrent cervical cancer following radiation therapy. Gynecol Oncol 1987;27:316.

Rutledge FN. Gynecologic oncology—1982–2002. 1982 Janeway lecture, American Radium Society. Am J Clin Oncol 1982;5:471.

Rutledge FN, Fletcher GH, McDonald EJ. Pelvic lymphadenectomy as an adjunct to radiation therapy in treatment for cancer of the cervix. Am J Roentgenol 1965;93:607.

Rutledge FN, Fletcher GH. Transperitoneal pelvic lymphadenectomy following supervoltage irradiation for squamous cell carcinoma of the cervix. Am J Obstet Gynecol 1958;76:321.

Rutledge FN, McGuffee VB. Pelvic exenteration: prognostic significance of regional lymph node metastasis. Gynecol Oncol 1987;26:374.

Rutledge FN, Smith JP, Wharton JT, O'Quinn AG. Pelvic exenteration: analysis of 29 patients. Am J Obstet Gynecol 1977;129:882.

Schmidt JD, Buchsbaum HJ. Transverse colon conduit diversion. Urol Clin North Am 1986;13:233.

Senekjian EK, Frey K, Herbst AL. Pelvic exenteration in clear cell adenocarcinoma of the vagina and cervix. Gynecol Oncol 1989;34:413.

Senekjian EK, Young JM, Weiser PA, et al. An evaluation of squamous cell carcinoma antigen in patients with cervical squamous cell carcinoma. Am J Obstet Gynecol 1987;157:433.

Shepherd JH. Pelvic exenteration, has it a role in 1987? A six year experience. Verh K Acad Geneeskd Belg 1989; 51(1).

Shingleton HM, Soong J-W, Gelder MS, Hatch KD, Baker VV, Austin JM Jr. Clinical and histopathologic factors predicting recurrence and survival after pelvic exenteration for cancer of the cervix. Obstet Gynecol 1989; 73:1027.

Shiromizu K, Ogaawa M, Kotake K, et al. Reconstruction of sigmoid vagina and conduit in total pelvic exenteration for recurrent cervical carcinoma. Jpn J Clin Oncol 1989;19:170.

Sohmer PR, Dawson RB. Transfusion therapy in trauma: a review of the principles and techniques used in the MIEMS program. Am Surg February 1979;45:109.

Sommers GM, Grigsby PW, Perez CA, et al. Outcome of recurrent cervical carcinoma following definitive radiation. Gynecol Oncol 1989;35:150.

Soper JT, Berchuck A, Creasman WT, Clarke-Pearson DL. Pelvic exenteration: factors associated with major surgical morbidity. Gynecol Oncol 1989a;36:93.

Soper JT, Larson D, Hunter VJ, Berchuck A, Clarke-Pearson DL. Short gracilis myocutaneous flaps for vulvovaginal reconstruction after radical surgery. Obstet Gynecol 1989b;74:823.

Spirtos NM, Ballon SC. Needle catheter jejunostomy: a controlled, prospective, randomized trial in patients with gynecologic malignancy. Am J Obstet Gynecol 1988; 158:1285.

Stanhope CR, Symmonds RE. Palliative exenteration. What, when, and why? Am J Obstet Gynecol 1985;152:12.

Stanhope CR, Webb MJ, Podratz KC. Pelvic exenteration for recurrent cervical cancer. Clin Obstet Gynecol 1990; 33(4):897.

Symmonds RE, Pratt JH, Webb MJ. Exenterative operations: experience with 198 patients. Am J Obstet Gynecol 1975;121:907.

Talledo OE. Pelvic exenteration—Medical College of Georgia experience. Gynecol Oncol 1985;22:181.

Tao LC, Pearson FG, Delarue NC, et al. Percutaneous fine needle aspiration biopsy. I. Its value to clinical practice. Cancer 1980;45:1480.

Terada K, Morley GW. Radical hysterectomy as surgical salvage therapy for gynecologic malignancy. Obstet Gynecol 1987;70:90.

Trelford JD, Goodnight J, Schneider P, Wolfe B, Sauder MT. Total exenteration, two or one ostomy. Surg Gynecol Obstet 1992;173:126.

Trelford JD, Silverton JS. Successful plastic procedures of the perineum. Gynecol Oncol 1979;7:239.

van der Brekel MW, Castelijns JA, Stel HV, et al. Occult metastatic neck disease: detection with US and US-guided fine needle aspiration cytology. Radiology 1991;180(2):457.

Wallace D, Hernandez W, Schlaerth JB, et al. Prevention of abdominal wound disruption utilizing the Smead-Jones closure technique. Obstet Gynecol 1980;56:226.

Webb MJ, Symmonds RE. Wertheim hysterectomy: a reappraisal. Obstet Gynecol 1979;54:140.

Wheeless CR Jr. Low colorectal anastomosis and reconstruction after gynecologic cancer. Cancer 1993(suppl);71:1664.

Wheeless CR Jr, Hempling RE. Rectal J pouch reservoir to decrease the frequency of tenesmus and defecation in low coloproctostomy. Gynecol Oncol 1989; 36:136.

Wheeless CR Jr, Julian CG, Burnett LS, Dorsey JH. Synthetic pelvic floor sling to decrease small bowel complications after total exenteration. Obstet Gynecol 1971; 38:779.

Willing SJ, Pursell SH, Koch SR, Tobin GR. Vaginal reconstruction with rectur abdominis myocutaneous flap: CT findings. Am J Radiol 1991;156:1001.

Youngs DD, Wise TN. Preparing a patient for surgery: consent, information, and emotional support. Clin Obstet Gynecol 1976;19:321.

Cancer of the Cervix by Hugh M. Shingleton and James W. Orr, Jr.
J. B. Lippincott Company, Philadelphia, © 1995.

13

Recurrent Cancer:
Radiation Therapy, Chemotherapy,
and Other Treatment

When metastatic disease occurs or when locally recurrent cervical cancer is not amenable to surgical resection, the physician, patient and family are faced with a difficult treatment decision in which the likelihood of cure is small. Most (60%) patients with recurrent cervical cancer do not receive treatment of curative intent (Kigawa et al 1992) but are managed with palliative strategies. In the United States at any particular time, as much as 60% of all radiation therapy can be categorized as palliative in intent (Chahbazian 1993).

RADIATION THERAPY
FOR PELVIC
DISEASE RECURRENCE

Although radiation treatment of metastatic disease sites can result in significant palliation, retreatment of radiorecurrent pelvic disease is rarely a primary consideration because normal tissue-tolerance doses are likely to have been delivered during primary therapy. For this reason, the use of a second course of teletherapy is usually accompanied by a dramatic increase in complications. The rates of short-term palliation, local control, or even cure are probably higher in those women retreated with irradiation for a late recurrence (Randall et al 1988). Keettel and colleagues (1968) summarized information that was available before publication of his report concerning reirradiation for recurrent carcinoma of the cervix and indicated that only 3% of reirradiated patients were 5-year survivors. Brunschwig

(1967) reported a 5.4% survival in 56 patients whose recurrence was treated with a second course of radiation therapy. Neither of these reports suggests a significant improvement in survival when compared with untreated patients. Jones and coworkers (1970) described minimal palliative effects and significant complications in patients who were treated with Maxitron or intracavitary application who had persistent disease or short tumor-free intervals after orthovoltage irradiation. This was particularly true of patients who had received adequate initial therapy. Patients most likely to benefit were those with late recurrent disease (5 to 20 years after initial therapy) who required retreatment with intracavitary radium alone. Nori and associates (1981) reported symptomatic relief in 70% of patients having recurrent cervical cancer treated with interstitial and external radiation therapy. The 1-year disease-free survival rate was 45%; 10% were 5-year survivors. Prempree and colleagues (1984) described successful radiation retreatment of patients having late recurrent cancers. Radiation retreatment was more successful when the recurrent tumor was small, minimally necrotic, and associated with minimal surrounding skin fibrosis.

Despite overall poor results, specific brachytherapy techniques may minimize complications. Interstitial or other forms of brachytherapy are better tolerated because normal tissue tolerance increases with smaller treatment volume. Randall and Barrett (1988) suggested the palliative and curative benefit of interstitial irradiation for small-volume centrally recurrent disease. Yamazaki and coworkers (1993) reported 5 patients having recurrent pelvic cancer who were treated with a remote high-dose afterloading interstitial implantation, employing a template technique. Three patients achieved complete local control and 2 obtained symptomatic control. Sharma (1991) reported the successful use of ^{125}I interstitial seed implants in 21 patients having recurrent gynecologic cancer. Success was excellent in those patients having small tumor volume (less than 41 cm[3]). Eight of 11 patients with cervical cancer had a complete local response. This patient subgroup may also be offered care with ultraradical surgery.

Intraoperative Radiation Therapy

Intraoperative electron beam irradiation (Goldson et al 1978) may prove beneficial in patients without central pelvic recurrence who have extrapelvic node spread (Table 13-1) or localized pelvic side wall recurrence (Delgado et al 1984). Electron beam therapy allows directed delivery of a therapeutic dose of radiation to an isolated volume of the lymphatic or side wall tissues without encompassing other organs. Intraoperative use allows an accurate determination of small field size, which can be visualized directly, avoiding the increased dosage after displacing normal structures such as small bowel, bladder, or rectum. Experimental studies indicate that peripheral nerve toxicity is the dose-limiting factor in intraoperative radiation therapy trials, with neuropathy occurring with doses of 20 Gy or more, with or without additional teletherapy.

Garton and colleagues (1993) reported 19 patients and summarized existing literature of patients treated with intraoperative radiation therapy for recurrent gynecologic malignancy—most of whom had cervical cancer. Actual local control, with or without central control at 5 years, was 71%. Actual control within the intraoperative radiation therapy field was 80%. The distant metastasis-free survival rate was also improved. Disease-free survival in patients having pretreatment microscopic residual disease was statistically and clinically different from those having macroscopic residual disease.

Monge and coworkers (1993) evaluated the clinical tolerance for intraoperative radiation therapy in 26 patients having recurrent gynecologic tumors—18 (69%) of whom had recurrent cervical cancers. Intraoperative radiation therapy–related toxicity included one episode of severe motor neuropathy. Local control rates were 33% and 77% in patients relapsing after full radiation therapy or those receiving full radiation therapy.

Hockel and Knapstein (1992) reported 10 patients who were treated by combined operative and radiation therapy and followed-up for 1 year. Eight of these patients had been treated primarily with irradiation; 5 (50%) patients were without evidence of disease with good performance status after 30, 25, 22, and 12 months. The authors concluded that the addition of intraoperative radiation therapy to surgical debulking achieves modest local control and long-term survival rates when tumor-free margins cannot be obtained in previously irradiated patients.

Unfortunately, most reported studies evaluating intraoperative radiation therapy combine primary and recurrent treatment and multiple primary disease sites,

TABLE 13-1
Results of Intraoperative Radiation Therapy for Primary and Recurrent Gynecologic Cancer*

| | | | | | SURVIVAL | | |
STUDY	PATIENTS (N)	RECURRENT	PRIMARY	EXTERNAL BEAM THERAPY	Patients (n)	(%)	FOLLOW-UP (MS)
Yordan, 1988	15	10	5	15	7	47	≥12
Delgado, et al 1984	19	3	16	16	9	47	10–36
Dosoretz, 1984	5	5	0	3	2	40	—
Calkins, 1985	3	3	0	3	3	100	—
Garton, et al 1993	21	19	2	14	12	38[†]	21.6–98.5
Monge, et al 1993	26	26	—	12	8	31	2–48

*Most are cervical cancer.
[†]Actuarial 2- and 5-year survivals were 58% and 33%, respectively; median survival, 9 months.

Modified from Garton GR, Gunderson LL, Webb MJ, et al. Intraoperative radiation therapy in gynecologic cancer: the Mayo Clinic experience. Gynecol Oncol 1993;48:328.

making it difficult to evaluate the role of this treatment method for recurrent disease. When additional studies confirm these reports, however, intraoperative therapy alone or combined with surgery or effective systemic therapy may benefit selected patients who have localized node recurrences either at the pelvic side wall or in the paraaortic nodes.

Radiation Therapy for Distal Metastasis

Isolated pulmonary metastases can be successfully resected (Mountain 1970); however, pulmonary metastases are rarely isolated, and systemic therapy is usually indicated. Localized radiation therapy may be of palliative benefit to a significant proportion of women, particularly those having large thoracic node metastases obstructing the superior vena cava or the trachea.

Bone metastases are relatively infrequent but result in significant dysfunction (Ratanatharathorn et al 1994) and frequently respond favorably to a palliative course of irradiation, with rapid relief of pain. Clinical experience with strontium 89, however, suggests that injection of 150 mCi may relieve pain in 80% of patients having bony metastasis (Robinson et al 1993). It is as effective as teletherapy (Bolger et al 1993), has minimal toxicity, offers durable palliation, prevents additional bone pain, and can be reused as necessary.

Grigsby and associates (1993) reported a retrospective analysis of 20 patients who developed their first recurrence exclusively in the paraaortic lymph nodes. Such recurrences were observed within the first 12 months in 45% of patients after initial diagnosis, and 75% were observed within the first 2 years. Sciatic pain, leg edema, and hydronephrosis were common manifestations. Patients were treated with external irradiation only to the paraaortic lymph nodes, and all patients died within 2 years of recurrence. Patients receiving more than 4500 cGy had a median survival of 14.2 months, compared with 7.1 months in those patients treated with less than 4500 cGy. The median survival for the entire group was 8.7 months; it was 7.5 months for those failing within 24 months of their original diagnosis and 17.8 months for those failing after 24 months of their original diagnosis. It appears that using radiation therapy in this clinical situation is appropriate.

Central nervous system metastasis, although rare, can be palliated with whole-brain radiation therapy; however, the optimal dose and rate of delivery remain controversial. Short time-dose fractionation schemes (e.g., 3000 cGy in 2 weeks or 2000 cGy in 1 week) are as beneficial as protracted therapy, with less expense and inconvenience to the patient (Borgelt 1980). Reports suggest the use of smaller daily fractions (180 to 200 cGy) to reduce neurotoxicity (Greenberg 1994). Administration of high-dose steroids to decrease cerebral edema probably increases the overall benefit and assists in more rapid symptomatic improvement.

CHEMOTHERAPY

Basic Principles

Most patients who have recurrent or persistent cervical cancer are not amenable to curative surgery or irradiation (Chung et al 1983). In these situations, chemotherapy offers the only hope for palliation or survival. The decision to employ cytotoxic therapy poses several difficult choices for the physician, all of which ultimately relate to no drug or drug combination being effective treatment for cervical cancer, regardless of histology. Although there are no exploitable pharmacologic differences between normal and malignant cells, chemotherapy is based empirically on a dissimilarity in response between them. Part of this differential response can best be explained by cell cytokinetics, pharmacokinetics, chemistry, and tumor cell biology.

Within each tumor are cell compartments: a proliferating cell compartment (those cells in the cell cycle); a nonproliferating clonogenic cell compartment (those cells that are in G_0 or resting); and a nonclonogenic cell compartment. Clonogenic cells have a capacity for proliferation and are referred to as malignant cells. Nonproliferating clonogenic cells can enter the proliferating compartment but are usually in a resting stage. Nonclonogenic cells are primarily stromal and connective tissue cells and a few differentiated or dying (nonreplicating) tumor cells. These nonclonogenic cells are of clinical importance because they comprise a large but variable portion of any tumor mass. This must be remembered when assessing tumor response to chemotherapeutic regimen because a simple decrease in size of the tumor mass during chemotherapy may only reflect the cytotoxic effect of therapy on the nonclonogenic cells (stroma, lymphocytes, fibroblasts, connective tissue). There is no consistent relation between the cytotoxic effects on clonogenic or nonclonogenic support cells and clonogenic tumor cells, making response data based on a decrease in tumor size a less than reliable estimate of therapeutic efficacy.

The movements between cell compartments cannot be determined in human tumors; however, there are three basic parameters that are of theoretic importance: cell transit time, tumor growth fraction, and the rate of cell loss in the primary tumor.

The cell cycle is classically divided into mitosis and interphase. The latter has been divided into three functionally distinct subdivisions (see Fig. 8-2 in Chap. 8). After mitosis, cells enter the G_1 phase (diploid DNA and minimal DNA synthesis). Synthesis of RNA and protein occurs at a stable rate until just before the S phase, when a burst of RNA synthesis occurs. On entry into the S phase, the DNA complement undergoes duplication. Phase G_2 is characterized by absent DNA synthesis while RNA and protein synthesis continues, preparing for cell division. The normal diploid number is restored during the M phase and the cell enters G_1. The length of G_1 largely determines the cell cycle time; it is variable, with a minimal but no maximal time period. The rapid "growth" of malignancies is thus not only due to rapid cell cycle times but also to the rapid entry of G_0 cells into the dividing cell pool.

Transit times through various phases of the cell cycle are obtained by close-labeled mitosis curves, in which the injection of tritiated thymidine is followed by multiple samplings of the tumor population as a function of time. The labeled fraction of mitotic cells can then be determined. Averette and associates (1976) performed DNA synthesis curves for invasive squamous cell carcinoma of the cervix and compared them with those for normal epithelium. Overall, little difference was reported in the synthesis phase and the G_2 phase between normal and neoplastic tissue. There was, however, a progressive shortening of the entire generation cycle, primarily due to a decrease in the postmitotic G_1 phase. Unfortunately, few other studies exist that indicate that cell cycle times for malignant cell lines are accelerated when compared with nonmalignant tissues.

The growth fraction includes that fraction of proliferating cells within a tumor that are in the S phase. In tumors with a low growth fraction, few cells are proliferating and chemotherapy has diminished efficacy. Tumors with a high growth fraction should be more responsive to cytotoxic agents, however. The general range of growth fraction in human tumors is 0.5 to 0.7; however, as the tumor enlarges, this number becomes smaller. Another important and widely variable factor in tumor biology is the rate of cell loss from the primary tumor. Cell loss is inferred because tumors often grow more slowly than their "potential" doubling time. This loss applies to those cells leaving the primary tumor, either because of cell death, movement of cells into other areas of the host, or removal secondary to immune reaction. Therefore, slow growth rates of human tumor cells may be explained by a small growth fraction, spontaneous cell loss due to cell death, cell migration, or cell exfoliation, and, in rare cases, a long cell cycle time, or by any combination of these factors.

Few reports have evaluated the role of cytometrically determined cell kinetic data as prognostic indicators in cervical cancer. Jakobsen and colleagues (1988) indicated that a high DNA index was associated with increased metastatic potential and reduced survival. Unfortunately, other reports have not confirmed this information (Quinn et al 1992).

Even fewer studies of cervical cancer cell kinetic-directed chemotherapy have been performed. O'Quinn and coworkers (1984) noted a reasonable clinical response in 11 patients who were treated with a kinetic-directed regimen. Additional clinical evaluation of a kinetic-directed regimen that allows the appropriate timing of cytotoxic drug administration is needed before it can benefit women with recurrent cervical cancer.

Clinical Results

The chemotherapeutic agents that were evaluated in patients having recurrent cervical cancer vary significantly in their route of administration, metabolism, method of action, and toxicity (Table 13-2).

The development of effective chemotherapy has been slow because many patients who have cervical cancer have early disease that is amenable to cure by either primary radical surgery or radical radiation therapy. Few studies contain an adequate number of patients and often group patients with different levels of disease, including those with isolated distant metastases, those with both pelvic recurrence and distant metastasis, and those with advanced untreated disease. Regimens treating different histologic types, using different drug dosages and schedules, make evaluation in drug trials almost impossible. Although reports demonstrating the potential effects of neoadjuvant chemotherapy have attracted interest, the effects of previous radiation therapy in patients having recurrent cervical cancer has hampered evaluation of chemotherapy benefits because pelvic fibrosis makes it extremely difficult to objectively evaluate response rates. The endarteritis that is associated with previous irradiation decreases blood supply, alters tumor perfusion, affects drug distribution, and interferes with drug-cycle scheduling by limiting bone marrow reserve. Additionally, pelvic disease recurrence may be associated with ureteral obstruction, resultant impaired renal function, and alteration of drug excretion. The effectiveness of chemotherapy in patients having recurrent or metastatic cervical cancer is also compromised by the development of drug resistance. For these reasons, drug-induced objective responses among patients who have advanced disease are most frequently observed in extrapelvic metastatic sites (Alberts et al 1991). Future studies likely will involve the use of specific radiologic techniques or serum tumor markers to delineate drug activity.

TABLE 13-2
Chemotherapeutic Agents Evaluated in Patients with Cervical Cancer

AGENT	ADMINISTRATION	METABOLISM	MAJOR TOXICITY
Adriamycin	Intravenous	Hepatic	Cardiac, myelosuppression, alopecia, nausea and vomiting, extravasation, radiation recall
Bleomycin	Intramuscular, intravenous, subcutaneous	Renal and peripheral	Pulmonary fibrosis, hyperpigmentation, alopecia, fever and chills, myelosuppression (mild)
Cis-diammine	Intravenous	Renal	Myelosuppression, neurotoxicity
Cis-diammine-dichloroplatinum	Intravenous	Renal	Renal toxicity (tubular), nausea and vomiting, neurologic, metabolic, myelosuppression (mild)
Cyclophosphamide	Oral or intravenous	Hepatic	Myelosuppression, nausea and vomiting, alopecia, hemorrhagic cystitis
Dibromodulcitol	Oral		Myelosuppression, gastrointestinal toxicity
Hexamethylmelamine	Oral	Hepatic	Nausea and vomiting, neuropathy, myelosuppression
Hydroxyurea	Oral	Peripheral	Myelosuppression, alopecia, radiation recall
Ifosfamide	Intravenous	Hepatic	Myelosuppression, cystitis
Melphalan	Oral	Peripheral	Myelosuppression, nausea and vomiting (mild), alopecia (rare)
Methotrexate	Oral, intravenous, intramuscular	Renal	Myelosuppression, stomatitis, hepatic toxicity, neurologic
Vincristine	Intravenous	Hepatic	Neurologic, myelosuppression (mild)

Single-Agent Cytotoxic Therapy

Little objective information is available on chemotherapeutic agents in the treatment of cervical cancer before 1976 (Table 13-3). Trials using drugs in different regimens suggested that with the exception of hydroxyurea, response rates varied between 0% and 25%. These data can be used only to suggest drug activity because they often represent combined retrospective trials, in which variable criteria for objective response and different dosing have been used. Generally, single-agent chemotherapy with these agents does not result in long-term benefit because the average median duration of response was 4 to 6 months, with little effect on survival (Thigpen et al 1981).

SQUAMOUS CELL CARCINOMA

The Gynecologic Oncology Group (GOG) and others have evaluated single agents and attempted to identify new active cytotoxic drugs for patients having recurrent or advanced squamous cell carcinoma through a systematic evaluation with defined tumor measurements and strict criteria for response. Forty-five cytotoxic drugs have been tested for use as a single cytotoxic agent, and few drugs with significant activity against cervical cancer have been described (Table 13-4).

The most effective single agent studied in recurrent squamous cell cancer is cisplatin (Table 13-5). When used in total doses of 50 to 120 mg/m^2 administered at 3- to 4-week intervals, objective response rates of about 25% are expected (Table 13-6). Few other standard cytotoxic drugs have been consistently associated with objective response rates of 25% or higher. Renal dysfunction was noted as being the dose-limiting toxicity of cisplatin in trials in the early 1970s; however, the use of intravenous hydration before and after therapy, in conjunction with osmotic diuretics, has reduced this problem significantly. Although cisplatin-induced renal toxicity can be an especially difficult problem in patients who have recurrent squamous cell carcinoma of the cervix, the risk of peripheral neuropathy also limits cisplatin dose intensity (Alberts et al 1989). Inherent rapidly acquired tumor cell resistance to the cytotoxicity of cisplatin is common and results in low overall objective and complete response rates in addition to short response durations and progression-free intervals (Alberts et al 1991). Prolonged cisplatin treatment appears to in-

TABLE 13-3
Single-Agent Chemotherapy in Cervical Carcinoma Before 1976

DRUGS	PATIENTS REPORTED (N)	OVERALL RESPONSE (%)
Alkylating agents		
Cyclophosphamide	188	15
Chlorambucil	44	25
Melphalan	20	20
Antimetabolites		
5-Fluorouracil	140	21
Methotrexate	77	16
Mitotic inhibitors		
Vincristine	44	23
Antibiotics		
Adriamycin	28	18
Bleomycin	172	10
Mitomycin C	18	22
Porfiromycin	78	22
Other agents		
Hexamethylmelamine	49	22
Hydroxyurea	14	0
6-Mercaptopurine	18	6
TOTAL	922	16.7

Modified from Thigpen T, Vance RB, Balducci L, Blessing J. Chemotherapy in the management of advanced or recurrent cervical and endometrial carcinoma. Cancer 1981;48:658.

duce multiple mechanisms of tumor resistance, including a rise in intracellular glutathione concentrations and increased DNA repair (Alberts et al 1991). Consequently, achievable doses may be insufficient to overcome the inherent drug resistance that is associated with cervical cancer.

Generally, response rates to cisplatin are higher in patients who have not received prior chemotherapy. Its activity is not confined to those patients having extrapelvic disease alone because 43% of patients having extrapelvic disease and 33% of patients having isolated pelvic disease have an objective response (Fig. 13-1). The duration of response is short: the median survival of chemotherapy-naive patients who are given cisplatin is about 7 months.

There is no apparent survival-related dose-response curve, and the low dose (50 mg/m^2) regimen is associated with the least toxicity. In the GOG study of cisplatin (Bonomi et al 1985), response rates in 444 patients depended on dose and schedule, with a 20.7% response rate at 50 mg/m^2, a 25% response rate at 20 mg/m^2 for 5 days, and a 31.4% response rate at 100 mg/m^2. Prolonged (24-hour) infusion lessens the emetic effects but does not affect efficacy. Unfortunately, there was no difference in complete response rates or survival among treatment groups. Therefore, doubling the cisplatin dose is insufficient to overcome the inherent resistance of cervical cancer cells.

Potter and colleagues (1989) reported 68 eligible patients who were treated with cisplatin as the primary chemotherapeutic agent for recurrent squamous cell carcinoma of the cervix. They reported an overall response rate of 40.2%. Women who had isolated chest disease had a 63% complete response rate and an overall response rate of 73%. No complete responses were noted in patients having localized pelvic disease recurrence or persistence; however, 21% of these patients had a partial response. Lesion size, clinical stage, patient age, and duration from primary treatment to recurrence did not affect response or survival. They concluded that isolated chest metastases were more likely to respond to cisplatin than were pelvic disease recurrences; however, location of recurrence did not significantly alter survival (mean, 22.7 months versus 14.1 months). Disease in other locations reduces the likelihood of response in the chest.

McGuire and coworkers (1989) reported a comparative trial of the platinum derivatives carboplatin and iproplatin in patients having advanced squamous cell carcinoma of the uterine cervix. This GOG study reported a response rate of 15% for carboplatin and 11% for iproplatin. A third of patients developed grade 3 or 4 neurotoxicity. Both of these drugs were considered to be inferior to cisplatin; however, the duration of patient survival appears similar for all three compounds.

TABLE 13-4
Single-Drug Therapy for Squamous Cell Carcinoma of the Cervix

DRUG	PRIOR THERAPY	RESPONSE (%)	DRUG	PRIOR THERAPY	RESPONSE (%)
ALKYLATING AGENTS			**ANTIMETABOLITES**		
Cyclophosphamide	Mixed	38/251 (15)	5-Fluorouracil	Mixed	29/142 (20)
Chlorambucil	Mixed	11/44 (25)	5-Fludarabine phosphate	Mixed	7/34 (21)
Melphalan	Mixed	4/20 (20)	5-Fludarabine phosphate	Mixed	0/20 (0)
Ifosfamide	No	7/46 (15)	Methotrexate	Mixed	17/96 (18)
Ifosfamide	Yes	3/27 (11)	6-Mercaptopurine	Mixed	1/18 (5)
Ifosfamide	Mixed	25/84 (29)	Dichloromethotrexate	No	3/37 (8)
Dibromodulcitol	No	16/55 (29)	Baker's antifol	Mixed	5/32 (16)
Dibromodulcitol	No	7/47 (15)	Trimetrexate	Yes	0/27 (0)
Galactitol	Mixed	7/36 (19)			
Semustine	Mixed	7/94 (7)	**PLANT ALKALOIDS**		
Lomustine	Mixed	3/63 (5)	Etoposide	Mixed	0/31 (0)
Yoshi 864	Yes	0/18 (0)	Teniposide	Yes	3/22 (14)
			Vincristine	Mixed	10/55 (18)
HEAVY METAL COMPLEXES			Vinblastine	Yes	0/33 (0)
Cisplatin	No	182/785 (23)	Vinblastine	Mixed	5/21 (24)
Cisplatin	Yes	8/30 (27)	Vinblastine	Yes	0/33 (0)
Carboplatin	No	27/175 (15)	Vindesine	Mixed	5/21 (24)
Iproplatin	No	19/177 (11)	Maytansine	Yes	1/29 (3)
ANTIBIOTICS			**OTHER AGENTS**		
Doxorubicin	No	12/61 (20)	Hydroxyurea	Mixed	0/14 (0)
Doxorubicin	Mixed	33/205 (16)	ICRF-159	Mixed	5/28 (18)
Mitoxantrone	Yes	2/26 (8)	Aminothiadiazole	Yes	1/21 (5)
Epirubicin	Mixed	5/27 (18)	AMSA	Yes	1/25 (4)
Epirubicin	Mixed	18/38 (48)	PALA	Yes	0/36 (0)
Esorubicin	Yes	0/28 (0)	Diaziquone	Yes	1/26 (4)
Menogaril	Yes	0/14 (0)	N-methylformamide	Yes	0/20 (0)
Piperazinedion	No	5/38 (13)	Spirogermanium	Yes	0/18 (0)
Echinomycin	Yes	2/28 (7)	Hexamethylmelamine	No	12/64 (19)
Porfiromycin	NO	17/78 (22)	Didemnin B	Mixed	0/24 (0)
			Didemnin	Mixed	0/16 (0)
			Amonafide	Yes	0/15 (0)
			CPT-11	Mixed	13/55 (25)

In another comparative trial, 89 patients who had recurrent measurable squamous cell carcinoma of the cervix were randomized to receive either carboplatin or iproplatin. The response rate for carboplatin was 26.1% and was 30% for iproplatin. The duration of response was 5.5 months for carboplatin and 6 months for iproplatin. Median survival was 7.5 months and 7.6 months, respectively (Lira-Puerto et al 1991).

Among new drugs, ifosfamide has attracted considerable attention, with two phase II trials suggesting response rates greater than 30% (Table 13-7). Sutton and associates (1989) reported the GOG experience, treating 24 patients with 1.2 g/m^2 of ifosfamide daily for 5 days. There were no complete responders and three partial responders for a response rate of 12.5%. Thus, the GOG data has not confirmed the same magnitude of activity (Thigpen 1989).

The GOG has evaluated dibromodulcitol (a halogenated sugar) given orally and reported a 29% response rate (Stehman et al 1989), suggesting marked activity; however, there are no confirmatory reports suggesting this degree of activity.

Single-agent doxorubicin has a reported 20% response rate and should be considered to be an active drug alone or in combination (Table 13-8) for the treatment of recurrent squamous cell cancer (Thigpen et al 1994).

TABLE 13-5
Active Single Agents in Cervical Carcinoma

DRUG	RESPONSE RATE (CR + PR %)
Platinum compounds	
Cisplatin	190/815 (23)
Carboplatin	27/175 (15)
Iproplatin	19/177 (11)
Doxorubicin	45/266 (17)
Ifosfamide	35/157 (22)
Dibromodulcitol	23/102 (23)

CR, complete response; PR, partial response.

Modified from Thigpen T, Vance RB, Khansur T. Carcinoma of the uterine cervix: current status and future directions. Semin Oncol 1994;21(2):43.

NONSQUAMOUS CELL TUMORS

Piperazinedione and *cis*-diaminedichloroplatinum (*cis*-platinum) have also been studied in nonsquamous recurrent or advanced carcinoma of the cervix, with respective response rates of 14% and 15% (Thigpen et al 1994).

A phase II trial (Sutton et al 1993) of ifosfamide and Mesna conducted in patients having recurrent or advanced nonsquamous cell carcinoma of the cervix reported a response rate of 15%. There was one complete response and five partial responders. The median duration of response was 4.2 months. Three responses occurred in patients who had pelvic disease only. No

response was observed in extrapelvic sites. Sutton and colleagues' conclusion was that ifosfamide possesses activity that compares favorably with that of other agents.

Morris and associates (1992) treated 10 patients having small cell carcinoma of the cervix with combination chemotherapy, using cisplatin (50 mg/m^2) and doxorubicin (50 mg/m^2) on day 1 and etoposide 75 mg/m^2 on days 1 through 3. Three of 7 patients who had measurable disease at the start of therapy had complete response.

CHEMOSENSITIVITY TESTING

In vitro chemotherapeutic testing has had limited predictive value in other tumors, and few reports have addressed its usefulness in cervical cancer. Parker and coworkers (1984) indicated that in vitro sensitivity testing was more accurate in predicting tumor resistance than in determining tumor susceptibility. Stratton and colleagues (1984), citing the problems with clonogenic assays, prospectively studied the subrenal capsule tumor implant assay and suggested that this assay was a clinically valid method to determine tumor susceptibility. Cohen and coworkers (1982) reported criteria for in vivo testing of *cis*-platinum, however. Preliminary results indicate that age, clinical stage, and differentiation of the tumor do not influence the in vivo response to *cis*-platinum; however, the in vivo response to a single dose may allow the physician to identify those who may benefit. Additional investigations that consider tumor heterogenicity and over-

TABLE 13-6
Gynecologic Oncology Group Studies of Single Agent Cisplatin

DOSE AND SCHEDULE	PRIOR THERAPY	RESPONSE (%)
Protocol 26C		
50 mg/m^2 every 3 weeks, 2-hour infusion	No	11/22 (5)
	Yes	2/12 (16)
Protocol 43		
50 mg/m^2 every 3 weeks, 2-hour infusion	No	31/150 (21)
100 mg/m^2 every 3 weeks, 2-hour infusion	No	52/166 (31)
20 mg/m^2/day × 5 days every 3 weeks, 2-hour infusion	No	32/128 (25)
Protocol 64		
50 mg/m^2 every 3 weeks, 2-hour infusion	No	28/164 (17)
50 mg/m^2 every 3 weeks, 24-hour infusion	No	184/798 (23)

Modified from Thigpen T, Vance RB, Khansur T. Carcinoma of the uterine cervix: current status and future directions. Semin Oncol 1994;21(2):43.

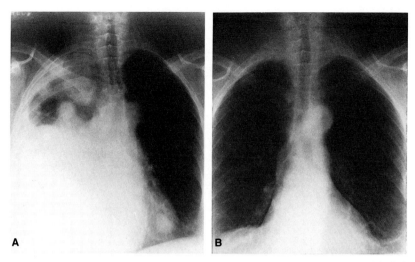

FIGURE 13-1. (**A**) This 65-year-old woman had extensive pulmonary recurrence, which dramatically responded to three courses of chemotherapy (**B**). (Shingleton JM, Orr JW Jr. Cancer of the cervix: diagnosis and treatment. New York, Churchill Livingstone, 1987.)

come the problems of evaluating tumor growth are necessary before routine use of this methodology.

Combination Therapy

Attempts to prolong remission and increase survival have prompted the study of various regimens of combination chemotherapy. There are numerous reported phase II trials of combination chemotherapy. The most commonly used drugs are bleomycin, 5-fluorouracil (5-FU), mitomycin C, methotrexate, cyclophosphamide, Adriamycin, and *cis*-platinum (Tables 13-9 through 13-11). Most studies (1) involve small patient numbers, with short follow-up; (2) employ variable methods of assessment of response, while

using different doses and schedules; and (3) do not provide for comparison across studies.

Cisplatin-based combination therapy has been extensively studied and associated with an overall objective response rate varying between 0% and 65%. Clinical complete response rates vary from 0% to 36% (Alberts et al 1991). Median duration of survival varies between 4 and 10.5 months. Thus, despite high objective response rates, survival is similar to that in reports using single-agent cisplatin (Alberts et al 1991, Buxton 1992).

Miyamoto and coworkers' (1978) report on a small group of patients who were treated with bleomycin and mitomycin C indicated a 93% response rate; 80% of patients were complete responders. Other trials using mitomycin C, vincristine, and bleomycin

TABLE 13-7
Single-Agent Activity of Ifosfamide in Cervical Carcinoma (Mesna Uroprotection Given in Each Regimen)

DOSE AND SCHEDULE	PATIENTS (N)	RESPONSE RATE (%)
No prior chemotherapy		
5 g/m^2 over 24 hr for 1 day	30	1 CR (33)
3.5 g/m^2 over 8 hr for 5 days	18	3 CR (50)
1.5 g/m^2 over 30 min for 5 days	30	6 CR (40)
Prior chemotherapy		
1.5 g/m^2 over 30 min for 5 days	9	0 CR (0)
1.5 g/m^2 over 30 min for 5 days	27	0 CR (11)

CR, complete response.

Modified from Thigpen T, Vance RB, Khansur T. Carcinoma of the uterine cervix: current status and future directions. Semin Oncol 1994;21(2):43.

TABLE 13-8
Gynecologic Oncology Group Protocol 23: A Randomized Trial
of Doxorubicin-Based Chemotherapy

REGIMEN	SITE OF DISEASE	RESPONSE RATE (%)
Doxorubicin	Pelvis	2 CR, 4 PR/38 (16)
	Extrapelvic	5 CR, 1 PR/23 (26)
	Overall	7 CR, 5 PR/61 (20)
Doxorubicin/Vincristine	Pelvis	1 CR, 5 PR/38 (16)
	Extrapelvic	0 CR, 3 PR/16 (19)
	Overall	1 CR, 9 PR/54 (7)
Doxorubicin/Cyclophosphamide	Pelvis	1 CR, 3 PR/28 (14)
	Extrapelvic	2 CR, 1 PR/11 (27)
	Overall	3 CR, 4 PR/39 (18)

CR, complete response; PR, partial response.

Modified from Thigpen T, Vance RB, Khansur T. Carcinoma of the uterine cervix: current status and future directions. Semin Oncol 1994;21(2):43.

have been associated with high response rates but are associated with considerable toxicity. Combination regimens containing *cis*-platinum have indicated a markedly increased response frequency but only an occasional report has demonstrated the benefit of combination chemotherapy in terms of increased response duration or survival. Buxton (1992) reported the results of a BIP (bleomycin, cisplatin, and ifosfamide) chemotherapy regimen and indicated that combination chemotherapy did not appear to confer survival advantage in patients having recurrent disease. Hoffman and associates (1991) reported 25 patients having recurrent squamous cell carcinoma that was treated with cisplatin, bleomycin, and mitomycin C. They indicated that this regimen had modest efficacy and represented no improvement over single-agent chemotherapy. Murad and colleagues (1994) reported a trial of bleomycin, carboplatin, and ifosfamide that was designed to evaluate tumor response. Objective responses were present in 60% of patients, and 8 patients (23%) had complete responses. Median overall survival duration was 11 months but fell to 4 months in those patients previously irradiated (Murad et al 1994).

Bonomi and coworkers (1989) reported the GOG's experience with 55 patients who were treated with cisplatin (50 mg/m^2) and 5-FU (1000 mg/m^2) for 5 days and found a 12.7% complete response rate and a 9.1% partial response rate. It was concluded that the addition of 5-FU did not add any significant advantage to the single-agent cisplatin treatment.

Although responding patients in the nonrandomized phase II trials had median survival durations of 1 to 2 years, the overall median duration of survival for all treated patients in each of these trials ranged between 4 and 10.5 months (Thigpen et al 1994). Thus, despite the relatively high objective response rates observed in some of these trials, most patients experience only partial tumor regression and survival durations were similar to those reported for single-agent platinum.

As expected, toxicity with a combination regimen may be increased. In one report, combined cisplatin, ifosfamide, and bleomycin chemotherapy was given to 14 patients having recurrent or metastatic cervical carcinoma; 2 patients suffered a septic death during the myelosuppressant phase (Tay et al 1992). Other reports confirm this risk (Manetta 1991).

Some regimens such as BOMP (bleomycin, On-

TABLE 13-9
Phase II Trials of Combinations of Cisplatin/5-FU

CISPLATIN/5-FU DOSE (MG/M^2) AND SCHEDULE	RESPONSE RATE (%)
No prior radiotherapy	
100 × 1/1000 × 5	7 CR, 13 PR/29 (69)
100 × 1/1000 × 5	4 CR, 9 PR/19 (68)
Prior radiotherapy	
100 × 1/1000 × 5	1 CR, 2 PR/16 (19)
100 × 1/1000 × 4*	8 CR, 6 PR/52 (27)
100 × 1/1000 × 5	0 CR, 2 PR/13 (15)
50 × 1/1000 × 5	7 CR, 5 PR/55 (22)
20 × 5/200 × 5	1 CR, 10 PR/18 (61)

*Allopurinol was added to cisplatin/5-FU in this trial.
CR, complete response; PR, partial response.

Modified from Thigpen T, Vance RB, Khansur T. Carcinoma of the uterine cervix: current status and future directions. Semin Oncol 1994;21(2):48.

TABLE 13-10
Ifosfamide-Based Combination Chemotherapy
for Cervical Carcinoma

COMBINATION	RESPONSE RATE (%)
No prior radiotherapy	
Ifosfamide/cisplatin 1.5 g/m^2 × 5, 20 mg/m^2 × 5	15/24* (62)
Ifosfamide/carboplatin 5 g/m^2 × 1300 mg/m^2 × 1	3 CR, 16 PR/32 (59)
BIP 30 mg × 1, 15 g/m^2 × 1, 50 mg/m^2 × 1	17/26* (65)
BIP 15 mg × 1, 15 g/m^2 × 1, 50 mg/m^2 × 1	3 CR, 6 PR/9 (100)
Prior radiotherapy	
BIP 30 mg × 1, 15 g/m^2 × 1, 50 mg/m^2 × 1	26/36* (72)
BIP 15 mg × 1, 1 g/m^2 × 1, 50 mg/m^2 × 1	1 CR, 4 PR/12 (42)
BIP 30 mg × 1, 5 g/m^2 × 1, 50 mg/m^2 × 1	0 CR, 3 PR/24 (13)

Uroprotection given with each regimen.
BIP, Bleomycin/ifosfamide/cisplatin chemotherapy.
*Data on CRs and PRs not available.
CR, complete response; PR, partial response.

Modified from Thigpen T, Vance RB, Khansur T. Carcinoma of the uterine cervix: current status and future directions. Semin Oncol 1994;21(2):43.

TABLE 13-11
Other Drug Combinations

COMBINATION	RESPONSE RATE (%)
Doxorubicin/cisplatin 60 mg/m^2, 50 mg/m^2 IV every 3 weeks	6/19* (32)
Interferon-alfa/13 *cis*-retinoic acid, 6 million U/d SC, 1 mg/kg/d orally	3 DR, 12 PR/32 (47)

CR, complete response; PR, partial response; IV, intravenously; SC, subcutaneously.
*Data on CRs and PRs not available.

Modified from Thigpen T, Vance RB, Khansur T. Carcinoma of the uterine cervix: current status and future directions. Semin Oncol 1994;21(2):43.

covin, mitomycin C, platinum; Surwit et al 1983, Belinson et al 1985) and BIP (bleomycin, ifosfamide, cisplatin) may be useful as primary or neoadjuvant therapy. Randomized prospective comparative trials have failed to define a distinct advantage of any drug regimen and emphasize the need to develop new active drugs or alternative effective methods of administration.

Gynecologic Oncology Group protocol 110 compares cisplatin alone with cisplatin plus ifosfamide (with Mesna) and dibromodulcitol.

Arterial Chemotherapy

Theoretically, arterial infusion of chemotherapeutic drugs could offer a distinct pharmacologic advantage because a higher concentration of the drug would perfuse the tumor. Reports using arterial infusion have not been encouraging, however. Morrow and associates (1977) evaluated a continuous pelvic arterial infusion of bleomycin in 20 patients having recurrent cervical cancer. Significant toxicity and little evidence of response was observed. Swenerton and coworkers (1979) infused bleomycin, mitomycin C, and vin-

cristine, with little response. Lifshitz and colleagues (1978) reported a 21% rate of tumor regression in 14 patients who were treated with intraarterial methotrexate and vincristine. Carlson and coworkers (1981) reported a 33% response rate in patients who were treated with pelvic infusion of *cis*-platinum. Hiraoka and associates (1980) developed a technique for pelvic vascular bed isolation in an attempt to increase the local concentration of chemotherapy; two patients who were treated with this technique using mitomycin C are long-term survivors. Kavanagh and coworkers (1984) reported that intraarterial vincristine, mitomycin C, bleomycin, and platinum produced objective responses in 12 of 25 (48%) previously untreated patients.

The effects of intraarterial infusion of cisplatin and bleomycin were evaluated by Kigawa and associates (1992) in 21 patients having locally recurrent cancer that failed previous radiation therapy. The response rate was 71.4%; the median duration of response was 21.1 months. In this study, both the G_1 and the proportion of S-phase cells were significantly increased in responding tumors but not in nonresponding tumors after arterial infusion. These findings suggest that the synchronization of the cancer cell cycle that is induced by these drugs is essential for tumor regression and that intrinsic tumor sensitivity is related to tumor cell or DNA uptake of the cytotoxic agents. Such differences between responders and nonresponders cannot be apparent until after treatment has begun. This methodology can be of benefit by determining response to future chemotherapy within 24 hours of first treatment rather than waiting for weeks after two to three courses of conventional cytotoxic therapy.

Alternative methods of therapeutic drug localization—using magnetically responsive drug-bearing microspheres—have been tested in animals with some success and need further testing in humans. Chemoembolization with sustained-release microcapsules may be beneficial in some of these patients (Kato et al 1981).

The place of hormonal alteration has not been defined, despite the suggestion of Gao and associates (1983) that the presence of progesterone receptors may be predictive of survival and Guthrie (1982) reporting long-term remissions using bromocriptine.

Access

Although not always a problem, venous access for drug administration and monitoring may become difficult, particularly in patients who are receiving multiagent therapy. Patient tolerance may be improved in these situations by establishing permanent access. Various methods (Fig. 13-2), including infusion ports and catheters, can be safely used (Rettenmaier et al 1985). We prefer bedside placement of a Groshong catheter,

which can be performed safely and cost-effectively (Holloway 1994). The use of indwelling ports has its own inherent risks, including infection or thrombosis (Raad et al 1994, Garrison 1994).

These catheters may also be used for nutritional support to maintain weight and other nutritional parameters (Nuutinen et al 1982). There is no reliable evidence that such support alters outcome in these patients, however.

TREATMENT OF SPECIAL PROBLEMS

Although rarely diagnosed in women who have gynecologic cancer, pericardial metastasis and effusion are often considered to be preterminal events (Rudoff et al 1989, Nelson et al 1993). Autopsy series suggest that only 6% of patients who die with cervical cancer have cardiac metastasis. Reports suggest that this problem may present in an unusual manner, however. Prayson

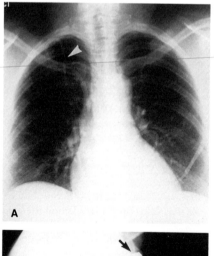
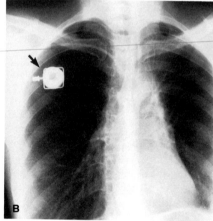
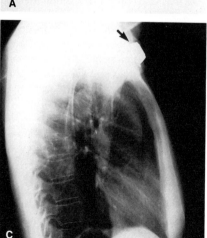

FIGURE 13-2. Long-term venous access for chemotherapy may be by (**A**) catheter (*arrow*) or (**B** and **C**) implanted ports (*arrows*). The cephalic, external, or internal jugular veins may be used for this purpose. (Shingleton JM, Orr JW Jr. Cancer of the cervix: diagnosis and treatment. New York, Churchill Livingstone, 1987.)

and Biscotti (1992) reported 1 patient who had recurrent cervical carcinoma who presented with cardiac tamponade related to extensive pericardial metastasis. She had a response to irradiation and chemotherapy at 16 months but eventually died 17 months after initial presentation. When faced with this situation, pericardiocentesis and aggressive treatment with irradiation or chemotherapy is justified if prolonging life is a goal.

Metabolic Problems

HYPERCALCEMIA

Significant metabolic problems such as hypercalcemia or uremia are not uncommon in patients who have recurrent cervical cancer. Hypercalcemia may be related to bone metastases but parathormone–related protein is thought to be the most common mediator of cancer-related hypercalcemia (Warrell 1993). When the physician elects to treat this complication, initial therapy should consist of but not depend on saline infusion with furosemide diuresis (Heggue et al 1985). In some situations, surgical resection of large tumor masses (Aboul-Hosn et al 1983) may result in the resolution of the hypercalcemia; however, technical problems usually preclude the use of surgery. Prostaglandin inhibitors are of little benefit and reduce serum calcium in fewer than 5% of patients who have cancer-related hypercalcemia. Intravenous phosphate loading is effective but it results in the unwanted side effects of renal failure, hypotension, and extraskeletal calcification. Steroid administration actively inhibits bone resorption, decreases interstitial absorption, and may result in short-term lowering of serum calcium levels.

Pharmacologic doses of calcitonin increase renal calcium excretion and inhibit bone absorption. Its action is rapid in onset and associated with minimal toxicity. Unfortunately, its hypocalcemic effect is relatively weak and fewer than 30% of patients who are treated with calcitonin alone achieve normocalcemia. Biphosphonates directly inhibit calcium release from bone and when given intravenously have a relatively significant effect on lowering serum calcium levels. Gallium nitrate, a potent inhibitor of bone resorption, has demonstrated a superior benefit in randomized studies comparing its hypocalcemic effect with that of calcitonin or etidronate (a biphosphonate; Warrell 1993).

If necessary, mitramycin (a drug that directly kills osteoclasts) can be used but should be reserved for patients without thrombocytopenia or renal or hepatic dysfunction who have not responded to biphosphonates or gallium nitrate.

In the rarest case, dialysis may be necessary to control hypercalcemia.

UREMIA

The incidence of uremia with recurrent cancer is apparently decreasing as new radiotherapeutic regimens result in superior pelvic control. Katz and Davies (1980) reported a decreased incidence of uremia from 28% to 7% over a 20-year interval. Their autopsy studies suggested less extensive ureteral involvement. Over this period of observation, the leading cause of death changed from renal failure to such conditions as myocardial infarction, pulmonary thromboembolism, pneumonia, cachexia, and sepsis.

The presence of ureteral obstruction, particularly when new, usually predicts recurrent tumor. In patients having histologic confirmation of recurrence, there is no evidence that urinary diversion by conduit is beneficial. Although it may allow return of normal renal function (Fukuoka et al 1983), it is not associated with prolonged survival, and patients often spend much of their remaining life in the hospital. When the stenosis is secondary to fibrosis, however, and recurrence is not established, percutaneous nephrostomies or ureteral stents placed without a general anesthetic may allow recovery of renal function and time for further evaluation and consideration of permanent diversion (Fig. 13-3). These stents may be internalized (Coddington et al 1984) for ease of management.

Urinary Fistulas, Bowel Fistulas, or Obstruction

Development of a late cancer-related urinary fistula is disconcerting to the patient and physician. Because simple nephrostomy diversion may not result in a dry patient, the question of a more permanent diversion by conduit or even nephrectomy should be considered. Although survival is short and morbidity and mortality are high, these risks must be weighed in relation to the patient's quality of life (Brin et al 1975, Fukuoka et al 1983, Meyer et al 1980). Generally, only patients who have a life expectancy of 4 months or more should be considered for this procedure.

Cancer-related small intestinal obstruction or fistula may be relieved by a simple bypass procedure, often with significant palliation. Conservative (long tube decompression) treatment of intestinal obstruction is less likely to be successful after irradiation or in the presence of recurrent cancer (Helmkamp et al 1985, Alvarez 1988). Extensive resections are not indicated. Because prior radiation therapy may render the ileocecal valve incompetent, complete isolation of the fistula segment may be necessary to prevent reflux and continued fistulous drainage.

Rectovaginal fistulas may be palliated by colostomy; however, use of an elemental diet to effect a "medical colostomy" may avoid the necessity for sur-

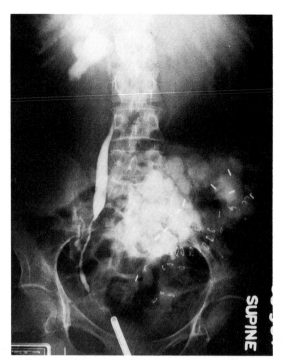

FIGURE 13-3. A retrograde dye study of a 59-year-old woman, demonstrating lower ureteral constriction. The contralateral kidney had no function. Intraoperative evaluation failed to demonstrate recurrent cancer, and she was successfully diverted with a transverse colon conduit. (Shingleton JM, Orr JW Jr. Cancer of the cervix: diagnosis and treatment. New York, Churchill Livingstone, 1987.)

gical intervention, especially in the nearly terminal patient.

Hemorrhage

Pelvic hemorrhage is a frightening experience. When present in patients who have recurrent cancer, a surgical approach is not the first line of therapy. Hypogastric artery ligation is difficult, usually morbid, and rarely necessary with the advent of arterial embolization (Schwartz et al 1975, Mann et al 1980). The decreased vascular resistance that occurs with hemorrhage results in preferential blood flow to bleeding sites and allows Gelfoam or steel coil embolization (Fig. 13-4). It is important to use arteriography to identify all vessels that may contribute to pelvic bleeding because frequently, vessels other than those originating from the hypogastric vessels are involved.

The use of the Nd:YAG laser (Schellhas et al 1983) or photoirradiation (Rettenmaier et al 1984) may play a role in the management of bleeding problems in these patients.

Patsner (1993) reported the potential benefit of topical acetone for control of life-threatening vaginal hemorrhage from recurrent gynecologic cancer.

Medical Pain Control

About 70% of all cancer patients experience significant pain (Grossman 1993). A fourth of cancer patients develop pain as a direct result of therapy. There are ample data to demonstrate that cancer pain is undertreated throughout the world. As many as 25% of all cancer patients die in severe pain, whereas as many as 60% to 70% of patients in the hospital or at home have inadequate pain relief during the final portion of their lives. The usual treatment regimen results in a 70% reduction of pain in less than half of patients. One of 8 patients who are treated report less than 30% relief. Resultant sleep disturbances, feelings of hopelessness, fear, and other problems often interfere with quality of life. The adequate relief of cancer pain can be achieved in 70% to 95% of patients with simple pharmacologic therapy (Beaver et al 1984, Portenoy 1993a, b, Grossman 1993). There is a wide array of effective options for the remaining 15% of patients who continue to have pain. Proper use of parenteral and intraspinal opioids, glucocorticoids, anti-inflammatory agents, or adjunctive medications, anesthetic, and neurosurgical procedures in addition to specific antineoplastic therapies should result in excellent pain control in 95% of patients who have pain due to cancer.

Unfortunately, oncologists seem reluctant to routinely assess pain and prescribe appropriate treatment (Grossman 1993). Studies document that physicians and nurses lack important opioid prescribing and monitoring skills. Clinicians commonly perceive that their patients underreport symptoms. This phenomenon could be attributed to stoicism, a desire to please the physician, the perception that pain is inevitable, concern that the physician could be distracted by reports of pain from the more important task of primary treatment, or the fear on the patient's part of possible serious side effects or addiction. The success of therapy for cancer pain depends on the ability of the clinician to assess the presenting problem, identify and evaluate pain syndromes, and formulate a plan for continuing care that is responsive to the changing needs of the patient. Only after consideration of the pain location, mechanism, extent of the tumor, physical and mental condition of the patient, and availability and practicality of the various methods of pain relief can appropriate therapy be selected. The aim of cancer pain management is to achieve and maintain an optimal balance between pain relief and adverse pharmacologic effects. Professional education in the area of cancer pain management often is inadequate. All of these issues are magnified in children, older patients, and individuals who have a history of drug abuse.

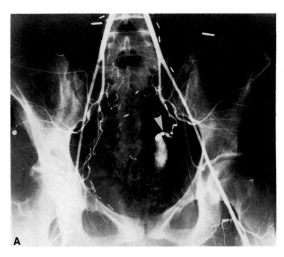
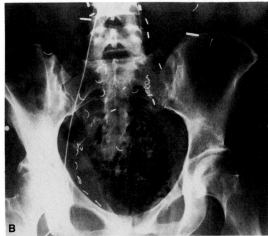

FIGURE 13-4. Control of hemorrhage in a patient with recurrent cancer. (**A**) The hypogastric artery (*arrow*) was easily demonstrated by arteriography as the site of hemorrhage. (**B**) Steel coil embolization promptly stopped the bleeding. (Shingleton JM, Orr JW Jr. Cancer of the cervix: diagnosis and treatment. New York, Churchill Livingstone, 1987.)

Pain is an entirely subjective phenomena. As such, it can only be experienced and quantified by the patient. Its assessment is further complicated when patients with chronic pain appear comfortable while they are actually experiencing considerable, even severe, unrelenting discomfort. Physicians and other healthcare personnel caring for cancer patients cannot provide adequate analgesia without knowing the degree of the patient's pain.

The cause of cancer-related pain is usually multifactorial. Such pain is the result of injury to somatic, visceral, and autonomic nerves. The damaged nerves produce a deafferentation pain, mediated by specific pathways in the central nervous system. Small, thin, myelinated nerve fibers (A-delta) and unmyelinated (C fibers) relay stimuli at different speeds to the dorsal root ganglia. After processing and relating to other inhibitory and exciting influences, they ascend through the neospinothalamic tract (pain intensity and localization) and paleospinothalamic (arousal and emotion) tract. Descending pathways from the medulla modulate pain transmission at the level of the dorsal root ganglia. Neurotransmitter substances (serotonin, substance P, dopamine, norepinephrine, and endogenous opioid peptides) are intimately involved in the processing and modulation of efferent and afferent pathways. Careful evaluation of pain and use of nonanalgesic regimens such as (1) local nerve blocks, (2) radiation therapy for bone metastases, (3) antibiotics for infections, (4) surgical procedures for bowel or ureteral obstruction, and (5) chemotherapy trials are appropriate. An attempt to relieve acute pain (thought to be related to the damage and increased excitability or sensitivity of peripheral axons or nerve membranes) is important and may be accomplished with medication. Chronic unrelenting pain secondary to deafferentation leads to central neuronal hyperactivity in the spinal cord or thalamus (Foley 1985), which is resistant to most forms of therapy. The particular problem of lower extremity pain and edema should be mentioned. Many consider this problem to be related to lymphatic obstruction; however, these patients may have primary or secondary venous thrombosis (Fig. 13-5) and are symptomatically relieved after systemic heparinization (Simon et al 1984). If no reversible component is present, it becomes necessary to prescribe alternative analgesia.

Three categories of analgesic medication are used in the treatment of cancer pain: nonsteroidal anti-inflammatory drugs (NSAIDs), opioid analgesics, and adjuvant analgesics. An adjuvant analgesic is defined as a drug that has a primary indication other than pain but can be an effective analgesic in specific circumstances (Portenoy 1993b). Drug selection generally proceeds in an approach known as the analgesic ladder, beginning with the use of a nonsteroidal anti-inflammatory drug for those patients having mild to moderate pain. This drug is often combined with an adjuvant analgesic when specific indication exists. Opioids are added when patients fail to obtain significant or satisfactory relief or for those who present with moderate to severe pain. Premature use can result in early development of tolerance and the necessity of large dosages to relieve pain in the later stages of disease. An adjuvant analgesic is again added if indicated. The World Health Organization has designated as-

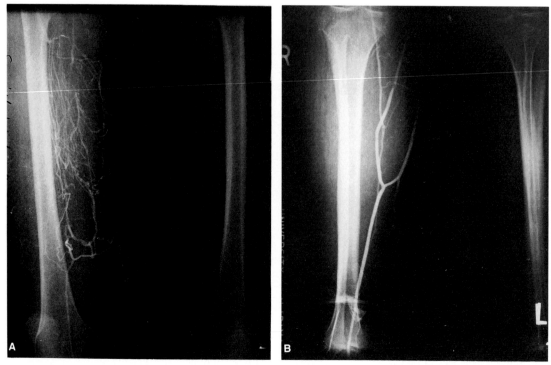

FIGURE 13-5. A 53-year-old woman with pelvic recurrence had extensive right unilateral leg edema and hip pain. (**A**) A venogram demonstrated total occlusion of the venous system. (**B**) She improved dramatically after 5 days of systemic anticoagulation (Shingleton JM, Orr JW Jr. Cancer of the cervix: diagnosis and treatment. New York, Churchill Livingstone, 1987.)

pirin, codeine, and morphine as the prototypical drugs for each of the three rings of the analgesic ladder.

NONSTEROIDAL ANTI-INFLAMMATORY DRUGS

Nonsteroidal anti-inflammatory drugs are believed to provide analgesia through a peripheral mechanism related to an inhibition of the enzyme cyclooxygenase (Table 13-12). This action presumably reduces tissue levels of prostaglandins, which serve as inflammatory mediators known to sensitize peripheral nociceptors. Information suggests, however, that these drugs have important central effects also.

The NSAIDs are comprised of numerous subclasses. Although there have been anecdotal suggestions that efficacy and side effect liability cluster within each subclass, the variability in response to different agents within a subclass (like the response to different subclasses) is so large that the analgesic response to any particular drug cannot be reliably predicted from the outcomes of previous trials. This variability suggests that the clinician must be familiar with several agents, so that the sequential trials can be undertaken in patients who do not initially obtain a favorable therapeutic response. The safe administration of these

agents requires familiarity with their potential adverse effects. Prudence is required when using these agents in specific patient subgroups that are at increased risk for adverse effects, including those (1) receiving concomitant corticosteroids, (2) who have a clotting disorder, (3) who have a propensity to peptic ulceration, or (4) who have impaired renal function.

Nonsteroidal anti-inflammatory drugs used alone are helpful for providing patients with mild to moderate pain relief and adequate analgesia when combined with opioid drugs in the treatment of more severe pain. They are particularly effective in patients who have bone pain and inflammatory lesions; however, their efficacy in neuropathic pain may be minimal.

The crude odds ratio for nonsteroidal anti-inflammatory agents, as a class, to result in neutropenia is 3. No single class of nonsteroidal anti-inflammatory agents nor any individual drug is associated with a unique risk, although the data on individual nonsteroidal agents is sparse. Even when excluding phenbutazone and indomethacin, an increased risk is observed (Strom et al 1993).

Dosing guidelines that minimize the risk of adverse effects are particularly important in the medically ill cancer population. Although these drugs are usually administered according to a fixed dosing regimen, the

TABLE 13-12
Selected Nonsteroidal Anti-Inflammatory Drugs
and Recommended Doses for Pain

Acid Source and Generic Name	Trade Name	Initial Oral Dose (mg)
Propionic acid		
Ibuprofen	Motrin	200–400
Naproxen	Naprosyn	250–500
Ketoprofen	Orudis	25–50
Indolacetic acid		
Indomethacin	Indocin	25
Sulindac	Clinoril	15–200
Pyrrolacetic acid		
Ketorolac tromethamine	Toradol	10*

*Intramuscular dose; initially, 30–60 mg; subsequently,
15–30 mg.

*Modified from Rummans TA. Nonopioid agents for treatment
of acute and subacute pain. Mayo Clin Proc 1994;69:481.*

availability of short half-life drugs (including aspirin, acetaminophen, and ibuprofen) allows "as needed" administration if it minimizes the dose and provides greater control for the patient.

Nonsteroidal anti-inflammatory drug analgesia is characterized by a ceiling dose, beyond which additional increments fail to yield greater pain relief, and by lack of demonstrable physical dependence or tolerance. Improved analgesia after an increase in dose implies that the ceiling has not been reached and further dose escalation can be considered. The contrary is also a possibility. The physician must remember that dose escalation is limited by the increasing risk of adverse effects and the lack of information about the safety of relatively high doses in the cancer population. Based on clinical experience and customary use, maximal doses of 1.5 to 2 times the standard recommended dose are prudent limits.

Although several weeks are needed to evaluate the efficacy of a dose when NSAIDs are used in the treatment of gross inflammatory lesions such as arthritis, clinical experience suggests that a briefer period, usually a week, is adequate for the same purpose in the treatment of cancer pain. Dose titration therefore usually proceeds at weekly intervals. Failure with one NSAID can be followed by success with another. In cancer patients having persistent mild pain, sequential trials of several NSAIDs may be useful to identify drugs that have a favorable balance between analgesia and side effects. Newer drugs (e.g., ketorolac tromethamine [Toradol]) have demonstrated effects comparable to opioid narcotics.

OPIOIDS

Relative analgesic potency is conventionally expressed as a dose that is equal as an analgesic to 10 mg of parenteral morphine. Equal analgesic dose information provides a useful guide for dose selection when the drug or route of administration is changed. Equal analgesic doses are not standard starting doses, nor do they constitute a firm conversion table for switching between opioids. For the patient who is opioid naive, with no evidence of renal failure, any of the available agonist opioids can be selected (Table 13-13). The chosen opioid should be administered by the least invasive and safest route that is capable of providing adequate analgesia. Noninvasive alternatives to the oral route in relatively nontolerant patients include the rectal, transdermal, nasal, and sublingual routes; for example, controlled-release morphine tablets can be administered rectally.

The development of expertise in the management of opioid analgesics is the single most important factor in successful treatment of cancer pain. Pharmacologic factors strongly influence the initial selection of an opioid and the choice of subsequent drugs if a change should become necessary. Based on the interaction with various opioid-receptor subtypes, opioid analgesics can be divided into agonist and agonist–antagonist classes. The agonist–antagonist drugs are seldom used in the management of cancer pain.

Codeine is the prototype for the "weak" opioids; however, propoxyphene, oxycodone, hydrocodone, dihydrocodone, and meperidine have also been used. None of these drugs have ceiling doses for analgesia but are customarily used orally at doses adequate to treat the nontolerant patient, usually with no more than moderate pain.

Meperidine is used by some clinicians but is not preferred because of its low oral potency. Its metabolite, normeperidine, can accumulate and produce central nervous system toxicity, including myoclonus, tremulousness, and even seizures. These events are most likely to become clinically evident in patients who have renal insufficiency and in those who require high doses for prolonged intervals. The metabolism of propoxyphene also yields a toxic metabolite, norpropoxyphene, with a clinical relevance of this compound limited at the doses that are employed during routine clinical practice.

In the United States, it has become common clinical practice to initiate opioid therapy with a combination product, usually one in which aspirin or acetaminophen is combined with either codeine, oxycodone, or propoxyphene. Patients are typically treated with a combination product until doses are reached that begin to exceed those that provide acceptable quantities of the coanalgesic. The administra-

TABLE 13-13
Characteristics of Narcotic Analgesics Commonly Used for Cancer Pain Relief

ANALGESIC	EQUI-ANALGESIC MILLIGRAM DOSE (MORPHINE, 10 MG IM)		ORAL: PARENTERAL POTENCY	ONSET OF ANALGESIA (MIN)	DURATION OF ANALGESIA (H)	CONTRAST TO MORPHINE
	IM	PO				
Morphine	10	30–60	0.17	30–60 (IM)	4–7	—
Fentanyl transdermal	0.1 (IV)	—	—	12–36	72	Days to reach steady state with transdermal use
Oxymorphone	1	10*	0.17	10–15 (IM)	3–6	Rapid onset; available as rectal suppository; no oral preparation
Hydromorphone	1.5	8	0.20	15–20 (IM or PO)	4–5	Short-acting; available as rectal suppository
Levorphanol	2	4	0.50	60–90 (IM or PO)	4–6	Long-acting; high oral potency; may accumulate
Butorphanol	2	—	—	30–60 (IM)	4	Nalorphine-like antagonistic properties; available in nasal spray
Heroin	5	30	0.17	—	5	Short-acting; illegal in the United States
Dezocine	10	—	—	30–60	3–4	Recently approved—little experience
Methadone	10	20	0.5	30–60 (IM or PO)	4–6	High oral potency
Nalbuphine	10	—	—	15 (IM)	3–6	Rapid onset; nalorphine-like antagonistic properties
Oxycodone	15	30	0.5	10–15 (PO)	3–6	Rapid onset; high oral potency
Alphaprodine	45	—	—	1–2 (IV)	0.5–1	Rapid-acting; short onset
Anileridine	30	50	0.5	15 (IM or		Rapid onset; short-
Pentazocine	60	180	0.3	20 (IM)	3	Shorter-acting nalorphine-like antagonistic properties; may precipitate withdrawal
Meperidine	75	300	0.25	30–50 (IM) 40–60 (PO)	2–4	Shorter-acting; metabolites may produce CNS excitation; avoid in renal failure
Codeine	130	200	0.65	15–30 (IM or PO)	4–6	High oral potency; constipation

*Rectal suppository.
IM, intramuscularly; *PO*, perorally; *IV*, intravenously.

tion of 2 tablets of an oxycodone acetaminophen combination product every 4 hours results in the administration of almost 4 g of acetaminophen per day, a dose that is safe for almost all patients. Three tablets administered every 4 hours provides almost 6 g of acetaminophen daily, a level that requires closer monitoring and may raise concern about hepatic toxicity in specific patients.

In most cases, failure of one of these combination products is followed by a switch to a pure agonist, usually given for severe pain. Morphine is usually considered to be the preferred drug for the treatment of severe cancer pain. Patients in the United States, however, have access to morphine, methadone, hydromorphone, narvophenol, and oxycodone as a single entity. Oxymorphone is available in rectal and parenteral formulations and fentanyl has become available in transdermal formulations.

Morphine administration results in an active metabolite, morphine 6-glucuronide. This metabolite binds to opioid receptors and produces potent analgesic effects; it appears in the plasma and cerebrospinal fluid of patients receiving morphine. High concentrations, particularly those in renal insufficiency, have been associated with toxicity. Because four to five half-lives are usually required to approach steady-state plasma concentration after any dose change, drugs with long half-lives may accumulate for many days after dosing is initiated or increased. The time required to approach steady state with these agents should be viewed as a period of increased risk, during which drug accumulation may result in delayed toxicity. For older and frail patients and particularly for patients who have major organ failure, drugs with long half-lives such as methadone and levorphanol are not recommended because they can be difficult to titrate and monitor. The active metabolites of propoxyphene (norpropoxyphene), meperidine (normeperidine), and morphine may accumulate in patients who have renal impairment and particular caution is required in using these agents for such patients. In most situations, morphine sulfate should be selected because of the short half-life and ease of titration in its immediate or least form. It is also available as a controlled-release preparation that allows a convenient 8- to 12-hour dosing interval once optimal dosage has been achieved.

The controlled-release oral morphine preparation requires 1 day to approach steady state. The new transdermal system for fentanyl usually requires 2 or more days. These intervals do not relate to the elimination half-lives of morphine or fentanyl, respectively, but to the absorption pharmacokinetics of the system by which each is delivered. The duration of analgesia after each dose can be another important factor in drug selection.

The large variability that characterizes the individual response to different opioid drugs suggests that prior experience with these agents should be considered when selecting a drug. For older patients and for those who have major organ failure, there are reasons to prefer short–half-life drugs that require relatively short periods to achieve stable plasma concentrations, including morphine and hydromorphone and oxycodone.

The success of cancer pain relief usually relates to the specific opioid selected. The oral route is preferred because of its relative safety, acceptability, and economy. Nonetheless, alternative routes are frequently needed, particularly for those patients having advanced disease. In the United States, rectal formulations are available for morphine, hydromorphone, and oxymorphone. The potency of opioids administered by this route is believed to be similar to oral dosing. Narcotic analgesics should be offered on a regular basis and not given "as necessary." This regimen not only relieves pain but reassures the patient by giving her confidence in the physician, thereby lowering the total analgesic dose by alleviating anxiety and apprehension.

Dose titration is essential at the start of therapy and is usually repeated as necessary during the patient's management. A patient who is relatively nontolerant, having had only some exposure to so-called weak opioids, should begin opioid treatment in a dose equivalent to 5 to 10 mg of intramuscular morphine every 4 hours. A useful approach to dose titration involves the concurrent use of a regular scheduled dose and a "rescue" dose. The rescue dose is a supplemental dose of the opioid that is offered on an as-needed basis. It can provide a means to treat "breakthrough" pain in patients who are already stabilized with a baseline opioid regimen and can be used to facilitate titration of the baseline regimen in patients having uncontrolled pain. The rescue dose can be offered every 2 hours as needed and more frequently in some patients. A quantity equivalent to about 5% to 15% of the total daily opioid intake is usually adequate.

Because the response to opioids increases linearly with the log of the dose, dose escalation of less than 30% to 50% is not likely to improve analgesia significantly. For example, in patients who have advanced cancer, the average daily opioid requirement is equivalent to 400 to 500 mg of intramuscular morphine. About 10% of patients require more than 2000 mg over 24 hours and some may require 3000 mg every 24 hours.

Studies in acute pain models have established the efficacy of transdermal fentanyl administration. There is, however, no evidence that the transdermal system provides benefits beyond optimal oral administration of other opioids in cancer patients. It is possible that indications (i.e., noncompliance) will evolve as further studies are completed. It should be emphasized that when using transdermal administration, the clinician must understand that there is a slow onset of effect after the patch is applied and a slow decay after its removal. During the initial titration phase, an alternative means of analgesia should be provided.

There is extensive experience with the use of infusion techniques to treat cancer pain, and intravenous opioid infusion is still used frequently in the hospital setting. The advent of ambulatory infusion devices can provide long-term subcutaneous opioid administration and provide a means to continue this approach indefinitely. Intraspinal administration of opioids has also achieved wide acceptance in the management of cancer pain.

Although opioid administration is associated with numerous potential side effects, the most common are constipation, nausea, and sedation. Constipation is so common that a prophylactic regimen should be given to all patients predisposed to this effect (e.g., older patients, those with intrinsic bowel disease, nonambulatory patients, and those concurrently taking other drugs with constipating effects). The frequency of opioid-induced nausea has been estimated to be 10% to 40%; opioid-induced vomiting occurs in 15% to 40% of patients. Clinical experience suggests that the size of the rescue dose should be equivalent to about 5% to 15% of the 24-hour baseline dose. Other important dose-limiting adverse effects include sedation, delirium, myoclonus, and respiratory depression. The occurrence of nausea should be aggressively managed with one of the various antiemetic drugs. Sedation precludes the use of an otherwise effective analgesic and can be managed by the addition of a psychostimulant, specifically dextroamphetamine or methylphenidate.

ADJUVANT ANALGESICS

Many drugs provide adjuvant analgesia (Table 13-14). The tricyclic antidepressants have been demonstrated to be analgesic in many types of chronic nonmalignant pain and are typically used to supplement an opioid regimen for patients who have cancer-related neuropathic pain syndromes, particularly those characterized by continuous dysesthesia, and patients with cancer pain accompanied with depression or insomnia. The likely mechanism is probably related to both the modulation of serotonin (an integral part of the descending endogenous pain pathway) or by treating depression, diminishing the perceived pain. These secondary amine drugs (desipramine, nortriptyline) are usually better tolerated but evidence of analgesic effects are stronger for the tertiary amine drugs (amitriptyline, doxepin, and imipramine). With all of these drugs, initial doses should be low (10 to 25 mg at night), then titrated upward.

Muscle relaxants and antispasmodics may be of use in situations associated with muscle spasm.

Studies have suggested that oral local anesthetic compounds may be effective in neuropathic pain. Mexiletine is the safest of these drugs and is used with continuous lancinating neuropathic pain.

The phenothiazine methotrimeprazine is analgesic and has been used clinically at times when employing opioid drugs is problematic or the pain is associated with vomiting, nausea, or anxiety.

Corticosteroids are important adjuvants in cancer pain, and their use can improve analgesia, mood, and appetite for the short term. They are most effective when pain is associated with inflammation or edema (e.g., tumor infiltration or nerve compression). If no benefit is noted after 1 week, the dose should be tapered and discontinued. If effective, the dose should be lowered to the lowest effective dose (Rummans 1994).

Adjunctive use of anticonvulsants may benefit patients having paroxysmal lancinating pain, often associated with a direct peripheral or central nervous system involvement.

Other adjuvant agents may be necessary to control the symptoms of depression, psychosis, or anxiety associated with recurrent incurable cancer. Fear, apprehension, anxiety, and depression accentuate cancer pain. Analgesic adjuvants such as anxiolytics or antidepressants may benefit selected patients. These drugs, however, have a lower potential than narcotics for controlling severe pain without producing undesired side effects.

Anecdotal evidence suggests that nonsteroidal anti-inflammatory drugs are particularly efficacious for bone pain, and corticosteroids are often advocated in difficult cases. Several surveys and controlled trials demonstrate that pamidronate and clodronate may relieve malignant bone pain. Newly developed radiopharmaceuticals that link a radioisotope with a biphosphonate compound are absorbed in areas of high bone turnover and apparently offer promise in controlling metastatic bone pain (strontium 89).

Anesthetic Techniques

Depending on the extent of disease, life expectancy, and cause of pain, there may be a place for a regional anesthetic or a neurosurgical procedure for those patients whose pain is uncontrolled; continuous epidural infusion of anesthetic agents by injection or infusion pump may give dramatic results (Malone et al 1985) and decrease narcotic intake and lower drug tolerance (Foley 1985; Table 13-15). The physician must not withdraw oral analgesics precipitously because withdrawal symptoms may ensue (Vincenti et al 1983).

Spinal analgesia is accomplished with epidural or

TABLE 13-14
Selected Adjuvant Drugs for Pain and Symptom Control

GENERIC NAME	TRADE NAME	INITIAL DOSE (MG)
TRICYCLIC ANTIDEPRESSANTS		
Amitriptyline HCl	Elavil	10–25
NortriptylineHCl	Pamelor	10–25
Imipramine	Tofranil	10–25
Desipramine HCl	Norpramin	10–25
Doxepin HCl	Sinequan	10–25
Trazodone HCl	Desyrel	25–100
CORTICOSTEROIDS		
Dexamethasone	Decadron	0.75
Methylprednisolone acetate	Depo-Medrol	4
Prednisone	Deltasone	5
Cortisone acetate	Cortone	25
ANTICONVULSANTS		
Phenytoin	Dilantin	100
Carbamazepine	Tegretol	100–200
Valproic acid	Depakene	250
Clonazepam	Klonopin	0.5–2
MUSCLE RELAXANTS		
Diazepam	Valium	5–10
Methocarbamol	Robaxin	500–1500
Cyclobenzaprine HCl	Flexeril	10
Baclofen	Lioresal	5–10
Orphenadrine citrate	Norgesic	25–50
ANTIPSYCHOTICS		
Phenothiazines		
Fluphenazine	Prolixin	0.5–5
Chlorpromazine	Thorazine	25–50
Butyrophenones		
Haloperidol	Haldol	0.5–5
SEROTONIN REUPTAKE INHIBITORS		
Fluoxetine HCl	Prozac	10–20
Sertraline HCl	Zoloft	25–50
Paroxetine HCl	Paxil	10–20
ANTISPASMODICS		
Belladonna and opium	B&O supprettes	30–60
Metoclopramide HCl	Reglan	10–25
Chlorpromazine	Thorazine	10–25

Modified from Rummans TA. Nonopioid agents for treatment of acute and subacute pain. Mayo Clin Proc 1994;69:481.

TABLE 13-15
Equivalent Daily Doses of Morphine

METHOD OF ADMINISTRATION	RELATIVE POTENCY (MG)*
Oral	300
Intravenous	20
Epidural	20
Intrathecal	1

*Relative approximations based on clinical observations.

Modified from Lamer TJ. Treatment of cancer-related pain: when orally administered medications fail. Mayo Clin Proc 1994;69:473.

subarachnoid delivery of appropriate analgesic agents by a percutaneous tunneled catheter, with or without an infusion port (Lamer 1994). Spinal analgesia, the most potent method of administration (Table 13-16), is indicated for patients who have opioid-sensitive pain that cannot be controlled with conventional oral, transdermal, or parenteral administration. Its use

provides intense analgesia, with less bothersome side effects. Its lack of efficacy in neuropathic pain and complications associated with available delivery systems are the only drawbacks.

Many somatic, visceral, and sympathetic nerves are amenable to neurolytic block (Table 13-17). Neurolytic nerve blocks using phenol cryotherapy or radiofrequency may be considered in patients who (1) have a limited life span, (2) have a favorable risk–benefit ratio, (3) have disease unresponsive to conventional antitumor treatment, and (4) exhibit a response to a prognostic blockade (Lamer 1994).

Surgical Pain Control

The use of neurodestructive procedures should be based on the careful evaluation of the likelihood and duration of analgesic benefit, the immediate risk of morbidity from the procedure, the anticipated length of hospital stay, and the risk of long-term neurologic sequelae.

Although clinical judgment is necessary to justify postoperative morbidity and mortality, neurosurgical procedures may be performed to control pain

TABLE 13-16
Anesthetic and Neurosurgical Analgesic Techniques for Pain Refractory to Systemic Pharmacotherapy

CLASS	TECHNIQUE	CLINICAL SITUATION
Regional analgesia	Spinal opioids and/or local anesthetics	Systemic opioid analgesia complicated by unmanageable supraspinally mediated adverse effects
Sympathetic blockade and neurolysis	Celiac plexus block	Refractory malignant pain involving the upper abdominal viscera, including the upper retroperitoneum, liver, small bowel, and proximal colon
	Lumbar sympathetic blockade	Sympathetically maintained pain involving the legs
	Stellate ganglion blockade	Sympathetically maintained pain involving the head, neck, or arms
Somatic neurolysis or pathway ablation	Chemical or surgical rhizotomy	Refractory brachial plexopathy or arm pain; intercostal nerve pain, chest wall pain; refractory bilateral pelvic or lumbosacral plexus pain in patients with urinary diversion who are confined to bed
	Trigeminal neurolysis	Refractory unilateral facial pain
	Transsacral neurolysis	Refractory pain limited to the perineum
	Cordotomy	Refractory unilateral pain arising in the torso or lower extremity
Other	Cingulotomy	Refractory multifocal pain
	Pituitary ablation	Refractory multifocal pain

Modified from Cherny NI. Strategies for managing cancer pain. Adv Oncol 1993;9(3):20.

TABLE 13-17
Neurolytic Nerve Blocks for Patients
With Cancer-Related Pain

TYPE OF PAIN	TYPE OF BLOCK
Perineal	Sacral nerve
Chest and abdominal wall	Intercostal nerve or paravertebral nerve
Causalgic	Neurolytic sympathetic
Visceral abdominal	Celiac plexus or splanchnic nerve
Visceral pelvic	Hypogastric plexus
Facial	Trigeminal nerve and its divisions

Modified from Lamer TJ. Treatment of cancer-related pain: when orally administered medications fail. Mayo Clin Proc 1994;69:473.

(Table 13-18). Neuroablative procedures, including neuroaugmentation, involve the stimulation or activation of endogenous pain-modulation or pain-suppression systems in the central nervous system. Dorsal rhizot-omy (sectioning of the sensory nerve roots to interrupt afferent pain fibers) may be useful when pain is localized to the abdominal wall or sacral or perineal area. Sacral rhizotomies carry little morbidity when the sacral roots S_2 and S_3 are preserved on one side to prevent urinary incontinence in patients who have intact bladders. Commissural myelotomy (interruption of

TABLE 13-18
Neurosurgical Procedures for Relief of Pain in Patients
With Cancer

Neuroaugmentative procedures
  Spinal cord stimulation
  Deep-brain stimulation
  Intracerebroventrical administration of opioids
Neuroablative procedures
  Peripheral procedures
    Neurectomy and neorotomy
    Dorsal rhizotomy
  Spinal cord procedures
    Percutaneous and open cordotomy
    Commissural myelotomy
    Lesioning of the dorsal root entry zone
  Cortical and brain stem procedures
    Stereotactic mesencephalotomy
    Mesencephalic spinothalamic tractotomy
    Trimeniothalamic tractotomy
    Pituitary ablation

crossing spinothalamic tracts) may also benefit those patients who have sacral pain or bilateral lower extremity pain. Dysesthesia and posterior column deficits after the procedure are transient, with satisfactory pain relief in more than 80% of patients; however, pain frequently recurs when the patient survives for longer than 1 year. Urinary incontinence and motor weakness are rare complications of myelotomy. Percutaneous cervical cordotomy is successful in more than 85% of patients; bilateral destruction of the spinothalamic tract, however, carries a significant risk of lower extremity paralysis or urinary incontinence. A phenol subarachnoid block may relieve pain in many patients who have a short (less than 3 months) life expectancy (Lifshitz et al 1976).

References

Aboul-Hosn H, Goldman M, Halsted G, Williams J. Hypercalcemia secondary to a cervical cancer: resolution by surgical resection. J Med Soc New Jersey 1983; 80:1025.

Alberts DS, Garcia D, Mason-Liddil N. Cisplatin in advanced cancer of the cervix: an update. Semin Oncol 1991; 18:11.

Alberts DS, Ignoffo R. Adriamycin-cyclophosphamide treatment of squamous cell carcinoma of the cervix. Cancer Treat Reports 1978;62:143.

Alberts DS, Martimbeau PW, Surwitz ON. Mitomycin-C, bleomycin, vincristine and *cis*-platin in the treatment of advanced, recurrent squamous cell carcinoma of the cervix. Cancer Clin Trials 1981;4:313.

Alberts DS, Mason-Liddil N. The role of cisplatin in the management of advanced squamous cell cancer of the cervix. Semin Oncol 1989;16(4):66.

Alvarez RD. Gastrointestinal complications in gynecologic surgery: a review for the general gynecologist. Obstet Gynecol 1988;72:533.

Averette HE, Weinstein GD, Ford JH Jr, et al. Cell kinetics and programmed chemotherapy for gynecologic cancer. I. Squamous cell carcinoma. Am J Obstet Gynecol 1976;124:912.

Baker LH, Opipari MI, Wilson H, et al. Mitomycin-C, vincristine, and bleomycin therapy for advanced cervical cancer. Obstet Gynecol 1978;52:146.

Bates R, Deppe G, Malone JM, et al. Combination chemotherapy for advanced adenocarinoma of the cervix. Cancer 1991;68:747.

Beaver WT, Foley KM, Cleeland CS, et al. Symposium on the management of cancer pain. Hospital Practice, Summer 1984.

Belinson JL, Stewart JA, Richards AL, McClure M. Bleomycin, vincristine, mitomycin C and cisplatin in the management of gynecological squamous cell carcinomas. Gynecol Oncol 1985;20:387.

Bloch B, Nel CP, Kriel A, Atad J, Goldberg G. Combination chemotherapy with cisplatin and bleomycin in advanced cervical cancer. Cancer Treat Reports 1984;68:891.

Boice CR, Freedman RS, Herson J, et al. Bleomycin and mitomycin-C (BLM-M) in recurrent squamous uterine cervical carcinoma. Cancer 1982;49:2242.

Bolger JJ, Dearnaley DP, Kirk D, et al. Strontium 89 (metastron) versus external beam radiotherapy in patients with painful bone metastases secondary to prostatic cancer: preliminary report of a multicenter trial. Semin Oncol 1993;20(3):32.

Bond WH, Arthur K, Banks AJ, et al. Combination chemotherapy in the treatment of advanced squamous cell carcinoma of the cervix. Clin Oncol 1976;2:173.

Bonomi P, Blessing J, Ball H, et al. A phase II evaluation of cisplatin and 5-Fluorouracil in patients with advanced squamous cell carcinoma of the cervix: a gynecologic oncology group study. Gynecol Oncol 1989;34:357.

Bonomi P, Blessing JA, Stehman FB, et al. Randomized trial of three displatin dose schedules in squamous cell carcinoma of the cervix: a Gyneclogic Oncology Group study. J Clin Oncol 1985;3:1079.

Borgelt B, Gelber R, Kramer S, et al. The palliation of brain metastases: final results of the first two studies by the radiation oncology group. Int J Radiat Oncol Biol Phys 1980;6:1.

Brin EN, Schiff J Jr, Weiss RM. Palliative urinary diversion for pelvic malignancy. J Urol 1975;113:619.

Brown DL, Mackey DC. Management of postoperative pain: influence of anesthetic and analgesic choice. Mayo Clin Proc 1993;68:768.

Brunschwig A. Surgical treatment of carcinoma of the cervix, recurrent after irradiation or combination or irradiation and surgery. Am J Roentgenol, Rad Ther Nuc Med 1967;99:363.

Buxton EJ. Experience with bleomycin, ifosfamide, and cisplatin in primary and recurrent cervical cancer. Semin Oncol 1992;19(2):9.

Calkins AR, Lester SG, Stehman FB, et al. Intraoperative radiotherapy in advanced, recurrent or metastatic malignancy. Indiana Med 1985;78:206.

Carlson JA Jr, Day TG, Allegra JC, et al. Methyl-CCNA, doxorubicin, and *cis*-diaminedichloroplatinum II in the management of recurrent and metastatic squamous carcinoma of the cervix. Cancer 1984;54:211.

Carlson JA Jr, Freedman RS, Wallace S, et al. Intra-arterial *cis*-platinum in the management of squamous cell carcinoma of the uterine cervix. Gynecol Oncol 1981;12:92.

Chahbazian C. Radiation therapy for the palliation of pain in advanced cancer. Am J Clin Oncol 1993;16(5):444.

Chan WK, Aroney RS, Levi JA, et al. Four-drug combination chemotherapy for advanced cervical carcinoma. Cancer 1982;49:2437.

Cherny NI. Strategies for managing cancer pain. Adv Oncol 1993;9(3):20.

Chung CK, Nahhas WA, Stryker JA, Mortel R. Treatment outcome of recurrent cervical cancer. J Surg Oncol 1983;24:5.

Coddington CC, Thomas JR, Hoskins WJ. Percutaneous nephrostomy for ureteral obstruction in patients with gynecologic malignancy. Gynecol Oncol 1984;18:339.

Cohen CJ, Deppe G, Yannopoulos K, Gusberg SB. Chemosensitivity testing with *cis*-platinum (II) diaminedichloride. 1. A new concept in the treatment of carcinoma of the cervix. Gynecol Oncol 1982;13:1.

Coleman RE, Clarke JM, et al. A phase II study of ifosfamide and cisplatin chemotherapy for metastatic or relapsed carcinoma of the cervix. Cancer Chemother Pharmacol 1990;27:52.

Conroy JF, Lewis GC, Bracy LW, et al. Low dose bleomycin and methotrexate in cervical cancer. Cancer 1976; 37:660.

Daghestani AN, Hakes TB, Lynch G, Lewis JL Jr. Cervix carcinoma: treatment with combination cisplatin and bleomycin. Gynecol Oncol 1983;16:334.

Day TG Jr, Warton JT, Gottlieb JA, Rutledge FN. Chemotherapy for squamous carcinoma of the cervix: doxorubicin-methyl-CCNA. Am J Obstet Gynecol 1978;132:545.

Deka AC, Deka BC, Patil RB, Joshi SG. Chemotherapy in recurrent or metastatic cervical cancer. Indian J Cancer 1979;16:32.

Delgado G, Goldson AL, Ashayeri E, et al. Intraoperative radiation in the treatment of advanced cervical cancer. Obstet Gynecol 1984;63:246.

DeMurua EO, George M, Pejovic MH, Dewaily J, Wolff JP. Combination cyclophosphamide, Adriamycin, and cisplatinum in recurrent and metastatic cervical carcinoma. Gynecol Oncol 1987;26:225.

dePalo GM, Bajetta E, Beretta G, Bonadonna G. Adriamycin plus bleomycin versus cyclophosphamide plus vincristine in advanced carcinoma of the uterine cervix. Tumori 1976;62:113.

Dosoretz DE, Tepper JE, Shim DS, et al. Intraoperative electron–beam irradiation in gynecologic malignant disease. Appl Radiol 1984;13:61.

Egashira K, Nakamura K, Terashima H, et al. MR imaging in uterine cervical cancer after radiotherapy. Radiat Med 1992;10:117.

Feun LG, Blessing JA, Barrett RJ, Hanjani P. A phase II trial of tricyclic nucleoside phosphate in patients with advanced squamous cell carcinoma of the cervix. Am J Clin Oncol 1993;16:506.

Fine S, Sturgeon JFG, Gospodarowicz MK, et al. Treatment of advanced carcinoma of the cervix with methotrexate, Adriamycin and cisplatin. Proc Am Soc Clin Oncol 1983;2:154(C-600).

Foley KM. The treatment of cancer pain. N Engl J Med 1985;313:84.

Forastiere AA, ed. Gynecologic cancer. New York: Churchill Livingstone, 1984.

Forney JP, Morrow CP, DiSaia PJ, Futoran RJ. Seven-drug polychemotherapy in the treatment of advanced and recurrent squamous carcinoma of the female genital tract. Am J Obstet Gynecol 1975;123:748.

Friedlander M, Kaye SB, Sullivan A, et al. Cervical carcinoma: a drug-responsive tumor experience with combined cisplatin, vinblastine and bleomycin therapy. Gynecol Oncol 1983;16:275.

Fukuoka M, Suzuki A, Fujii S, Okamura H. Palliative urinary diversion in patients with advanced cervical cancer. Eur J Obstet Gynecol Reprod Biol 1983;16:293.

Gao YL, Twiggs LB, Leung BS, et al. Cytoplasmic estrogen and progesterone receptors in primary cervical carcinoma: clinical and histopathologic correlates. Am J Obstet Gynecol 1983;146:299.

Garrison RN, Wilson MA. Intravenous and central catheter infections. Surg Clin North Am 1994;74:557.

Garton GR, Gunderson LL, Webb MJ, et al. Intraoperative radiation therapy in gynecologic cancer: the Mayo Clinic experience. Gynecol Oncol 1993;48:328.

Glover DD, Lowry TF, Jacknowitz AI. Brompton's mixture in alleviating pain of terminal neoplastic disease: preliminary results. South Med J 1980;73:278.

Goldson AL, Delgado G, Hill LT. Intraoperative radiation of the para-aortic nodes in cancer of the uterine cervix. Obstet Gynecol 1978;52:713.

Greenberg BR, Hannigan J, Gerretson L, et al. Sequential combination of bleomycin and mitomycin-C in advanced cervical cancer. An American experience: a northern California oncology group study. Cancer Treat Reports 1982;66:163.

Greenberg BR, Kardinal CG, Pajak TF, Bateman JR. Adriamycin versus Adriamycin and bleomycin in advanced epidermoid carcinoma of the cervix. Cancer Treat Reports 1977;61:1383.

Greenberg MS. Handbook of neurosurgery, 3rd ed. Lakeland, FL, Greenberg Graphics, 1994.

Grigsby PW, Vest ML, Perez CA. Recurrent carcinoma of the cervix exclusively in the para-aortic nodes following radiation therapy. Int J Radiat Oncol Biol Phys 1993;28:451.

Grossman SA. Is pain undertreated? Adv Oncol 1993;9(3):9.

Guthrie D. Treatment of carcinoma of the cervix with bromocriptine. Br J Obstet Gynaecol 1982;89:853.

Guthrie D, Way W. The use of Adriamycin and methotrexate in carcinoma of the cervix. Obstet Gynecol 1978;52:349.

Haid M, Homesley H, White DR, et al. Adriamycin-methotrexate combination chemotherapy of advanced carcinoma of the cervix. Obstet Gynecol 1977;50:103.

Hakes T, Nikrui M, MaGill G, Ochoa M. Cervix cancer. Treatment with combination vincristine and high doses of methotrexate. Cancer 1979;43:459.

Hanjani P, Bonnell S. Treatment of advanced and recurrent squamous cell carcinoma with combination doxorubicin and cyclophosphamide. Cancer Treat Reports 1980;64:1363.

Hannigan EV, Dinh TV, Doherty MG. Ifosfamide with mesna in squamous carcinoma of the cervix: phase II results in patients with advanced or recurrent disease. Gynecol Oncol 1991;43:123.

Heggue G, Carpenter JT. Hypercalcemia of malignancy. Intern Med 1985;6:71.

Helmkamp BF, Kimmel J. Conservative management of small bowel obstruction. Am J Obstet Gynecol 1985;152:677.

Hirabayashi K, Okada E. Combination chemotherapy with 254-S, ifosfamide, and peplomycin for advanced or recurrent cervical cancer. Cancer 1993;71:2769.

Hiraoka O, Nakai T, Shimuzu C. Modified pelvic vascular bed isolation chemotherapy: theoretical basis, surgical procedure and two clinical case reports. Gynecol Oncol 1980;9:134.

Hockel M, Knapstein PG. The combined operative and radiotherapeutic treatment (CORT) of recurrent gynecologic tumors infiltrating the pelvic wall (abstract). 23rd Annual Meeting, Society of Gynecologic Oncologists, 1992.

Hoeg JM, Slatopolsky E. Cervical carcinoma and ectopic hyperparathyroidism. Arch Intern Med 1980;140:569.

Hoffman MS, Kavanagh JJ, Roberts WS, et al. A phase II evaluation of cisplatin, bleomycin, and mitomycin-C in patients with recurrent squamous cell carcinoma of the cervix. Gynecol Oncol 1991;40:144.

Holloway RW, Orr JW Jr. Experience with the Groshong catheter on a gynecologic oncology service (abstract). Annual Meeting, American College of Obstetrics and Gynecology, Orlando, FL, May 9, 1994.

Jacobs AJ, Blessing JA, Munoz A. A phase II trial of Didemnin B (NSC 325319) in advanced and recurrent cervical carcinoma: a Gynecologic Oncology Group study. Gynecol Oncol 1992;44:268.

Jakobsen A, Bichel P, Kristensen GB, Nyland M. Prognostic influence of ploidy level and histopathologic differentiation in cervical carcinoma stage IB. Eur J Cancer Clin Oncol 1988;24(6):969.

Jobson VW, Muss HB, Thigpen JT, et al. Chemotherapy of advanced squamous carcinoma of the cervix: a phase I-II study of high-dose cisplatin and cyclophosphamide. A pilot study of the Gynecologic Oncology Group. Am J Clin Oncol 1984;7:342.

Jones TK Jr, Levitt SH, King ER. Retreatment of persistent and recurrent carcinoma of the cervix with irradiation. Radiology 1970;95:167.

Junor E, Davies J, Habeshaw T, et al. Carboplatin-based combination chemotherapy for advanced carcinoma of the cervix. Cancer Chemother Pharmacol 1991;27:481.

Kaern J, Trope C, Abeler V, Iversen T, Kjorstad K. A phase II study of 5-fluorouracil/cisplatinum in recurrent cervical cancer. Acta Oncol 1990;29:25.

Kato T, Nemoto R, Mori H, et al. Arterial chemoembolization with microencapsulated anticancer drug. JAMA 1981;245:1123.

Katz HJ, Davies JNP. Death from cervix uteri carcinoma: the changing pattern. Gynecol Oncol 1980;9:86.

Kavanagh J, Wallace S, Delclos L, Rutledge F. Update of the results of intra-arterial (IA) chemotherapy for advanced squamous cell carcinoma of the cervix. Proc Am Soc Clin Oncol 1984;25:C-671.

Keettel WC, VanVoorhis LW, Latourette HB. Management of recurrent carcinoma of the cervix. Am J Obstet Gynecol 1968;102:671.

Kigawa J, Kanamori Y, Ishihara H, et al. Response rate and cell-cycle changes due to intra-arterial ifusion chemotherapy with cisplatin and bleomycin for locally recurrent uterine cervical cancer. Am J Clin Oncol 1992;15:474.

Krebs HB, Girtanner RE, Nordqvist RB, et al. Treatment of advanced cervical cancer by combination of bleomycin and mitomycin-C. Cancer 1980;46:2159.

Kredentser DC. Etoposide (VP-16), ifosfamide/mesna, and cisplatin chemotherapy for advanced and recurrent carcinoma of the cervix. Gynecol Oncol 1991;43:145.

Kumar L, Bhargara VL. Chemotherapy in recurrent and advanced cervical cancer. Gynecol Oncol 1991;40:107.

Lamer TJ. Treatment of cancer-related pain: when orally administered medications fail. Mayo Clin Proc 1994;69:473.

Leichman LP, Baker LH, Stanhope CR, et al. Mitomycin C and bleomycin in the treatment of far advanced cervical cancer: a Southwest oncology group pilot study (abstract). Cancer Treat Reports 1980;64:1139.

Lele SB, Piver MS, Barlow JJ. Cyclophosphamide, Adriamycin and platinum chemotherapy in treatment of advanced and recurrent cervical carcinoma. Gynecol Oncol 1983;16:15.

Lifshitz S, Debacker LJ, Buchsbaum HJ. Subarachnoid phenol block for pain relief in gynecologic malignancy. Obstet Gynecol 1976;48:316.

Lifshitz S, Railsback LD, Buchsbaum HJ. Intra-arterial pelvic infusion chemotherapy in advanced gynecologic cancer. Obstet Gynecol 1978;52:476.

Lira-Puerto V, Silva A, Morris M, et al. Phase II trial of carboplatin or iproplatin in cervical cancer. Cancer Chemother Pharmacol 1991;28:391.

Lira-Puerto VM, Hidalgo IN, Morales FR, Tenorio F. Bleomycin, methotrexate and cyclophosphamide in advanced squamous cell carcinoma of the uterine cervix. Proc Am Soc Clin Oncol 1979;20:319 (C-117).

Llorens AS. Chemotherapy of squamous cell carcinoma of the cervix. Obstet Gynecol 1980;55:373.

Long HJ, Wieand HS, Foley JF, et al. Phase II evaluation of menogaril in patients with advanced cervical carcinoma. Invest New Drugs 1991;9:349.

Look KY, Blessing JA, Muss HB, Partridge EE, Malfetano JH. 5-Fluorouracil and low-dose Leucovorin in the treatment of recurrent squamous cell carcinoma of the cervix. A phase II trial of the Gynecologic Oncology Group. Am J Clin Oncol 1992;15(6):497.

Macia M, Novo A, Ces J, et al. Neoadjuvant and salvage chemotherapy with cisplatin (CDDP) and 5-Fluorouracil (5-FU) in cervical carcinoma. Eur J Gynaecol Oncol 1993;XIV:192.

Majima H. Combination chemotherapy of disseminated cervix carcinoma with bleomycin (BLM) and mitomycin-C (MMC). Proc Am Soc Clin Oncol 1977;18:320(C-216).

Malfetano J, Keys H, Kredentser D, et al. Weekly cisplatin and radical radiation therapy for advanced, recurrent, and poor prognosis cervical carcinoma. Cancer 1993;71:3703.

Malfetano JH, Blessing JA, Homesley HD, Hanjani P. A phase II trial of gallium nitrate (NSC#15200) in advanced or recurrent squamous cell carcinoma of the cervix. A Gynecologic Oncology study. Invest New Drugs 1991;9:109.

Malone BT, Beye R, Walker J. Management of pain in the terminally ill by administration of epidural narcotics. Cancer 1985;55:438.

Malviya VK, Liu PY, Alberts DS, et al. Evaluation of amonafide in cervical cancer, phase II. Am J Clin Oncol 1992;15:41.

Manetta A. Bleomycin, ifosfamide, and cisplatin (BIP) in patients with recurrent and advanced cervical cancer (letter; comment). Gynecol Oncol 1991;42:104.

Mann WJ, Jander HP, Partridge EE, et al. Selective arterial embolization for control of bleeding in gynecologic malignancy. Gynecol Oncol 1980;10:279.

McGuire WP, Arseneau J, Blessing JA, et al. A randomized comparative trial of carboplatin and iproplatin in advanced squamous carcinoma of the uterine cervix: a Gynecologic Oncology Group study. J Clin Oncol 1989;7:1462.

Meier W, Eiermann W, Stieger P, et al. Squamous cell carcinoma antigen and carcinoembryonic antigen levels as prognostic factors for the response of cervical carcinoma to chemotherapy. Gynecol Oncol 1990;38:6.

Melzack R, Mount BM, Gordon JM. The Brompton mixture versus morphine solution given orally: effects on pain. Can Med Assoc J 1979;120:435.

Meyer JE, Yatsuhashi M, Green TH Jr. Palliative urinary diversion in patients with advanced pelvic malignancy. Cancer 1980;45:2698.

Miyamoto T, Takabe Y, Watanabe M, Terasima T. Effectiveness of a sequential combination of bleomycin and mitomycin-C on an advanced cervical cancer. Cancer 1978;41:403.

Moertel CG, Ahmann DL, Taylor WF, et al. A comparative evaluation of marketed analgesic drugs. N Engl J Med 1972a;286:813.

Moertel CG, Ahmann DL, Taylor WF, et al. Relief of pain by oral medication: a controlled evaluation of analgesic combinations. JAMA 1972b;229:55.

Monge RM, Jurado M, Azinovic I, et al. Intraoperative radiotherapy in recurrent gynecologic cancer. Radiother Oncol 1993;28:127.

Morris M, Gershenson CM, Eifel P, et al. Treatment of small cell carcinoma of the cervix with cisplatin, doxorubicin, and etoposide. Gynecol Oncol 1992;47:62.

Morrow CP, DiSaia PJ, Mangan CF, et al. Continuous pelvic arterial infusion with bleomycin for squamous cell carcinoma of the cervix recurrent after radiation therapy. Cancer Treat Reports 1977;61:1403.

Mountain CF. Surgical management of pulmonary metastases. Postgrad Med 1970;48:128.

Murad AM, Triginelli SQ, Ribalta JCL. Phase II trial of bleomycin, ifosfamide, and carboplatin in metastatic cervical cancer. J Clin Oncol 1994;12(1):55.

Muss HB, Blessing JA, Hanjani P, et al. Echinomycin (NSC 526417) in recurrent and metastatic nonsquamous cell carcinoma of the cervix. A phase II trial of the Gynecologic Oncology Group. Am J Clin Oncol 1992;14(4):363.

Nelson BE, Rose PG. Malignant pericardial effusion from squamous cell cancer of the cervix. J Surg Oncol 1993;52:203.

Nori D, Hilaris BS, Kim HS, et al. Interstitial irradiation in recurrent gynecological cancer. Int J Radiat Oncol Biol Phys 1981;7:1513.

Nuutinen LS, Kauppila A, Ryhanen P, et al. Intensified nutrition as an adjunct to cytotoxic chemotherapy in gynaecological cancer patients. Clin Oncol 1982;8:107.

O'Quinn AG, Barranco SC, Costanzi JJ. Tumor cell kinetics-directed chemotherapy for advanced squamous carcinoma of the cervix. Gynecol Oncol 1984;18:135.

Obasaju CK, Cowan RA, Wilkinson PM. Recurrent cervical cancer treated with cisplatin and methotrexate. Clin Oncol 1993;5:203.

Omura GA. Current status of chemotherapy for cancer of the cervix. Oncology 1992;6(4):27.

Papavasikiou C, Pappas J, Aravantinos D, et al. Treatment of cervical carcinoma with Adriamycin combined with methotrexate. Cancer Treat Reports 1978;62:1387.

Parker RL Jr, Welander CE, Homesley HD, et al. Use of the human tumor stem cell assay to study chemotherapy sensitivity in cancer of the cervix. Obstet Gynecol 1984;64:412.

Patsner B. Topical acetone for control of life–threatening vaginal hemorrhage from recurrent gynecologic cancer. Eur J Gynecol Oncol 1993;14:33.

Petrilli ES, Castaldo TW, Ballon SC, et al. Bleomycin-mitomycin C therapy for advanced squamous carcinoma of the cervix. Gynecol Oncol 1980;9:292.

Piver MS, Barlow JJ, Dunbar J. Doxorubicin, cyclophosphamide and 5-fluorouracil in patients with carcinoma of the cervix or vagina. Cancer Treat Reports 1980;64:549.

Piver MS, Barlow JJ, Lele SB, Maniccia M. Weekly *cis*-diamminedichloroplatinum II as induction chemotherapy in recurrent carcinoma of the cervix. Gynecol Oncol 1984;18:313.

Piver MS, Barlow JJ, Xynos FP. Adriamycin alone or in combination in 100 patients with carcinoma of the cervix or vagina. Am J Obstet Gynecol 1978;131:311.

Portenoy RK. Cancer pain management. Semin Oncol 1993a;20:19.

Portenoy RK. Pathophysiology of cancer pain. Adv Oncol 1993b;9(3):15.

Potter ME, Hatch KD, Potter MY, Shingleton HM, Baker VV. Factors affecting the response of recurrent squamous cell carcinoma of the cervix to cisplatin. Cancer 1989;63:1283.

Prayson RA, Biscotti CV. Recurrent cervical squamous cell carcinoma presenting with cardiac tamponade. Am J Cardiovasc Pathol 1992;4(1):69.

Prempree T, Amornmarn R, Villasanta U, et al. Retreatment of very late recurrent invasive squamous cell carcinoma of the cervix with irradiation. II. Criteria for patient selection to achieve the success. Cancer 1984;54:1950.

Quindlen EA. Management of pain: neurosurgical approaches. In DeVita DT Jr, Hellman S, Rosenberg SA, eds. Cancer: principles and practice of oncology. Philadelphia: JB Lippincott, 1982.

Quinn CM, Wright NA. The usefulness of clinical measurements of cell proliferation in gynecologic cancer. Int J Gynecol Pathol 1992;11:131.

Raad II, Luna M, Khalil S, et al. The relationship between the thrombotic and infectious complications of central venous catheters. JAMA 1994;271:1014.

Ramm K, Vergote I, Trope C. Bleomycin-ifosfamide-cisplatinum (BIP) in recurrence of previously irradiated cervical cancer (abstract). Eur J Cancer (Suppl) 1991;2:127.

Randall ME, Barrett RJ. Interstitial irradiation in the management of recurrent cracinoma of the cervix after previous radiation therapy. NC Med J 1988;49:306.

Ratanatharathorn V, Powers WE, Steverson N, et al. Bone metastasis from cervical cancer. Cancer 1994;73:2372.

Rettenmaier MA, Berman ML, DiSaia PJ, et al. Photoradiation therapy of gynecologic malignancies. Gynecol Oncol 1984;17:200.

Rettenmaier MA, Micha JP, Kucera PR, Berman ML, DiSaia PJ. A simplified method for right arterial catheter insertion. Gynecol Oncol 1985;21:207.

Robinson RG, Preston DF, et al. Clinical experience with strontium 89 in prostatic and breast cancer patients. Semin Oncol 1993;20(3):44.

Rosenthal CJ, Khulpateea N, Boyce J, et al. Effective chemotherapy for advanced carcinoma of the cervix with bleomycin, cisplatin, vincristine and methotrexate. Cancer 1983;52:2055.

Rosenthal CJ, Platica O, Khulpateea N, et al. Effective combination chemotherapy in advanced squamous cell carcinoma. Proc Am Soc Clin Oncol 1979;20:371.

Rudoff J, Percy R, Benrubi G, Ostrowski ML. Case report: recurrent squamous cell carcinoma of the cervix presenting as cardiac tamponade: case report and subject review. Gynecol Oncol 1989;34:226.

Rummans TA. Nonopioid agents for treatment of acute and subacute pain. Mayo Clin Proc 1994;69:481.

Schellhas HF, Weppelmann G. The neodymium:YAG laser in the treatment of gynecologic malignancies. Lasers Surg Med 1983;3:225.

Schwartz PE, Goldstein HM, Wallace S, Rutledge FN. Control of arterial hemorrhage using percutaneous arterial catheter techniques in patients with gynecologic malignancies. Gynecol Oncol 1975;3:276.

Scott I, Bergin CJ, Muller NL. Mediastinal and hilar lymphadenopathy as the only manifestation of metastatic carcinoma of the cervix. Can Assoc Radiol J 1986;37(1):52.

Sharma SK, Forgione H, Isaacs JH. Iodine–125 interstitial implants as salvage therapy for recurrent gynecologic malignancies. Cancer 1991;67:2467.

Simon NL, Orr JW Jr, Hatch KD, Shingleton HM. Lower extremity edema due to deep vein thrombosis in patients with recurrent cervix cancer. Gynecol Oncol 1984;19:30.

Sivanesaratnam V. The role of chemotherapy in cervical cancer—a review. Singapore Med J 1988;29:397.

Slayton RE, Blessing JA, Rettenmaier M, Ball H. A phase II clinical trial of diaziquone (AZQ) in the treatment of patients with recurrent adenocarcinoma and adenosquamous carcinoma of the cervix. A Gynecologic Oncology Group study. Invest New Drugs 1989;7:337.

Sommers GM, Grigsby PW, Perez CA, et al. Outcome of recurrent cervical carcinoma following definitive radiation. Gynecol Oncol 1989;35:150.

Sorbe B, Frankendal B. Combination chemotherapy in advanced carcinoma of the cervix. Cancer 1982;50:2028.

Stehman FB, Blessing JA, McGehee R, Barrett RJ. A phase II evaluation of mitolactol in patients with advanced squamous cell carcinoma of the cervix: a gynecologic oncology group study. J Clin Oncol 1989;17(12):1892.

Stehman FB, Blessing JA, McGehee R, Barrett RJ. A phase II evaluation of mitolactol in patients with advanced squamous cell carcinoma of the cervix: a Gynecologic Oncology Group study. J Clin Oncol 1989;7:1892.

Stratton JA, Kucera PR, Micha JP, et al. The subrenal capsule tumor implant assay as a predictor of clinical response to chemotherapy: 3 years of experience. Gynecol Oncol 1984;19:336.

Strom BL, Carson JL, Schinnar R, et al. Nonsteroidal anti-inflammatory drugs and neutropenia. Arch Intern Med 1993;153:2119.

Surwit EA, Alberts DS, Aristizabel S, et al. Treatment of primary and recurrent, advanced squamous cell cancer of the cervix with mitomycin-C + vincristine + bleomycin (MOB) plus cisplatin (PLAT). Proc Am Soc Clin Oncol 1983;24:C596.

Sutton GP, Blessing JA, Adcock L, Webster KD, DeEulis T. Phase II study of ifosfamide and mesna in patients with previously treated carcinoma of the cervix. A Gynecologic Oncology Group study. Invest New Drugs 1989;7:341.

Sutton GP, Blessing JA, DiSaia PJ, McGuire WP. Phase II study of ifosfamide and mesna in nonsquamous carcinoma of the cervix: a Gynecologic Oncology Group study. Gynecol Oncol 1993;49:48.

Sutton GP, Blessing JA, McGuire WP, et al. Phase II trial of ifosfamide and mesna in patients with advanced or recurrent squamous carcinoma of the cervix who had never received chemotherapy: a Gynecologic Oncology Group study. Am J Obstet Gynecol 1993;168:805.

Swenerton KD, Evers JA, White GW, et al. Intermittent pelvic infusion with vincristine, bleomycin and mitomycin C for advanced recurrent carcinoma of the cervix. Cancer Treat Reports 1979;63:1379.

Tattersall MHN, Ramirez C, Coppleson M. A randomized trial of adjuvant chemotherapy after radical hysterectomy in stage IB–IIA cervical cancer patients with pelvic lymph node metastases. Gynecol Oncol 1992;46:176.

Tay SK, Lai FM, Soh LT, et al. Combined chemotherapy using cisplatin, ifosfamide and bleomycin (PIB) in the treatment of advanced and recurrent cervical carcinoma. Aust NZ J Obstet Gynaecol 1992;32:3.

Thigpen JT. Chemotherapy for gynecologic tumors. Curr Opin Oncol 1989;1:105.

Thigpen T, Shingleton HM. Phase II trial of *cis*-platinum in treatment of advanced squamous cell carcinoma of the cervix. Am Soc Clin Oncol Abstracts, C-102.

Thigpen T, Vance RB, Balducci L, Blessing J. Chemotherapy in the management of advanced or recurrent cervical and endometrial carcinoma. Cancer 1981;48:658.

Thigpen T, Vance RB, Khansur T. Carcinoma of the uterine cervix: current status and future directions. Semin Oncol 1994;21(2):43.

Trope C, Johnsson JE, Grundsell H, Mattsson W. Adriamycin methotrexate combination chemotherapy of advanced carcinoma of the cervix: a third look. Obstet Gynecol 1980;55:488.

Trope C, Johnsson JE, Simonsen E, et al. Bleomycin-mitomycin C in advanced carcinoma of the cervix. Cancer 1983;51:591.

Vermorben JB, Oosterom AT, et al. Phase II study of vincristine (V), bleomycin (B), mitomycin-C (M), and cisplatin (P) in disseminated squamous cell carcinoma of the uterine cervix. Third NCI-EORTC symposium on new drugs in cancer therapy, Brussels, Belgium, European Organization for Research on Treatment of Cancer, October 15–17, 1981:A9.

Vincenti E, Chiaranda M, Ambrosini A, et al. New trends for pain relief in gynaecologic oncology. Eur J Gynaecol Oncol 1983;4:122.

Vogl SE, Zaravinos T, Kaplan BH. Toxicity of *cis*-diamminedichloroplatinum II given in a 2-hour outpatient regimen of diuresis and hydration. Cancer 1980;45:11.

von Maillot K, Ranger IM. Chemotherapy for advanced recurrent carcinoma of the cervix. A report on the treatment of 22 patients. Arch Gynecol 1982;231:253.

Wallace JH Jr, Hreshchyshyn MM, Wilbanks GD, et al. Comparison of the therapeutic effects of Adriamycin alone versus Adriamycin plus vincristine versus Adriamycin plus cyclophosphamide in the treatment of advanced carcinoma of the cervix. Cancer Treat Reports 1978;62:1435.

Warrell RP. Metabolic emergencies. In DeVita VT, Hellman S, Rosenberg SA, eds. Cancer: principles and practice of oncology, 4th ed. Philadelphia: JB Lippincott, 1993:2128.

Wheelock JB, Krebs HB, Goplerud DR. Bleomycin, vincristine, and mitomycin C (BOM) as second-line treatment after failure of *cis*-platinum based combination chemotherapy for recurrent cervical cancer. Gynecol Oncol 1990;37;21.

Wojcik EM, Selvaggi SM, Johnson SC, et al. Factors influencing fine-needle aspiration cytology in the management of recurrent gynecologic malignancies. Gynecol Oncol 1992;46:281.

Wynant HP, Morelle V, Fonteyne E, Carpentier P. Ureterosigmoidostomy: reevaluation of a forgotten continent urinary diversion. Acta Urol Belg 1991;59(4):103.

Yamazaki H, Inoue T, Ikeda H, et al. High-dose rate remote afterloading intestinal radiotherapy employing the template technique for recurrent cancer in the pelvic area. Strahlenther Onkol 1993;169:481.

Yarbro JW, ed. The management of pain in the cancer patient. Semin Oncol 1993;20(2):1.

Yordan EL, Jurado M, Kiel K, et al. Intraoperative radiation therapy in the treatment of pelvic malignancies: a preliminary report. Baillieres Clin Obstet Gynaecol 1988;2:1023.

Cancer of the Cervix by Hugh M. Shingleton and James W. Orr, Jr.
J. B. Lippincott Company, Philadelphia, © 1995.

14

Social, Psychological, and Sexual Aspects of Cervical Cancer and Its Treatment

The diagnosis of cancer evokes a bleak image of physical pain, suffering, debility, and untimely death to the patient, her family, and friends. Although confrontation with death is the key issue for many patients, the struggle of everyday living assumes equal importance for others (Fig. 14-1).

Reaction and adjustment to the diagnosis of cancer is analogous to the phases of dying described by Kuebler-Ross (1969). Initially, the woman may deny the seriousness of her symptoms and consequently delay seeking professional help. When she does report the symptom or symptoms to her physician, her anxiety may be further heightened because she is aware of delay and may wonder whether this has compromised her opportunity for cure. The shock and disbelief that she experiences after hearing the diagnosis may compromise her understanding of the physician's statements concerning treatment and prognosis. Anger and hostility may follow because she feels betrayed by her body, guilty because of her delay, and frightened about the future. The physician, as the bearer of bad news, may become the target of her rage. Bargaining is evident in some women who cooperate excessively with the healthcare provider: the unspoken expectation is that they will be cured in exchange for their good behavior. Disappointment over the loss of physical well-being is to be expected and may be followed by depression. During diagnosis, staging, and treatment, the physician must follow certain steps in an attempt to calm the patient and her family, to dispel the gloom and hopelessness, and to ensure that they understand the nature of the illness and its treatment. These initial steps are:

1. The physician, the nurse, the patient and the patient's partner or family member should participate in the initial discussion regarding diagnosis, treatment, and progress.
2. The setting must be quiet, private, and comfortable.
3. In an unhurried discussion, the patient is asked to state her understanding of her situation and is encouraged to guide the conversation with her questions.
4. The physician should be factual, optimistic within reason, and alert to cues.
5. After the physician leaves, the nurse can repeat, reinforce, or expand the key elements of the discussion.
6. Instructions concerning the options and the initiation of treatment must be clear and concise, preferably in writing.
7. The patient should have appropriate lines of communication available to rediscuss important issues if necessary.

Some patients' reactions are more understandable in terms of their previous histories. The relation between squamous cell carcinoma of the uterine cervix and sexual behavior is well established and may contribute to many of the patient's fears and anxieties. A woman who has strong religious feelings who develops cervical cancer after having experienced an abortion, an extra-

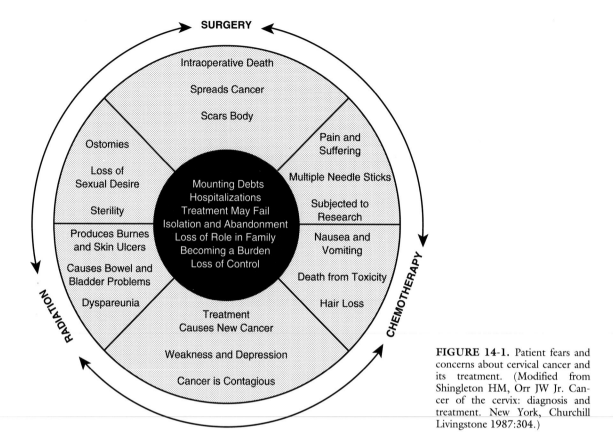

FIGURE 14-1. Patient fears and concerns about cervical cancer and its treatment. (Modified from Shingleton HM, Orr JW Jr. Cancer of the cervix: diagnosis and treatment. New York, Churchill Livingstone 1987:304.)

marital affair, or a venereal infection may interpret her disease as punishment for sin or wrongdoing. The compliant, passive woman who endures treatment as though she is "getting what she deserves" may be a candidate for counseling. The highly anxious or guilt-ridden patient often cannot process information effectively and may appear uncooperative when actually she needs support. Some women who develop this disease in the absence of "risk factors" need additional counseling regarding the malignant process. Because of the site of the malignancy, the physician should discuss the effect of the disease and treatment on each woman in terms of her self-image and sexuality. Surgery may shorten the vagina; irradiation is likely to cause vaginal stricturing and resultant dyspareunia (Schover et al 1989). Any gynecologic surgery, not just cancer treatment, disturbs sexual function; because of her excessive dependence on her sexual partner, a woman who is treated for cervical cancer may try to adapt to him in an attempt to meet his sexual needs during her illness and treatment. Their lessened sexual response is not based solely on dyspareunia; indeed, the frequency of dyspareunia tended to be low and decreased with time (Wiejmar Schultz et al 1991). One review (Andersen 1987) addressed psychologic response and sexual dys-

function related to pelvic cancer in women and documented the effect of cancer diagnosis and symptoms on women's sexuality (Table 14-1).

With the diagnosis of cancer, the woman's life, activities, responsibilities, and interdependent relationships are invaded. She may have responsibilities and strong emotional ties to her children, her spouse, her parents, and others. She may be working and active in a church, a club, or other professional, political, or social organizations. Her creativity may be expressed in homemaking and childbearing as well as in her career. Just as one cannot separate the body from the mind, neither must a woman be separated by disease from her family and society.

The diagnosis of cancer and its treatment disrupts an individual's daily activities and requires great energy for her to cope with associated stress. Previously successful adaptive behaviors may fail, anxiety is generated, and self-esteem may be lost (Corney et al 1992). The physician's primary goal of medical, surgical, or radiation therapy intervention must be to eradicate the cancer with minimal physical and psychologic trauma to quickly return the individual to her normal (or nearly normal) life. Women find it difficult to ask for more help when "the hospital has saved (their) life"

TABLE 14-1
Percentage of Women With Gynecologic Cancer and Matched Healthy Women
Reporting Sexual Dysfunction

		CANCER PATIENTS	
DYSFUNCTION	HEALTHY WOMEN	Before Symptoms	After Symptoms
Inhibited desire	17%	12%	56%
Inhibited excitement	7%	10%	49%
Inhibited orgasm	10%	7%	37%
Dyspareunia	0%	5%	37%

Modified from Andersen BL. Psychological responses and sexual outcomes of gynecologic cancer. In Lurain JR, Sciarra JJ (eds). Gynecology and obstetrics, Philadelphia, JB Lippincott, 1987;4:1; with permission.

(Wilson-Barnett 1991). The healthcare team must offer emotional support to such women even when it is not requested.

If cure is not a realistic expectation, the cancer patient must be assisted in functioning well for the duration of her illness. Fundamental to achieving this goal is an understanding of what the disease means to the patient and the development of a sense of rapport and trust among the healthcare team, the patient, and her family. The physician must approach specific areas, such as pain control, with a reassuring attitude.

Attention is usually focused on the effect of cancer on the psyche, although psychologic factors as a cause of cancer have received attention in the literature for centuries. Although one can correlate certain personality characteristics with the development of cancer, any actual causative effect remains unproved. Severe emotional trauma (e.g., the loss of a spouse or child, with its attendant grief and depression) has been implicated in both the development and the acceleration of the course of cancer. It has been suggested that cancer patients can use this relation between psyche and cancer to their advantage, shifting the effect in a positive way (Simonton et al 1980). Some patients visualize the destruction of cancer cells by their own white blood cells. Although the scientist may probably dismiss the validity of this notion of controlling the disease, the benefit in terms of the patient's perception of control of her own body may be important.

SURGICAL TREATMENT

The loss of control that accompanies anesthesia and surgery often makes patients feel helpless. The unspoken fears of "never waking up" and of intolerable pain are frequently present. The importance of addressing these fears during a preoperative counseling session

with the patient cannot be overemphasized. When hysterectomy is part of the treatment for cervical cancer, familiarity with the psychologic implications of the procedure is also important. The attendant anatomic and physiologic changes are obvious to the clinician but not so readily apparent to the patient.

Many women believe that the uterus is the source of their femininity and strength and consequently may feel "less of a woman" without it. Well-meaning friends and family members are often sources of misinformation. The woman who is facing hysterectomy or other cancer treatment may be told that the loss of the uterus leads to premature aging, senility, and even insanity. Such misunderstandings can often be clarified during a preoperative visit, and details of the operative procedure can be described. Questions directed to the patient facilitate discussion:

- What does your uterus mean to you?
- How will hysterectomy change your life?
- What is the most important function of your uterus?
- What are your thoughts about losing your uterus?

The effects of oophorectomy—including vasomotor symptoms, loss of libido, reduction of vaginal lubrication, and decreased sensation in the lower genital tract—may be disruptive. The patient should be informed that many of these symptoms may be alleviated by the administration of exogenous estrogen. In specific situations, young women can be told that normal ovaries may be conserved. The risks of reoperation (3% to 8%) and other potential problems should be detailed, however.

In premenopausal women, the cessation of menses and loss of fertility caused by the hysterectomy must be addressed. Women who view their menses as a cleansing function are less likely to accept this change than are the women who dislike the process or who have experienced significant menstrual discomfort. Knowing that contraception is absolute allows some women to feel relief and to experience increased sexual enjoyment. Others feel a loss of identity that is associated with loss of the ability to reproduce.

If surgery is perceived by the patient as being mutilating, it is likely to be damaging rather than restorative. The woman who expects hysterectomy to decrease her sexual excitability or enjoyment often exhibits a self-fulfilling prophecy when she experiences decreased libido postoperatively. Women who depend on their gynecologic illness to secure relief from sexual commitments to their partners may develop anxiety if they believe that the removal of the reproductive organs will lead to the expectation that they will become more responsive sexually. Thus, surgery may constitute a threat to the marital relationship in differing ways.

Many patients and spouses believe that genital cancer is contagious; therefore, whatever sexual relationship was previously experienced may cease. Guilt that is associated with prior sexual activity and a belief that this may have caused the cancer becomes a deterrent to positive adjustment and recovery. During and after treatment, marital discord and abandonment of the woman by her mate are common. The importance of educating the woman and her partner cannot be overemphasized. Generally, the single most significant factor in postoperative sexual adjustment is the degree of pretreatment sexual satisfaction. The woman who experienced a good sexual relationship before surgery is more likely to resume such a relationship postoperatively, whereas those having preoperative sexual dysfunction are likely to continue or develop a worsened sexual relationship after surgery.

Surgical resection of the proximal vagina may create problems with sexual function in some women, particularly in the immediate postoperative period. Kenter and coworkers (1989) believed this to be a problem in about a fourth of women. Most women can be assured that the shortening of the vagina does not necessarily affect sexual activities. The interruption of sensory nerve pathways to the vagina and perineum by pelvic operations may result in decreased sensation, however, and in rare cases lack of orgasm. Postoperative dyspareunia may be lessened and sensation enhanced by a change in coital position or the addition of lubrication. For example, if the female lies supine with the thighs adducted the male senses greater depth. If the female is superior and astride, she may control or limit depth of thrusting by her partner (Hubbard et al 1985).

To facilitate satisfactory sexual function, the physician may encourage extended foreplay and clitoral stimulation because orgasm is still possible. Other expressions of affection, such as fondling or oral–genital sex, may be helpful in reassuring the woman that she is still a sexual being with the ability to love and be loved in a physical way. If successful, her increased feelings of self-worth serve to combat any tendency toward depression. Careful evaluation of postoperative sexual function is important because in many situations, sexual counseling may be beneficial (Capone et al 1980).

Bladder dysfunction usually complicates postoperative recovery for patients after radical hysterectomy. Although the catheter is in place, many women hesitate to leave home for fear that others will notice the catheter. Some women become excessively preoccupied with voiding, measuring, and recording residual urine. These anxieties can potentially delay their postoperative recovery. A more serious difficulty is encountered in the occasional patient who has persistent bladder dysfunction that requires intermittent self-catheterization. This may be viewed by the woman as humiliating and disabling in terms of gainful employment. The involuntary loss of urine that may occur after surgery presents another set of social, personal, and medical problems. Careful reassurance regarding continued care is important in these situations. Most women can be assured, however, that bladder sensation ultimately returns to normal and that there is little risk of long-term disability.

Some patients have difficulty relinquishing the "sick" role. The patient who enjoyed the love and concern that others expressed during her treatment may suddenly feel the loss of this support when she completes treatment. She fears recurrence and may attribute every ache and pain to cancer. This situation should be discussed with the patient, with the understanding that this connection of every symptom to cancer becomes less prominent with the passage of time. Cancer patients initially realign their life goals toward survival. Once it appears that this goal will be achieved, they may again be faced with many of the problems that they experienced before the diagnosis was made. In effect, they have focused all their energies on enduring the ordeal of cancer and its treatment, only to find that the successful outcome returned them to a previous existence in which unhappiness may have prevailed. They receive no sympathy from friends and relatives, who tell them to be grateful, and their sense of isolation may become painful.

RADIATION TREATMENT

It is paramount to discuss the patient's ideas about radiation therapy and its effects before the initiation of treatment. Some people believe that radiation therapy can cause cancer, that exposure to an irradiated patient may be harmful to others. Some women have difficulty viewing radiation therapy as first-line treatment, believing that it is actually the last resort because the tumor could not be removed surgically. The physician should always be prepared to answer the question, "Why can't you operate?" Patients want the diseased organ removed so that the whole idea of cancer can be dismissed and forgotten. It becomes the physician's responsibility to discuss the options of treatment and the reason that a surgical procedure may not be the most appropriate method of treatment in a particular situation. The time element can also be stressful. Radiation therapy is usually delivered over a 5- or 6-week interval, compared with an operation, which can be performed in a few hours. In addition, an immediate statement of the likelihood of a successful result cannot be provided to patients who are treated by irradiation, whereas surgically treated patients are relieved when told that the cancer has been removed and had not spread.

Radiation therapy as primary treatment for cervical carcinoma is associated with a variety of symptoms and disturbances of body functions. As curative doses of irradiation are delivered to the pelvis, the normal tissues of the bladder and rectum are affected, and the patient may experience hematuria, urinary urgency, frequency, dysuria, nocturia, tenesmus, diarrhea, or rectal bleeding. These effects and the associated fatigue, anorexia, nausea, and vomiting lead some patients to perceive the treatment as damaging. Because most people seek medical attention to feel better or to obtain relief, they may lose sight of the long-term goal of cure as long as symptoms persist.

The likelihood of transient skin changes in the radiation field, such as desquamation and ulceration of the lower abdomen or back, should be mentioned during pretreatment counseling. Subcutaneous fibrosis, increased pigmentation, and hair loss may develop in the radiation field, and patients should also be informed of these probabilities. Such changes are often of little significance medically but may be of major importance to the patient, who feels disfigured and senses a loss of sexual attractiveness. These skin changes represent tangible evidence that she is indeed different and the acceptance of them by her partner is of great importance to her.

Anatomic and functional vaginal alterations after radiation therapy can present a major problem for many women. Many symptoms persist for years or even for a lifetime. After irradiation, the vaginal epithelium thins and the vagina shortens and may become stenotic, inelastic, or partially obliterated. Lubrication may not occur with sexual excitement. Vaginal bleeding, discharge, and dyspareunia may accompany attempts at vaginal intercourse. Such direct vaginal effects of radiation therapy occur in most women (Abitbol 1974). Estrogen replacement (topical or systemic)

may improve the elasticity of the vaginal epithelium. Vaginal administration of estradiol may be more active locally because it does not require absorption and metabolism. Vaginal dilation during and after completion of the treatment program may maintain or promote patency. When this cannot be accomplished by sexual intercourse, use of a mechanical device (obturator) may be helpful. Many women may equate the use of such a dilator with masturbation, a practice that may not be acceptable. When sexual intercourse has been abandoned, the reasons for abstinence should be explored with the patient and her spouse. If a woman suspects a link between sexual intercourse and the development of her cancer, she may avoid that activity to "prevent" recurrent disease. Postcoital bleeding or discharge, with or without dyspareunia, may raise fears of recurrence because these often were the symptoms the woman experienced before diagnosis and treatment.

The patient should be made aware of the safety precautions employed during her hospitalization for intracavitary irradiation placement, especially those that restrict visiting privileges of family and friends. Such preparation lessens the sense of isolation that may otherwise be experienced.

The duration of radiation treatment may make other demands on the patient and her family. The financial burden of transportation to a treatment facility, time away from home, loss of income, expense of child care, and cost of meals and lodging can be heavy. The support of a governmental or charitable agency may be needed because many of these women are from low-income situations.

ULTRARADICAL SURGERY FOR RECURRENT CANCER

The choices of further therapy for women who have persistent or recurrent cancer are somewhat limited because most who have recurrent or persistent tumor are incurable. The only chance for long-term survival in those women who have central pelvic recurrence is pelvic exenteration, a radical operation that in itself is life-threatening. Because the operation may require urinary and fecal diversion and removal of the entire vagina, the woman's lifestyle may be completely changed. Unfortunately, the alternative to the surgery is death within 1 to 2 years. Fortunately, continent urinary diversion, rectal reanastomosis, and vaginal reconstruction can be offered to many women in this clinical situation. Three procedures, however, carry potential risks, which must be explained. The woman must, with the help of her physicians and family, carefully assess the quality of her life and decide whether she is willing to accept the surgical risks and the potential lifestyle changes to survive. Most women choose surgery because they desire to remain a part of their families and their communities as long as possible. Some are not willing to endure more pain or to accept the disfiguration, and they should not be coerced into accepting the surgery because they are likely to be seriously dissatisfied with the results. The physician must decide whether the patient can benefit from the procedure based on the potential for resection of the tumor and the general medical and psychiatric health of the woman.

It has been suggested that some women who have a previous or current psychiatric problem are extremely poor candidates for an exenteration because of their marginal ability to cope with their environment. There is no psychologic test available to predict the effect of surgery on the psyche and in our experience, several such patients have done well after exenteration. It may be important to allow a counselor or the therapist to participate in discussions, both before and after the surgery. This is particularly important when the patient has a specific therapist who is aware of her previous psychiatric history.

Many times, the physician is concerned that the exenteration candidate does not fully comprehend the extent and effects of the surgical procedure. This may be due to (1) limited educational background, (2) use of defense mechanisms such as denial, or (3) a sense of well-being that is achieved through religious beliefs. Although there may be no way to assure complete patient understanding, we believe that if a patient can give a reasonably accurate description of the extent of the operation, the physician has met his or her responsibility of informed consent. Many patients require time to make their decisions. Repetition of the risk–benefit information may be necessary to ensure understanding by the patient and her family. A family that is united in favor of the decision serves as a source of support for the patient postoperatively; however, the final decision ultimately rests with the woman, even though her decision may be contrary to the wishes of her family or physician.

The loss of the vagina after exenteration is a major threat to women who are sexually active, particularly to those who are accustomed only to vaginal intercourse. Women who have used other forms of sexual expression may find loss of the vagina less of an assault to their sexuality. In contrast, the patient who indicates that sexual activity is not important to her may be denying her sexuality to her physician for fear of embarrassing herself or her "rescuer." She may be expressing an inability to cope with any issue beyond survival or she may be responding to fear of an additional surgical procedure aimed at vaginal reconstruction. This problem may be minimized by the surgeon's willingness to perform exenteration and concurrent vaginal reconstruction and by his recogni-

tion of the need for the woman to express her sexuality in a physical way after the surgery. Lamont and associates (1978) suggested that a sexual counselor should be involved during preoperative assessment, during the hospital stay, and during the recovery period after hospitalization.

An important factor in patient acceptance of exenteration relates to the woman's role in the family. If she is employed outside the home, important income may be lost and other members of the family may not be able or willing to assume her financial or in-home responsibilities. This is particularly true when she has young children. The social worker can be a valuable member of the healthcare team in identifying resources available to the family during the absence of the woman from her usual environment. To allow these considerations to create a prolonged delay of the surgery may be shortsighted, however, because the surgical procedure may be her only chance of long-term survival.

Postoperative adjustment to exenteration depends on (1) severity of the physical insult, (2) duration of convalescence, (3) preoperative concept of self, (4) previous ability to cope with crises, (5) availability of family support, and (6) the relationship with the physician and other healthcare professionals. It is clear that a complicated recovery is more stressful to all concerned. Patients who are doing well medically in the early postoperative period may nonetheless suffer an emotional decline and physical deterioration; grieving is an appropriate response to loss of body parts, separation from home and loved ones, and disruption of an independent lifestyle. Excessive anxiety and depression, however, may indicate that the physical changes related to the operation have exacerbated a preexisting psychiatric problem. Alternatively, when the patient's preoperative concept of self was based on internal values more than external physical factors, she may better tolerate the postoperative changes in her body. Some women perceive themselves as being less than complete after exenteration; however, others are acutely aware of their diseased parts and may experience an improved sense of self after successful removal of the cancerous tissues.

An essential component of the exenteration patient's ability to recover a positive self-image is her attitude toward the urinary and fecal diversions. The need for radical surgery is not always clear to patients because the organs removed may have caused few or no symptoms. Although continent urinary diversion and rectal reanastomosis decrease problems, the creation of an ostomy is associated with new problems, real or imagined. Patterns of clothing selection may need to be altered. The patient must learn new skills to manage leakage, odor, flatus, and excoriation of the peristomal skin. A period of experimentation in the use of ostomy equipment must follow surgery. At this time, persistence, flexibility, attention to detail, and a sense of humor can be the patient's best defense against frustration. The whole idea of soilage or fecal contamination is repulsive to women who feel that it is not socially acceptable for one to eliminate feces through an opening in the abdominal wall. Many patients live in relative isolation without disclosing information about the ostomies to their friends and acquaintances. The support of an enterostomal therapist is mandatory in preoperative selection of stoma sites, assistance in psychologic rehabilitation, and teaching the patient how to contain and manage the diverted urinary or fecal stream. A visit by an active previous exenteration patient can assist in preoperative counseling and is helpful to the early postoperative patient in establishing a goal of recovery—that is, an image of ability instead of the perception of disability that may be the patient's mindset. Later, participation in ostomy groups can be beneficial in overcoming isolation and fears of social embarrassment. As previously noted, continent conduits (Penalver et al 1989, Hohenfellner et al 1990) and rectal reanastamosis (Hatch et al 1990, Partridge 1991) as improvements in exenteration techniques promise to lessen some of the difficulties for women undergoing such surgery.

Postoperative depression is common but when beyond the normal magnitude of the grieving process, depression becomes counterproductive and constitutes a significant threat to recovery. Sleep disturbances, failure to eat, and reluctance to ambulate or participate in self-care activities impede progress and can precipitate major physical complications. Individuals who have a previous history of depression are more likely to experience postoperative depression, although even patients with no previous history usually exhibit some depressive symptoms. Psychiatric intervention and antidepressants may be necessary if the patient is to successfully negotiate the rehabilitation process.

Every individual has patterns of coping with stress that have been developed through trial and error. It is helpful to identify those patterns preoperatively so that their use may be encouraged after surgery. The woman should be encouraged to begin a favorite hobby again as soon as possible, particularly if it is an activity that has provided relaxation or release of tension. The individual who copes by being in charge and controlling her environment must be given as many opportunities as possible for making choices and maintaining control. For example, if she prefers to bathe in the evening, arrangements should be made so that this can be accomplished according to her wishes.

Personal support is vital after exenteration. The husband is the key figure in most cases but a parent, child, sibling, or friend may play the central role. The husband (or significant support person) is extremely important and he must be included in teaching, planning, and gauging progress after surgery. In the ab-

sence of family support, alternate figures assume more importance. Close friends or nurses may develop a strong relationship with the patient and assist with her postoperative care, rehabilitation, and support. The specific identity of the individual who actually assists the patient in her struggle toward recovery is not important as long as someone is available for such assistance.

Occasionally, patients may have difficulty escaping from the dependent role imposed by exenteration. Some women enjoy the attention they receive and feel special, in contrast to the preoperative feeling of isolation. Others may lack the courage to risk failure in their attempts to regain the ability to function independently. Another group may have been dependent even without the imposed physical disability. A preoperative assessment of the value the patient assigns to her own independence may be helpful in her postoperative care.

The ideal relationship between the physician and patient is one of trust, warmth, and closeness. The physician who remains distant loses considerable advantage in influencing the patient's recovery.

CHEMOTHERAPY

Chemotherapy is the only alternative treatment available for those women who have received maximal tolerated doses of irradiation and are not candidates for pelvic exenteration. Administration of chemotherapy in patients having cancer of the cervix excludes cure as a realistic objective. Palliation, with reduction in tumor mass, relief of symptoms, and extended survival, is the goal. For those patients whose disease remains stable, it is often difficult to say whether chemotherapy had any positive effect.

Continued treatment in the absence of measurable response may have a positive psychologic effect because the patient may believe that something is being done to help her while she waits for a "miracle." She may not yet have concluded that the best days of her life are past, that she will never feel any better, or that medical treatment has failed. There is an element of specialness in the treatment process as the patient is the subject of conferences and the object of attention by the entire healthcare team. These women may also enjoy the attention showered on them by friends and family and an intense caring relationship with the physician and the oncology nurse.

Women who demand all that medical science has to offer are likely to find their needs met because the clinician usually responds to the challenge. In contrast, women who are not assertive may be denied aggressive management. Potentially beneficial treatment should be offered to all, and treatment decisions should not depend on demands for or resistance to treatment on the part of the patient or her family.

In these situations, few individuals decline participation in clinical cancer trials. Some patients genuinely want to contribute to the advancement of knowledge and in a sense make their deaths more meaningful. Some women are fearful of being involved in these investigational protocols and may not understand the benefit of such programs. It is important that the physician assure the patient who agrees to enter a protocol study that her participation is valuable. It is an unusual opportunity to enhance or reinforce the feeling of self-worth of a patient.

The patient who accepts treatment with a chemotherapeutic agent must be informed and must agree to the possible side effects of a particular regimen. The toll that these drugs can exact is significant, including the real possibility of death secondary to toxicity. Hair loss caused by many of the agents is upsetting to some women, not only because it changes their appearance but also because it is tangible evidence that a serious problem exists. It alters the simplest of tasks: personal grooming. The price these women pay for hope is high; however, others are willing to accept any bodily insult to remain alive. Interestingly, when asked in retrospect, most patients would resubmit themselves to these risks, even for a 1% chance of cure.

It is important that the physician consider the chemotherapy patient's plight. She is subjected to a form of therapy that may not be helpful but usually produces unwanted symptoms. The outcome of the disease and the effect of the therapy are equally unknown to her. A situation ensues that aggravates her sense of guilt because she is no longer able to provide for her family and is only placing her family under a financial burden. At every visit she fears yet must be prepared for the words that indicate that treatment has failed. Family members, including her partner, may begin to withdraw as her suffering becomes too great for them to bear and they begin the process of separation that will culminate in her death.

The patient and her family need assistance in coping with this extraordinary amount of stress. The oncology nurse and social worker are key individuals in assisting the patient and her family. The social worker has the ability to tap community resources to meet specific needs in individual circumstances. The minister or priest can give spiritual guidance, assist the family in setting priorities, and help keep hope alive.

THE DYING PATIENT

Despite all efforts, a significant number of cervical cancer patients are not successfully treated. When all forms of therapy have failed, the focus of physician and patient must change to preparation for the death of the patient. The physician may share the woman's sense of failure but must reassure her that she will not be abandoned. The goals of treatment are to keep her pain-free and comfortable, to assist her in remaining functional for as long as possible, and to keep the family informed so that shared time is well spent. The physician, the patient, and her family must accept each small victory over a symptom or a complaint while acknowledging a loss of control over the disease process.

Communication is vital in the care of the terminal patient. All healthcare professionals must clearly understand the goals and objectives regarding any given patient. The patient and her family may ask the same question (how long?) in different ways to many people, hoping to receive a more promising reply. In their distress and denial, the family may insist that a piece of information has never been provided to them when actually it simply was not heard. The spokesperson for the family usually comes forward and makes his or her presence known to the clinician. This individual can be an ally and should be regarded as such. Separate communication with numerous members of the family is not advised and is often disruptive. The physician meets his or her responsibility best when meeting with the group or with the designated spokesperson and encouraging family members to communicate with each other at this time of great pain.

It is important to determine where the death will occur (Seale 1991). For many patients and families, death at home is perceived as comforting because it provides an opportunity for the patient and family to have uninterrupted time together. Even when death at home is chosen, the link between the patient and the treatment center needs to be maintained. During times of stress, the family and the patient need a person to contact who can advise them and provide the supplies and medication required. Special hospital beds may be made available through community agencies, and visiting nurses can assist with care on an intermittent basis.

Hospital admission for terminal care and death are chosen by some because of the inability to provide skilled nursing care in the home or for other family reasons (Mor et al 1990). The medical staff must always be available to arrange admission at any time.

Hospice Care

The concept of hospice care for the terminally ill originated in England and is used in some other parts of the world, including the United States (Lukoshok 1990). In Great Britain, these patients are admitted to facilities having a home-like atmosphere; whenever possible, patients are allowed to return to their homes. Caring for patients in their own homes has been the focus of the American hospice movement (Stoddard

1989). The goals of hospice care include pain control, with or without impairment of the patient's mental faculties; increased involvement of family members in patient care, with the support of a professional nursing staff; and development of the remaining capabilities of the patient (Feinsinger 1991). The nurses also work with family members to aid their adjustment to the loss, both before and after the death of the patient. The hospice adds a dimension of compassion to care of the dying patient.

References

Abitbol MM, Davenport JH. The irradiated vagina. Obstet Gynecol 1974;44:249.

Andersen BL. Psychological responses and sexual outcomes of gynecologic cancer. In Lurain JR, Sciarra JJ, eds. Gynecology and obstetrics, vol 4. Philadelphia: JB Lippincott, 1987.

Capone MA, Good RS, Westie KS. Psychosocial rehabilitation of gynecologic oncology patients. Arch Phys Med Rehabil 1980;61:128.

Corney RH, Everett H, Howells A, Crowther ME. Psychosocial adjustment following major gynecological surgery for carcinoma of the cervix and vulva. J Psychosom Res 1992;36:561.

Feinsinger R. Symptom control during the last week of life on a palliative care unit. J Palliat Care 1991;7:5.

Hatch KD, Gelder MS, et al. Pelvic exenteration with low rectal anastomosis: survival, complications, and prognostic factors. Gynecol Oncol 1990;38:462.

Hohenfellner R, Müller SC, Riedmiller H, Thüroff JW. Continent urinary diversion: the Mainz pouch technique. In Knopstein PG, Friedberg V, Sevin B-U, eds. Reconstructive surgery in gynecology. New York: Thieme Medical Publishers, 1990.

Hubbard JL, Shingleton HM. Sexual function of patients after cancer of the cervix treatment. Clin Obstet Gynecol 1985;12:247.

Kenter CG, Ansink AC, Heintz APM, Aartsen EJ, Delemarre JFM, Hart AAM. Carcinoma of the uterine cervix stage I and IIA: results of surgical treatment: complications, recurrence and survival. Eur J Surg Oncol 1989;15:55.

Kuebler-Ross E. On death and dying. New York: Macmillan, 1969.

Lamont JA, Petrillo AD, de Sargeant EJ. Psychosexual rehabilitation and exenteration surgery. Gynecol Oncol 1978;6:236.

Lukoshok H. Hospice care under Medicare—an early look. Prev Med 1990;19:730.

Mor V, Masterson-Allen S. A comparison of hospice vs. conventional care of the terminally ill cancer patient. Oncology 1990;4:85.

Partridge EE. Pelvic exenteration. In Lurain JR, Sciarra JJ, eds. Gynecology and obstetrics, vol 4. Philadelphia: JB Lippincott, 1991.

Penalver MA, Bejany DE, Averette HE, et al. Continent urinary diversion in gynecologic oncology. Gynecol Oncol 1989;34:274.

Schover LR, Fife M, Gershenson DM. Sexual dysfunction and treatment for early stage cervical cancer. Cancer 1989;63:204.

Seale C. A comparison of hospice and conventional care. Soc Sci Med 1991;32:147.

Simonton OC, Matthews-Simonton S, Sparks TF. Psychological intervention in the treatment of cancer. Psychosomatics 1980;21:226.

Stoddard S. Hospice in the United States: an overview. J Palliat Care 1989;5:100.

Wiejmar Schultz WCM, van de Weil HBM, Bouma J. Psychosexual functioning after treatment for cancer of the cervix:a comparative and longitudinal study. Int J Gynecol Cancer 1991;1:37.

Wilson-Barnett J. Providing relevant information for patients and families. In Corney R, ed. Developing communication and counselling skills in medicine. London: Routledge, 1991.

INDEX

Page numbers followed by *f* indicate figure; *t* following a page number indicates a table.